Textbook of
Pharmacology, Pathology and Genetics
for Nurses–II

Textbook of Pharmacology, Pathology and Genetics for Nurses–II

As per the Revised INC Syllabus for BSc Nursing

SECOND EDITION

Suresh Sharma MSc (N) PhD FNRS RN (USA)
Professor and Principal
College of Nursing
All India Institute of Medical Sciences (AIIMS)
Jodhpur, Rajasthan, India

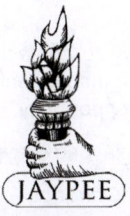

JAYPEE BROTHERS MEDICAL PUBLISHERS
The Health Sciences Publisher
New Delhi | London

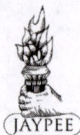

Jaypee Brothers Medical Publishers (P) Ltd

Headquarters
Jaypee Brothers Medical Publishers (P) Ltd
EMCA House, 23/23-B
Ansari Road, Daryaganj
New Delhi 110 002, India
Landline: +91-11-23272143, +91-11-23272703
+91-11-23282021, +91-11-23245672
Email: jaypee@jaypeebrothers.com

Corporate Office
Jaypee Brothers Medical Publishers (P) Ltd
4838/24, Ansari Road, Daryaganj
New Delhi 110 002, India
Phone: +91-11-43574357
Fax: +91-11-43574314
Email: jaypee@jaypeebrothers.com

Overseas Office
J.P. Medical Ltd
83 Victoria Street, London
SW1H 0HW (UK)
Phone: +44 20 3170 8910
Fax: +44 (0)20 3008 6180
Email: info@jpmedpub.com

Website: www.jaypeebrothers.com
Website: www.jaypeedigital.com

© 2022, Jaypee Brothers Medical Publishers

The views and opinions expressed in this book are solely those of the original contributor(s)/author(s) and do not necessarily represent those of editor(s) and publisher of the book.

All rights reserved. No part of this publication may be reproduced, stored or transmitted in any form or by any means, electronic, mechanical, photocopying, recording or otherwise, without the prior permission in writing of the publishers.

All brand names and product names used in this book are trade names, service marks, trademarks or registered trademarks of their respective owners. The publisher is not associated with any product or vendor mentioned in this book.

Medical knowledge and practice change constantly. This book is designed to provide accurate, authoritative information about the subject matter in question. However, readers are advised to check the most current information available on procedures included and check information from the manufacturer of each product to be administered, to verify the recommended dose, formula, method and duration of administration, adverse effects and contraindications. It is the responsibility of the practitioner to take all appropriate safety precautions. Neither the publisher nor the author(s)/editor(s) assume any liability for any injury and/or damage to persons or property arising from or related to use of material in this book.

This book is sold on the understanding that the publisher is not engaged in providing professional medical services. If such advice or services are required, the services of a competent medical professional should be sought.

Every effort has been made where necessary to contact holders of copyright to obtain permission to reproduce copyright material. If any have been inadvertently overlooked, the publisher will be pleased to make the necessary arrangements at the first opportunity.

Inquiries for bulk sales may be solicited at: jaypee@jaypeebrothers.com

Textbook of Pharmacology, Pathology and Genetics for Nurses–II

First Edition: 2016
Second Edition: **2022,** Reprint: 2024
ISBN: 978-93-5465-569-2

Printed at India by Rajkamal Electric Press, Kundli, Haryana.

Dedicated To

My Mother

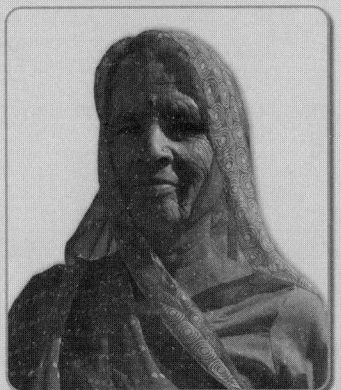

Late Smt Bhagwati Devi Sharma
(09/05/1947–17/02/2015)

My mom, I born through you, I grew with your feedings, you were my first teacher, who taught me to become, what I am today….while breathing in air, I can feel your presence…... I feel blessed every moment and at every step of my life… I feel proud to be your son. Mom your unconditional love and belief in my capabilities provided me the power and energy to carry out such endless tedious tasks.

Contributors and Reviewers

Aminder Singh MD
Associate Professor
Department of Pathology
Dayanand Medical College and Hospital
Ludhiana, Punjab, India

Anshuman Darbari MS MCh
Additional Professor (CTVS)
Department of CTVS
All India Institute of Medical Sciences
Rishikesh, Uttarakhand, India

Ashi Chug MDS
Additional Professor
Department of Dentistry and Maxillofacial Surgery
All India Institute of Medical Sciences
Rishikesh, Uttarakhand, India

Frahanul Huda MS
Additional Professor
Department of General Surgery
All India Institute of Medical Sciences
Rishikesh, Uttarakhand, India

Gagandeep Singh MD
Assistant Professor
Department of Microbiology
All India Institute of Medical Sciences
New Delhi, India

Hemlata MSc (N)
Tutor
College of Nursing
All India Institute of Medical Sciences
Jodhpur, Rajasthan, India

Jagdeesh Goyal MD
Professor
Department of Pediatrics
All India Institute of Medical Sciences
Jodhpur, Rajasthan, India

Jaison Joseph MSc (N)
Assistant Lecturer
College of Nursing
Pandit BDS University of Health Sciences
Rohtak, Haryana, India

Joyce Joseph MSc (N)
Assistant Professor
College of Nursing
All India Institute of Medical Sciences
Raipur, Chhattisgarh, India

Jyoti Arora MS
Professor
Department of Anatomy
Vardhman Mahavir Medical College and Safdarjang Hospital
New Delhi, India

Kumar Satish Ravi MD
Additional Professor
Department of Anatomy
All India Institute of Medical Sciences
Rishikesh, Uttarakhand, India

Maneesh Sharma MSc (N)
Assistant Professor
College of Nursing
All India Institute of Medical Sciences
Rishikesh, Uttarakhand, India

Manisha Bisht MD, DM
Additional Professor
Department of Pharmacology
All India Institute of Medical Sciences
Rishikesh, Uttarakhand, India

Mayank Mishra MD
Additional Professor
Department of Pulmonary Medicine
All India Institute of Medical Sciences
Rishikesh, Uttarakhand, India

Mohd Salahuddin Ansari MD
Professor
Department of Anatomy
Aligarh Muslim University
Aligarh, Uttar Pradesh, India

Monil Singhai MD
Joint Director
National Center for Disease Control
New Delhi, India

Nancy Kurien MSc (N)
Tutor
College of Nursing
All India Institute of Medical Sciences
Jodhpur, Rajasthan, India

Neena Sood MD
Former Professor and Head
Department of Pathology
Dayanand Medical College and Hospital
Ludhiana, Punjab, India

Neha Singh MD
Additional Professor
Department of Pathology
All India Institute of Medical Sciences
Rishikesh, Uttarakhand, India

Nipin Kalal MSc (N)
Assistant Professor
College of Nursing
All India Institute of Medical Sciences
Jodhpur, Rajasthan, India

Parul Saini MSc (N)
Assistant Professor
Faculty of Nursing
SGT University, Gurugram, Haryana, India

Poonam Arora MD
Associate Professor
Department of Anesthesiology
All India Institute of Medical Sciences
Rishikesh, Uttarakhand, India

Persuna Jelly MSc (N)
Assistant Professor
Faculty of Nursing
All India Institute of Medical Sciences
Rishikesh, Uttarakhand, India

Priya Sharma MSc (N)
Tutor
College of Nursing
All India Institute of Medical Sciences
Jodhpur, Rajasthan, India

Puneet Dhamija MD DM
Additional Professor
Department of Pharmacology
All India Institute of Medical Sciences
Rishikesh, Uttarakhand, India

Rajeev Goyal MD
Associate Professor
Department of Biochemistry
Lady Hardinge Medical College
New Delhi, India

Raj Kumar MS MCh PhD
Former Director
All India Institute of Medical Sciences
Rishikesh, Uttarakhand, India

Rajneesh K Arora MS MCh
Additional Professor
Department of Neurosurgery
All India Institute of Medical Sciences
Rishikesh, Uttarakhand, India

Ram Nawal Rao MD
Professor
Department of Pathology
Sanjay Gandhi Postgraduate Institute of Medical Sciences
Lucknow, Uttar Pradesh, India

Ravi Kant MD
Additional Professor
Department of Medicine
All India Institute of Medical Sciences
Rishikesh, Uttarakhand, India

Shaina Sharma MSc (N)
Nursing Tutor
College of Nursing
All India Institute of Medical Sciences
Rishikesh, Uttarakhand, India

Sohinder Kaur MS
Director Professor
Department of Anatomy
Lady Hardinge Medical College
New Delhi, India

Subodh Kumar MD
Additional Professor
Department of Pulmonary Medicine
All India Institute of Medical Sciences
Gorakhpur, Uttar Pradesh, India

Suresh Sharma MSc (N) PhD FNRS RN (USA)
Professor and Principal
College of Nursing
All India Institute of Medical Sciences (AIIMS)
Jodhpur, Rajasthan, India

Vandana Mehta MS
Professor
Department of Anatomy
Vardhman Mahavir Medical College and Safdarjang Hospital
New Delhi, India

Vasantha Kalyani MSc (N)
Professor-cum-Principal
College of Nursing
All India Institute of Medical Sciences
Deoghar, Jharkhand, India

Preface to the Second Edition

Pharmacology, pathology, and genetics are the diverse, important part of health sciences in the study of disease. New research in pharmacology, pathology and genetics allows easier, faster diagnosis, treatment, and care of patient suffering with diverse disease conditions. Nurses today are not merely restricted to providing bedside care to sick and injured hospitalized patients; they have more challenging expansions and extensions of their role in healthcare delivery system. Nurses are actively involved in treatment and care of sick and injured people either as acute care nurse practitioners or as family health nurse practitioners. In view of this, gradually widening horizon of nursing, it is crucial for nurses to acquire knowledge of pharmacokinetics, pharmacodynamics, drug doses, routes, adverse effects, and nurses' role in administration of common drugs. In addition, also to understand disease etiology, genetic basis of disorders, pathogenesis, morphological and histopathological changes, clinical presentation, diagnostic methodologies, and their interpretation in various diseases.

Furthermore, understanding molecular and clinical human genetic principles and concepts for nursing practice is relevant in assisting nurses to understand disease, assess risk for disease, provide a scientific foundation for the care they provide and promote health and wellness among patients and their families. Today, a foundational knowledge of the principles, practices, and psychosocial implications of genetics is essential to basic nursing care.

There is scarcity of comprehensive, simple, and lucid literature about pharmacology, pathology and genetics, which nurses can easily understand, interpret, and utilize in nursing care practices. Therefore, it is a modest attempt to bring much needed simple, comprehensive and learner friendly content of pharmacology, pathology and genetics. This title *Textbook of Pharmacology, Pathology and Genetics for Nurses-II* is not intended to be exhaustive of the pharmacology, pathology, and genetic issues important for nurses. Instead, it is meant to provide insight, food for thought, into some of the human response, care delivery, and professional issues nurses will be required to grapple with today and in the coming years regarding these disciplines. This book will be ready reference for the nursing faculty and students in the subject of pharmacology, pathology, and genetics since it is based on syllabus prescribed by Indian Nursing Council, AIIMS, PGIMER, JIPMER, RAKCON (DU) and other national and international universities.

Suresh Sharma

Preface to the First Edition

Pharmacology, Pathology and Genetics are the diverse, important part of health sciences in the study of disease. New research in pharmacology, pathology and genetics allows easier, faster diagnosis, treatment and care of patient suffering with diverse disease conditions. Nurses today are not merely restricted to provide bedside care to sick and injured hospitalized patients; they have more challenging expansions and extensions of their role in healthcare delivery system. Nurses are actively involved in treatment and care of sick and injured people either as acute care nurse practitioners or as family health nurse practitioners. In view of this, gradually widening horizon of nursing, it is crucial for nurses to acquire knowledge of pharmacokinetics, pharmacodynamics, drug doses, routes, adverse effects and nurses role in administration of common drugs. In addition, also to understand disease etiology, genetic basis of disorders, pathogenesis, morphological and histopathological changes, clinical presentation, diagnostic methodologies and their interpretation in various diseases.

Furthermore, understanding molecular and clinical human genetic principles and concepts for nursing practice is relevant in assisting nurses to understand disease, assess risk for disease, provide a scientific foundation for the care they provide and promote health and wellness among patients and their families. Today, a foundational knowledge of the principles, practices, and psychosocial implications of genetics is essential to basic nursing care.

There is scarcity of comprehensive, simple and lucid literature on the subject of pharmacology, pathology and genetics, which nurses can easily understand, interpret and utilize in nursing care practices. Therefore, it is a modest attempt to bring much needed simple, comprehensive and learner-friendly content of pharmacology, pathology and genetics. *Textbook of Pharmacology, Pathology and Genetics for Nurses* is not intended to be exhaustive of the pharmacology, pathology and genetic issues important for nurses. Instead, it is meant to provide insight, food for thought, into some of the human response, care delivery, and professional issues nurses will be required to grapple with today and in the coming years in regard to these disciplines. This book will be ready reference for the nursing faculty and students in the subject of pharmacology, pathology and genetics since it is based on syllabus prescribed by Indian Nursing Council, AIIMS, PGIMER, JIPMER, RAKCON (DU) and other national and international universities.

Suresh Sharma

Contents

SECTION 1: PHARMACOLOGY-II

1. **Drugs Used in Disorders of Ear, Nose, Throat and Eye**   3
   Hemlata, Nipin Kalal, Suresh Sharma
   Antihistamines *3*
   Topical Application for
   Eye, Ear, Nose and Buccal Cavity *5*

2. **Drugs Used on Urinary System**   11
   Farhanul Huda, Hemlata, Suresh Sharma
   Renin-Angiotensin
   Aldosterone System *11*
   Diuretics and Antidiuretics *12*
   Alkalinizers *28*

3. **Drugs Acting on Nervous System**   33
   Raj Kumar, Suresh Sharma,
   Rajneesh Arora, Poonam Arora, Hemlata
   Basis and Applied Pharmacology
   of Commonly Used Drugs *33*
   Analgesics and Anesthetics *33*
   Non-Selective COX Inhibitors *33*
   Preferential COX-2 Inhibitors *37*
   Selective COX Inhibitors *38*
   Analgesic-Antipyretics with
   Poor Anti-inflammatory Action *38*
   Opioids and Other Central
   Analgesics *39*
   Anesthesia *42*
   General Anesthesia *42*
   Classification *43*
   Hypnotics and Sedatives *52*
   Skeletal Muscle Relaxants *55*
   Peripherally Acting Muscle Relaxants *55*
   Centrally Acting Muscle Relaxants *62*
   Antipsychotics *63*
   Antidepressants *74*
   Antianxiety Drugs *81*
   Anticonvulsants *86*
   Drugs for Neurodegenerative
   Disorders and Miscellaneous Drugs *92*
   Stimulants, Ethyl Alcohol and Treatment
   of Methyl Alcohol Poisoning *94*

4. **Drugs Used for Hormonal Disorders and Supplementation, Contraception and Medical Termination of Pregnancy**   112
   Prasuna Jelly, Hemlata, Suresh Sharma
   Estrogen and Progesterone *112*
   Oral Contraceptive and Hormone
   Replacement Therapy *119*
   Vaginal Contraceptives *125*
   Drugs for Infertility and Medical
   Termination of Pregnancy *126*
   Uterine Stimulants and Relaxants *129*
   Uterine Relaxants (Tocolytics) *131*

5. **Drugs Used for Pregnant Women During Antenatal, Labor and Postnatal Period**   135
   Hemlata, Suresh Sharma
   Tetanus Prophylaxis *135*
   Iron and Vitamin K1
   Supplementation *136*
   Oxytocin, Misoprostol *136*
   Ergometrine *140*
   Methyl Prostaglandin E2 Alpha *141*
   Magnesium Sulfate *144*
   Calcium Gluconate *145*

6. **Miscellaneous Drugs**   148
   Vasantha Kalyani, Hemlata, Suresh Sharma
   Drugs Used for Deaddiction *148*
   Drugs Used in CPR and Emergency *148*
   IV Fluids and Electrolyte
   Replacement *153*
   Common Poisons, Drugs
   Used for Treatment of Poisoning *153*

Vitamins and Minerals
Supplementations 161
Vaccines and Sera (Universal
Immunization Program Schedule) 167
Anticancer Drugs: Chemotherapeutic
Drugs Commonly Used 171
Notes on Individual Drugs 171
Nursing Responsibilities 176
Patient Education 176
Causes for Failure of Chemotherapy 177
Superinfection 177
Chemoprophylaxis 178
Immunosuppressants
and Immunostimulants 178

7. **Introduction to Drugs Used in Alternative Systems of Medicine** 183

   Raj Kumar, Hemlata, Suresh Sharma

   Ayurveda, Homeopathy,
   Unani, and Siddha, etc. 183
   Department of AYUSH Under
   the Ministry of Health and Family
   Welfare 190
   Drugs Used in Common Ailments 190

8. **Fundamental Principles of Prescribing** 193

   Suresh Sharma

   Prescriptive Role of Nurse Practitioners:
   Introduction 193
   Legal and Ethical Issues
   Related to Prescribing 194
   Principles of Prescribing 198
   Steps of Prescribing 198
   Prescribing Competencies 202

SECTION 2: PATHOLOGY-II

9. **Kidney and Urinary System** 209

   Aminder Singh, Nancy Kurien, Suresh Sharma

   Glomerulonephritis 209
   Pyelonephritis 216
   Renal Calculi 219
   Cystitis 221
   Renal Cell Carcinoma 223
   Renal Failure 225

10. **Male Genital System** 229

    Aminder Singh, Nancy Kurien, Suresh Sharma

    Cryptorchidism 229
    Testicular Atrophy 231
    Prostatic Hyperplasia 231
    Carcinoma of Penis 233
    Carcinoma of Prostate 234

11. **Female Genital System** 237

    Neena Sood, Nancy Kurien, Suresh Sharma

    Carcinoma Cervix 237
    Carcinoma Endometrium 238
    Uterine Fibroids 240
    Vesicular Mole (Hydatidiform Mole) 242
    Choriocarcinoma 243
    Ovarian Cysts 244
    Ovarian Tumors 245

12. **Breast** 251

    Aminder Singh, Joyce Joseph, Suresh Sharma

    Fibrocystic Changes 251
    Fibroadenoma 251
    Breast Cancer 252

13. **Central Nervous System** 256

    Neena Sood, Nancy Kurien, Suresh Sharma

    Meningitis 256
    Encephalitis 257
    Stroke 258
    CNS Tumors 264
    Metastatic CNS Tumors 266

SECTION 3: CLINICAL PATHOLOGY

14. **Examination of Body Cavity Fluids** 271

    Neena Sood, Nancy Kurien, Suresh Sharma

    Cerebrospinal Fluid Analysis 271
    Examination of Sputum 273
    Analysis of Gastric Constituents 275
    Analysis of Duodenal Contents 276
    Analysis of Peritoneal Fluid 277
    Analysis of Pericardial Fluid 278
    Analysis of Semen 279
    Urine Examination 282
    Fecal Examination 287

SECTION 4: GENETICS

15. Introduction to Genetics — 293
Suresh Sharma, Sohinder Kaur
- Concept of Genetics 293
- Basic Genetic Terms 294
- Practical Applications of Genetics in Nursing 295
- Review of Cellular Division 302
- Genes 316
- Protein Biosynthesis 325
- Genetic Code 327
- Naming Genes 328
- Chromosome 329
- Chromosomal Aberrations/Chromosomal Mutation 332
- Patterns of Inheritance 336
- Sex-linked Inheritance 341
- Mendelian Theory of Inheritance 348
- Multiple Allots and Blood Groups 348
- Facts about Transmission of Genetic Disorders 351
- Mechanism of Inheritance 352
- Gene Mutation (Errors of Transmission) 353

16. Emerging Paradigm of Genetics in Nursing — 362
Suresh Sharma
- Genetic Nursing Practice Milestones 363
- Roles of Nurses in Genetics 364
- Importance of Genetics in Nursing Curriculum 364
- Barriers and Approaches for Implementation of Genetics in Nursing 367
- Assumptions Regarding Genetics and Health Care in Future 368

17. Maternal and Prenatal Genetics — 371
Suresh Sharma, Vandana Mehta
- Genetics and Infection 371
- Consanguinity Atopy 375
- Prenatal Nutrition and Food Allergies 378
- Role of Prenatal Nutrition in Prevention of Genetic Disorders 380
- Maternal Age 381
- Maternal Drug Therapy 384
- Effects of Radiation, Drugs and Chemicals 389
- Prenatal Testing and Diagnosis 396
- Noninvasive Tests 398
- Invasive Tests 400
- Preimplantation Prenatal Diagnosis 408
- Infertility 410
- Spontaneous Abortions 417
- Neural Tube Defects 420
- Down Syndrome 426

18. Neonatal and Children Testing or Screening — 434
Suresh Sharma, Jyoti Arora
- Meaning and Purpose 434
- Newborn Screening 435
- Genetic Testing and Screening in Children 437
- Congenital Abnormalities 441
- Developmental Delay 442
- Dysmorphism 446
- Role of Nurses in Genetic Testing for Neonates and Children 447

19. Genetic Conditions of Adolescents and Adults — 450
Suresh Sharma, Kumar Satish Ravi
- Genetic Statistics 450
- Naming Genetic Conditions 450
- Common Genetic Conditions 451
- Therapeutic Approaches for Genetic Disorders 484
- Nursing Management in Genetic Disorders 486

20. Services Related to Genetics — 496
Suresh Sharma, Mohd Salahuddin Ansari
- Genetic Testing 496
- Gene Therapy 503
- Genetic Counseling 510

Index — 515

INC Syllabus

PHARMACOLOGY—II

Including Fundamentals of Prescribing Module

Description: This course is designed to enable students to acquire understanding of Pharmacodynamics, Pharmacokinetics, principles of therapeutics and nursing implications. Further it develops understanding of fundamental principles of prescribing in students.

Competencies: On completion of the course, the students will be able to
- Explain the drugs used in the treatment of ear, nose, throat and eye disorders.
- Explain the drugs used in the treatment of urinary system disorders.
- Describe the drugs used in the treatment of nervous system disorders.
- Explain the drugs used for hormonal replacement and for the pregnant women during antenatal, intra natal and postnatal period.
- Explain the drugs used to treat emergency conditions and immune disorders.
- Discuss the role and responsibilities of nurses towards safe administration of drugs used to treat disorders of various systems with basic understanding of pharmacology.
- Demonstrate understanding about the drugs used in alternative system of medicine.
- Demonstrate understanding about the fundamental principles of prescribing.

COURSE OUTLINE

T–Theory

Unit	Time (Hrs)	Learning Outcomes	Content	Teaching/ Learning Activities	Assessment Methods
I	4 (T)	Describe drugs used in disorders of ear, nose, throat and eye and nurses' responsibilities	**Drugs used in disorders of ear, nose, throat and eye** • Antihistamines • Topical applications for eye (chloramphenicol, gentamycin eye drops), ear (soda glycerin, boric spirit ear drops), nose and buccal cavity-chlorhexidine mouthwash • Composition, action, dosage, route, indications, contraindications, drug interactions, side effects, adverse effects, toxicity and role of nurse	• Lecture cum discussion • Drug study/ presentation	• Short answer • Objective type

Unit	Time (Hrs)	Learning Outcomes	Content	Teaching/ Learning Activities	Assessment Methods
II	4 (T)	Describe drugs acting on urinary system and nurse's responsibilities	**Drugs used on urinary system** • Pharmacology of commonly used drugs ▪ Renin angiotensin system ▪ Diuretics and antidiuretics ▪ Drugs toxic to kidney ▪ Urinary antiseptics ▪ Treatment of UTI – acidifiers and alkalinizers • Composition, action, dosage, route, indications, contraindications, drug interactions, side effects, adverse effects toxicity and role of nurse	• Lecture cum discussion • Drug study/ presentation	• Short answer • Objective type

III	10 (T)	Describe drugs used on nervous system and nurse's responsibilities	**Drugs acting on nervous system**
			• Basis and applied pharmacology of commonly used drugs
			• Analgesics and anaesthetics
			▪ Analgesics: Non-steroidal anti-inflammatory (NSAID) drugs
			▪ Antipyretics
			▪ Opioids and other central analgesics
			  – General (techniques of GA, pre anesthetic medication) and local anesthetics
			  – Gases: Oxygen, nitrous, oxide, carbon-dioxide and others
			• Hypnotics and sedatives
			• Skeletal muscle relaxants
			• Antipsychotics
			▪ Mood stabilizers
			• Antidepressants
			• Antianxiety drugs
			• Anticonvulsants
			• Drugs for neurodegenerative disorders and miscellaneous drugs
			• Stimulants, ethyl alcohol and treatment of methyl alcohol poisoning
			• Composition, action, dosage, route, indications, contraindications, drug interactions, side effects, adverse effects toxicity and role of nurse
				• Lecture cum discussion
				• Drug study/ presentation
					• Short answer
					• Objective type

INC Syllabus

Unit	Time (Hrs)	Learning Outcomes	Content	Teaching/ Learning Activities	Assessment Methods

IV	5 (T)	Describe drugs used for hormonal disorder and supplementation, contraception and medical termination of pregnancy and nurse's responsibilities	**Drugs used for hormonal, disorders and supplementation, contraception and medical termination of pregnancy**
			• Estrogens and progesterones
			   ▪ Oral contraceptives and hormone replacement therapy
			• Vaginal contraceptives
			• Drugs for infertility and medical termination of pregnancy
			   ▪ Uterine stimulants and relaxants
			• Composition, actions dosage route indications contraindications, drugs interactions, side effects, adverse effects, toxicity and role of nurse
				• Lecture cum discussion
				• Drug study/ presentation
					• Short answer
					• Objective type

V	3 (T)	Develop understanding about important drugs used for women before, during and after labour	**Drugs used for pregnant women during antenatal, labor and postnatal period** • Tetanus prophylaxis • Iron and Vit K1 supplementation • Oxytocin, misoprostol • Ergometrine • Methyl prostaglandin F2-alpha • Magnesium sulphate • Calcium gluconate	• Lecture cum discussion • Drug study/ presentation	• Short answer • Objective type

VI	10 (T)	Describe drugs used in deaddiction, emergency, poisoning, vitamins and minerals supplementation, drugs used for immunization and immunesuppression and nurse's responsibilities	**Miscellaneous drugs**
			• Drugs used for deaddiction
			• Drugs used in CPR and emergency-adrenaline, chlorpheniramine, hydrocortisone, dexamethasone
			• IV fluids and electrolytes replacement
			• Common poisons, drugs used for treatment of poisoning
			   ▪ Activated charcoal
			   ▪ Ipecac
			   ▪ Antidotes
			   ▪ Anti-snake venom (ASV)
			• Vitamins and minerals supplementation
				• Lecture cum discussion
				• Drug study/ presentation
					• Short answer
					• Objective type

Unit	Time (Hrs)	Learning Outcomes	Content	Teaching/ Learning Activities	Assessment Methods
			• Vaccines and sera (universal immunization program schedules) • Anticancer drugs: Chemotherapeutic drugs commonly used • Immuno-suppressants and immunostimulants		
VII	4 (T)	Demonstrate awareness of common drugs used in alternative system of medicine	**Introduction to drugs used in alternative systems of medicine** • Ayurveda, Homeopathy, Unani and Siddha etc. • Drugs used for common ailments	• Lecture cum discussion • Observational visit	• Short answer • Objective type
VIII	20 (T)	Demonstrate understanding about fundamental principles of prescribing	**Fundamental principles of prescribing** • Prescriptive role of nurse practitioners: Introduction • Legal and ethical issues related to prescribing • Principles of prescribing • Steps of prescribing • Prescribing competencies	• Completion of module on fundamental principles of prescribing	• Short answer • Assignments evaluation

PATHOLOGY—II AND GENETICS

Placement: IV Semester

Theory: 1 Credit (20 hours) (includes lab hours also)

Description: This course is designed to enable students to acquire knowledge of pathology of various disease conditions, understanding of genetics, its role in causation and management of defects and diseases and to apply this knowledge in practice of nursing.

Competencies: On completion of the course, the students will be able to:
- Apply the knowledge of pathology in understanding the deviations from normal to abnormal pathology.
- Rationalize the various laboratory investigations in diagnosing pathological disorders.
- Demonstrate the understanding of the methods of collection of blood, body cavity fluids, urine and feces for various tests.
- Apply the knowledge of genetics in understanding the various pathological disorders.
- Appreciate the various manifestations in patients with diagnosed genetic abnormalities.
- Rationalize the specific diagnostic tests in the detection of genetic abnormalities.
- Demonstrate the understanding of various services related to genetics.

COURSE OUTLINE

T–Theory

Unit	Time (Hrs)	Learning Outcomes	Content	Teaching/Learning Activities	Assessment Methods
I	5 (T)	Explain pathological changes in disease conditions of various systems	**Special pathology: Pathological changes in disease conditions of selected systems** • **Kidneys and urinary tract** ▪ Glomerulonephritis ▪ Pyelonephritis ▪ Renal calculi ▪ Cystitis ▪ Renal cell carcinoma ▪ Renal failure (acute and chronic) • **Male genital systems** ▪ Cryptorchidism ▪ Testicular atrophy ▪ Prostatic hyperplasia ▪ Carcinoma penis and Prostate. • **Female genital system** ▪ Carcinoma cervix ▪ Carcinoma of endometrium ▪ Uterine fibroids ▪ Vesicular mole and Choriocarcinoma ▪ Ovarian cyst and tumors • **Breast** ▪ Fibrocystic changes ▪ Fibroadenoma ▪ Carcinoma of the breast • **Central nervous system** ▪ Meningitis. ▪ Encephalitis ▪ Stroke ▪ Tumors of CNS	• Lecture • Discussion • Explain using slides, X-rays and scans • Visit to pathology lab, endoscopy unit and OT	• Short answer • Objective type
II	5 (T)	Describe the laboratory tests for examination of body cavity fluids, urine and faeces	**Clinical Pathology** • Examination of body cavity fluids: ▪ Methods of collection and examination of CSF	• Lecture • Discussion • Visit to clinical lab and biochemistry lab	• Short answer • Objective type

Unit	Time (Hrs)	Learning Outcomes	Content	Teaching/Learning Activities	Assessment Methods
			and other body cavity fluids (sputum, wound discharge) specimen for various clinical pathology, biochemistry and microbiology tests • **Analysis of semen:** ▪ Sperm count, motility and morphology and their importance in infertility • **Urine:** ▪ Physical characteristics, analysis, culture and sensitivity • **Faeces:** ▪ Characteristics ▪ Stool examination: Occult blood, ova, parasite and cyst, reducing substance etc. ▪ Methods and collection of urine and faeces for various tests		

GENETICS COURSE OUTLINE

T–Theory

Unit	Time (Hrs)	Learning Outcomes	Content	Teaching/Learning Activities	Assessment Methods
I	2 (T)	Explain nature, principles and perspectives of heredity	**Introduction:** • Practical application of genetics in nursing • Impact of genetic condition on families • Review of cellular division: Mitosis and meiosis • Characteristics and structure of genes • Chromosomes: Sex determination	• Lecture • Discussion • Explain using slides	• Short answer • Objective type

Unit	Time (Hrs)	Learning Outcomes	Content	Teaching/ Learning Activities	Assessment Methods
			• Chromosomal aberrations • Patterns of inheritance • Mendelian theory of inheritance • Multiple allots and blood groups • Sex linked inheritance • Mechanism of inheritance • Errors in transmission (mutation)		
II	2 (T)	Explain maternal, prenatal and genetic influences on development of defects and diseases	**Maternal, prenatal and genetic influences on development of defects and diseases** • Conditions affecting the mother: Genetic and infections • Consanguinity atopy • Prenatal nutrition and food allergies • Maternal age • Maternal drug therapy • Prenatal testing and diagnosis • Effect of radiation, drugs and chemicals • Infertility • Spontaneous abortion • Neural tube defects and the role of folic acid in lowering the risks • Down syndrome (Trisomy 21)	• Lecture • Discussion • Explain using slides	• Short answer • Objective type

III	2 (T)	Explain the screening methods for genetic defects and diseases in neonates and children	**Genetic testing in the neonates and children**
			• Screening for
			  ▪ Congenital abnormalities
			  ▪ Developmental delay
			  ▪ Dysmorphism
				• Lecture
				• Discussion
				• Explain using slides
					• Short answer
					• Objective type

IV	2 (T)	Identify genetic disorders in adolescents and adults	**Genetic conditions of adolescents and adults** • Cancer genetics: Familial cancer • Inborn errors of metabolism • Blood group alleles and hematological disorder • Genetic haemochromatosis • Huntington's disease • Mental illness	• Lecture • Discussion • Explain using slides	• Short answer • Objective type
V	2 (T)	Describe the role of nurse in genetic services and counselling	**Services related to genetics** • Genetic testing • Gene therapy • Genetic counseling • Legal and ethical issues • Role of nurse	• Lecture • Discussion	• Short answer • Objective type

SECTION 1

PHARMACOLOGY-II

CHAPTERS

- Drug Used in Disorders of Ear, Nose, Throat and Eye
- Drugs Used on Urinary System
- Drugs Acting on Nervous System
- Drugs Used for Hormonal Disorders and Supplementation, Contraception and Medical Termination of Pregnancy
- Drugs Used for Pregnant Women During Antenatal, Labor and Postnatal Period
- Miscellaneous Drugs
- Introduction to Drugs Used in Alternative Systems of Medicine
- Fundamental Principles of Prescribing

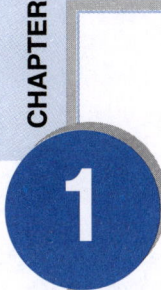

CHAPTER 1

Drugs Used in Disorders of Ear, Nose, Throat and Eye

Hemlata, Nipin Kalal, Suresh Sharma

Hearing and maintaining equilibrium and balance are the two basic sensory functions of the ear. Topical medications in the form of eardrops are the most common therapy for ear problems. Otitis media, or ear irritation, is a frequent pharmacological indication. Ophthalmic pharmacology has emerged as a distinct stream of pharmacology in recent years. Ocular therapies have grown greatly in scope, and additional medications have been created. Drugs that are often used for therapeutic and diagnostic reasons in ENT and eye disorders are briefly discussed.

ANTIHISTAMINES

Antihistamines are the drugs which alter the effect of histamines by occupying its receptors. For details *see* Chapter 4 Page No. 89 (Volume 1). Following are the antihistamines used for the ENT and eye disorders.

Drugs Used in Eye Disorders

The ophthalmic antihistamines are used to treat the allergic disorders of eyes and prevent conjunctivitis. It inhibits the histamine-mediated inflammatory responses. It is considered as the gold standard for the treatment of allergies.

Examples—antazoline sulfate, azelastine hydrochloride, olopatadine, epinastine hydrochloride, ketotifen.

Indication

- Allergic conjunctivitis
- Seasonal and perennial conjunctivitis
- Corneal inflammation

Dose: 1–2 drops twice daily until the cessation of symptoms

Contraindication

Hypersensitivity.

Side Effects

- **Ocular side effects:** Local irritation and stinging are possible, visual disturbances, keratitis, edema, and photophobia
- **Systemic side effects (rare):** Headache, pruritus and skin reactions, drowsiness and dry mouth reported

Patient Education
- Advise about the safety during home usage of the drug.
- Instruct the patient not to drive or use any machinery while on treatment.
- Instruct the patient to avoid sharing of the drug.

Nursing Consideration
- Check the right of medication before administering
- Ensure proper administration of eye drops and eye ointment **(Figs. 1.1A and B)**
- Evaluate the sign for side effects as there can be rebound vasodilation after prolonged use, severe renal impairment, pregnancy and breastfeeding.
- Ensure the regular usage of the drugs as these drugs act quickly but consider oral antihistamines if symptoms are severe or not limited to the eye. They may be used concurrently with a mast cell stabilizer (ketotifen has mast cell stabilizing properties too). Antazoline preparations are available over-the-counter (OTC).

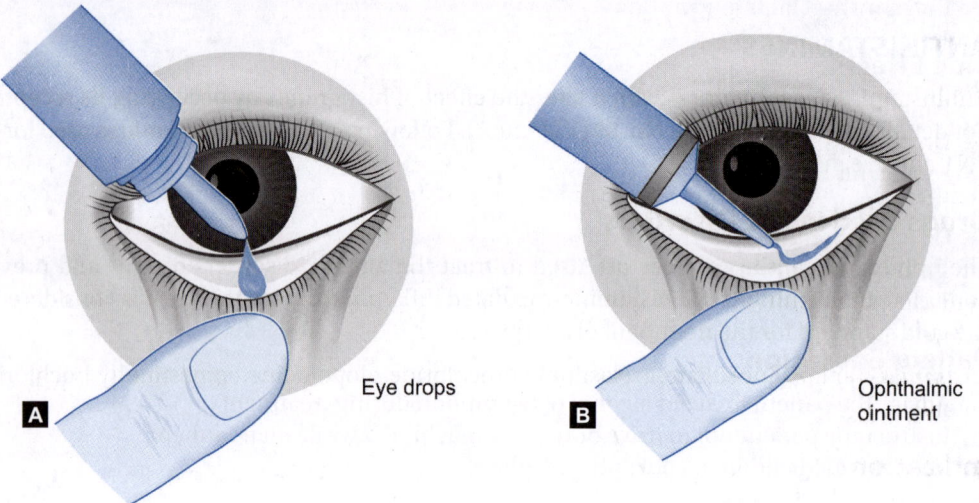

Figs. 1.1A and B: Method of instillation of ophthalmic (A) Eye drops and (B) Ointment.

Drugs used in ENT Disorders

The antihistamines are used to treat the allergic disorders of ear, nose and throat, i.e., allergic rhinitis.

Examples—olopatadine, acrivastine, levocetirizine, and fexofenadine.

Indication
- Allergic rhinitis
- Surgical intervention
- Sore throat
- Otitis media with effusion

Drug and its Dose
See **Table 1.1**.

Table 1.1: Drug, dose and frequency of antihistamines used in common ENT disorders.

Drug name	Dosage	Frequency
Levocetirizine	2–2.5 mg/day in night (HS)	Once a day
Cyproheptadine	0.5 mg/kg/day	Twice or thrice a day
Cetirizine	10 mg/day	Once a day
Diphenhydramine	25–50 mg	Once a day

Contraindication
- Hypersensitivity
- End stage renal disease
- Newborn
- Pregnant and lactating mothers

Side Effects
- Fatigue
- Drowsiness
- Headache
- Dry mouth
- Urinary retention
- Tachycardia
- Taste perversion

Patient Education
- Advise the patient to avoid alcohol consumption during treatment
- Instruct the patient not to drive or use any machinery while on treatment.
- Keep the medication in cool and dark place.

Nursing Consideration
- Check the right of medication before administering
- Check for any contraindications of the drug
- Ensure the safe administration of the drug **(Figs. 1.2A and B)**
- Evaluate the sign for side effects as there can be rebound vasodilation after prolonged use, severe renal impairment, pregnancy and breastfeeding.

TOPICAL APPLICATION FOR EYE, EAR, NOSE AND BUCCAL CAVITY

Topical Application for Eye

Chloramphenicol
Chloramphenicol is a broad-spectrum antibiotic used to treat the bacterial eye infections, i.e., conjunctivitis.

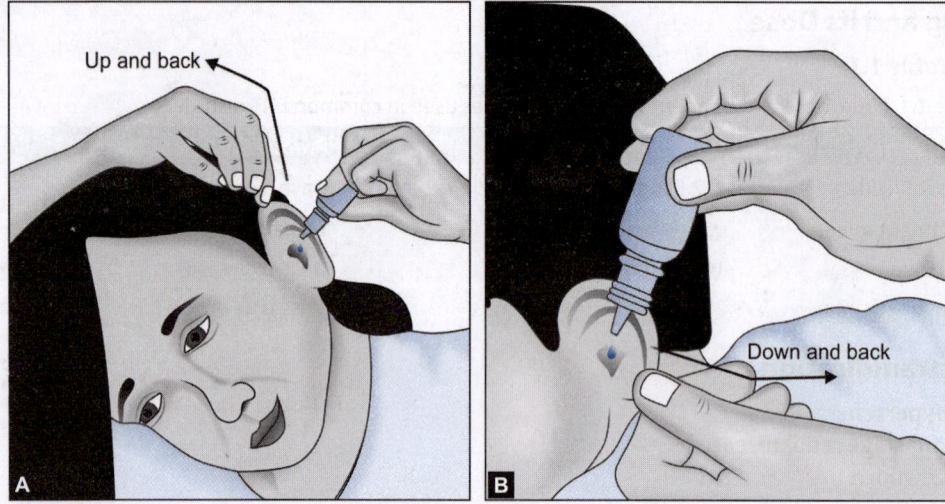

Figs. 1.2A and B: Method of administration of ear drop in (A) Adult and (B) Child.

Action

It inhibits the formation of peptide bond and protein synthesis in bacteria, by diffusing in the bacterial cell membrane.

Indication

Bacterial conjunctivitis

Dosage

Ointment—1 cm of ointment every 3–4 hourly for 5 days.

Contraindication

- Hypersensitivity
- Porphyria

Side Effects

- Blurring of vision
- Burning sensation
- Redness

Toxicity

- Gray baby syndrome
- Abdominal distension

Patient Education

- Advise the patient to avoid usage of the contact lenses during treatment
- Instruct to clean the hands before administering the drugs
- Avoid prolong usage. Keep the medication in cool and dark place

Nursing Consideration
- Check the right of medication before administering
- Check for any contraindications of the drug
- Administer the drug as shown in **Figure 1.1B**
- Evaluate the sign for side effects of rash, itching, dizziness and dyspnea
- Monitor the liver and kidney function test

Gentamycin

Action
It is an aminoglycoside antibiotic which inhibits the formation of bacterial protein synthesis resulting in defective cell membrane. It binds the 30 S ribosomal subunits.

Indication
- Bacterial conjunctivitis
- Blepharitis

Dosage
- **Ointment 0.3% conc:** 1 cm of ointment every 3–4 hourly for 5 days
- **Drops:** 2 drops in infected eye 4–5 days in a day

Contraindication
- Hypersensitivity
- Chronic kidney disease

Side Effects
- Auditory and vestibulary dysfunction
- Site irritation
- Burning sensation

Patient Education
- Advise the patient to avoid usage of the contact lenses during treatment
- Instruct to clean the hands before administering the drugs. Keep the medication in cool and dark place.

Nursing Consideration
- Check the right of medication before administering
- Check for any contraindications of the drug
- Administer the drug as shown in **Figures 1.1A and B**
- Monitor the liver and kidney function test

Topical Application for Ear

Soda Glycerine
It is also known as glycerol. Soda bicarb glycerine is used in ear infection to soften the dry ear wax. It is the safest drug.

Action

It is an aminoglycoside antibiotic which inhibits the formation of bacterial protein synthesis resulting in defective cell membrane. It binds the 30 S ribosomal subunits.

Indication

Softened the ear wax (Cerumen)

Dosage

Drops: 3–4 drops in infected ear twice daily for 3–5 days.

Contraindication

- Hypersensitivity
- Recent Ear surgery
- Pregnancy and lactation

Side Effects

- Dryness in ear
- Stomach cramps
- Flatulence

Patient Education

- Instruct to clean the hands before administering the drugs
- Keep the medication in cool and dark place

Nursing Consideration

- Check the right of medication before administering
- Check for any contraindications of the drug
- Administer the drug as shown in **Figures 1.2A and B**

Boric Spirit Drop

Boric spirit contains boric acid and alcohol. It inhibit the bacterial and fungal growth.

Action

It is an aminoglycoside antibiotic which inhibits the formation of bacterial protein synthesis resulting in defective cell membrane. It binds the 30 S ribosomal subunits.

Indication

- Bacterial or fungal infection
- Chronic suppurative otitis media

Dosage

Drops 4%: 3–4 drops in infected ear twice daily for 10 days.

Contraindication

- Hypersensitivity
- Recent ear surgery

Side Effects
- Nausea and vomiting
- Headache
- Drowsiness
- Loss of coordination
- Dysnea.

Patient Education
- Instruct to clean the hands before administering the drugs
- Keep the medication in cool and dark place
- Instruct the patient avoid consumption of alcohol while on medication

Nursing Consideration
- Check the right of medication before administering
- Check for any contraindications of the drug
- Administer the drug as shown in **Figures 1.2A and B.**

Topical Application for Nose and Buccal Cavity
Chlorhexidine Mouthwash
Chlorhexidine mouthwash is an antiseptic agent with topical antibacterial. Its antibacterial activity helps in managing the gingival inflammation and bleeding. It is used in the case of plague or bad breath by the action of reducing bacterial species associated with buccal cavity infections.

Indication
- Periodontitis
- Gingivitis
- Mouth wash (oral care) to remove order
- Oral rinse before dental work
- Sore throat

Dosage
Mouthwash: 1/2 ounce (15 mL) undiluted for 30 sec twice a day

Contraindication
Hypersensitivity

Side Effects
- Staining on tooth or tongue surface
- Alter taste
- Formation of tartar
- Throat irritation

Patient Education
- Instruct the patient do not swallow the mouthwash
- It should be used after brushing.

- Do not rinse the mouth immediately
- Avoid eating after the mouth wash to prevent stain
- Keep the medication in cool and dark place

MULTIPLE CHOICE QUESTIONS

1. **Which of the following is the correct technique for ear drop instillation in an adult?**
   a. Down and back
   b. Up and back
   c. Down and forward
   d. Up and forward
2. **Drug chloramphenicol belong to which of the following?**
   a. Antibiotic
   b. Antiviral
   c. Antifungal
   d. Antihistamine
3. **Which of the following is not an indication for chlorhexidine mouthwash?**
   a. Conjunctivitis
   b. Periodontitis
   c. Gingivitis
   d. Sore throat
4. **Indication for boric spirit drop**
   a. Keratitis
   b. Conjunctivitis
   c. Chronic suppurative otitis media
   d. Rhinitis

Answer Key

1. b
2. a
3. a
4. c

FURTHER READING

1. Griffin, Glenn, Cheryl AF. "Antihistamines and/or decongestants for otitis media with effusion (OME) in children." The Cochrane database *of systematic reviews vo*l. 2011,9 CD003423. 7 Sep. 2011, doi:10.1002/14651858.CD003423.pub3
2. Kimchi N, Bielory L. The allergic eye: recommendations about pharmacotherapy and recent therapeutic agents. *Curr Opin Allergy Clin Immunol.* 2020;20(4):414-420. doi:10.1097/ACI.0000000000000669
3. National Center for Biotechnology Information. PubChem Compound Summary for CID 5959, Chloramphenicol;.2002.
4. National Center for Biotechnology Information. PubChem Compound Summary for CID 753, Glycerol; 2002.
5. National Center for Biotechnology Information. PubChem Compound Summary for CID 9552079, Chlorhexidine; 2002.
6. Oong GC, Tadi P. Chloramphenicol. [Updated 2021 Nov 17]. In: StatPearls [Internet]. Treasure Island (FL): StatPearls Publishing; 2022

CHAPTER 2

Drugs Used on Urinary System

Farhanul Huda, Hemlata, Suresh Sharma

Urinary system includes kidney, ureter and urinary bladder. This system plays an important role in maintaining the normal blood pressure. The diseases, such as chronic kidney disease, cardiac disease affect the sodium and water reabsorption later, it cause edema. This system based on the physiology of renin-angiotensin-aldosterone system (RAAS).

RENIN-ANGIOTENSIN ALDOSTERONE SYSTEM

The RAAS regulates the systemic vascular resistance and blood volume. This system cause chronic alteration in order to raise the blood volume. It is composed of three main compounds —renin (release by kidney), angiotensin II (converted from angiotensin I via ACE inhibitor) and aldestrone (release by adrenal gland). This system increase blood volume in response to decreased renal blood pressure, and hypotension.

The schematic presentation of RAAS system mechanism is explained in **Figure 2.1**. RAAS system activates as soon as hypotension or renal blood flow decrease, the sympathetic nervous

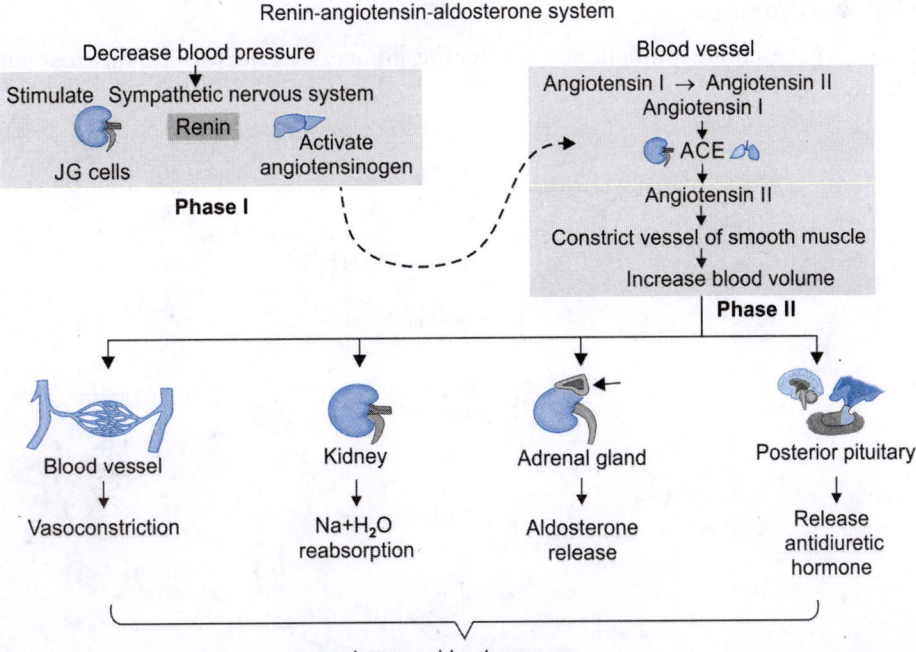

Fig. 2.1: Schematic presentation of renin-angiotensin-aldosterone system (RAAS) mechanism.
(JG cells: juxtaglomerular cells)

system activates. It acts on afferent arterioles of kidney, to activate the juxtaglomerular cells (JG cells). This JG cells contain prorenin gets activated and cleavages into renin. Renin released into the blood and targets the liver, which produce angiotensinogen. The renin cleavage the angiotensinogen into angiotensin I (precursor of angiotensin II). ACE inhibitor (found in the vascular endothelium of lung and kidney) convert the angiotensin I into angiotensin II.

This conversion constricts the smooth muscles and cause increase in blood volume by acting on blood vessels, kidney, adrenal gland and posterior pituitary gland. Blood vessel gets constricted and raises the blood volume. The kidney activates and causes sodium and water reabsorption. The adrenal gland release aldosterone cause sodium and potassium excretion at the distal and collecting tubule of kidney. The posterior pituitary release antidiuretic hormone (ADH) cause water reabsorption in the kidney. This angiotensin II decreases the baroreceptor reflex, and increases the blood pressure. This is the counterproductive goal of RAAS.

DIURETICS AND ANTIDIURETICS

Diuretics/Natriuretics

The diuretics act by inhibiting tubular reabsorption to cause net loss of Na^+ and water from urine **(Fig. 2.2)**; just 1% decrease in tubular reabsorption would more than double urine output.

Classification

The diuretics are classified into three group **(Fig. 2.3)**.

High Efficacy Diuretics

Drugs name: Furosemide, bumetanide, piretanide, ethacrynic acid, torsemide, azosemide.

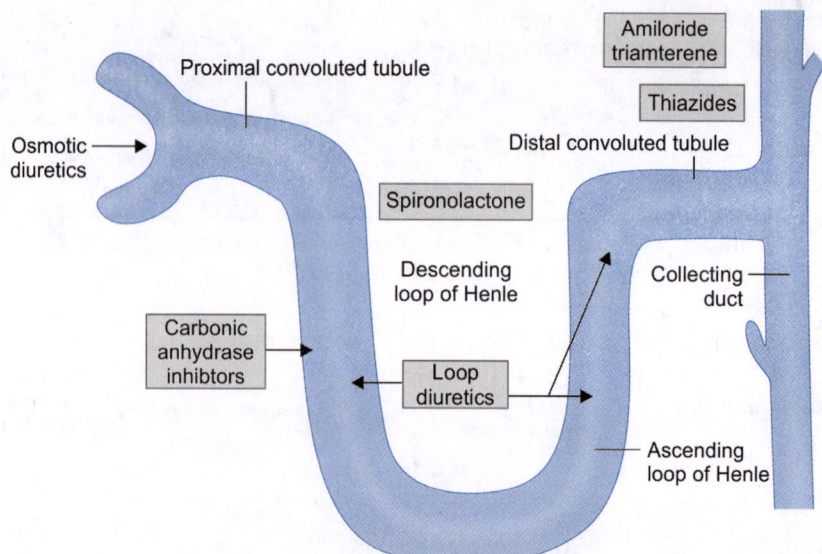

Fig. 2.2: Site of action of diuretics.

CHAPTER 2: Drugs Used on Urinary System

High efficacy diuretics
- Sulfamoyl derivatives—furosemide, bumetanide, piretanide, ethacrynic acid, torsemide, and azosemide

Moderate efficacy diuretics
- Thiazides; benzothiadiazine—chlorothiazide, hydrochlorothiazide, polythiazide, bendroflumethiazide, cyclopenthiazide
- Thiazide-related agents—chlorthalidone, clopamide, indapamide, metolazone, xipamide.

Low efficacy diuretics
- Potassium sparing diuretics—triamterene, amiloride, spironolactone
- Carbonic anhydrase inhibitors—acetazolamide, methazolamide, dorzolamide
- Osmotic diuretics—mannitol, urea, glycerol, Isosorbide
- Methylxanthines—theophylline

Fig. 2.3: Classification of diuretics.

Mechanism of action (Inhibit Na^+, K^+, $2Cl^-$ Symporter)

Frusemide (Loop diuretics) acts by inhibiting $NaCl^-$ reabsorption in the thick ascending limb of the Henle's loop **(Fig. 2.2)**. It blocks the Na^+, K^+, and Cl^- symporter in the thick ascending limb of the Henle's loop because of which it is called is a loop diuretic. It greatly increases the excretion of Na^+ and Cl^- in the urine. As a large amount of $NaCl^-$ is absorbed in this segment, loop diuretics are highly efficacious. Diuretic response increases with dose and overenthusiastic treatment can cause dehydration.

Other Actions

- Loop diuretics also enhance the excretion of K^+, Ca^{++} and Mg^{++} (but Ca^{++} is reabsorbed in the distal tubule—hence no hypocalcemia).
- They increase reabsorption of uric acid in the proximal tubule.
- On long-term use, they also alter renal hemodynamics to reduce fluid and electrolyte reabsorption in the proximal tubule; loop diuretics enhance renin release.
- Frusemide is also a weak carbonic anhydrase inhibitor hence it increases the excretion of HCO_3 and phosphate.

Intravenous furosemide causes venodilation and reduces left ventricular filling pressure. It thus relieves pulmonary congestion in congestive heart failure (CHF) and in pulmonary edema even before the onset of diuresis. **Table 2.1** depicts the dose for high efficacy diuresis.

Table 2.1: Dose for high efficacy diuresis.

S. No.	Name of the drugs	Dose	Route
1.	Furosemide (Lasix)	20–80 mg/day up to 600 mg/day 20–40 mg	Oral/intramuscular/intravenous
2.	Torsemide	2.5–5 mg/day increased to 10 mg/day 4–6 weeks	Oral
3.	Bumetanide	1 mg IV loading dose then 0.5–2 mg/day PO divided q 12 h	Intravenous, oral

Pharmacokinetics

Furosemide is rapidly absorbed orally, highly bound to plasma proteins, metabolized in the liver and excreted by the kidneys. Given intravenously frusemide acts in 2–5 minutes, while following oral use, it takes 20–40 minutes. Plasma t½ half life is 1½ hours and duration of action is 4–6 hours. Loop diuretics reach the ascending limb of Henle's loop as they are secreted by the organic acid transport system.

Indications

- Acute CHF
- Acute pulmonary edema
- Edema associated with CHF
- Edema associated with renal or liver disease
- Hypertension
- Acute renal failure
- Cerebral edema
- Acute hypercalcemia and hyperkalemia

Contraindications

Anuria, severe renal failure, hepatic coma, pregnancy and lactation.

Side Effects

- Hypotension and volume depletion, as well as hypokalemia because of enhanced secretion of K^+.
- They may also produce alkalosis due to enhanced H1 secretion.
- Dose-related ototoxicity, more often in individuals with renal impairment. These effects are more pronounced with ethacrynic acid than with furosemide. These agents should be administered cautiously in the presence of renal disease or with the use of other ototoxic agents, such as aminoglycosides.
- These agents can cause hypersensitivity reactions.
- Ethacrynic acid produces gastrointestinal (GI) disturbances.

Nursing Responsibilities

- Administer drug during day time to avoid sleep disturbance
- Do not mix parenteral solution with highly acidic solutions with pH below 3.5
- Monitor serum electrolytes, hydration, liver and renal function periodically
- Administer potassium rich diet to patient
- Check for any contraindication

Patient Education

- Educate about the role of diuretics
- Instruct patient to weight regularly
- Instruct patient to eat potassium rich diet
- Advice patient to avoid taking drug at bedtime

Other high efficiency diuretics

- *Bumetanide* is similar to furosemide but is 40 times more potent than furosemide. It induces very rapid diuresis and highly effective in pulmonary edema. Bumetanide is more lipid-soluble; oral bioavailability is 80%–100% and is better tolerated.

- *Torsemide*—oral absorption is more rapid and more complete. The elimination $t_{1/2}$ (3.5 hours) and duration of action (4–8 hours) are longer. It is used in edema and hypertension.
- *Ethacrynic acid* is more likely to cause adverse effects particularly ototoxicity and hence is not commonly used.

Moderate Efficacy Diuretics

Drug Name

- **Thiazides;** benzothiadiazines—chlorothiazide, hydrochlorothiazide, polythiazide, bendroflumethiazide, cyclopenthiazide.
- **Thiazide related agents:** Chlorthalidone, clopamide, indapamide, metolazone, xipamide.

Mechanism of Action (Inhibit Na^+/Cl^- Cotransport)

Thiazides act on the early distal tubule. Thiazides have a moderate efficacy because 90% of the filtered sodium is already reabsorbed before reaching the distal tubule. This group of drugs blocks Na^+/Cl^- cotransport system in the early distal tubule. They also inhibit carbonic anhydrase activity and increase bicarbonate loss. Thiazides also enhance excretion of Mg^+ and K^+ (in distal segments, Na^+ in the lumen is exchanged for K^+ which is then excreted). But they inhibit urinary excretion of Ca^{++} and uric acid resulting in hypercalcemia and hyperuricemia. The action begins in 1 hour of administration but duration of action is 6–48 hours.

Table 2.2 depicts the doses for moderate efficacy diuretics.

Indications

- Edema
- Hypertension
- Diabetes insipidus
- Hypercalciuria
- Liver cirrhosis

Contraindications

Contraindicated with allergy to thiazides, sulfonamides; fluid or electrolyte imbalance; renal disease (can lead to azotemia); liver disease (risk of hepatic coma); anuria.

Table 2.2: Doses for moderate efficacy diuretics.

S. No.	Name of the drugs	Dose	Route	Action duration (in hours)
1.	Hydrochlorothiazide	Adult—25–100 mg/day	Oral	6–12
2.	Chlorothiazide	Adult—0.5 –1 g (10–20 mL/day)	Oral/intravenous (IV)	48
3.	Metolazone	5–10 mg/day	Oral/IV	12–24
4.	Xipamide	20–40 mg/day maximum 80 mg/day	Oral/IV	12
5.	Indapamide	2.5–5 mg/day	Oral/IV	12–24
6.	Clopamide	10–60 mg/day	Oral/IV	12–18

Adverse Effects
- **CNS:** Dizziness, vertigo, paresthesias, weakness, headache, drowsiness, fatigue
- **CV:** Orthostatic hypotension, venous thrombosis, volume depletion, cardiac arrhythmias, chest pain
- **Dermatologic:** Photosensitivity, rash, purpura, exfoliative dermatitis, hives, alopecia
- **GI:** Nausea, anorexia, vomiting, dry mouth, diarrhea, constipation, jaundice, hepatitis, pancreatitis
- **Genitourinary:** Polyuria, nocturia, impotence, loss of libido
- **Hematologic:** Leukopenia, thrombocytopenia, agranulocytosis, aplastic anemia, neutropenia
- **Other:** Muscle cramps, muscle spasms, fever, gouty attacks, flushing, weight loss, rhinorrhea, electrolyte imbalances, and hyperglycemia.

Nursing Responsibilities
- Give with food or milk if GI upset occurs
- Mark calendars or provide other reminders of drug for alternate day or 3–5 days/week therapy
- Reduce dosage of other antihypertensives by at least 50% if given with thiazides; readjust dosages gradually as blood pressure (BP) responds
- Administer early in the day so increased urination will not disturb sleep
- Measure and record weights to monitor fluid changes.

Patient Education
- Advice patient to record intermittent therapy on a calendar, or use prepared, dated envelopes.
- Instruct patient to take drug early so increased urination will not disturb sleep.
- Instruct patient drug may be taken with food or meals if GI upset occurs.
- Advice patient to check the weight on a regular basis, at the same time and in the same clothing; record weight on your calendar.
- Advice patient that they may experience these side effects: Increased volume and frequency of urination; dizziness, feeling faint on arising, drowsiness (avoid rapid position changes; hazardous activities, such as driving; and alcohol); sensitivity to sunlight (use sunglasses, wear protective clothing, or use a sunscreen); decrease in sexual function; increased thirst (sucking on sugarless lozenges and frequent mouth care may help); gout attack (report any sudden joint pain).
- Instruct patient to report weight change of more than 3 pounds in 1 day, swelling in your ankles or fingers, unusual bleeding or bruising, dizziness, trembling, numbness, fatigue, muscle weakness or cramps.

Low Efficacy Diuretics

a. Potassium sparing diuretics (Aldostrone Antagonist)

Drugs name: Triamterene, amiloride, spironolactone

Mechanism of action (Conserve K⁺)

Potassium-sparing diuretics act as aldostrone antagonist by reduce Na^+ reabsorption and reduce K^+ secretion in the distal part of the nephron (collecting tubule). These are not potent

Table 2.3: Doses for potassium-sparing diuretics.

S. No.	Name of the drug	Dose	Route
1.	Spironolactone, triamterene amiloride	Adult: 25–200 mg/qdm single or divided dose child 5 mg qd, may be increased to 10–20 mg qd	Oral
2.	Triamterene	Adult: 100 mg bid (not exceed 300 mg/day)	Oral
3.	Amiloride	Adult: 5–10 mg/day PO q Day or divided q 12 h	Oral

diuretics when used alone; they are primarily used in combination with other diuretics. It enhances the excretion of calcium by a direct action on the renal tubules. **Table 2.3** depicts the doses for potassium-sparing diuretics.

Indications
- Diagnosis and maintenance of primary hyperaldosteronism
- Adjunctive therapy in edema associated with CHF, nephrotic syndrome, hepatic cirrhosis when other therapies are inadequate or inappropriate
- Treatment of hypokalemia or prevention of hypokalemia in patients who would be at high risk if hypokalemia occurred—digitalized patients, patients with cardiac arrhythmias
- Essential hypertension, usually in combination with other drugs.

Contraindications
- Allergy
- Hyperkalemia
- Renal disease
- Anuria
- Use cautiously with pregnancy and lactation.

Adverse effects
- **CNS:** Dizziness, headache, drowsiness, fatigue, ataxia, confusion
- **Dermatologic:** Rash, urticaria
- **GI:** Cramping, diarrhea, dry mouth, thirst, vomiting
- **GU:** Impotence, irregular menses, amenorrhea, postmenopausal bleeding
- **Hematologic:** Hyperkalemia, hyponatremia, agranulocytosis
- **Other:** Carcinogenic in animals, deepening of the voice, hirsutism, gynecomastia.

Nursing responsibilities
- Give daily doses early so that increased urination does not interfere with sleep.
- **Make suspension as follows:** Tablets may be pulverized and given in cherry syrup for young children. This suspension is stable for 1 month if refrigerated.
- Measure and record regular weight to monitor mobilization of edema fluid.
- Avoid giving food rich in potassium.
- Arrange for regular evaluation of serum electrolytes and blood urea nitrogen BUN.
- Mark calendars of edema outpatients as reminders of alternate day or 3-5-day/week therapy.

Patient education
- Advice patient to take the drug early because of increased urination.
- Advice patient to weigh yourself on a regular basis, at the same time and in the same clothing, and record the weight on your calendar.

- Instruct patient to avoid foods that are rich in potassium (fruits, Sanka); avoid licorice.
- Advice patient that he/she may experience these side effects—increased volume and frequency of urination; dizziness, confusion, feeling faint on arising, drowsiness (avoid rapid position changes, hazardous activities—driving, using alcohol); increased thirst (suck on sugarless lozenges; use frequent mouth care); changes in menstrual cycle, deepening of the voice, impotence, enlargement of the breasts can occur (reversible).
- Advice patient to report weight change of more than 3 pounds in 1 day, swelling in your ankles or fingers, dizziness, trembling, numbness, fatigue, enlargement of breasts, deepening of voice, impotence, muscle weakness or cramps.

b. Carbonic Anhydrase Inhibitors

Drug name: Acetazolamide, methazolamide, dorzolamide.

Mechanism of Action
- Carbonic anhydrase is an enzyme that catalyzes the formation of carbonic acid, which spontaneously ionizes to H^+ and HCO^-. This HCO^- combines with Na^+ and is reabsorbed.
- Carbonic anhydrase inhibitors block sodium bicarbonate reabsorption and cause HCO^- diuresis.
- Carbonic anhydrase is present in the nephron, eyes, gastric mucosa, pancreas and other sites. **Table 2.4** depicts the dose for carbonic anhydrase inhibitors.

Drug name: Acetazolamide

Acetazolamide is sulfonamide derivative, which is acarbonic anhydrase inhibitor and enhances the excretion of sodium, potassium, bicarbonate and water. The loss of bicarbonate leads to metabolic acidosis.

Pharmacokinetics

Acetazolamide is well absorbed orally and excreted unchanged in urine. Action of single dose lasts 8–12 hours.

Indications
- Glaucoma
- To alkaline urine
- Epilepsy
- Acute mountain sickness
- Periodic paralysis
- Hyperphosphatemia

Adverse effects
- Acidosis, hypokalemia, drowsiness, paresthesia, fatigue, abdominal discomfort
- Hypersensitivity reaction—fever, rashes

Nursing responsibilities
- Check electrolytes level periodically
- Check vital signs regularly
- Check weight of patient daily
- Check for the signs of metabolic acidosis

Table 2.4: Dose for carbonic anhydrase inhibitors.

Name of the drug	Dose	Route
Acetazolamide	250 mg	Oral

c. Osmotic Diuretics

Drug name: Mannitol is a pharmacologically inert substance due to low molecular weight of 182.

Mechanism of action: Mannitol when given IV (orally not absorbed), gets filtered by the glomerulus, but not reabsorbed. It causes water to be retained in the proximal tubule and descending limb of Henle's loop by osmotic effect resulting in water diuresis. There is also some loss of sodium. It can be given in large amount to raise tubular fluid and plasma osmolarity.

Dose

Intravenous as 10%, 20% in 100, 350 and 500 mL vacuum.

Indications
- Increased intracranial or intraocular tension (acute congestive glaucoma, head injury, stroke)
- Acute renal failure to maintain glomerular filtration rate (GFR)
- To counteract low osmolarity of plasma/extracellular fluid (ECF) due to hemodialysis or peritoneal dialysis.

Adverse effects

Dehydration, ECF volume expansion, headache and allergic reactions.

Nursing considerations
- Assess electrolytes level periodically
- Check vital signs regularly
- Check weight of patient daily
- Administer the drug at faster speed until and unless it is contraindicated.

Drugs name: Isosorbide and glycerol

These are orally active osmotic diuretics, which may be used to reduce intraocular or intracranial tension. Intravenous glycerol can cause hemolysis.

Dose: 0.5–1.5 g/kg as oral solution.

d. Methylxanthines

Drugs name: Theophylline and Caffeine have mild diuretic effect.

Mechanism of action: Methylxanthines are alkaloids found in high concentration in coffee, tea and chocolates. They inhibit the tubular fluid reabsorption along the renal proximal tube.

Antidiuretics

Antidiuretics (inhibit the water excretion without affecting salt excretion) are drugs that reduce urine volume, particularly in diabetes insipidus (DI).

Classification (Fig. 2.4)

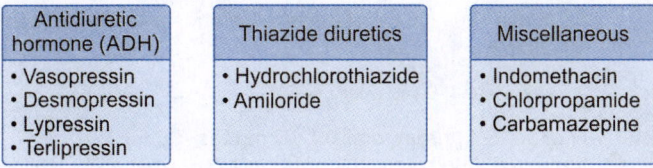

Fig 2.4: Classification of antidiuretics.

I. Antidiuretic Hormone

Antidiuretic hormone (ADH) is a nonapeptide secreted by the posterior pituitary along with oxytocin. It is synthesized in the supraoptic and paraventricular nuclei of the hypothalamus, transported along the hypothalamo-hypophyseal tract to the posterior pituitary and is stored there. ADH is released in response to two stimuli—dehydration and rise in plasma osmolarity.

Mechanism of Action

Antidiuretic hormone enhances water reabsorption by acting on the collecting duct. ADH activates the V2 receptors present on the cell membrane of the collecting duct and increases the water permeability of these cells. ADH causes vasoconstriction and raises BP mediated by V1 receptors. It also acts on other smooth muscles to increase peristalsis in the gut and contracts the uterus. Vasopressin is given parenterally as injection—subcutaneous (SC)/intramuscular (IM)/IV. **Table 2.5** depicts the doses for antidiuretic hormone.

Indications

- Diabetes insipidus of pituitary origin—desmopressin is the preparation used. It should be used lifelong.
- Bleeding esophageal varices—ADH constricts mesenteric blood vessels (V1 receptors) and may help. Analogs, such as desmopressin, terlipressin and lypressin can be used.
- Before abdominal radiography—expels gases from the bowel.
- Hemophilia and von Willebrand's disease—ADH may release factor VIII and prevent bleeding.
- Nocturia/bedwetting in children—Intranasal or oral desmopressin is used.

Contraindications

- Individuals suffering from vascular disease
- Especially disease of coronary arteries

Adverse Effects

- When used intranasally ADH can cause nasal irritation, allergy, rhinitis and atrophy of nasal mucosa.
- Other effects include nausea, abdominal cramps and backache (due to contractions of the uterus).

Table 2.5: Doses for antidiuretic hormone.

S. No.	Drug	Dose
1.	Lypressin	Injections 20 IU/mL, 10 IU [intramuscular (IM) or subcutaneous (SC)] or 20 IU diluted in 100–200 mL of dextrose solution and infused intravenous (IV) in 10–20 min
2.	Terlipressin	2 mg, repeat 1–2 mg every 4–6 h
3.	Desmopressin	IV or SC; 2–4 µg/day, oral; 0.1–02 mg tds Intranasal; Adult—10–40 µg/day in 2–3 divided doses, children—5–10 µg/day at bed time

Nursing Responsibilities
- Monitor 24 output of the patient
- The ADH therapy is lifelong required, such as in DI.
- Assess any nasal irritation, atrophy of nasal mucosa in local application.

II. Thiazide Diuretics

Diuretic thiazides paradoxically exert an antidiuretic effect in DI. High-ceiling diuretics are also effective, but are less desirable because of their short and brisk action, e.g., hydrochlorothiazide, amiloride.

Mechanism of Action

Diuretics thiazides paradoxically exert an antidiuretic effect in DI. Thiazide reduces urine volume in both pituitary origin as well as renal DI by an unknown mechanism.

Indications
- Diabetes insipidus
- Nephrogenic (DI)
- Mobilization of edema fluid

Dosage

Hydrochlorothiazide 50–150 mg in daily divided dose.

Contraindications
- Hypokalemia
- Renal producing impairment
- Hypersensitivity

Side Effects
- Depletion of K^+
- Inhibition of insulin secretion
- Risk of atherosclerosis
- Hyperglycemia

Nursing Responsibilities
- Monitor I and O serum electrolyte and BP
- Assess for effects of hypokalemia
- Moderate restriction of Na^+ Cl^- intake has been shown to enhance the antidiuretic effect
- Monitor the client for hyperglycemia

III. Miscellaneous

a. Chlorpropamide

Chlorpropamide has a long duration of action oral hypoglycemic, found to reduce urine volume in DI of pituitary origin, but not is renal DI it sensitize the kidney to ADH action its efficacy depends on small amount of the circulating home one. It is not active when ADH is totally absent. It also directly prone salt reabsorption in the ascending limb C-may contributes to its antidiuretic action.

Mechanism of action
The principle action is B-cells of islets stimulate insulin secretion, reducing plasma glucose cone.

Doses
Initially 250 mg/day (100–125 mg/day in old patients) maintenance 100–500 mg/day (usual 250 mg/day) depending on condition.

Indication
To lower blood glucose level.

Contraindications
Mild renal impairment, liver dysfunction, fever, infection or trauma.

Side effects
Hypoglycemia, nausea, vomiting, diarrhea or constipation, headache, weight gain, cholestatic jaundice, dilutional hyponatremia, intolerance to alcohol.

Nursing responsibilities
- Carefully observe the patient for signs of hypoglycemia
- Patient should be taught the cause of hypoglycemia reactions and how to avoid having excessive response to oral hypoglycemia drugs
- Watch for signs of hyperglycemia and ketoacidosis
- Patients should learn not to skip planned meals or snacks

b. Carbamazepine
Carbamazepine is an antiepileptic anticonvulsant, drug which reduces urine volume in DI of pituitary origin. It has been shown to stimulate ADH secretion. However, it is not valuable in the treatment of DI.

Mechanism of action
Carbamazepine has a stabilizing influence on neuronal membrane. It can inhibit voltage dependents Na^+ channel. Probably of greater importance is its ability to facilitate Na^+ extrusion from nerve cells and to prevent intracellular accumulation of this cation during repetitive stimulation. Thus, it selectively inhibits high frequency discharge, which little effect on onward neuronal discharge. Influence of CA^{2+} during depolarization is also decreased.

Indications
- Partial and generalized epileptic seizures
- Preventing pain of trigeminal neuralgia

Doses
On the 1st day of epilepsy treatment, a total dose of 200 mg is administered for trigeminal neuralgia the uncial dose is 100 mg.

Contraindications: Abnormalities in liver function.

Side effects
- Sedation, dizziness, vertigo, diplopia and ataxia
- Hypersensitivity reactions are realizes, hepatitis
- Water retention and hyponatremia
- Vomiting
- Diarrhea
- Acute intoxication causes coma, convulsions

Nursing responsibilities
- Treatment is started with a single drug selected for its known effectiveness in controlling the kind of seizures.
- Small doses are administered first and dosage is gradually reused at intervals of 5–7 days, until the patient's seizures are controlled.
- If the drug is effective, but causes minor signs and symptoms of over dosage, its dose is slowly reduced to a level that the patient can tolerate.
- Also instruct the patient never discontinue drug therapy abruptly.
- Pay attention to the patient's emotional needs and make sure that he understands the nature of his/her illness.

c. Clofibrate

Clofibrate is a hypolipidemic drugs, it has been found to enhance the secretion of ADH from pituitary and exerts a beneficial effect in nephrogenic diabetes insipidus (NDI). This action may causes water attention when used as hypolipidemic.

Indications
- Reducing cholesterol and triglyceride level
- Myocardial infarction
- To lower pressure lipil level
- Neurogenic diabetes insipidus.

Contraindications
Liver and kidney disorder and in pregnant/lactating women.

Doses
- 0.5–1 g bd
- Atromid-S, Lipomid, Dechostrol 0.5 g capsule 00 2 g daily is 2 day.

Side effects
- Increased appetite, weight gain, diarrhea
- Paid abdomen skin rashes, neuralgia
- Cardiac dysrhythmia.

Nursing responsibilities
- Patient checking deliberate should have serum transaminases determine periodically.
- Be aware of various specific medical disorders from which patients taking drugs of this type may also be suffering in order to keep these conditions under control.
- Patient should be advised to take nicotinic acid with meals or plenty of fluids to lessen symptoms of GI irritation, such as heartburn.
- Be sure that patients who are going to begin drug therapy understand that they must continue other non-drug measurers that help to reduce the risk of cardiovascular disease.

IV. Drugs toxic to Kidney

Drugs are used to manage the disease, such as hypertension, DM, and chronic kidney disease, etc. These agents are discussed in previous chapters based on different classification. Depending upon the mechanism of action, indication and contraindication drugs are being prescribed. The drugs which cause nephrotoxicity are contraindicated in managing the disease relayed to urinary system. It is very important to review the drugs mechanism, adverse effect and other factor before prescribing to the patient. **Table 2.6** shows the drugs which are toxic

Table 2.6: List of nephrotoxic drugs.

List of nephrotoxic drugs		
• Acyclovir	• Enalaprilat	• Mesalamine
• Ambisome	• Foscarnet	• Methotrexate
• Amikacin	• Gadopentetate dimeglumine	• Nafcillin
• Amphotericin B	• Gadoxetate disodium	• Piperacillin/tazobactam
• Captopril	• Ganciclovir	• Piperacillin
• Carboplatin	• Gentamicin	• Sirolimus
• Cefotaxime	• Ibuprofen	• Sulfasalazine
• Ceftazidime	• Ifosfamide	• Tacrolimus
• Cefuroxime	• Iodixanol and	• Ticarcillin/clavulanic acid
• Cidofovir	• Iohexol	• Tobramycin
• Cisplatin	• Iopamidol	• Topiramate
• Colistimethate	• Ioversol	• Valacyclovir
• Cyclosporine	• Ketorolac	• Valganciclovir
• Dapsone	• Lisinopril	• Vancomycin
• Enalapril	• Lithium	• Zonisamide

to kidney and should not be used in managing the disease of urinary system. **Figure 2.5** shows impairment caused by nephrotoxic drugs.

V. Urinary Antiseptics

Urinary antiseptics are substances, which prevent bacterial infection in urinary tract. They cannot be used to treat systemic infections because effective concentrations are not achieved in plasma with safe doses. Furthermore, effective antibacterial concentrations reach the renal pelvis and bladder. Treatment with such drugs can be thought of as local therapy only in the kidney and bladder. Their usefulness is limited to lower urinary tract infections (UTIs), e.g., methenamine, nitrofurantoin.

I. Methenamine

Methenamine is a urinary antibacterial agent whose action depends on its hydrolysis to ammonia and formaldehyde in an acidic urine. Methenamine is most often used in the form of an acid salt (hippurate, mandelate) which helps to maintain a low urinary pH.

Mechanism of Action

The mechanism of action of methenamine is given in **Figure 2.6**.

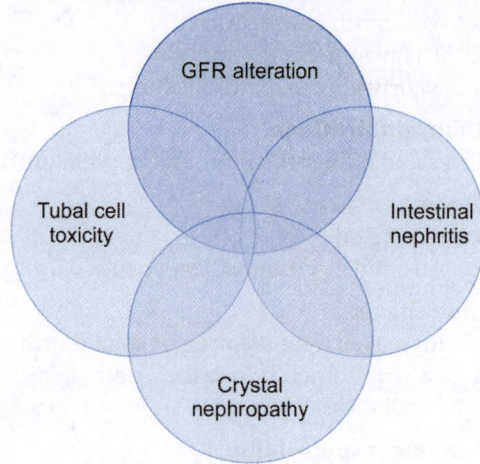

Fig. 2.5: Effect of nephrotoxic drugs.

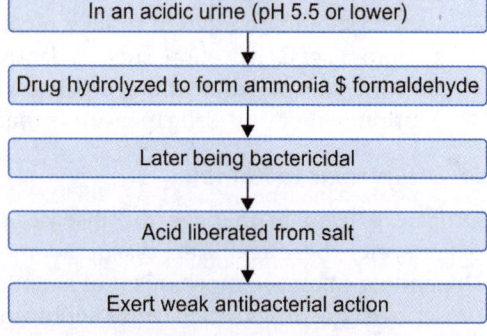

Fig. 2.6: Mechanism of methenamine.

Indications
- Treatment of chronic bacteriuria associated with cystitis, pyelonephritis.
- Prophylaxis before urinary instrumentation.
- Adjunctive treatment of patients with anatomic abnormalities of urinary tract.

Table 2.7 depicts the doses for methenamine.

Adverse Effects
Cramping, vomiting, diarrhea, stomatitis, anorexia, urinary urgency, bladder irritation, dysuria, proteinuria, hematuria, hypersensitivity reactions, and abdominal pain.

Contraindications
Renal insufficiency, severe hepatic disease and severe dehydration.

Nursing Considerations
- Do not use alone for acute infections.
- Use cautiously in pregnant or nursing mothers and in patients with gout.
- Monitor intake—output. Provide adequate fluids.
- Monitor urinary pH provide supplementary acidification if urinary pH exceeds 5.5.
- Recognize that methenamine is not suitable for prevention of urinary infections in patients with indwelling catheters.
- Be aware that methenamine can interfere with laboratory urine determination.
- To minimize GI distress, administer drug with food around the clock at regular intervals.

Dietary precaution
Advise patient to avoid excessive intake of alkalinizing foods, such as milk or citrus fruits.

II. Nitrofurantoin
A synthetic nitrofuran derivative, nitrofurantoin is a specific urinary antibacterial agent.

Mechanism of action
Bacteriostatic in low concentrations and bactericidal in higher concentrations. Its probable mechanism to interfere with carbohydrate metabolism by inhibition of acetyl coenzyme-A, may also impair bacterial cell wall formation.

Uses
- Treatment of UTI due to susceptible organisms.
- Prophylaxis against recurrent bacteriuria.

Dosage
- **Oral:** Adults: 50–100 mg four times a day, chronic therapy 25–50 mg four times a day.
- **Children:** 5–7 mg/kg/day in four divided doses.

Table 2.7: Doses for methenamine.

S. No.	Drugs	Dose
1.	Methenamine	Tablet 0.5 g (Adults—1 g four times a day, children—500 mg four times a day)
2.	Methenamine hippurate (Hiprex, Urex)	Tablet 1 g (Adults—1 g twice a day, children—0.5–1 g twice a day)
3.	Methenamine mandelate (Mandelamine)	Tablet 0.5 g–1 g (Adults—1 g four times a day, children—0.5 g four times)

- **Prophylaxis of recurrent infections:** 50 mg daily at bedtime least for 6 months.
- **IV infusion:** over 120 lb 180 mg twice a day.

Infusion solution is prepared by adding 20 mL 5% dextrose injection to the vial containing 180 mg nitrofurantoin sodium, each ml of this solution is added to at least 25 ml of parentral fluid, final solution is administered at rate of 2–3 ml/min.

Adverse effects
- **GI:** Diarrhea, abdominal pain, pancreatitis, parotitis.
- **Pulmonary:** Chills, cough, chest pain, pulmonary infiltration, diffuse interstitial pneumonitis or fibrosis.
- **Dermatologic:** Rash, pruritus, urticaria, angioedema, alopecia.
- **Hematologic:** Hemolytic anemia, megaloblastic anemia, leukopenia, granulocytopenia, eosinophilia, thrombocytopenia, agranulocytosis.
- **Allergic:** Drug fever, asthmatic attack, cholestatic, jaundice, arthralgia, anaphylaxis.
- **Neurologic:** Dizziness, drowsiness, paresthesia, headache, peripheral neuropathy.

Contraindications
Anuria, oliguria, significant renal impairment, pregnancy at term, infants under 3 months.

Nursing responsibilities
- Administer oral drug with meals or milk to reduce GI distress and possibly to improve absorption.
- Ensure that drug is taken at evenly spaced intervals.
- Instruct patient to rinse mouth thoroughly after use of oral suspension to prevent staining of teeth.
- Be alert for signs of urinary tract superinfection.
- Protect drug from strong light
- Note that drug can cause false positive tests for serum glucose, bilirubin, alkaline phosphate, BUN levels.

Other drugs
- Other drugs used in UTI are sulfonamides, cotrimoxazole, nalidixic acid, fluoroquinolones, ampicillin, cloxacillin, carbenicillin, aminoglycosides, tetracyclines and cephalosporins
- Urinary analgesic—phenazopyridine (Pyridium) has analgesic actions on the urinary tract. It relieves burning symptoms of dysuria and urgency.

VI. Treatment of UTI- Acidifiers and Alkalinizers

Acidifiers
- Acidifiers are the agents or drugs, which are used to treat acid-base imbalance in the body or for the treatment of metabolic alkalosis acidifiers are the agents, which are used to neutralize the pH which has been increased due to certain causes, such as excess alkali intake.
- **Metabolic alkalosis:** It is a process in which plasma bicarbonate level is increased. This is usually the result of increase loss of acid from the stomach or kidneys, potassium depletion accompanying diuretic therapy, excessive alkali intake, or severe adrenal gland hyperactivity. If alkalosis is severe it may cause apathy, confusion, tetany.

Classification
- Ammonium chloride
- Ascorbic acid

- Calcium chloride
- Phenazopyridine.

I. Ammonium Chloride

Ammonium chloride is primarily used as a systemic and urinary acidifier to treat metabolic alkalosis, to correct chloride depletion and to assist in urinary excretion of certain basic drugs. The drug has been used as an expectorant and is found in a number of over-the-counter cough preparations, although its efficacy is subject to considerable doubt and its use in this manner should be discouraged.

Mechanism of action
Ammonium chloride may increase flow of respiration, fluid by reflex irrigation of the gastric mucosa.

Indications
- Metabolic alkalosis
- Hypochloremia
- Adrenal gland hyperactivity

Contraindications
Severe renal, hepatic and pulmonary diseases

Doses
- **Expectorants—adults:** 200–400 mg every 4 hourly
- Children—50–75 mg/kg in divided doses
- Urinary acidification—3–12 g a day in divided doses at 4–6 hours intervals

Side effects
- Metabolic acidosis (vomiting, thirst, weakness, hyperventilation, lethargy, drowsiness, confusion)
- Headache
- Hyperglycemia
- Hypokalemia
- Hypocalcemia
- Too rapid IV administration can result in arrhythmias, tonic convulsions and coma.

Nursing responsibilities
- Note rate and depth of respiratory rate during drug therapy, hyperventilation, weakness and shortness of breath are possible early signs of acidosis
- Use cautions in patients with chronic heart disease and in small children
- Do not use enteric-coated tablets or expectorants, because gastric irrigation, the desired action is stimulated
- Avoid administration of milk or other alkaline solution with NH_4Cl.

II. Ascorbic Acid

Vitamin C or ascorbic acid is an essential dietary substance that plays a major role in many metabolic reactions as well as the formation and maintenance of collagen and intracellular ground substances. It is also used as supplement to treat metabolic alkalosis or alkali excess.

Mechanism of action
Ascorbic acid acts as an acidifier, which helps to neutralize the alkali excess, thus helps to reduce the pH toward its normal values.

Uses
- Prevention and treatment of scurvy and other vitamin C deficiency states
- Deep burns and delayed wound healing
- Acidification of urine, usually in conjunction with a urinary anti-infective

Contraindications
Use of sodium ascorbate injection in patients with Na restricted or calcium ascorbate in patient's receiving digitalis drugs.

Interactions
- Large doses of ascorbic acid lower urinary pH and thus may reduce excretion of acidic drugs (e.g., salicylate, barbiturates) and increases excretion of basic drugs (e.g., quinidine, atropine, tricyclic antidepressants, phenothiazine)
- Ascorbic acid in large doses may enhance the absorption of oral iron.

Table 2.8 depicts the route and dose for ascorbic acid.

Adverse reactions
Usually with large doses: Diarrhea, precipitation of oxalate or urate renal stones, soreness at IM or SC injection site and dizziness or faintness with too rapid IV injection.

Nursing responsibilities
- Use cautiously in patients with glucose-6-phosphate dehydrogenase deficiency, hyperuricemia, or renal impairment and pregnant women.
- Be aware that large doses may result in false readings in certain laboratory tests, i.e., urine glucose, serum uric acid and urinary steroids determinations.
- Inject slowly IV or avoid dizziness and possibly fainting.
- Do not inject calcium ascorbate SC and avoid IM injections in infants, as tissue necrosis can occur.

ALKALINIZERS

Alkalinizers are the agents or drugs, which are used to neutralize the pH, which has been decreased due to certain causes, such as metabolic acidosis.

Metabolic Acidosis

It is a process that causes a decrease in pH of body as a result of retention of acids, or a loss of bicarbonate buffers. It may be categorized by presence or absence of an abnormal anion gap.
- The anion gap met: Acidosis include diabetic, alcoholic and lactic acidosis, the acidosis of renal failure and acidosis that result from consumption of excess acids, such as salicylates, methanol or ethanol.

Table 2.8: Route and dose for ascorbic acid.

Route	Dose of ascorbic acid
Oral	Treatment of deficiency state: 100–500 mg/day as needed Prophylaxis; 50–100 mg/day Urinary acidification 4–12 g/day of ascorbic acid in divided doses every 4 hours
IM, SC, IV	Up to 2 g/day as needed for severe deficiency states; maintenance dose is 100–250 mg once or twice a day

- **Non-anion gap met:** Acidosis occurs in diarrhea, renal tubular acidosis and multiple myeloma among other conditions.

Classification
- Sodium bicarbonate
- Sodium acetate
- Sodium citrate
- Potassium citrate
- Acetazolamide

I. Sodium Bicarbonate
Sodium bicarbonate the acting systemically.

Mechanism of Action (Fig. 2.7)

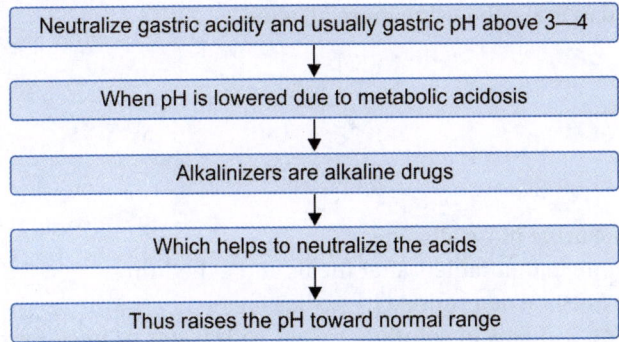

Fig. 2.7: Mechanism of sodium bicarbonate.

Indications
- Treatment of GI symptoms associated with hyperacidity (e.g., heartburn, acid indigestion)
- Treatment of hyperacidity associated with gastritis, peptic ulcer and esophagitis
- Metabolic Acidosis

Contraindications
Cardiac and renal patients, hypertension

Dose
About 0.3–2 g as needed one to four times a day

Significant Adverse Reactions
- Systemic alkalosis
- Sodium overload
- Milk-alkalosis syndrome
- Rebound hypersecretion

Nursing Responsibilities
- Administer alkalinizers in liquid form if possible, because efficacy is greater than with tablet or capsule formulations.

- If given in a tablet form instruct patient to chew before swallowing and follow with water.
- Note that food acts as a buffer to gastric acid for approximately 60 minutes and that the presence of food can enhance the action of alkalinizers. Thus, alkalinizers taken on an empty stomach have action of 30 minutes, whereas if they are taken 1 hour after meals, their duration is approximately 3 hours.
- During chronic therapy, administer alkalinizers 1 hour before or 3 hours after meals.

II. Potassium Citrate and Sodium Citrate

Potassium citrate may be used to control uric acid and cystine kidney stones.

Uses

- Effective in reducing pain and frequency of micturation when these are caused by highly acidic urine
- Widely used to treat urinary calculi (kidney stones) and in patient with cystinuria
- Citrates are used to make the urine more alkaline.

Contraindications

- Cardiac diseases
- Hypertension

Dose

- **Tablets:** To make urine more alkaline
- **Adults:** At first, one to four tablets after meals and at bedtime
- **Children:** Dose must be determined by pediatrician.
- **Solution—adults:** 2-3 tsps of solution; mixed with water or juice four times a day, after meals and at bed time
- **Children:** 1-3 tsps of solution. Mixed with water or juice, four times a day after meals.

Nursing Responsibilities

- Advice the patient to keep this drug as a stand by for emergency treatment of acute pain, but should not use it routinely.
- Milk should be avoided with drug, so as to avoid milk alkali syndrome.
- Flush nasogastric (NG) tube with water after administration
- Drink plenty of fluids
- Instruct client to take drug as directed not to exceed maximum dose
- Antacids should be taken at least 2 hours apart from other drugs as drug interactions may occur
- Warn clients not to use if diagnosed with heart disease.

III. Acetazolamide

Acetazolamide is a carbonic anhydrase inhibitor. The drug has been employed as a mild diuretic also, for relief of migraine, headache and chronic open-angle glaucoma.

Mechanism of Action

It inhibits the enzyme carbonic anhydrase, reducing formation of H^+ and HCO^- ions, appears to retard excessive or abnormal discharges from central neurons.

CHAPTER 2: Drugs Used on Urinary System

Uses
- Adjunctive treatment of absence seizures
- Metabolic acidosis

Dosage: 8–30 mg/kg/day in divided doses; usual range is 100–400 mg/day in combination with anticonvulsants.

Contraindications
- Renal and hepatic dysfunction
- Acidosis
- Adrenal insufficiency
- Narrow angle glaucoma
- Sulfa allergy
- Severe pulmonary obstruction
- Early pregnancy

Adverse Reactions
Polyuria, hematuria, glycosuria, drowsiness, hepatic dysfunction, confusion, myopia, urticaria, rash.

Nursing Responsibilities
- Cautions patient to report signs of hypokalemia (muscle weakness, cramping, cardiac irregularities) and metabolic acidosis (nausea, vomiting, abdominal pain, weakness, malaise, dehydration) and adjust dosage as needed.
- Use parenteral solution within 24 hours after reconstitution, because it contain no preservatives
- Observe diabetic patients closely because acetazolamide may alter antidiabetic drug requirements by increasing blood glucose level.

MULTIPLE CHOICE QUESTIONS

1. **Acetazolamide should not be given in:**
   a. Sulfonamide hypersensitivity
   b. Glaucoma
   c. High altitude sickness
   d. COPD
2. **Potassium-sparing diuretics include:**
   a. Spironolactone
   b. Triamterene
   c. Amiloride
   d. Bumetanide
3. **The antidiuretic action of Desmopressin is due to activation of............................?**
   a. V 1a receptor
   b. V 2 receptor
   c. V 1b receptor
   d. V1 and V2 receptor
4. **Aldosterone works on:**
   a. Proximal tubule
   b. Distal tubules
   c. Loop of Henle
   d. Collecting duct
5. **Potassium-sparing diuretics acts on:**
   a. Na⁺ K⁺ pump
   b. Aldosterone receptor
   c. Carbonic anhydrase
   d. Na⁺ Cl⁻ symporter

Answer Key
1. a   2. a   3. b   4. d

FURTHER READING

1. Bell M, Jackson E, Mi Z, McCombs J, Carcillo J. Low-dose theophylline increases urine output in diuretic-dependent critically ill children. Intensive Care Med. 1998;24(10):1099-1105. doi:10.1007/s001340.
2. Berridge MJ. Unlocking the secrets of cell signaling. Ann rev physiology. 2005;67:1.
3. Cabrera-Vera TM, et al. Insights into G protein structures, function, and regulation, endocr Rev. 2003;24:765.
4. Davies MA, Samuels Y. Analysis of the genome to personalize therapy for melanoma. Oncogene 2010;295545.
5. Feng XH, Derynck R. Specificity and versatility in TGF-beta signaling through smads. Ann rev Cell Dev Biol 2005;21:659.
6. Fountain JH, Lappin SL. Physiology, Renin Angiotensin System. Pubmed Shelf. Stat Pearls Publishing. Treasure Island (FL) 2022 Jan. Pg 1-14.
7. Galandrin S, Olingy-Longpre G, Bouvier M. The evasive nature of drug efficacy: Implications for drug discovery, trends Pharmacology science. 2007;28:423.
8. Ginty DD, Segal RA. Retrograde neurotrophin signaling. Trk-ing along the axon. Curr Opin Neurobiol. 2002;12268.
9. Givelli O, et al. Orphan GPCRs and their ligands. Pharmacology ther. 2006;110:525.
10. Goldstein SL, Mottes T, Simpson K, et al. A sustained quality improvement program reduces nephrotoxic medication-associated acute kidney injury. Kidney Int. 2016;90(1): 212-21.
11. Gouaux E, MacKinnon R. Principles regulation of lymphocyte activation by tyrosine kinases and phosphatases. J Clin Invest. 2002;109:9.
12. Kenakin T. Principles: Receptor theory in molecular pharmacology. Trends pharmcol sci. 2004;25:186.
13. Mosesson Y, Yarden Y. Oncogenic growth factor receptors: implications for signal transduction therapy. Semin cancer Biol. 2004;14:262.
14. Osswald H, Schnermann J. Methylxanthines and the kidney. Handb Exp Pharmacol. 2011;(200):391-412. doi:10.1007/978-3-642-13443-2_15.
15. Pawson T. Dynamic control of signaling by modular adaptor proteins. Curr opin cell Biol. 2007;19:112.
16. Rajagopal S, Rajagopal K, lefkowitz RJ: Teaching old receptors new tricks-biasing seven-transmembrane receptors. Nat Rev drug discov. 2010;9:373.
17. Roden DM, George AL Jr. The genetic basis of variability in drug responses, nat rev drug discov. 2002;1:37.
18. Rosenbaum DM, Rasmussen SG, Kobilka BK. The structure and function of G-protein-coupled receptors. Nature. 2009;1:674.
19. Sharma SK. Textbook of Pharmacology, Pathology and Genetics for Nurses. Jaypee Publications. 2016;206-17.
20. Small KM, McGraw DW, Liggett SB. Pharmacology and physiology of human adrenergic receptor polymorphisms. Ann rev pharmacol toxicol. 2003;43:381.
21. Sorking A, von Zastrow M. Endocytosis and signaling: Intertwining molecular networks. Nat Rev Mol Cell Biol. 2009;10:609.
22. Yuan TL, Cantley LC. PI3K Pathway alterations in cancer: Variations on a theme. Oncogene. 2008;27:5497.
23. Yu FH, et al. Overview of molecular relationship in the voltage-gated ion channel super family. Pharmcol Rev. 2005;57:387.

CHAPTER 3

Drugs Acting on Nervous System

Raj Kumar, Suresh Sharma, Rajneesh Arora, Poonam Arora, Hemlata

BASIS AND APPLIED PHARMACOLOGY OF COMMONLY USED DRUGS

Nervous system enables the interaction of individual to its surrounding. Its sensory component detect the stimuli, while the motor component provide control on cardiac, skeletal muscle, also it control the glandular secretions. It helps the individual to respond to the stimuli by the process of Receiving, Storing, and Processing.

The nervous system is broadly classified into two categories **(Fig. 3.1)**. Further, the Autonomic system is divided into Sympathetic and Parasympathetic system.

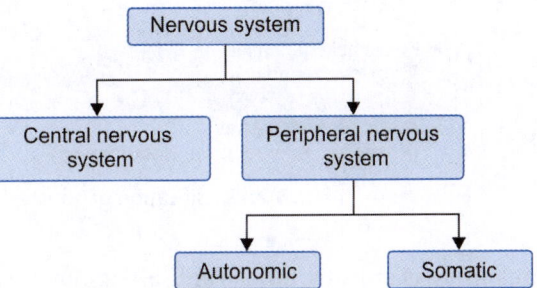

Fig 3.1: Classification of nervous system.

ANALGESICS AND ANESTHETICS

Analgesic: Nonsteroidal Anti-inflammatory Drugs (NSAIDs)

- Nonsteroidal anti-inflammatory drugs are also called non-narcotic, non-opioid or Aspirin-like analgesics as they do not depress the central nervous system (CNS) and do not produce physical dependence.
- Anti-inflammatory agents are drugs that alleviate symptoms of inflammation, but do not necessarily deal with the cause.
- Analgesics are drugs used to relieve pain also known as pain killers.
- Antipyretic activity results in lowering the temperature, and is considered to involve the hypothalamus.

Classification

The classification of nonsteroidal anti-inflammatory drugs is presented in **Figure 3.2**.

NON-SELECTIVE COX INHIBITORS

Salicylates

Aspirin

Aspirin is a salicylate that helps to relieve headaches, muscular and joint pains, and reduces inflammation. Acetyl salicylic acid (ASA) has been considered the drug of choice in the

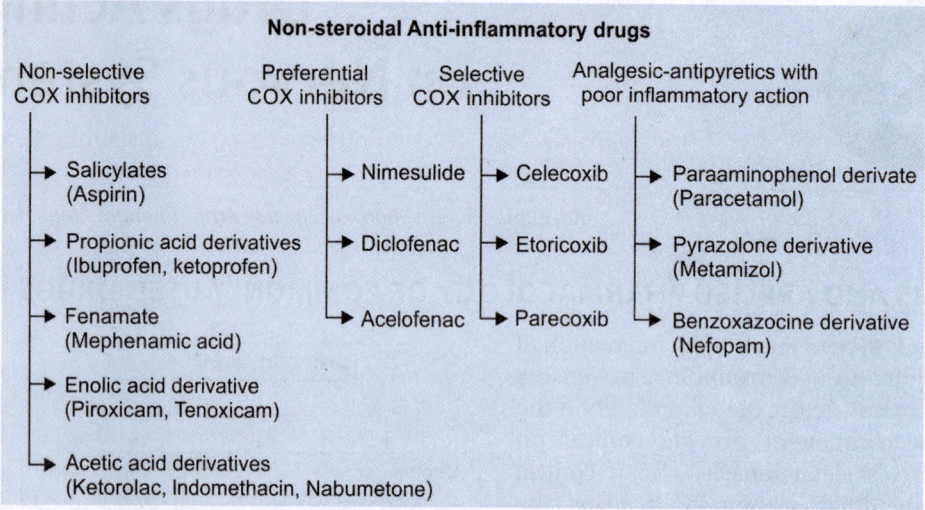

Fig. 3.2: Classification of nonsteroidal anti-inflammatory drugs.

treatment of arthritis, but it's anti-inflammatory action occurs only when given in large doses (3–4 g/day), but at larger doses it produces side effects that are the main disadvantages when they are used for treatment of arthritis conditions. Nonsteroidal anti-inflammatory drugs (NSAIDs) tend to be more appropriate for arthritis conditions. It is available in form of tablets.

Mechanism of Action

Aspirin inactivates cyclooxygenase irreversibly and inhibits prostaglandin synthesis and platelet aggregation.

Indications

Used for pain, fever, inflammatory conditions such as rheumatic fever, rheumatoid arthritis, osteoarthritis, dysmenorrhea and symptomatic relief of the common cold pain and fever. It is used for reducing the risk of recurrent transient ischemic attacks (TIA/stroke), or Myocardial infarctions (MI/heart attack) at low doses.

Contraindications

In patients with history of hypersensitivity to drug; with history of asthma, peptic ulcer and those with bleeding disorders. It is also contraindicated in children with chickenpox, influenza and in lactating mothers.

Dose

Adult
- 0.3–0.6 g 6–8 hourly for *minor aches and pain*
- 4–5 g or 75–100 mg/kg/day in divided doses for 1–3 days and after 4–7 days dose is reduced to 50 mg/kg/day in case of *acute rheumatic fever*
- 3–5 g/day in case of *rheumatoid arthritis*
- 60–100 mg/day in case of *post MI and post stroke*.

Child
Not recommended, unless for certain conditions.

Adverse Effects
Dizziness, cinchonism (ringing in the ear), skin eruptions, epigastric discomfort, peptic ulceration and bleeding, increase bleeding tendency, hypersensitivity reactions.

Salicylate overdose
Salicylate overdose can be fatal, particularly in children. Acute lethal dose is approximately 10–30 g for adults, and 4 g in children. It requires immediate hospitalization. Patient presents with symptoms of confusion, rapid deep breathing, sweating, tinnitus (noises in the ear), and deafness followed in severe cases by unconsciousness. Vomiting should be induced if possible (patient is conscious) with syrup of ipecac. Activated charcoal can also be given as it decreases absorption if given within 2 hours after ingestion. Chronic salicylate toxicity may occur when > 100 mg/kg/d is ingested for 2 or more days. It is more difficult to recognize and is associated with increased morbidity and mortality. Compared to acute poisoning, hyperventilation, dehydration, systemic acidosis and severe CNS manifestations occur more frequently and treatment includes supportive measures.

Nursing responsibilities
- Take with or after food to avoid gastrointestinal (GI) disturbances (including ulcers)
- The drug is hydrolyzed in the stomach, and primarily absorbed in the stomach and upper small intestine. Peak level is within 15 minutes to 2 hours, so patient should expect the drug effect to be noticed within 15 minutes from taking the medication
- The ASA should not be used for self-medication of pain for longer than 10 days in adults or 5 days in children, unless directed by a physician
- The ASA preparations should not be used if a strong vinegar-like odor is present
- Avoid ASA for at least 1 week prior to surgery
- Patients should inform the dentist or doctor of taking this medication before doing any laboratory or dental work
- Avoid alcohol while taking this medication since it increases the risk of GI ulceration and bleeding.

Propionic Acid Derivatives

Ibuprofen
Ibuprofen (IBP) is a propionic acid derivative. Comparable to Aspirin (ASA) in its analgesic action, but higher doses are required for anti-inflammatory effect. It has been reported to have less GI symptoms than Aspirin in equi-effective doses. Cross-sensitivity with ASA and other NSAIDs has been reported. IBP inhibits platelet aggregation and prolongs bleeding time, but does not affect prothrombin or whole blood clotting times.

Dose: Table 3.1 shows dosage and plasma half-life of propionic acid derivatives.

Table 3.1: Dosage and plasma half-life of propionic acid derivatives.

Drug	Plasma half-life	Dosage
Ibuprofen	2–4 hr	400–600 mg (5–10 mg/kg) tds
Naproxen	12–16 hr	250 mg bd-tds
Ketoprofen	2–3 hr	50–100 mg bd-tds
Flubiprofen	4–6 hr	50 mg bd-qid

Pharmacokinetics
Ibuprofen is well-absorbed orally metabolized by liver and excreted in urine as well as bile.

Indications
Ibuprofen can be used in dysmenorrhea, rheumatoid arthritis, osteoarthritis and other musculoskeletal disorders where pain is more prominent than inflammation. They can also be used in soft tissue injury, fractures, vasectomy, tooth extraction, postpartum and postoperatively to suppress swelling and inflammation.

Contraindications
In patients who are hypersensitive where urticaria, severe rhinitis, bronchospasm, angioedema are precipitated by ASA or other NSAIDs. It is also contraindicated in patients with active peptic ulcer or bleeding abnormalities.

Adverse effects
Gastrointestinal disturbances are most common, i.e., heartburn, nausea and dyspepsia, abdominal distress, gastritis and ulceration. Also, dizziness, drowsiness, jaundice, and fatigue may occur. Side effects are dose related. Incidence or aggravations of epilepsy and parkinsonism have been reported with use of NSAIDs.

Nursing responsibilities
- Drug should be cautiously used in pregnancy, lactating women, patients with renal and liver disease.
- Patients with history of cardiac decompensation should be observed closely for evidence of fluid retention and edema.
- Instruct patient to report immediately any passage of dark tarry stool, coffee-ground emesis, blood or protein in urine. This can be an indication for GI bleeding. Medication should be stopped and patient should be re-evaluated.
- Caution if skin rash, itching, visual disturbances or persistent headache should occur.
- Caution in hypertension, chronic renal failure and patients with SLE. Advise patient not to drink alcohol, to avoid increased risk of GI ulceration and bleeding.

Fenamate
Mephenamic Acid
Mephenamic acid has an analgesic, antipyretic and weaker anti-inflammatory drug, which inhibits synthesis of prostaglandins. It is absorbed orally and excreted in urine as well as bile. It is indicated in patients with muscle, joint and soft tissue pain. It is also effective in dysmenorrhea and at some extent in rheumoid and osteoarthritis. Its dosage is 250–300 mg tds. Diarrhea, epigastric distress, skin rashes, dizziness and other CNS manifestations are its common adverse effects.

Enolic Acid Derivative
Piroxicam
Piroxicam is long-acting and has good anti-inflammatory, analgesic and antipyretic activity. No clinically significant drug interactions are seen and is better tolerated as it is less ulcerogenic. Dosage of drug is 20 mg od. It is used for rheumatoid arthritis, osteoarthritis, ankylosing spondylitis, acute musculoskeletal pain and postoperative pain. Gastrointestinal intolerance, rashes, pruritus and edema are its common side effects.

Acetic Acid Derivatives
Ketorolac
- It has both analgesic and anti-inflammatory action. It inhibits prostaglandin synthesis and relieves pain. It is rapidly absorbed after oral and IM administration and is excreted in urine.
- It is frequently used in dosage of 15–30 mg IV or IM every 4–6 hours (maximum 90 mg/ day) postoperative, dental and acute musculoskeletal pain. Orally it is used in dose of 10–20 mg 6 hourly for short-term management of pain. It can also be used in renal colic, migraine and pain due to bony metastasis. Its common side effects are nausea, abdominal pain, dyspepsia, ulceration, loose stools, drowsiness, headache, dizziness, nervousness and pain at injection site.

Indomethacin
- It is a very potent arylacetic acid NSAIDs derivative. As it has higher potential to cause serious side effects when used in high doses so it should be carefully used. It has equal or a little superior action than naproxen, but higher incidence of side effects. It relieves only inflammatory or tissue injury related pain. It inhibits prostaglandin synthesis; well absorbed orally and excreted by kidney. It can be used in dosage of 25–30 mg bd-qid in case of ankylosing spondylitis, acute exacerbations of destructive arthropathies, psoriatic arthritis and rheumatoid arthritis. It is most common drug used for medical closure of patent ductus arteriousus—three 12 hourly IV injections of 0.1–0.2 mg/kg. It is contraindicated in machinery operators, drivers, psychiatric patients, epileptics, renal disease, pregnant women and in children.
- Gastrointestinal and CNS side effects are common like gastric irritation, nausea, anorexia, gastric bleeding, frontal headache, mental confusion, ataxia, hallucination, depression and psychosis. Increased risk of bleeding is also common.

PREFERENTIAL COX-2 INHIBITORS
Nimesulide
Nimesulide weakly inhibits prostaglandin synthesis and has analgesic, antipyretic and anti-inflammatory action. It is used in painful inflammatory conditions like sports injury, sinusitis, ear, nose and throat disorders, dental surgery, low backache, postoperative pain and arthritis. It is completely absorbed orally and excreted in urine. Side effects of drug are heartburn, nausea, loose motions, rashes, pruritus and dizziness. As it causes hepatic failure so is banned in many countries like US, Switzerland, Spain, etc.

Diclofenac Sodium
Diclofenac sodium is acetic acid derivative and has analgesic, antipyretic, and anti-inflammatory properties. At therapeutic doses it has little effect on platelet aggregation. Patients not responding to IBP can be given diclofenac instead. Do not co-administer with other NSAIDs or salicylates. It is used in rheumatoid and osteoarthritis, bursitis, toothache, dysmenorrhea, renal colic and postoperative inflammatory conditions. Dosage is 50 mg tds, then bd oral, 75 mg deep IM.

Adverse Effects

Mild epigastric pain, nausea, headache, dizziness, and rashes are the adverse effects. Gastric ulceration and bleeding are less common. It also increases the risk of heart attack and stroke.

SELECTIVE COX INHIBITORS

Celecoxib

Celecoxib is similar to diclofenac and has anti-inflammatory, analgesic and antipyretic effects. Abdominal pain, dyspepsia, mild diarrhea, rashes, edema and rise in blood pressure (BP) are its common side effects. It is mainly used for rheumatoid and osteoarthritis in a dose of 100–200 mg bd.

Etoricoxib

Etoricoxib is used in dosage of 60–120 mg od for osteo/rheumatoid/acute gouty arthritis, ankylosing spondylitis, dysmenorrhea, acute dental surgery pain. Side effects are dyspepsia, abdominal pain, pedal edema, hypertension, dry mouth, taste disturbances and paresthesia.

ANALGESIC-ANTIPYRETICS WITH POOR ANTI-INFLAMMATORY ACTION

Antipyretics

Para-aminophenol Derivatives

Paracetamol

Paracetamol has analgesic, good antipyretic and weak anti-inflammatory properties. It is equivalent to Aspirin in relieving pain and reducing fever, but it has little effect on platelet function, does not affect bleeding time and generally produces no gastric bleeding or ulcers. It reduces fever by direct action on the hypothalamus heat-regulating center with consequent peripheral vasodilatation, sweating and dissipation of heat. It is easily absorbed orally and is well metabolized by the hepatic microsomal enzymes. It is safe and well-tolerated drug. Nausea and rashes occasionally occur due to its intake.

Indications

Paracetamol is used for pain and fever and is good substitute for ASA, when ASA is not tolerated or is contraindicated.

Contraindications

Hypersensitivity and patients with severe liver and kidney damage.

Dosage forms

Paracetamol is available in tablets, capsules, suspension and suppositories.

Nursing Responsibilities

- Do not exceed recommended doses
- Chronic excessive use (> 4 g/d) eventually may lead to transient hepatotoxicity
- If pain or fever persists for more than 3 days consult a physician
- Use caution when patients are taking other drugs that might affect the liver

Acute Paracetamol Poisoning

Acute paracetamol poisoning occurs if large dose (>150 mg/kg or 10 g in an adult) is taken. Acute poisoning symptoms include nausea, vomiting, drowsiness, confusion, liver tenderness, low blood pressure, cardiac arrhythmia, jaundice and acute hepatic and renal failure.

Antidote: *N-acetylcysteine*
Treatment: Immediately refer to emergency room, induce vomiting or gastric lavage is to be done. Oral N-acetylcysteine (150 mg/kg IV infusion over 15 min) is a specific antidote for toxicity. Follow special directions for administration of N-acetylcysteine antidote and monitor the patient for several days.

OPIOIDS AND OTHER CENTRAL ANALGESICS

Opioid Analgesics

Opioid analgesics are mainly centrally acting (brain and spinal cord), which are used for severe pain. The drugs used to alleviate moderate to severe pain are either opiates (derived from the opium poppy) or opiate-like (synthetic drugs). These drugs are together as opioids. Classification of opioids is presented in **Figure 3.3**.

Morphine

Pharmacological Actions

- **Central nervous system:** It is strong analgesic and depresses respiratory center in dose dependent manner. It has calming effect. Cough center, temperature regulating center and vasomotor centers are depressed by morphine.
- **Cardiovascular system:** It causes vasodilatation due to depression of vasomotor center and histamine release.
- **Gastrointestinal tract:** Gastrointestinal secretions are decreased due to reduction in movement of water and electrolytes from mucosa to the lumen. This results in constipation.
- **Urinary bladder:** Tone of sphincter muscle and detrusor muscle increased, which causes urinary urgency and difficulty in micturition.

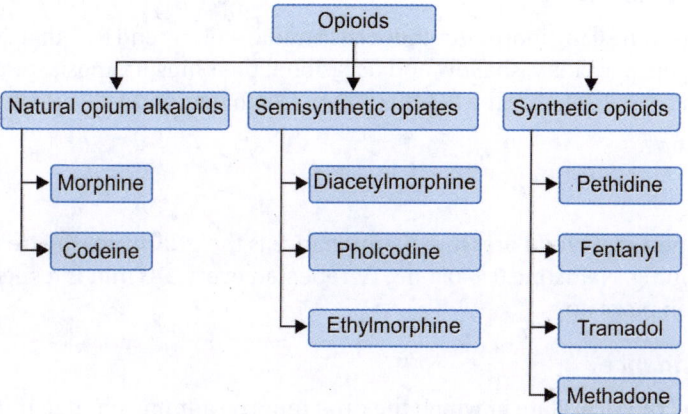

Fig. 3.3: Classification of opioids.

- **Bronchial smooth muscle:** Therapeutic doses have no effect. High doses may produce constriction.

Mechanism of Action

Opioids generally produce inhibition of neuronal activity and inhibit the release of neurotransmitters. They activate descending inhibitory systems.

Pharmacokinetics

Morphine is readily absorbed from all sites of administration and distributed to all tissues. Morphine is poorly transported across the blood-brain barrier; it is metabolized in liver and excreted in urine.

Indications

- Chronic pain arising from terminal illness can be relieved by opioid drugs
- Postoperative pain
- Diagnostic procedures
- Orthopedic manipulations
- Myocardial infarction
- Preanesthetic medication (fentanylderivatives)
- Dyspnea
- Cough suppression (codeine, dextromethorphan)
- Diarrhea and dysentery

Contraindications

- Decreased respiratory reserve: Emphysema, severe obesity, asthma
- Biliary colic
- Head injury
- Reduced blood volume
- Hepatic insufficiency
- Convulsant states

Acute Morphine Poisoning

Toxicity develops with 50 mg morphine-induced intramuscularly and its lethal dose is about 250 mg. Stupor or coma, flaccidity, shallow and occasional breathing, cyanosis, pinpoint pupil, fall in BP, shock and convulsions are the manifestation. Death may occur due to respiratory failure.

Antidote- Naloxone.

Treatment

Respiratory support and blood pressure maintenance is the priority for the treatment of Acute Morphine Poisoning. Naloxone 0.4–0.8 mg IV repeated every 2–3 min is a specific antagonist till the respiration picks up.

Physical Dependence

It is an abnormal physical state in which the drug must be administered to maintain 'normal' function. Physical dependence is manifested by 'withdrawal symptoms' when administration of the drug is stopped. Physical dependence is a powerful reinforcement for continued drug taking behavior.

Symptoms

- 8–12 hours: Lacrimation, rhinorrhea, yawning, sweating
- 12–14 hours: Restless sleep
- 48–72 hours: Symptoms peak, dilated pupils, anorexia, gooseflesh (cold turkey), restlessness, irritability, tremor, nausea/vomiting, intestinal spasm and diarrhea, muscle spasm
- 7–10 days symptoms end

Other Opioids

Codeine

Codeine is less potent than morphine and is mainly used as antitussive. It is effective orally and is well-absorbed. It produces less respiratory depression and is less constipating. Codeine has less addiction liability and tolerance is uncommon. It is less potent than morphine (1–6 hr) as an analgesic (60 mg codeine = 10 mg morphine). Duration of action is 4–6 hours. 10–30 mg is the antitussive dose. Constipation is the most common side effect.

Meperidine or Pethidine

Meperidine or pethidine has similar properties like morphine, but is less potent than morphine. High doses of pethidine produce excitation and convulsions, it has less smooth muscle spasm than morphine and has little antitussive action. It also has anti-cholinergic effects, which can cause dry mouth and blurring of vision.

Fentanyl

Fentanyl is 100 times more potent than morphine in analgesia and respiratory depression. It has shorter duration of action. It is also used in anesthesia. It has mild effects on the cardiovascular system. It slightly reduces heart rate and BP. Hence it is found to be safer than other opioids in cardiovascular surgeries.

Pentazocine

Pentazocine is mixed agonist and antagonist and is less potent than morphine. It will precipitate withdrawal in dependent individuals and may produce dysphoria. Pentazocine can be given both orally and parenterally. It undergoes first pass metabolism. Its dose is 50–100 mg oral; 30–60 mg IM (Fortwin). It is a commonly used opioid analgesic especially in postoperative and chronic pain. Sedation, sweating, dizziness, nausea, dysphoria with anxiety, nightmares and hallucinations are its common adverse effects.

Opioid Antagonists

Naloxone

Naloxone eliminated first pass metabolism [half-life (t1/2) 60–100 min]. Readily reverses the coma and respiratory depression of opioid overdose. Rapidly displaces all receptor bound opioid molecules; therefore it is very effective reversing heroin overdose. Given orally it undergoes first pass metabolism and is metabolized by the liver. Hence it is given intravenously in dosage of 0.4 mg IV. Duration of action is 3–4 hours.

Naltrexone

Naltrexone is another pure opioid antagonist and is more potent than naloxone. Orally it is effective and has a longer duration of action of 1–2 days. It is used for 'opioid blockade' therapy in post addicts.

ANESTHESIA

- The term 'anesthesia' is derived from the Greek word 'anaistheris' meaning 'no sensation'.
- Anesthesia is an artificially induced state of partial or total loss of sensation with or without loss of consciousness.
- Anesthesia agents can produce muscle relaxation, block transmission of pain, impulses, and suppress reflexes. It can also temporarily decrease memory retrieval a recall.
- The depth and effects of anesthesia are monitored by observing changes in respiration, oxygen saturation and end tidal CO_2 levels, heart rate, urine output and BP.

Classification

Classification of anesthesia is shown in **Figure 3.4**.

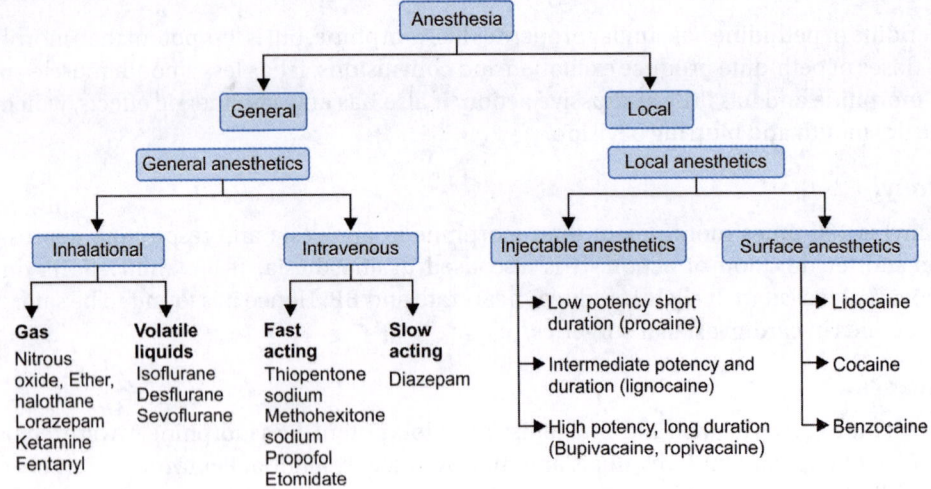

Fig. 3.4: Classification of anesthesia.

GENERAL ANESTHESIA

Definition

- General anesthetics are agents that in sufficient amounts are capable of producing analgesia, decreases muscle reflex activity and immediately loss of consciousness
- General anesthetics are drugs that are led to bring about a state in which painful surgical procedures can be performed painlessly and safely.

Stages of General Anesthesia

Stage of Analgesia
Stage of analgesia is from the beginning of inhalation of the anesthetic to loss of consciousness. Consciousness becomes progressively clouded. The patient's awareness of sensory stimulus is disrupted; hearing and other perceptions are distorted. Feeling of floating and numbness. Analgesia (loss of pain sensation) may be profound with some anesthetics, for example, ether, methoxyflurane. Complete loss of consciousness marks the end of this stage.

Stage of Delirium or Excitement
Stage of delirium or excitement is from loss of consciousness to beginning of surgical anesthesia. Patient is unconscious, but may show signs of psychomotor excitement, which are the result of drug-induced depression of inhibitory areas of the CNS, respiratory and cardiovascular reflexes may be hyperactive. It may be associated with excitement—shouting, crying and violent behavior.

Surgical Anesthesia
This begins with a shift from irregular to regular breathing and a loss of eyelid reflexes. Artificially divided into four planes to indicate increasing depth of anesthesia:
- Plane-1: Eyeball movements; regular breathing
- Plane-2: Eyeball fixed, breathing less, deep or full; skeletal muscle tone reduced
- Plane-3: Chest breathing shallow; abdominal respiration deeper, no wink response when the cornea is touched
- Plane-4: Chest breathing stops; abdominal breathing become increasingly shallow.

Medullary Paralysis
Respiration ceases. Cardiovascular collapse may occur if respiration arrest is not corrected by resuscitative measures.

CLASSIFICATION

Inhalation Anesthetic

Mechanism of Action
Mechanism of inhalation anesthetic is presented in **Figure 3.5**.

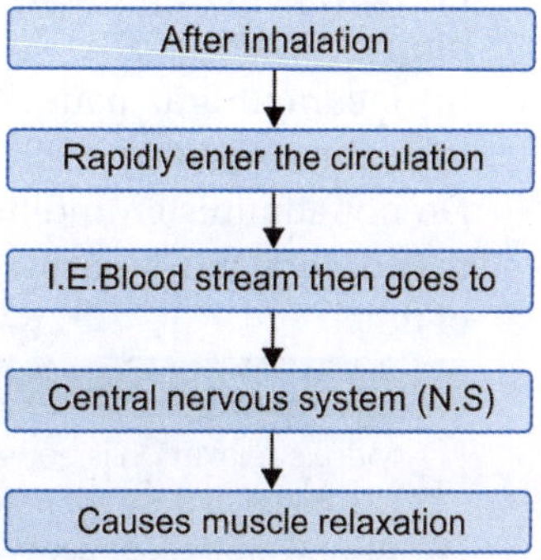

Nitrous oxide (N_2O): It is colorless, sharp and sweet odorless, non-inflammable and non-irritating gas. It produces light anesthesia with minimal muscle relaxation. It does not cause significant depression of respiration or vasomotor center. It has little effect on respiration, heart and BP. N_2O (50%) has been used with O_2 for dental and obstetric analgesia. Prolonged exposure to gas can depress bone marrow and can cause peripheral neuropathy.

Fig. 3.5: Mechanism of action of inhalation anesthetic.

After inhalation → Rapidly enter the circulation → I.E. Blood stream then goes to → Central nervous system (N.S) → Causes muscle relaxation

Ether: It is highly volatile liquid and can be inflammable and explosive. It is a potent and reliable anesthetic, good analgesic, muscle relaxant and does not depress cardiovascular and respiratory functions in therapeutic doses.

Halothane: It is nonirritating, noninflammable, volatile liquid with sweet odor. It is a direct myocardial depressant. Cardiac output and BP start falling and heart rate may decrease and it also causes respiratory depression. Pharyngeal and laryngeal reflexes are abolished early. It is preferred in asthmatic patients. It also causes intestinal and uterine contractions.

Indications

- Anesthesia, especially in patients with CVS complications, reduced arterial tension or impending shock
- Obstetrical analgesia
- Induction (basal) anesthesia
- Dental analgesia

Contraindications

- Simultaneous use of adrenergic agents
- Asthmatic condition
- Use of electrocautery equipment during administration

Adverse Reactions

Postoperative nausea, vomiting, headache, bradycardia, confusion, convulsions and cyanosis are its adverse reactions. Malignant hyperthermia is also possible

Nursing Responsibilities

- During administering gases as inhalation anesthetic, use adequate precautions to prevent explosion when drug is present.
- Be alert for sign of arrhythmias and have proper materials and equipment on hand to quickly treat arrhythmias if occurs.
- Position patient properly to reduce danger of aspiration of vomit during administering nitrous oxide.
- In pneumothorax patients, use cautions because pulmonary pressure may be elevated with nitrous oxide.
- Do not administer undiluted (without oxygen) N_2O for more than few breaths. Hypoxia may occur if nitrous oxide is used in greater concentrations (more than 80%) for any length of time.

Nursing Alerts!

- Muscle relaxation is generally sufficient for most operations. If additional relaxation is desired, use minimal doses of neuromuscular blocking agents
- Always pretreat patients with anti-cholinergic agents prior to ether anesthesia to reduce the volume of secretions produced by the anesthetics
- During recovery, nausea and vomiting are common. Turn patient's head toward one side to avoid aspiration of the vomitus
- Have vasopressors available to treat hypotension if it develops
- As with any general anesthetic, remember that the sense of hearing is one of the earliest to return during recovery avoid remarks that may be upsetting to the patient during this time, even though he may still be unconscious.

Intravenous Anesthetics

Mechanism of Action

After injection of general anesthesia it goes into circulation and rapidly taken up by brain where it causes anesthetic effect. It is rapidly redistributed to other parts of the body. Therefore within 5 minutes after injection barbiturate level of brain has decline to about one half of its peak refined shortly (30–45 sec) after injection.

Thiopentone Sodium

Thiopentone sodium is generally used for induction because of rapid onset of action. When it is injected IV (3–5 mg/kg) as a 2.5% solution it produces unconsciousness in 15–20 seconds. It is poor analgesic and weak muscle relaxant. Immediately after injection BP falls due to vasodilation. If hypovolemia, shock or sepsis is present then cardiovascular collapse may occur. It can also be used for rapid control of convulsions. Laryngospasm can occur after administration of drug, which can be prevented by atropine premedication and administration of succinylcholine immediately after thiopentone.

Methohexitone Sodium

Methohexitone sodium is three times more potent but similar to thiopentone. It has quicker and brief action usually within 5–8 minutes.

Propofol

Propofol is used as an IV anesthetic for induction and maintenance. Its action starts within 15–45 seconds and lasts for 5–10 minutes. It does not cause bronchospasm and preferably suited for outpatient surgery. In subanesthetic doses (25–50 µg/kg/min) is the choice of drug for sedating intubated patients in intensive care units.

Benzodiazepines

Benzodiazepines like diazepam, lorazepam and midazolam are used to induce or supplement anesthesia. They cause sedation, amnesia and reduce anxiety, which are beneficial in such patients. The BZDs may be employed alone in procedures like endoscopies, reduction of fractures, cardiac catheterization and cardioversion. The BZDs are also used as preanesthetic medication.

Ketamine

Ketamine is also called dissociative anesthesia. It can cause profound analgesia, immobility and amnesia with light sleep. Patient unable to process sensory stimuli but can open his/her eyes and can do swallowing. Respiration is not depressed, but heart rate, cardiac output and BP are elevated. A dose of 1–2 mg/kg IV or 3–5 mg/kg IM is given. It can be used for short surgeries and burn dressing.

Indications

- Induction anesthesia
- Short surgical procedures with minimal painful stimuli

- Induction of a hypnotic stage
- Supplementation of other anesthetics
- Aid to narcoanalysis and narcosynthesis in psychiatric disorders
- Production of tranquilization and analgesia for diagnostic and minor surgical procedures, e.g., Treatment of burns

Contraindications
- Latent or manifest porphyria
- Absence of suitable veins for IV administration
- Status asthmaticus
- Hypotension
- Severe cardiovascular disease
- Addison's disease
- Myxedema
- Increased blood urea
- Increased intracranial pressure
- Myasthenia gravis

Side Effects
Pain at injection site, intensified muscle tone, hallucinations, confusion, transient venous pain, myoclonic skeletal muscle movement, respiratory depression, hypotension, tachycardia, arrhythmias, laryngospasm and hiccough are its common side effects.

Nursing Responsibilities
- Use only clear, colorless diffusions.
- Be alert for signs of excess pain or swelling at injection site.
- Follow diluting instructions carefully, sterile water for injection is the preferred diluents.
- Note that solutions in sterile water are stable for up to 6 weeks at room temperature, but solutions in saline or dextrose are stable only for 24 hours.
- Have appropriate resuscitative equipment and respiratory aids on hand in case of extreme respiratory depression.
- Monitor vital signs during administration and if possible, give small test dose initially to determine sensitivity.
- If shivering or facial twitching occurs, warm patient with blankets.
- Give IV injection slowly to minimize the occurrence of muscle rigidity.
- Closely monitor patient postoperatively because drug may have extended action due to slow metabolism.
- Recognize that fluids and vasodepressor agents may be needed to manage hypotension and have these agents available.

Local Anesthetics
Mechanism of Action
Mechanism of actions of local anesthesia is presented in **Figure 3.6**.

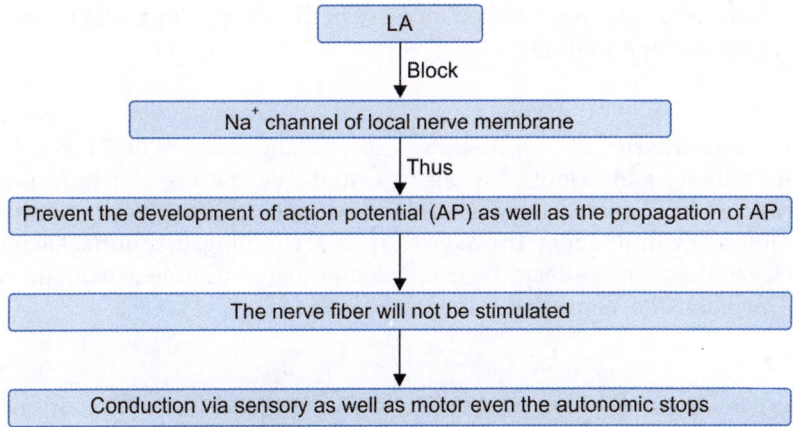

Fig. 3.6: Mechanism of action of local anesthesia.

Indications
- Relief of pain, soreness, irritation and itching associated with various skin and mucous membrane disorders, e.g., minor burns, rashes, wound, allergic conditions, fungus infection, skin ulcers, hemorrhoids, fissures.
- Production of corneal and conjunctival anesthesia to facilitate ophthalmic procedures; such as gonioscopy, tonometry, removal of foreign bodies and minor ocular surgery.
- Production of infiltration nerve block, spinal epidural or caudal anesthesia in surgery, obstetrics or dental work.
- Management of cardiac arrhythmias

Contraindications
- Topical history of allergic reactions
- Injection history of hypersensitivity, severe infection and heart block
- Procaine is contraindicated in methemoglobinemia

Common Side Effects
Topical: Sensitization reactions, stinging or burning in the eyes, allergic contact dermatitis with fissuring of fingertips, urinary and cutaneous lesion, edema, anaphylactic swelling, irritation, sloughing, and neurosis.

Injection: (Mainly due to systemic reaction). CNS stimulation (dizziness, blurred vision, confusion, irritability, convulsions, tremors) followed by CNS depression, muscle twitching, drowsiness, unconsciousness, bradycardia, myocardial depression.

Epidural or caudal injection: May provoke penile nerve block, urinary retention, incontinence, paresthesias, headache or backache.

Notes on Individual Compounds
Cocaine
Cocaine is good surface anesthetic and rapidly absorbed from buccal mucous membrane. It stimulates CNS and effect mood and behavior of an individual. It also stimulates vagal center

and causes nausea and vomiting. Marked increase in BP is seen along with pyrexia. It can be induced during ocular anesthesia.

Lidocaine

Lidocaine can be used as surface anesthetic or injectable anesthetic. When injected it can block nerve within 3 minutes and vasodilation occurs at that area. It is used for surface application, infiltration, nerve block, epidural, spinal and intravenous regional block anesthesia. It also works as an anti-arrhythmic agent. Drowsiness, mental clouding, dysphoria, altered taste and tinnitus are its common side effects. Its overdose may cause muscle twitching, convulsions, arrhythmias, hypotension, coma and respiratory arrest.

Bupivacaine

Bupivacaine has longer duration of action and can be used for infiltration, nerve block, epidural and spinal anesthesia.

Uses of Local Anesthesia

Surface Anesthesia

Surface anesthesia can be applied topically on mucous membrane and abraded skin. Loss of motor functions is not seen. Its onset and duration depends on the site, drug its concentration and form, e.g., lidocaine (10%) sprayed in the throat acts in 2–5 minutes and produces anesthesia for 30–45 minutes. It is used for tonometry, surgery, nasal lesions, stomatitis, sore throat, tonsillectomy, endoscopies, intubation, gastric ulcer, burns and proctoscopy.

Infiltration Anesthesia

Infiltration anesthesia is infiltrated under the skin at the time of operation to block sensory nerve endings. Its onset of action is fast. It is used in minor operations where area to be anesthetized is less like in case of incisions, excisions, episiotomy, hydrocele, etc.

Conduction Block

Area distal to injection is anesthetized and paralyzed in this after injecting local anesthesia (LA). **Field block:** Subcutaneous injection of a LA solution proximal to the site to be anesthetized, blocks nerve transmission in the region distal to the injection. Sites such as forearm, scalp, anterior abdominal wall and lower extremity are used for field block.

Nerve Block

Injection of a solution of a LA about/around individual peripheral nerves or nerve plexuses produces larger areas of anesthesia with a smaller amount of the drug than conduction, surface and infiltration anesthesia. Anesthesia starts a few centimeters distal to the injection.

Spinal Anesthesia

In this LA is injected in subarachnoid space between L2 and L3 or L3 and L4. Its primary site of action is cauda equina in which lower portion of body is anesthetized and paralyzed. It is used for operations on the lower limbs, pelvis, lower abdomen, e.g., prostatectomy, fracture, obstetric problems and cesarean. It is safer than GA and produces good analgesia and muscle relaxation without loss of consciousness. Respiratory paralysis, hypotension,

CHAPTER 3: Drugs Acting on Nervous System

headache, cauda equina syndrome, septic meningitis and nausea vomiting are its common complications.

Epidural Anesthesia

Local anesthesia is injected into the spinal extradural (SA) space. It acts on nerve roots while small amounts diffuse into SA space. It is technically more difficult and comparatively larger volumes of the anesthetic are needed.

Intravenous Regional Anesthesia

This type of anesthesia is useful for rapid anesthetization of an extremity. Limb is elevated to ensure venous drainage through gravity and a tourniquet is applied to prevent the re-entry of the blood. A dilute solution of the local anesthetic is then injected intravenously. It diffuses into extravascular tissues. Onset of anesthesia is in 2 minutes. Because of the pain produced by the tourniquet, this type of anesthesia is used for procedures lasting less than 1 hour. About 25% of the drug enters into the systemic circulation. This type of anesthesia is generally used on the upper limbs though it can also be used on the legs and the thighs.

Nursing Responsibilities

- Do not inject local anesthetic into areas of infection because effectiveness in greatly diminished and systemic toxicity may be enhanced
- Use lowest dose resulting in effective anesthesia to minimize danger to systemic effects
- Give injection slowly to decrease danger in case of allergic reactions
- Place patient receiving spinal anesthesia in proper position to avoid diffusion of drug toward respiratory muscles
- Counsel patients receiving spinal or epidural anesthesia that sensation in lower areas of body may not return for an hour or two. Be prepared to assist movement as needed
- Use caution in giving solutions with vasoconstrictors in patient with peripheral vascular diseases of hypertension
- Do not autoclave solutions of local anesthetics containing epinephrine
- Discard unused portions of solutions not containing preservations

Gases: Oxygen, Nitrous Oxide, Carbon Dioxide and Others

The three vital respiratory gases – Oxygen (O_2), Carbon dioxide (CO_2) and Nitrous oxide (NO) help in the tissue perfusion by intersecting the Human red blood cells (RBCs). It is used as inhalation form of General Anesthesia.

Oxygen

Oxygen is a vital gas to support the life. It is non-combustible, colorless, tasteless and odorless gas. It is used as a medicine in the patient with decrease oxygen level as medical oxygen therapy.

Drug Class

It is a general anesthetic and inhalation agent

Formulation

It is used in respiratory system as inhalation of medical gas

Indications

The therapeutic use includes:
- Respiratory failure (Chronic or Acute)
- Aspiration
- Altered mental status
- Suspected hypoxemia
- Pulmonary injury
- Decrease in SpO2
- Carbon monoxide poisoning
- Postoperatively
- Hemodynamic insufficiency
- Minimize cardiopulmonary overload

Contraindications

- Unfavorable ventilation response to oxygen treatment
- May not required in case of Asthma, Bronchitis, Acute heart failure, Pulmonary embolism.

Toxicity

Oxygen toxicity occurs due to high FiO_2 while delivery oxygen therapy. This can cause alveolar damage and intestinal edema. Prolonged use can cause Fibroblasts and can cause irreversible pulmonary fibrosis. It can induce hypercapnic respiratory failure.

Nitrous Oxide

It is colorless, sharp or sweet odor, non-inflammable and non-irritating gas. It produces light anesthesia with minimal muscle relaxation. It does not cause significant depression of respiration or vasomotor center. It has little effect on respiration, heart and BP. N_2O (50%) has been used with O_2 for dental and obstetric analgesia. Prolonged exposure to gas can depress bone marrow and can cause peripheral neuropathy. It is a vasodilating agent.

Drug Class

It is a general anesthetic and inhalation agent.

Formulation

It is used in respiratory system as inhalation of medical gas. In comparison to other anesthetic agent it has minimal effect on hemodynamic and respiratory system.

Indications

The therapeutic use includes:
- Hypoxic respiratory failure (Near term neonates)
- Conjunction with ventilatory support
- Pulmonary heart disease
- Persistent pulmonary hypertension
- Treatment of cystic fibrosis

CHAPTER 3: Drugs Acting on Nervous System

Contraindications
- Hypersensitivity
- Critically ill patients
- Pregnancy (First trimester)
- Pneumothorax
- Middle ear surgery
- Cardiac disease
- Psychiatric disorders

Adverse Effects
- Respiratory depression
- Postoperative nausea and vomiting
- Diffusion hypoxia
- Collapse lung

Carbon Dioxide

It is colorless, odorless gas and faint acid taste. It is non-toxic and non-combustible. It is used as insufflation gas for minimal invasive surgeries. It enlarges as stabilize the body cavities for better visibility in case of Endoscopy, Laparoscopy, etc.

Drug Class
It is a general anesthetic and inhalation agent.

Formulation
It is a pure gas used as inhalation of medical gas. It is also used for sterilization of equipments.

Indications
- Insufflation gas in minimal invasive surgery
- Cryotherapy
- Respiratory stimulant in anesthesia
- Cardiac surgery.

Contraindications
- Hypersensitivity
- Increase cranial pressure
- Intracranial bleeding
- Head injury
- Coma

Adverse Effects
Toxicity cause cortical and subcotical depression.

Nursing Consideration
- Check for rational usage
- Administer after the prescription

- Place the No smoking board while administering oxygen
- Ensure humidification of the oxygen
- Check for the sign of toxicity
- Ensure proper equipment used for the administration
- Monitor oxygen saturation while procedure
- Ensure safe storage of the nitric oxide gas

HYPNOTICS AND SEDATIVES

Sedative-Hypnotics

Sedative: A drug that subdue excitement and calm the subject without inducing sleep through drowsiness may be produced. Sedation refers to decrease responsiveness to any level of stimulation is associated with some decrease in motor activity.

Hypnotics: A drug that induce or maintain sleep similar to normal arousable sleep. This is not to be confused with hypnosis meaning a 'trance like state' in which the subjects become passive and highly suggestible.

Classification (Fig. 3.7)

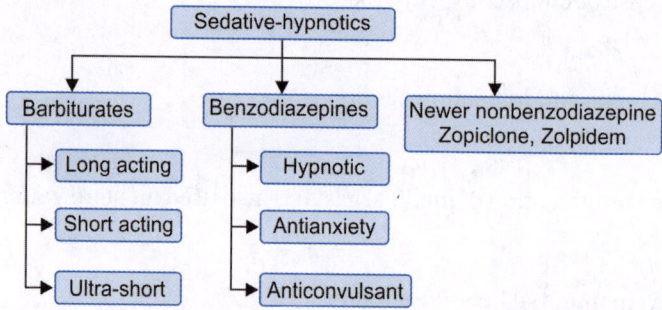

Fig. 3.7: Classification of sedative-hypnotics.

Barbiturate

The clinically useful barbiturates have been categorized in to four groups based upon their duration of action:
- Long-acting (6–8 hr): Phenobarbitone.
- Short-acting (2–4 hr): Pentobarbitone, butobarbitone.
- Ultra short-acting (10–30 min): Methohexitone, thiopentone.

Mechanism of Action of Barbiturates is Presented in Figure 3.8

Pentobarbital (Nembutal) Phenobarbitone: (Refer antiepileptics) Pharmacological action
- CNS: They produce dose dependent effects, sedation, sleep, anesthesia, coma. Hypnotics decreases time to get into sleep and increases the duration of sleep. Sedatives if administered at day time can produce drowsiness, reduction in anxiety and excitability. Barbiturates have anticonvulsive properties also.

CHAPTER 3: Drugs Acting on Nervous System

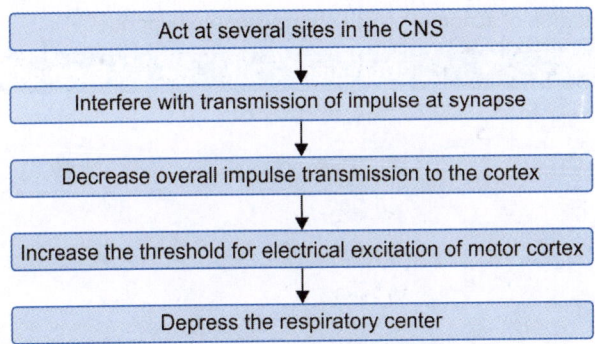

Fig. 3.8: Mechanism of action of barbiturates.

- Respiratory system: It gets depressed by the higher doses of barbiturates.
- CVS: They produce slight decrease in BP and heart rate. They can also produce reflex tachycardia.
- Skeletal muscles: When used in anesthetic doses it can reduce muscle contraction.
- Kidney: Decrease in BP can cause increase in ADH release and thus reduces the urine output.
- Pharmacokinetics: Drug is metabolized in liver and excreted in urine.

Preparation

Capsules—30 mg, 50 mg, 100 mg; Elixir—20 mg/5 mL; Suppositories 30 mg, 60 mg, 120 mg, 200 mg; injection—50 mg/mL.

Usual Dosage Range

- **Oral:**
  - Sedation adult 30 mg, three to four times/day; child 2 mg/kg to 6 mg/kg/day
  - Hypnosis adult 100 mg
- **Rectal:** adult 150–200 mg; child 25–80 mg
- **IM:** adult 150–200 mg; child 25–80 mg.

Nursing Responsibilities

- Be aware that use for prolonged periods of time, even at therapeutic levels is associated with a high incidence of addiction.
- Counsel chronic users to note and report that appearance of sore throat, fever, bruising, rash, jaundice are signs of possible hematologic toxicity.
- When giving IV administer slowly to prevent respiratory depression and hypotension.
- Recognize that barbiturates given to patients in severe pain produce anxiety and restlessness and may intensify the person's reaction to the painful stimuli. Always given in combination with an analgesic in the presence of pain.

Benzodiazepines (Refer Antiepileptics)

They produce lower degree of neuronal depression than barbiturates. Higher doses of hypnotics can cause respiratory depression, but in lower doses it does not affect other body parts doses, duration of action of some of the commonly used hypnotics is presented in **Table 3.2**.

Table 3.2: Dose and duration of action of some commonly used hypnotics.

Hypnotic	Dose (mg)	Duration of action (hours)
Long-acting		
Diazepam	5–10	24–48
Chlordiazepoxide	10–20	24–48
Nitrazepam	5–10	24
Alprazolam	0.25–0.5	24
Short-acting		
Triazolam	0.125–0.25	< 6
Midazolam	7.5–10	< 6
Lorazepam	1–2	12–18
Temazepam	10–20	12–18
Newer agents		
Zolpidem	5–10	< 4
Zaleplon	5–20	< 4
Zopiclone	7.5–10	< 4

Mechanism of Action

Benzodiazepines enhance the effect of Gamma-Aminobutyric Acid (GABA) by increasing GABA affinity for the GABA receptor. Binding of GABA to site opens the chloride channel, resulting in hyperpolarized cell membrane that prevents further excitation of cell.

Indications

Benzodiazepines (BZDs) can be used as antianxiety, muscle relaxant and anti-convulsion drug. It also helps to fasten sleep, reduce intermittent awakening and increase total sleep time.

Adverse effects: Benzodiazepines are generally well tolerated. The common side effects in-clued drowsiness, confusion, amnesia, lethargy, weakness, headache, blurred vision, ataxia, day time sedation and impaired motor coordination such as driving skills, therefore, while on BZDs driving should be avoided. In some patients it may cause paradoxical irritability and anxiety.

Benzodiazepine Antagonist

Flumazenil

Flumazenil reverses the depressant and stimulants effects of benzodiazepines. It is absorbed orally on IV injection it starts its action in seconds and lasts for 1–2 hours. It is used to reverse BZD anesthesia effects within 1 minute of an IV injection of flumazenil. In case of BZD overdose flumazenil 0.2 mg/min can be injected till the patient gains consciousness. It is safe and well-tolerated drug by patients with little agitation and discomfort.

Newer Non-benzodiazepine

Zopiclone

Zopiclone is the first non-BZD hypnotics and is indicated for less than 2 weeks for treatment of insomnia. It is given in dosage of 7.5 mg tablet, one tablet at bedtime for not more than 2–4 weeks. It can cause bitter or metallic taste, psychological disturbances, dry mouth and impaired judgment.

Zolpidem

Zolpidem increases the duration of sleep, but does not have anticonvulsant, antianxiety and muscle relaxant effects. Presently it is one of most prescribed hypnotics. Its dosage is 5–10 mg (maximum 20 mg) at bedside, dose should be decreased to half in case of elderly and patients with liver disease. Side effects are less and even large doses do not depress respiration.

SKELETAL MUSCLE RELAXANTS

Muscle relaxants consist of group of drugs that are used to reduce muscular spasm and also to relax the muscles during surgery. They act peripherally at neuromuscular junction or centrally in the cerebrospinal axis. Centrally acting muscle relaxants are used mainly for painful muscle spasms and spastic neurological conditions.

Classification

Based on their site of action, skeletal muscle relaxants may be classified as follows **(Fig. 3.9)**.

PERIPHERALLY ACTING MUSCLE RELAXANTS

Neuromuscular Blocking Agents

Non-depolarizing (Competitive) Blockers (Table 3.3)

Mechanism of action

Non-depolarizing blockers receptors sites at neuromuscular junction.

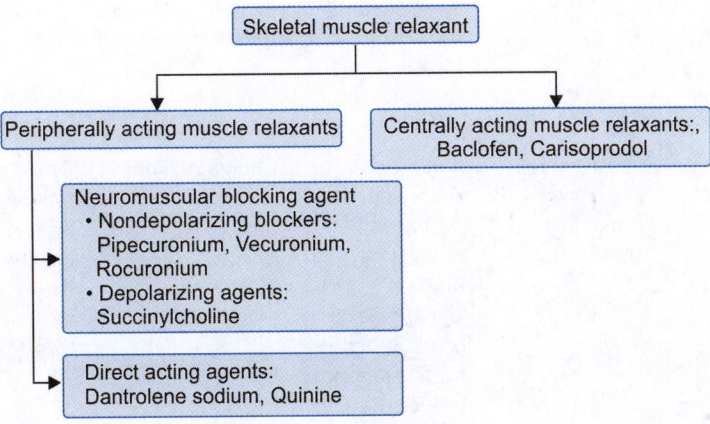

Fig. 3.9: Classification of muscle relaxants.

Table 3.3: Mechanism of action, doses, routes and side effects of non-depolarizing (Competitive) blocker muscle relaxants.

Types	Commonly used drugs	Mechanism of action	Dose and route	Side effects

Peripherally acting muscle relaxants:
• Neuromuscular
• Blocking agents
  ▪ Non-depolarizing blockers
  ▪ Depolarizing blockers
• Directly acting agents
	Pipecuronium, vecuronium, atracurium, rocuronium Succinylcholine (SCh) Dantrolene sodium, quinine	Non-depolarizing blockers bind to nicotinic receptors on the motor end plate and block the actions of acetylcholine (ACh)
		The neuromuscular effects of SCh are like those of ACh SCh stimulates the nicotinic receptors and depolarizes the skeletal muscle membrane. These agents directly affect the skeletal muscle contractile mechanism It inhibits the muscle contraction by preventing the calcium release from the sarcoplasmic reticulum
			Adults: 20–80 mg IV injection
			Children: 1–2 mg/kg IV injection
			Adults: 20–80 mg IV injections IM: 2.5 mg/kg to a maximum of 150 mg
			Children: 1–2 mg/kg IV injection
			Adults: Initially 25 mg orally once daily increase gradually in 25 mg to a maximum of 100mg two to four/day; maintain each dose for 4–7 days before increasing
			Children: Initially 0.5 mg/kg orally twice a day; increase by 0.5 mg/kg increments to a maximum of 3 mg/kg two to four times/day
				Erythema, itching, urticaria, wheezing, hypotension, tachycardia, respiratory depression, apnea
				Muscle weakness, bronchospasm, apnea, hypotension, arrhythmias, intraocular pressure
				GI : Constipation, bleeding, cramping, anorexia, gastric irritation
				
				CNS: Headache, lightheadedness, insomnia, seizures, confusion, nervousness
				CVS: Tachycardia, phlebitis, blood pressure
				Urinary : Crystal urea, incontinence, nocturia, urinary retention, impotence

Centrally acting muscle relaxants	Carisoprodol, diazepam, baclofen, Tizanidine	It depresses the spinal polysynaptic reflexes by depressing these spinal reflexes, centrally acting muscle relaxants reduce the muscle tone	Adults: 20–500 mg three to four times/day Children: 125 g – 500 mg three to four times/day	Drowsiness, fatigue, dizziness, blurred vision, insomnia, confusion, hypotension, flushing, dysuria enuresis, thrombocytopenia

Normal Process (Fig. 3.10)

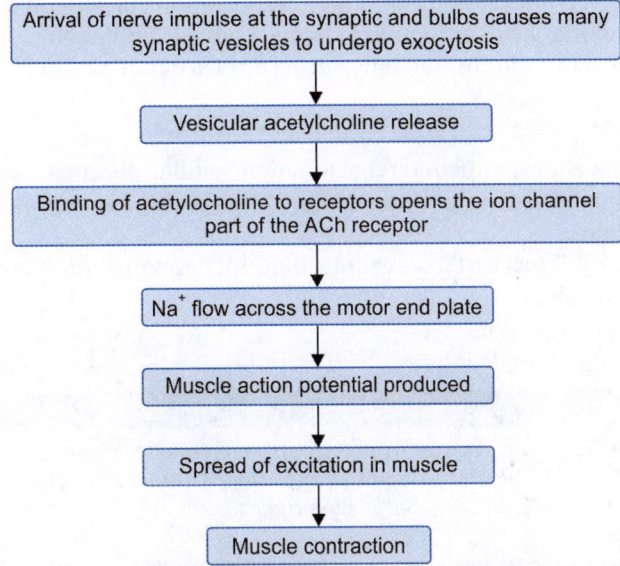

Fig. 3.10: Normal process of muscle contraction.

Mechanism of Action of Muscle Relaxant (Fig. 3.11)

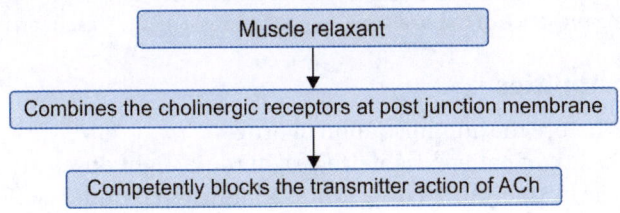

Fig. 3.11: Mechanism of action of muscle relaxants.

Notes on Individual Compounds

Pipecuronium: It is a muscle relaxant with a slow onset and longer duration of action, so recommended for prolonged surgeries. It comes in preparation of Arduan 4 mg/2 mL injection. Hypotension and bradycardia may occur due its cardiovascular action. It can be eliminated through liver and kidney.

Vecuronium: It comes in preparation of Norcuron 4 mg; dissolve in 1 mL solvent applied and Neovec 4 mg, 10 mg vial. It has shorter duration of action and excreted mainly in bile. Due to lack of histamine releasing and ganglionic action it has cardiovascular stability. It is most common drug used for routine surgeries and in intensive care units.

Rocuronium: It has rapid onset and intermediate duration of action. It can be used as an alternative to succinylcholine (SCh) for tracheal intubation. 0.3–0.6 mg/kg/h can be infused IV to facilitate mechanical ventilation in intensive care units. Rocunium, Curomid 50 mg/5 mL, 100 mg/10 mL vials are its preparations.

Indications
- Relaxation of skeletal muscles during surgery as an adjunct to general anesthesia.
- Facilitation of endotracheal intubation or in mechanical ventilation.
- Reduce intensity of muscle contractions during electro or chemo shock therapy.

Contraindications
- Myasthenia gravis, shock, impaired renal function, cardiac diseases, hypertension, hyperthyroidism, sensitivity to drug; patients in those histamine releases prove a definite hazard, sensitivity to iodides.
- Dose initially: 0.4–0.5 mg/kg IV bolus injection; maintenance dose is 0.08–0.1 mg/kg at 15–30 minute intervals.
- Adults: 20–80 mg IV injection.
- Children: 1–2 mg/kg IV injection.

> **Nursing Alerts!**
> - Recognize that drugs should be used only by personnel skilled in respiratory management. Equipment for endotracheal intubation and respiratory assistance must be readily available
> - Administer only electron an adequate analgesia because drug has no effect on consciousness or pain threshold
> - Do not administer drug IM, because severe tissue injury can result. Monitor vital signs continually until recovery from drug effects is complete
> - As all antidepolarizing blockers, treat overdosage edrophonium or neostigmine, fluid replacement and vasopressors if needed and respiratory assistance
> - Perform renal function tests and electrolyte determinations before use because effects may be increased in the presence of hypokalemia, hypermagnesia or decreased renal clearance capacity

Nursing Responsibilities
- Check vital signs before the administration of drug.
- Check for 5 R's, i.e., right patient, right drug, right route, right dose, and right time.
- Reduce initial dose by one-third if drug is first administered under isoflurane or enflurane anesthesia.
- Do not give before unconsciousness has been attained.
- Do not mix injection with alkaline solution in the same syringe or administer simultaneously during IV infusion through the same needle, because atracurium may be inactivated.
- Inform patients that tachycardia may occur immediately following administration, but will decline gradually.
- Recognize that drug can interfere the physical signs of anesthesia.
- Monitor fluid intake and output to determine serial status because renal dysfunction may greatly prolong and intensify drug effects.
- Critically observe patient during diagnostic test for myasthenia because very small doses can produce an exaggerated response.

Adverse Reactions
Erythema, itching, urticaria, wheezing, hypotension, tachycardia, respiratory depression, apnea, hypotension, profound muscle weakness, circulatory depression and increased secretions.

Deploraized Blockers

Succinylcholine (SCh) (Suxamethonium and decamethonium) are its examples.

Mechanism of Action (Fig. 3.12)

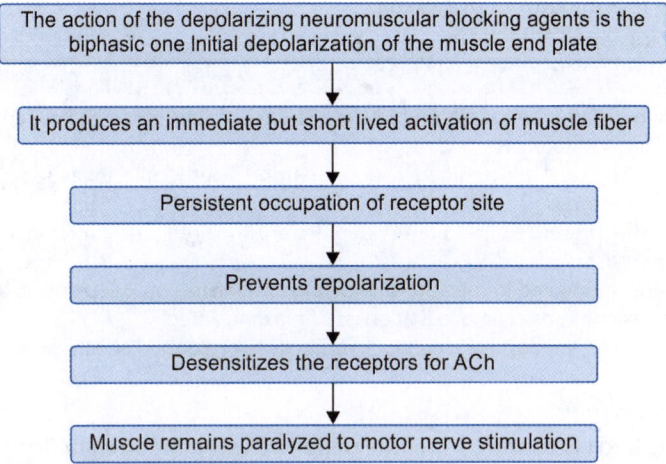

Fig. 3.12: Mechanism of action of depolarized blocker muscle relaxant.

Notes on Individual Compounds

Succinylcholine: It is most common muscle relaxant for passing tracheal tube. Excellent intubation conditions can be obtained within 1–1.5 minutes of administration of drug. Continues IV infusion can be done for longer duration muscle relaxation. Change in BP and HR, arrhythmias and hyperkalemia are its common complications so should be used for young children. Midarine, Scoline, Myorelex, Entubate 50 mg/mL injection 2 mL are its preparations. Risk of aspiration is increased in patients with gastroesophageal reflux disease (GERD) and in the obese.

Indications

- Skeletal muscle relaxation as an adjunct to general anesthesia
- Reduce the intensity of muscle contractions during shock therapy
- Facilitate intubation procedures
- Assist mechanical respiration
- Reduce initial muscle fasciculations.

Contraindications

- History of malignant hyperthermia.
- Severe respiratory depression.
- Acute narrow angle glaucoma.
- Penetrating eye injury.
- Deficiency of plasma pseudocholinesterase.

Adverse Reactions

Muscle weakness, bronchospasm, apnea, hypotension, arrhythmias, intraocular pressure.

Dose

- Adults: 2–80 mg IV injections test dose of 10 mg may be given initially to determine patient's sensitivity.
- IV: 2.5 mg/min of a 0.1% or 0.2% solution.
- 1M: 2.5 mg/kg to a maximum of 150 mg.
- Children: 1–2 mg/kg IV injection.

Nursing Alerts!

- Be aware that overdosage can cause complete respiratory paralysis for which O_2 artificial respiration is the only effective antidote
- The action of the drug can be intensified by dehydration, hypothermia, renal disease, carcinomas and electrolyte imbalances
- Use cautiously in the presence of respiratory depression, impaired renal function, severe burns, fractures, muscle spasm
- Monitor vital signs during and immediately following administration. Keep airway clear of secretions
- Be aware that transient apnea can occur at onset of maximal effect
- Do not use together an antidepolarizing blockers because prolonged effects can occur

Nursing Responsibilities

- Check the drug and check the 5 Rs' of the patient: Right patient, right drug, right dose, right route, right time.
- Inform patient that muscle pain and stiffness may be present for sometime following recovery.
- Make sure proper facilities are available for treatment of respiratory distress.
- To avoid patient distress, administer only after unconsciousness has been attained anesthetic.
- Monitor body temperature during administration.
- When the drug is given IM, inject deep into muscle, preferably the deltoid.
- Do not administer if facilities for artificial respiration and O_2 are not immediately available.

Mechanism of Action of Direct Acting Blocking Muscle Relaxants Agents (Fig. 3.13)

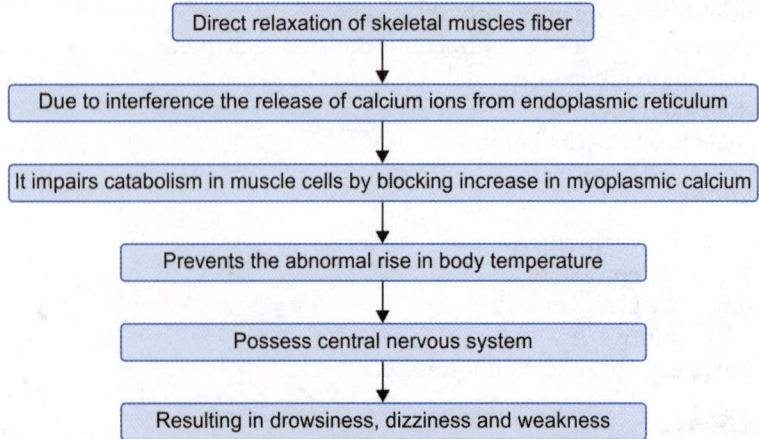

Fig. 3.13: Mechanism of action of direct acting blocking muscle relaxant agents.

Notes on Individual Compounds

Dantrolene sodium: It acts slowly, but adequately absorbed from GIT. It penetrates brain and produces some sedation. Orally 25–100 mg qid can be used to reduce spasticity in upper motor neuron disorders, hemiplegia, paraplegia, cerebral palsy and multiple sclerosis. It can be used IV 1 mg/kg repeated as required in case of malignant hyperthermia.

Quinine: It reduces muscle tone in myotonia congenita. It can be used to abolish nocturnal leg cramps at bedtime in 200–300 mg of dosage.

Indications

- Relief of muscle spasticity associated chronic neurologic disorders, e.g., cerebral palsy, stroke, spinal cord injury or multiple sclerosis.
- Emergency treatment of malignant hyperthermia.
- Preoperative prophylaxis of malignant hyperthermia in high-risk patient.

Contraindications

Hepatic disease, children under five conditions in increase spasticity is necessary to sustain upright posture or balance.

Dose

- Adults: Initially 25 mg orally once daily increase gradually in 25 mg to a maximum of 100 mg two to four time/day; maintain each dose for 4–7 days before increasing.
- Children: Initially 0.5 mg/kg orally twice a day; increase by 0.5 mg/kg increments to a max of 3 mg/kg two to four times/day.

Nursing Alerts!

- Recognize that the drug has a potential for serious hepatotoxicity, especially long-term therapy
- Use only in conjunction appropriate and frequent monitoring of hepatic function
- Ask patient to be alert for appearance of skin rash, itching, black or bloody stools and yellowish skin discoloration and report these developments immediately
- Discontinue drug if no observable benefit occurs in 45 days because the danger of liver damage increases prolonged use
- Use cautiously in the presence of impaired pulmonary function, cardiac impairment caused by myocardial disease, hepatic dysfunction and in pregnant or lactating women
- Caution patient that drowsiness is likely to occur in early stages of therapy and to avoid hazardous situations

Nursing Responsibilities

- Use the lowest effective dose in all cases and closely observe the patient for any sign of developing toxicity.
- Advice patient to avoid prolonged exposure to sunlight, because photosensitivity reactions can occur.
- Watch for signs of exacerbation of spasticity, an indication that the drug is providing some benefits.

Adverse Reactions

- GI: Constipation, bleeding, cramping, anorexia, gastric irritation.
- CNS: Headache, light headedness, insomnia, seizures, confusion, nervousness.
- CVS: Tachycardia, phlebitis, high BP.
- Urinary: Crystal urea, incontinence, nocturia, urinary retention, impotence.

CENTRALLY ACTING MUSCLE RELAXANTS

Mechanism of Action (Fig. 3.14)

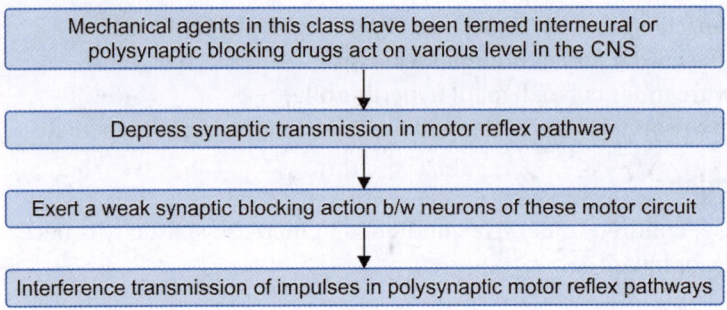

Fig. 3.14: Mechanism of action of centrally acting muscle relaxants.

Notes on Individual Compounds

Carisoprodol: It is used to relieve muscle spasm in case of musculoskeletal disorders. It also has some analgesic, antipyretic and anticholinergic properties. It can be used as carisoma 350 mg tab; one tablet Tds-qid, Somaflam 175 mg + ibuprofen 400 mg tablet.

Diazepam: It lies under the classification of BZDs which act on brain to reduce the muscle tone. It is particularly useful in spinal injuries and tetanus. It can be combined with analgesics to reduce muscle spasm in rheumatic disorders. Its dose is 5 mg tds orally and 10–40 mg IV in tetanus.

Baclofen: It depresses polysynaptic and monosynaptic reflexes in spinal cord to produce muscle weakness. It can be used in many neurological disorders like multiple sclerosis, spinal disorders and flexor spasms to reduce spasticity. It can be used in dosage of 10 mg bd to 25 mg tds. Lioresal, Liofen 10 mg, 25 mg tab are its preparations.

Tizanidine: It inhibits polysynaptic reflexes to decrease muscle tone and frequency of muscle spasms without reducing strength of muscle. It can be used to decrease spasticity in neurological disorders and to decrease painful muscle spasms of spinal origin. Dry mouth, night time insomnia and hallucinations are its side effects. It can be used in dosage of 2 mg tds; maximum 24 mg/day.

Indications

- Relief of pain and discomfort of muscle spasm associated acute musculoskeletal disorders, e.g., inflammatory states peripheral injury, connective tissue disorders.
- Alleviation of spasticity resulting from multiple sclerosis, spinal cord disease and other neurologic conditions.

Contraindications
- Patient with stroke or rheumatic disorders
- Children under 12 years age
- Pregnant women, nursing mothers
- Hyperthyroidism, arrhythmias, congestive heart failure, acute recovery phase of myocardial infarction
- In anemia, renal or hepatic impairment.

Adverse Effects
- Drowsiness, fatigue, dizziness, anorexia, hiccups, bleeding, abdominal pain.
- Ataxia, headache, blurred vision, insomnia, confusion, irritability, paresthesias.
- Tachycardia, hypotension, flushing, petechiae, thrombophlebitis, chest pain, palpitations.
- Urinary retention, dysuria, enuresis.
- Leucopenia, pancytopenia, thrombocytopenia, agranulocytosis, hemolytic anemia.
- Abnormal liver function tests, jaundice.

Dose
- Adults: 20–500 mg three to four times/day; reduce gradually as improvement is noted.
- Children: 125–500 mg three to four times/day; may crush and mixed food or other vehicle.

Nursing Alerts!
- Caution patient against engaging in any hazardous activity while taking these drugs because drowsiness is common and often marked
- Advise patient to avoid concomitant use of other CNS depressants while taking one of these drugs
- Use drugs cautiously in presence of hepatic or renal dysfunction, respiratory depression and in young children, pregnant or lactating women and the elderly or debilitated
- Inform use to immediately report signs of developing hepatotoxicity (e.g. abdominal pain, with fever, nausea, diarrhea) or blood dyscrasias (e.g. fever, sore throat, malaise, mucosal ulceration, petechiae)

Nursing Responsibilities
- Advice patient to take last dose at bedtime, because drowsiness may aid sleep.
- Be aware that due to CNS effects the compounds, prolonged use may lead to dependence. Abrupt termination of the drug in these patients may evolve withdrawal symptoms.

ANTIPSYCHOTICS
- Over a span of several decades the antipsychotic drugs are proving effective in controlling a broad range of mental and emotional disorders. These various chemical agents have revolution used the treatment of mental illness with increased use of these drugs, their action and side effects of have also increased.
- Antipsychotic appear to act principally at lower brain contours to improve the disturbed thought process of the psychotic individual and therefore create a more favorable mental state for other form of psychotherapy.

Definition

The antipsychotic drugs represented by several chemically distinct groups of compounds are capable of improving the mood and calming the disturbed behavior of psychotic patient without causing marked sedation or habituation psychotropic drugs can also be defined as chemical that affect the brain and nervous system alter feeling and emotion.

Mechanism of Action

Dopamine 1 (DA1) and dopamine 2 (DA2) are two dopamine receptors. Mechanism of action of antipsychotic drugs is presented in **Figure 3.15**.

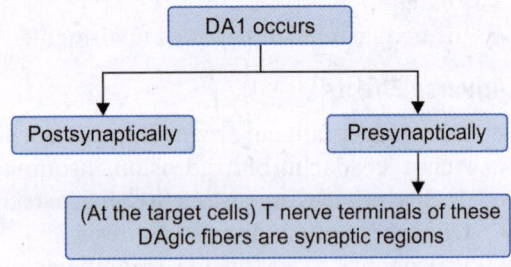

Fig. 3.15: Mechanism of action of Dopamine 1.

Classification (Fig. 3.16)

High-potency Antipsychotic Drugs

- Fluphenazine (Prolixin)
- Haloperidol (Haldol)
- Thiothixene (Navane)
- Trifluoperazine (Stelazine)

Moderate-potency Antipsychotic Drugs

- Loxapine (Loxitane)
- Molindone (Moban)
- Perphenazine (Trilafon)

Low-potency Antipsychotic Drugs

- Chlorpromazine (CPZ) (Thorazine)
- Mesoridazine (Serentil)
- Thioridazine (Mellaril)

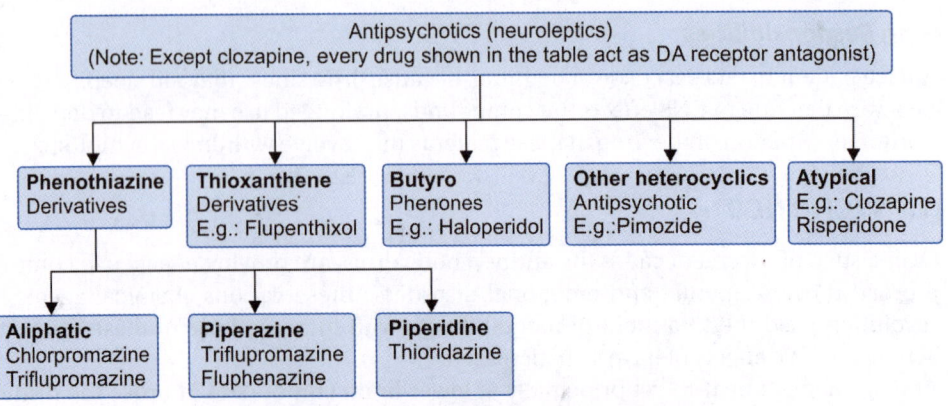

Fig. 3.16: Classification of antipsychotic drugs.

Notes on Individual Compounds

Chlorpromazine

Pharmacological action

CNS: It reduces irrational behavior, agitation and aggressiveness and controls psychotic symptomatology. It lowers seizure threshold and can precipitate fits in untreated epileptics. It has D2 receptor blocking action.

Local anesthetic: Like procaine it has local anesthetic action but has irritation action so not used for the same.

CVS: Neuroleptics produce orthostatic hypotension due to α-blockade action and reflex tachycardia. It also has a direct myocardial depressant effect like quinidine and some antiarrhythmic actions also. In higher doses it directly depresses heart and produce electrocardiographic (ECG) changes.

Skeletal muscle: In site of action in basal ganglia or medulla oblongata it reduces certain types of spasticity. However, it does not have direct effect on muscle fibers.

Pharmacokinetics: Single dose effects usually last for 6–8 hours. The elimination t½ is variable, but mostly is in the range of 18–30 hours. Therapeutic effects may be seen at 30–200 ng/mL. After discontinuing the drugs metabolites are excreted in urine and bile for months.

Triflupromazine: It is mainly used as antiemetic and is more potent than CPZ. When injected it produces muscle dystonias in children.

Thioridazine: It has anticholinergic action and incidence of extrapyramidal side effects is low. It can cause cardiac arrhythmias and eye damage are common risks.

Penfluridol: It is used for chronic schizophrenia and social adjustment. Dosage is 20–60 mg oral (maximum 120 mg) once weekly.

Atypical antipsychotics:

Clozapine: It is an effective antipsychotic and it has very low incidence of extrapyramidal side effects (EPS). Sedation is low and no endocrine side effects, no galactorrhea and gynecomastia are seen with its use. It is effective in patients not responding to chlorpromazine (resistant cases). The most important disadvantage with clozapine is that it may cause agranulocytosis in some patients, which can be fatal.

Risperidone: It is most commonly used antipsychotics. It blocks alpha adrenergic and histamine H1 receptors and is effective against both positive and negative symptoms of schizophrenia.

Dose (Table 3.4)

Adverse Reactions

CNS: Hyperpyrexia, lowering of convulsive threshold hyperactivity, confusion, bizarre dream, insomnia, depression, cerebral edema.

Neuromuscular: Extrapyramidal reaction, dystonias, akathisia, pseudoparkinsoinism, tardive dyskinesia, hyperreflexia.

Cardiovascular: Tachycardia, fainting, ECG changes, cardiac arrest.

Table 3.4: Doses of antipsychotics drugs.

Drugs	Dosage
Phenothiazines • Chlorpromazine (Thorazine) • Triflupromazine (Vesprin)	Adults • Initially 50–150 mg IM • Maintenance 10–200 mg every 4–6 hr orally or IM • As required children (over 12)
Eiperazines	Adult • 20 mg 3 times (80–120 mg day in hospitalized patient) children • 0.8–1.6 mg 1 kg/day
Thioridazine	Adult • Psychosis • Initially 50–100 mg three times/day; maintenance 200–800 mg day • In 2–4 divided dose • Depressive neuroses • Initially 25 mg three times/day • Maintenance 20–200 mg/day in three to four divided doses Children (1–2 years)
Thioxanthenes Thiothixene (Navane)	Adults • Oral Initially 25–50 mg three to four times/day, increase to optimal level (maximum 600 mg/day) • IM 25–50 mg three to four times/day; substitute oral therapy as soon as possible Children • Oral 10–25 mg, 3–5 mg two to three times/day • IM over 12 years, same as adult dose • Oral initially 2–5 mg two to three times/ day, maintenance 20–60 mg/ day in divided doses • IM 4 mg to four times/day (usual range 16–25 mg/day)
Dibenzoxazepine • Clozapine (Clozaril)	• Initially 10 mg orally twice a day, increase to optimal level (usually 60–100 mg/day) (maximum 250 mg/day) • IM 12.5–50 mg every 4–6 hours to control acutely agitated patient
Butyrophenone • Olanzapine (Zyprexa)	• Oral 0.5–5 mg two to three times/day depending on symptom (maximum 100 mg/day) • IM 2–5 mg; repeat at 2–4 hours intervals as needed

Hematologic: Blood dyscrasias, agranulocytosis leukopenia, leukocytosis, anemias, thrombocytopenia, pancytopenia.

Hypersensitivity: Urticaria, itching, eczema photosensitivity, contact dermatitis, angioneurotic edema, anaphylactic reaction, dermatitis, cholestatic jaundice.

Endocrine: Abnormal lactation, breast engorgement, gynecomastia, changes in libido, amenorrhea, glycosuria and hyperglycemia, increased appetite.

Extrapyramidal Side Effects (Table 3.5)

Table 3.5: Extrapyramidal side effects of antipsychotic drugs.

Side effects	Nursing interventions
Peripheral nervous system effects	
Constipation	Increase fluid intake, encourage high dietary and provide laxatives as necessary
Dry mouth	Advise client to use sugarless hard candy or gum, sips of water frequently
Nasal congestion	Suggest over-the-counter nasal decongestants that are safe for use with antipsychotic agents
Blurred vision	Ask client to avoid dangerous tasks This symptom will usually last only a short time at the beginning of treatment Eye drops should be used for the short-term need
Mydriasis	Advise client to report any eye pain immediately
Photophobia	Advise client to wear sunglasses when in sunlight
Orthostatic hypotension	Advise client to get out of chair or bed slowly, to sit before standing, and rise slowly Observe to see if change to another antipsychotic is advisable
Tachycardia	This is usually a reflex response to hypotension When intervention for hypotension is effective, reflex tachycardia usually decreases with clozapine, hold the dose if pulse rate is > 140
Urinary retention	Encourage client to void when urge is present and void frequently. Catheterize for residual urine Client should closely monitor output. Older men with benign prostatic hyperplasia are particularly susceptible to urinary retention
Urinary hesitation	Provide privacy, encourage client to take the time to avoid run water in sink or pour warm water over perineum
Sedation	Help client to get up, get dressed and begin the say early
Weight gain	Advise client to maintain appropriate diet
Agranulocytosis	• There is a high incidence of agranulocytosis for client who are taking clozapine; white cell counts (NBC) need to be monitored weekly • If the WBC < 3,500 cells/mm³ prior to therapy, no treatment should begin • After treatment has begun a WBC < 3,000 cells mm³ and a granulocyte count of <1,500 cells/mm³ indicate that treatment should be interrupted to monitor for infection • If WBC is < 2,000 cells/mm³ and granulocyte count is <1,000 cells/mm³, halt therapy and do not begin treatment with the drug again, if infection develops, antibiotics should be prescribed
Central nervous system effects	
Akathisia	Usually develops within the first 2 months. There is an uncontrollable need to move. Occurs most often with high-potency antipsychotics Treatment is usually with anxiety or psychotic agitation, it is likely that antipsychotic dosage would be increased, thereby making akathisia more intense

Contd...

Contd...

Side effects	Nursing interventions
Dystonias	• Acute: Usually occur early in treatment and are dangerous and severe • Oculogyric crisis or torticollis are the most common occurrences • Treatment includes antiparkinson drug or antihistamine immediately and offer reassurance • Obtain an order of IM administration when client begins treatment with antipsychotics or if in acute state of dystonias, call physician immediately • For less acute dystonias, notify the physician when an order for an antiparkinson drug is warranted
Drug-induced parkinsonism	A chronic nervous disease characterized by a fine, slowly spreading tremor, muscular, weakness and rigidity, and a peculiar gait induced by some antipsychotic medications. Assess for three major symptoms tremors, rigidity and bradykinesia. Report to physician immediately, antiparkinson drugs will be indicated
Tardive dyskinesia	Develops in 15–20% of clients during long-term therapy. The risk is related to duration of treatment and dosage size. For many clients symptoms are irreversible. Assess for signs using the Abnormal Inventory Movement Scale (AIMS). Anticholinergic agents will worsen it, so use is contraindicated
Neuroleptic malignant seizures	This is fatal side effect of antipsychotic medications. Routinely take client's temperature and encourage adequate water intake. Also routinely assess for rigidity, tremor, and similar symptoms
Seizures	Occur in approximately 1% of clients taking antipsychotic medications. Clozapine causes an even higher rate, up to 5% of clients taking 600–900 mg/day. For dosages of clozapine greater than 600 mg/day a normal electroencephalogram (EEG) should be performed. If a seizure occurs, it may be necessary to discontinue clozapine

Indications

- Management of acute and chronic psychosis, either organic or drug induced.
- Control of the manic phase of manic-depressive psychosis.
- Relief of severe nausea and vomiting.
- Control of intractable hiccups.
- Relief of anxiety, apprehension and agitation associated with a variety of somatic disorders or prior to surgery.
- Facilitation of alcohol withdrawal adjunctive treatment of tremors and acute intermittent porphyria.
- Control of aggressive in disturbed children.

Contraindications

- Bone marrow depression
- Blood dyscrasis
- Parkinsonism
- Jaundice
- Liver damage
- Renal insufficiency
- Cerebral arteriosclerosis
- Coronary disease

CHAPTER 3: Drugs Acting on Nervous System

- Circulatory collapse
- Mitral insufficiency
- Severe hypotension
- Chronic alcoholism
- Subcortical brain damage.

Nursing Alerts!

- Use these drugs very cautiously in patient with glaucoma, prostatic hypertrophy, epilepsy, diabetes, severe hypertension, ulcers, cardiovascular disease, chronic respiratory disorders, liver impairment, in pregnant or lactating women, in children under 6 months of age, and in persons exposed to extreme heat, phosphorus insecticides or pesticides
- Caution against operating dangerous machinery during initial stages of therapy because drowsiness is common
- Observe carefully for early signs of blood dyscrasias (fever, sore throat, mucosal ulceration, fatigue, upper respiratory infection) and advise physician
- Note signs of developing jaundice (fever, sore throat, mucosal ulceration, fatigue, upper respiratory infection)
- Caution against abrupt stoppage of therapy particularly with high doses, because gastritis, vomiting, dizziness, tremors, insomnia and psychotic behavior may occur, withdraw drug gradually over several weeks (e.g. 10–25% reduction in dosage every 2 week)
- Critically observe for appearance of fine worm-like movement of the tongue, an early sign of retardive dyskinesia which usually develops after long-term (6–24 months) treatment. Because the symptoms (significant adverse reactions) are difficult to treat, prompt cessation of therapy at the initial sign of the developing syndrome can prevent worsening of symptoms. Be aware that antiparkinsonian drugs do not alleviate these symptoms and may, in fact worsen them
- Monitor renal function of patients on long-term therapy. If serum creatinine if elevated, discontinue the drug
- Advise periodic breast examination in patient on chronic therapy, especially those with previous breast cancer of a family history of breast cancer
- Observe for sign of dizziness and weakness indication of orthostatic hypotension. Monitor BP before each dose during the initial treatment period. Advise patient to change position gradually, set up slowly, and lie down immediately if dizziness occurs. Caution against prolonged standing and lengthy hot showers or baths because hypotension is likely to develop
- Keep patient in recumbent position for at least 1 hour after parenteral administration and monitor blood pressure closely. Marked hypotension can be treated by placing patient in head-low position and if necessary, by using volume expanders and repressor agents such as level arterial or dopamine. Do not use epinephrine because reversal of effects can occur, leading to worsened hypotension.

Nursing Responsibilities

- Periodically evaluate patient on long-term therapy, and make dosage adjustment as necessary. Doses should be keep as low as possible, and drug-free periods should be employed where possible to minimize incidence of untoward reactions, particularly dyskinesia and other involuntary movement episodes to extreme heat, phosphorus insecticides or pesticides.
- Caution against operating dangerous machinery during initial stages of therapy because drowsiness is common.
- Observe carefully for early signs of blood dyscrasias (fever, sore throat, mucosal ulceration, fatigue, upper respiratory infection) are common early in therapy and usually disappear others such as orthostatic hypotension, extrapyramidal reactions, and sedation may be minimized by selection of proper agent.

- Be alert for the onset of acute dystonic reactions. These reactions are very frightening to many patients. Remain with the patient to provide reassurance, and notify the physician promptly.
- Do not use antiparkinsonian medication to prevent extrapyramidal reaction. If symptoms appear during antipsychotic therapy, attempt to eliminate by dosage reduction first. If unsuccessful, titrate dose of antiparkinsonian drug carefully so that the smallest dose to relieve the extrapyramidal symptoms is employed.
- Caution patient to avoid direct sunlight while taking these drugs, because photosensitivity reactions can occur. Use of sunscreen lotion is recommended.
- Note the children with acute illnesses (e.g. mumps, measles, severe infection) or who are dehydrated are more susceptible than adults to development of dystonias (i.e. neck spasms, eye rolling, dysphagia, convulsions). Be prepared to discontinue drug and consult physician.
- Monitor fluid intake and output bowel function during prolonged therapy and observe for abdominal distention. Urinary retention and constipation can occur. Increase fluid intake and roughage in the diet condition. Reduced dosage or change the drug if above conditions persists. Avoid use of proprietary laxative unless prescribed because many contain anticholinergics and many interact with phenothiazines.
- Observe diabetic patient for sign of altered carbohydrate metabolism such as glycosuria, weight loss and polyphagia. Dosage alterations or dietary changes may be warranted.
- Alert patient to the possible occurrence of endocrine changes caused by the antipsychotic drug. Menstrual irregularities, gynecomastia, breast engorgement, impotence and altered libido are possible. Provide reassurance to the patient and attempts minimize. Change by dosage adjustment or use of an alternate drug.
- Encourage frequent rinsing of the mouth, adequate fluid intake and use of gum or hard candy to alleviate mouth dryness. Stress meticulous oral candidiasis, especially with use of the oral concentrate.
- Warn patients that drug may discover the urine (pink to red-brown). This is not serious and does not necessitate interruption of therapy.
- Emphasize the need to maintain a regular dosage schedule, especially during initial stages, because beneficial effects sometimes require several weeks to become manifest. Periodically re-evaluate the patient's status and stress the need for regular follow-up care.
- Avoid drug contact with skin or mucous membrane, because contact dermatitis can occur.
- Dispense oral liquid preparation in dark bottles, because solutions are light sensitive.
- Do not use discolored indictable solution or mix other solution in same syringe. Inject deeply IM. Avoid subcutaneous injection because tissue irritation is common.
- Note the phenothiazines may interfere with laboratory tests for pregnancy. I-131 uptake, urinary catecholamines, urine ketones, bilirubin and steroids.

Mood Stabilizers

Mood stabilizers are the drugs used to treat mood disorders, generally characterized by rapid unstable mood shifts alternating between mania (emotional highs) and depression (lows). These are a diverse group of drugs used primarily in the treatment of bipolar disorders (manic depressive illness) and other conditions related thematically through the presence of mood abnormalities (e.g. mood swings), volatility (including violence and explosiveness), impulsivity, impulsive aggression and affectively unstable personality disorders (e.g.

CHAPTER 3: Drugs Acting on Nervous System

borderline personality disorder). In general, in bipolar disorder, mood stabilizers are more effective in the manic, than the depressive phase of illness.

Since long **Lithium (Li)** has been the drug of choice in this class due to its high efficacy in treating rapid alterations between manic and depressive phases. Other atypical anti-convulsants and anti-psychotics and have also been effective in treatment of bipolar disorder.

Since about one-third of patients either do not respond or cannot tolerate lithium, anticonvulsant mood stabilizers have provided important new alternatives in the treatment of bipolar and related disorders. The drug of choice is Li (used as lithium carbonate), but more or less other drugs (listed later) can also be used as mood stabilizers where lithium is not a good choice to be made.

The anticonvulsants, in addition, have the ability to prevent seizures (epilepsy).

Classification

There is no specified classification, yet we can group mood stabilizers in three classes:
- **Lithium:** This is an alkali metal and is the oldest and best known mood stabilizer.
- **Anticonvulsants:** These are atypical drugs used as mood stabilizers with good results; these include carbamazepine, sodium valproate, lamotrigine and gabapentin.
- **Antipsychotics:** These drugs have been recently tried as mood stabilizers; these include risperidone, topiramate and olanzapine.
- Though this is a generic classification including antipsychotics and anticonvulsants, the fact that mood stabilizers are a diverse kind of drugs with its own particular therapeutic action justifies including these drugs, as they have the mood stabilizing properties.

Lithium

Lithium has been used for over 50 years as a mood stabilizer. The US Food and Drug Administration (FDA) has authorized the therapeutic use of Li. It has been shown superior in controlling depression, mania and long-term mood stability.

Mechanism of Action

The precise action is not yet precisely known. Many hypotheses have been put forward to understanding the working:
- However, lithium ion (Li^+) substitutes for the sodium ion (Na+), thereby compromising the ability of neurons to release, activate or respond to neurotransmitters.
- Lithium also stabilizes calcium (Ca^{2+}) channels and decreases neuronal activity via effects on secondary messenger systems, all of which may add to its therapeutic profile.

Based on recent findings it has been put forward that Li^+ inhibits hydrolysis of inositol-1-phosphate in neurons. As a result, the supply of free inositol for regeneration of membrane phosphatidylinositides is reduced. The inositides are the source of Inositol-3-phosphate (IP3) and Diacylglycerol (DAG) which directly lead to Ca^{2+} mobilization and protein kinase C activation that produces response in neurons.

The mechanism of action of lithium can be summarized in **Figure 3.17**.

Indications

- Bipolar disorder
- Manic depressive psychosis

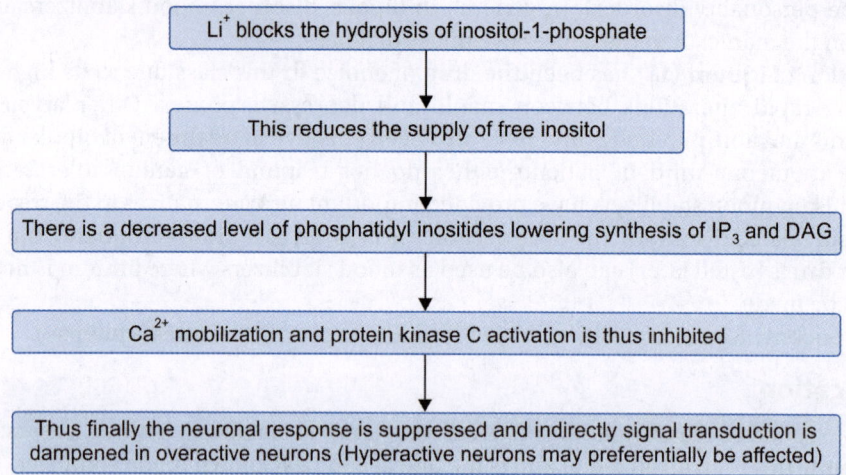

Fig. 3.17: Mechanism of action of lithium.

- Recurrent mania
- Cyclic depression
- Acute hypomania.

Contraindications

Lithium is not to be or may not be used in following conditions:
- **Pregnancy:**
  - It is to be used in extreme caution in pregnancy and lactation.
  - Research has shown Li to affect the fetus adversely.
  - Exposure to Li during first trimester is associated with slightly increased risk of Ebstein's anomaly.
  - Lithium is also excreted in the milk of lactating mother.
- **Cardiovascular diseases:** It disrupts the cardiac conduction system.
- **Kidney disorders (renal impairment):** Li inhibits action of ADH on distal tubules and may cause diabetes insipidus like state, thus is to be avoided in renal impairment.
- Thyroid disorders.
- **Severe dehydration:** It inhibits the reabsorption of water leading to excessive urination and thirst.
- **Psoriasis:** It can worsen the situation.
- Hepatic disorders.
- **Obesity:** Weight gain is common in Li therapy.
- Diabetes.
- Brain trauma.

Examples

- Lithium carbonate (Li_2CO_3)
- Lithium chloride (LiCl)-LiCl causes gastric irritation and thus less preferred

Dosage

- Adults: 900–1,800 mg per day (in divided doses 300–600 mg tid).
- Dosage should be maintained to achieve therapeutic blood levels of Li^+ at 0.6–1.2 mEq/L.
- Dosage should be increased gradually to 900–1,800 mg/day starting from 300 mg/day.
- Children: 15–20 mg in 2–3 divided doses to achieve blood levels of 0.4–0.5 mEq/L.

Side Effects/Adverse Reactions

Common side effects of Li^+ on different systems are:
- **CNS:** May cause headache, drowsiness, dizziness, ataxia, tremors, seizures, confusion, slurred speech and restlessness; it is reported to alter electroencephalography (EEG) pattern in children.
- **Cardiovascular:**
  - May cause hypotension, circulatory collapse edema.
  - It disrupts the cardiac conduction system and causes changes in ECG.
  - Can also cause arrhythmias.
- **Dermatological:** It can induce or exacerbate acne and psoriasis, drying of hair, alopecia, pruritus.
- **Endocrine:** Hypothyroidism, goiter and hyperglycemia.
- **Gastrointestinal:** Dry mouth, metallic taste, nausea and diarrhea.
- **Genitourinary:** Polyuria, albuminuria, renal toxicity and edema.
- **Systemic:** Hyponatremia and leukocytosis.
- **Others:** Weight gain, tinnitus and blurred vision.

Interactions of other Drugs

- Diuretics increase Li^+ levels in body, e.g., furosemide and chlorothiazide.
- NSAIDs may increase Li^+ in body, e.g., ibuprofen and celecoxib.
- Antihypertensive drugs may worsen the side effects of Li, e.g., Ca^{2+} channel blockers and angiotensin-converting enzyme (ACE) inhibitors.
- Antipsychotics may worsen the side effects and some are neurotoxic with Li^+, e.g., haloperidol, quetiapine, chlorpromazine, etc.
- Some may decrease the amount of Li^+, e.g., caffeine and theophylline.

Nursing Responsibilities

- Assess the client's mood and behavior before and during the course of Li therapy and monitor the mood changes.
- Assess for minor Li toxicity such as vomiting, diarrhea, poor coordination, weakness and major Li toxicity, i.e., tremors, tinnitus and severe thirst.
- Prepare the patient for expected side effects in non-anxious manner.
- Discuss which side effects should subside (nausea, dry mouth, diarrhea, thirst, mild tremor, weight gain, insomnia, lightheadedness and bloatedness). Identify the side effects that require immediate notification of physician (e.g. severe hand tremor, muscle weakness, vomiting, sedation and vertigo).
- Monitor serum Li^+ levels weekly two three times for first 2 months and afterwards once weekly.
- Serum Li^+ levels must be maintained within 0.6–1.2 mEq/L.

- Therapeutic and toxic levels are very close so careful monitoring must be done.
- Monitor sodium and fluid intake; decreased Na⁺ and fluid intake may lead to excessive Li+ levels in the body; increased Na⁺ and fluid intake decreases Li⁺ retention.
- Monitor urine for albuminuria, glycosuria, and uric acid during the beginning of treatment; assess for signs of urinary dysfunction and monitor serum creatinine levels (must be less than 1.2 mg/dL).
- Monitor input and output, and promote fluid intake of 2,000–3,000 mL per day to prevent retention.
- Assess the weight and check for edema in legs, ankles and wrists; monitor for weight gain.
- Administer reduced dosage to elderly, as they have decreased renal and cardiovascular function.

Patient Education

- Educate and inform the client about symptoms of minor toxicity and major toxicity, provide a written document detailing these effects.
- Teach the client and family that a long-term treatment may be required, which is best decided by the physician.
- Tell the client about blood Li levels and establish a confidence that blood samples may be drawn frequently for monitoring as therapeutic and toxic levels are pretty close.
- Advise client to monitor urine specific gravity.
- Advise client that contraception is necessary and if client plans to become pregnant then she must inform the physician; Li can cause defects in fetus.
- Advise client that Li should be taken regularly in spaced doses; never double the dose if missed it can lead to toxicity of lithium.
- Advise to take Li with food to prevent stomach upset; Li should not be taken with coffee, tea or cola as they decrease Li levels; also avoid alcohol.
- Advise not to operate machinery, drive or do other activities that may be dangerous if you are not alert.
- Client should not start on a low or high sodium diet without consultation.
- Advice patient to maintain a consistent dietary sodium intake but to increase in perspiration.
- Discuss any medication taken in past or taking, with the physician, also report any allergies.
- Advise to drink enough water especially in hot weather and after physical activities; suggest drinking 10–12 glasses of water per day to reduce thirst and to maintain normal fluid balance.
- Tell other doctors that you are taking Li.
- Advice patient to elevate feet to prevent or relieve ankle edema.

ANTIDEPRESSANTS

These are group of drugs which are used for the treatment of depression disorders. They are also called *mood elevators*. They may relieve the depression effects of temporary situational stress. Like other psychiatric drugs, antidepressants were discovered by accident. The first antidepressants, imipramine, a tricyclic and iproniazid, a monoamine oxidase inhibitor (MAOIs), were discovered in the 1950s. These drugs were found to have the side effects of improving patient's mood. However the newer selective serotonin reuptake inhibitors (SSRI's) were early examples of rational drug design.

- Antidepressants are the medication that prevent or relieve depression. It is used to correct neurochemical imbalances that affect moods.
- Antidepressants are used most widely for serious depressions, but they can also be helpful for some milder depressions. Antidepressants, although they are not 'uppers' or stimulants, take away or reduce the symptoms of depression and help the depressed person feel the way he/she did before he became depressed.
- Antidepressants are also used for disorders characterized principally by anxiety. They can block the symptoms of panic, including rapid heartbeat, terror, dizziness, chest pains, nausea and breathing problems. They can also be used to treat some phobias.

Mode of Action (Fig. 3.18)

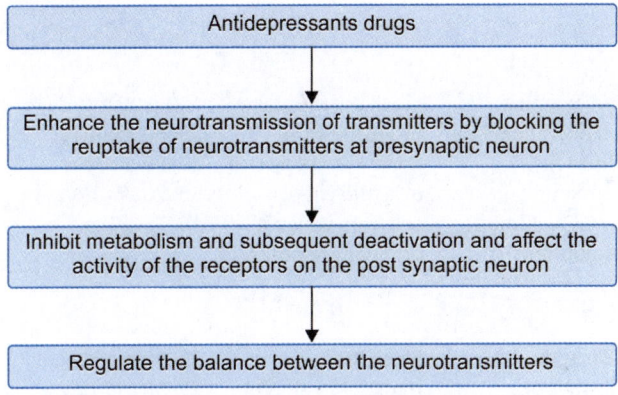

Fig. 3.18: Mechanism of action of antidepressants.

Classification

Classification of antidepressants along with commonly used drugs, mechanism of action, dosages, routes of administration and side effects is presented in **Table 3.6**.

Table 3.6: Classification of antidepressants.

Types	Commonly used drugs	Mechanism of action	Dose and route	Side effects
Tricyclic antidepressants	Amitriptyline (Endep), desipramine (Norpramin), imipramine (Tofranil or Depsonil), nortriptyline (Aventyl), protriptyline (Vivactil), doxepin (Spectra)	Block reuptake of norepinephrine and serotonin by neuron	25–50 mg/day 25–50 mg/day 25–50 mg/day 25–50 mg/day 10 mg/day 25–50 mg/day	Orthostatic hypotension, sweating, palpitations, increased blood pressure

Contd...

Contd...

Types	Commonly used drugs	Mechanism of action	Dose and route	Side effects
Monoamine oxidase inhibitors	Isocarboxazid (Marplan), phenelzine sulfate (Nardil), tranylcypromine sulfate (Parnate), Eldepryl	Increase amount of norepinephrine to release catecholamine and Release of larger amount of norepinephrine to react with receptor	10–60 mg/day 15 mg/day 10 mg/day 5 mg/day	Orthostatic hypotension, weight gain, edema, constipation, urinary hesitancy, vertigo, weakness, fatigue, change in cardiac rate and rhythm, sexual dysfunction
Selective serotonin reuptake inhibitors	Fluvoxamine (Luvox) fluoxetine (Prozac), paroxetine (Paxil), sertaline (Zoloft), citalopram	Block the reuptake of serotonin (5-hydroxytryptamine) into presynaptic cell from which it originally released	100–200 mg/day 20–60 mg/day 20–50 mg/day 50–200 mg/day 10–75 g/day	Nervousness, over activation, drowsiness, headache, insomnia, indigestion, irritability, anxiety, sleeplessness
Atypical antidepressants	Mianseril (Tetradep), maprotiline (Ludiomil), mirtazapine	Block the transporter site for norepinephrine and serotonin	25–50 mg/day 25–50 mg/day 15–30 mg/day	Dry mouth, constipation, sedation, lightheadedness

Tricyclic Antidepressants

Tricyclic antidepressants are heterocyclic compounds used primarily as antidepressants. The TCAs were first discovered in the early 1950s. They are named after their chemical structure, which contains three rings of atoms.

Mechanism of Action (Fig. 3.19)

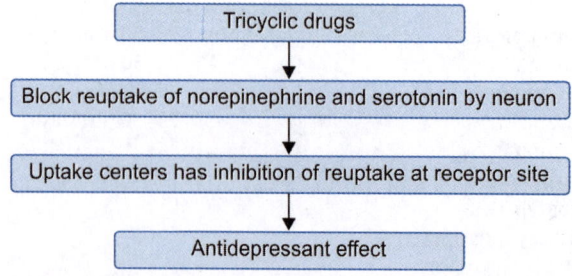

Fig. 3.19: Mechanism of action of tricyclic antidepressants.

Indications

- **Major depression episodes:** Unipolar and bipolar depression, melancholia
- **Secondary depression**: Depression associated with organic syndrome or disease
- **Panic disorder**: Panic attack
- Generalized anxiety
- Eating disorder
- Pain
- **Others:** Childhood enuresis, peptic ulcers, grief reaction, adjustment disorders.

Contraindications

- Arrhythmias
- Myocardial infarction
- Hyperthyroidism
- Impaired renal and hepatic function
- Pregnancy: Safety in pregnancy and lactation is not yet established so avoid breastfeeding
- Not recommended for children under 12 years
- History of past seizures
- Benign prostatic hyperplasia (BPH)
- Elderly or debilitated patient.

Side Effects

- **Anticholinergic effects:** Dry mouth, constipation, urinary retention, blurred vision.
- **Cardiac effects:** Postural hypotension, tachycardia, arrhythmias, cardiac ECG changes, heart failure.
- **Neurological effects:** Drowsiness, sedation, delusions, delirium, tremors, speech blockage, paresthesias, ataxia, akathisia, tardive dyskinesia.
- **GI effects:** Nausea, vomiting, loss of appetite, jaundice, weight gain.
- **Allergic effects:** Skin rashes, jaundice, agranulocytosis, leukocytosis, eosinophilia.
- **Other side effects:** Galactorrhea, gynecomastia, hyperglycemia, hypoglycemia.

Special Considerations while Administration

- Caution the client to be careful working around machines, driving cars and crossing streets because of possible altered reflexes, drowsiness and dizziness.
- Refrain the client from drinking alcohol as it can block the affect of antidepressant drugs.
- Advice the client to take full dose at bedtime to reduce the experience of side effects during day time.
- Sudden stopping of TCAs can give rise to symptoms like: nausea, altered heartbeat, nightmares, cold sweats.
- Inform the client and relatives that mood elevation may take place for 7–28 days.

Monoamine Oxidase Inhibitors

These drugs are not widely used as they have dangerous side effects. They can cause death due to severity of interaction. These drugs are generally used when the TCAs fail.

Mechanism of Action (Fig. 3.20)

Indications

- Panic disorder or anger
- Social phobia
- Generalized anxiety disorders
- Obsessive compulsive disorder (OCD)
- Post-traumatic stress disorder
- Bulimia nervosa
- Parkinson disease
- Hypersomnia.

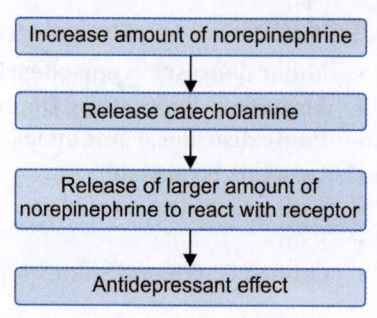

Fig. 3.20: Mechanism of action of monoamine oxidase inhibitors.

Contraindications

- Known hypersensitivity
- Pheochromocytoma (adrenal gland tumor)
- Congestive cardiac failure
- Severe hepatic and renal impairment
- Hypertension
- Not use in pregnancy and during lactation
- Not use in age above 65 years.

Common Side Effects

- Orthostatic hypotension
- Weight gain
- Edema
- Constipation
- Urinary hesitancy
- Vertigo
- Weakness
- Fatigue
- Change in cardiac rate and rhythm
- Sexual dysfunction.

Adverse Effects

- Intracranial hemorrhage
- Hyperpyrexia
- Convulsions
- Coma
- Tremors
- Dryness of mouth
- Blurred vision
- Death.

Alcohol particularly beer and wine (Chianti, sherry, scotch), aged cheese, chicken liver, broad beans, orange pulp, smoked fish, sour cream, yoghurt, bananas, spinach, tomatoes, plums, eggplant, coffee, chocolates, colas or tea, raisins should be avoided while using MAOIs.

Overdose of MAOIs can cause hyperthermia, hypertension, tachycardia, dilated pupils, hyperactive reflexes and involuntary movement of face and jaw.

Selective Serotonin Reuptake Inhibitors

Selective serotonin reuptake inhibitors (SSRIs) have antidepressant effects as comparable to other classes of antidepressants effects without significant cardiovascular, anticholinergics and sedative effects. These drugs are specific to serotonin and have little or no ability to block the other receptors. They are fairly safe in overdose.

Mechanism of Action

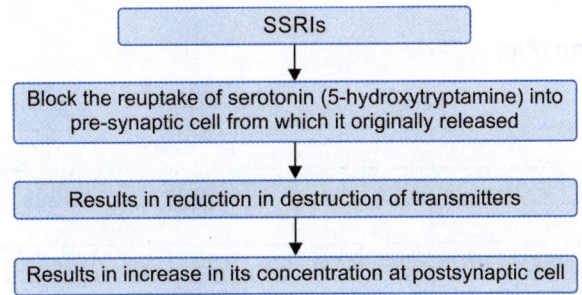

Fig. 3.21: Mechanism of action of selective serotonin reuptake inhibitor.

Indications
- Bulimia nervosa
- Hypochondriasis
- Premenstrual dysphoric disorder.

Contraindications
- With simultaneous use of MAOIs
- People taking pimozide (a diphenylbutylpiperidine derivative), analgesics, tramadol hydrochloride.

Side Effects
- Nervousness
- Over activation
- Drowsiness
- Headache
- Insomnia
- Indigestion
- Irritability
- Anxiety
- Sleeplessness.

Special Considerations while Administration
- Tell the client that these side effects are of short-term.
- If the patient cannot tolerate one of the SSRIs or receives only minimal effectiveness, several choices can be considered.
- Patients should start at a low dose, which is increased over a period of 5–10 days.

- Patients should see their doctor every 1–2 weeks until substantial improvement occurs; it may take 4–8 weeks before a patient experiences the effects of any antidepressant.
- Side effects usually diminish within 1–4 weeks (exceptions may be weight gain and sexual dysfunction).

Atypical Antidepressants

Atypical antidepressants contain four rings of atoms, are a closely related group of antidepressant compounds.

Mechanism of Action (Fig. 3.22)

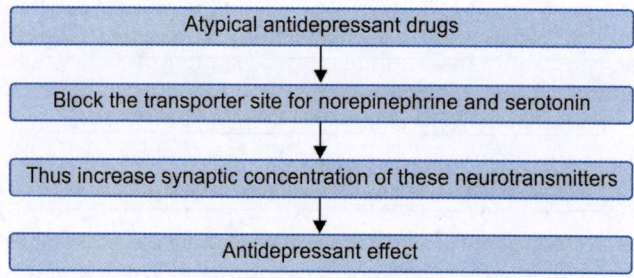

Fig. 3.22: Mechanism of action of atypical antidepressants.

Indications
- Obsessive compulsive disorder.
- Major depressive disorder.
- Post-traumatic stress disorder.
- Generalized anxiety.
- Panic disorder with agoraphobia.

Side Effects
- Dry mouth.
- Constipation.
- Sedation.
- Light headedness.
- Tetracyclic drugs are less likely to cause sexual dysfunction, significant long-term weight gain and sleep disturbances.

Amoxapine can lead to cause: Agitation, delirium, convulsions, hyperactive deep tendon reflexes, bowel and bladder paralysis and even death.

Nursing Consideration
- Antidepressants can cause side effects, but most of them are mild and go away after taking the medicine for a few weeks.
- Taking an antidepressant for at least 6 months after gives better feeling and can help keep away from getting depressed again.
- Patients should start at a low dose, which is increased over a period of 5–10 days.
- Patients should see their doctor every 1–2 weeks until substantial improvement occurs.

CHAPTER 3: Drugs Acting on Nervous System

- It may take 4–8 weeks before a patient experiences the effects of any antidepressant.
- Side effects usually diminish within 1–4 weeks (exceptions may be weight gain and sexual dysfunction).
- Antidepressants should be taken only in the amount prescribed and should be kept in a secure place away from children.
- Patients who become symptom-free have the best chance for complete recovery compared to patients whose symptoms merely improve.
- If no improvement occurs, an alternative drug may be tried. More than 80% of patients respond to some antidepressants, although specific drugs are helpful for only about half of patients. This suggests that if one medication fails, another has a good chance of being helpful.
- When used with proper care, following the doctor's instructions, antidepressants are useful medications that can control many of the physical symptoms of depression, while work on changing the life stressors that contributed to its cause.

ANTIANXIETY DRUGS

- **Anxiety:** State of uneasiness characterized by apprehension and worry about possible events.
- It is a collection of unpleasant feelings identical to a fearful feelings experienced under conditions of actual danger.

Types

- Exogenous anxiety.
- Endogenous anxiety.

Anti-anxiety agents are the drugs which are used to treat anxiety. Also called as anxiolytics and minor tranquilizers. A comprehensive classification of antianxiety drugs is presented in **Table 3.7**.

Table 3.7: Antianxiety drugs.

Types	Commonly used drugs	Mechanism of action	Dose and route	Side effects
Benzodiazapine	Clonazepam (Klonopin) Diazepam (Valium) Lorazepam (Ativan) Clobazam	It enhances the effect of gamma-aminobutyric acid (GABA) by increasing GABA affinity for the GABA receptor. Binding of GABA to site opens the chloride channel, resulting in hyperpolarized cell membrane that prevents further excitation of cell	Adults 0.5–5 mg tds, children 0.02–0.2 mg/kg/day 0.2–0.5 mg/kg slow intravenous (IV); maximum 100 mg/day. 0.1 mg/kg IV at the rate of 2 mg/min. Start with 10–20 mg at bed time up to 60 mg/day	Sedation, dullness, lack of concentration, irritability, behavioral abnormalities

Contd...

Contd...

Types	Commonly used drugs	Mechanism of action	Dose and route	Side effects
Azapirones	Buspirone (Buspar) Ispapirone	Buspirone does not affect GABA receptors, it seems to produce various effects in the midbrain and act as a midbrain modulator possibly due to its high affinity for serotonin receptor	PO 5–10 mg tid	Dizziness, light headedness, insomnia, tachycardia, palpitation, headache
Antihistamines	Hydroxyzine (Atarax)	Causes central nervous system (CNS) depression	Adult: PO 25–100 mg tid or qid; intra-muscular (IM) 25–100 mg	Drowsiness, dry mouth, dizziness, blurred vision, hypotension
Propanediols	Meprobamate (Miltown)	Causes CNS depression	Sedative: PO 1.2–1.6 mg in 3–4 divided doses Hypnotic: PO 400–800 mg	Drowsiness, dizziness, vertigo, slurred speech, weakness, headache, tachycardia, hypotension, nausea, vomiting

Benzodiazepines

Benzodiazepines most commonly used nowadays and is the drug of choice used to treat anxiety disorders. It includes: Diazepam, chlordiazepoxide, alprazolam, clonazepam, lorazepam and oxazepam. It has high-therapeutic index (hence less suicidal potentials). It has lower abuse liability, mild tolerance, less marked dependence and withdrawal symptoms. Diazepam is used as a muscle relaxant.

Mechanism of Action (Fig. 3.23)
Pharmacotherapeutic

- Generalized anxiety
- Sedative and hypnotic effects
- Seizures disorder
- Major depression
- Skeletal muscle spasm
- Insomnia
- Alcohol withdrawal symptoms
- Panic attack
- Preoperative anxiety.

CHAPTER 3: Drugs Acting on Nervous System

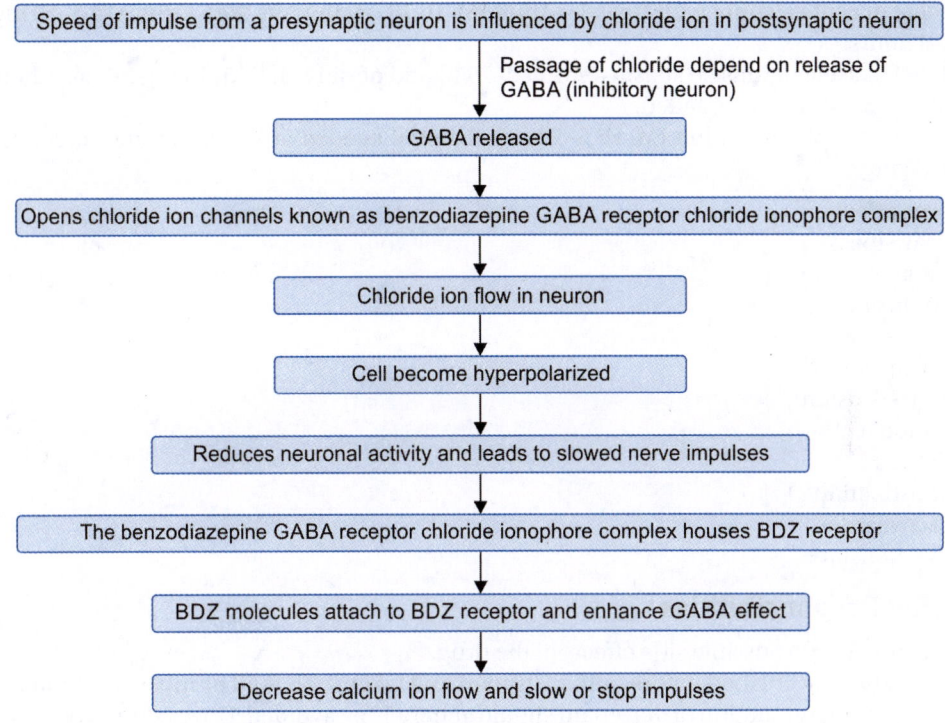

Fig. 3.23: Mechanism of action of benzodiazepines.

Adverse Drug Reaction

- Dependence if duration of therapy exceeds 3 months
- Birth defect if taken early in pregnancy
- Excitement (destructive behavior)
- Nausea, vomiting, diarrhea
- Epigastric pain
- Urinary incontinence
- Impairment of driving skills
- Blurring of vision.

Notes on Individual Drugs

Diazepam

Diazepam is available in the forms of tablet, injection and oral solutions. It is rapidly absorbed from GI tract metabolized in liver and excreted primarily in urine. It is used in anxiety, alcohol withdrawal, skeletal muscle spasm and status epilepticus and is contraindicated in pregnancy and hypersensitivity.

Dosage

- Anxiety—Adult oral tablet 2–10 mg bid to qid oral capsule 15–30 mg.
- Moderate anxiety—IM, IV 2–5 mg, repeat in 3–4 hours if needed.
- Severe anxiety—IM, IV 10 mg, repeat in 3–4 hours if needed.

- Relief in acute alcohol withdrawal—Adult IM, IV 10 mg initially then reduce to 5-10 mg in 3-4 hours.
- Relief in skeletal muscle spasm—Adult 2-10 mg tid or qid IM, IV 5-10 mg initially then 5-10 mg in 3-4 hours if needed.
- Status epilepticus—Adult IM, IV 5-10 mg, repeat if needed at 10-15 minutes intervals up to 30 mg.

Adverse effects
- Drowsiness
- Fatigue
- Confusion
- Headache
- Slurred speech
- Blurred vision
- Diplopia
- Nausea
- Constipation
- Tachycardia
- Hypotension.

Nursing Responsibilities
- Monitor for the possible side effects of the drug.
- Tablet may be crushed before administration and taken with fluid or mixed with food.
- Abrupt discontinuation of diazepam should generally be avoided. Doses should be tapered to termination.
- Suicidal tendencies may be present in anxiety states accompanied by depression. Observe necessary preventive measures.
- Monitor intake and output ratio, including bowel elimination.

Alprazolam

Alprazolam is available in form of tablet and oral solution. It is oxidized in liver and renal elimination occurs. It is used in anxiety associated with depression and panic disorder and contraindicated in pregnant or breastfeeding mother, pulmonary depression and hypersensitivity. PO 0.25-0.5 mg tid is used in anxiety disorder.

Adverse effects
- Light headedness
- Dizziness
- Depression
- Headache
- Insomnia
- Restlessness
- Tachycardia
- Sedation.

Nursing responsibilities
- Alprazolam may be administered without regard to meals.
- Drowsiness and sedation are the most common side effects. Monitor especially the elderly or debilitated who may require supervised ambulation or side rails.

- Instruct the client on long-term therapy not to quit taking the drug abruptly. Abrupt withdrawal can be life-threatening. Symptoms include depression, insomnia, increased anxiety, tremors, vomiting and sweating.
- Provide family education.
- The client should:
  - Not stop taking drug abruptly.
  - Not consume other CNS depressants.
  - Not take non-prescription medication without approval from physician.
  - Carry a card or piece of paper at all times stating the name of medication being taken.

Lorazepam

Lorazepam is available in form of tablet, injections and oral suspension. It is rapidly absorbed from GI tract not metabolized in liver and excreted in urine. Short-lived anxiety state, obsessive and compulsive disorder and insomnia are its indications. It is contraindicated in hypersensitivity, pregnancy and nursing mother, children < 12 years, shock and coma. It is used in PO 2–6 mg/day in divided doses.

Adverse effects
- Sedation
- Dizziness
- Weakness
- Depression
- Restlessness
- Confusion
- Blurred vision.

Nursing responsibilities
- When higher oral dosage is required the evening dose should be increased before the day time dose.
- IM lorazepam is injected undiluted, deep into a large muscle mass.
- Supervise ambulation of elderly patient for at least 8 hours after lorazepam injection to prevent falling or injury.
- Regimen should be terminated gradually over a period of several days.

Buspirones hydrochloride

Buspirones hydrochloride is first anxiolytic in new class of agents and is less sedating. They are available in form of tablets and used PO 5–10 mg tid in case of generalized anxiety states. It is contraindicated in breastfeeding patient, impaired renal or hepatic functions and hypersensitivity.

Adverse drug reactions
- Dizziness
- Light headedness
- Insomnia
- Tachycardia
- Palpitation
- Headache.

Nursing responsibilities
- Instruct the patient to take the last dose of buspirone several hours before bedtime to prevent insomnia.
- Advise the patient to ask the physician to recommend an analgesic if headache occur.
- Monitor the patient for adverse reaction and drug interactions during buspirone therapy.
- Help the patient to explore alternative methods for inducing sleep if insomnia occurs such as warm bath or quiet meditation.

ANTICONVULSANTS

Table 3.8: Comprehensive classification of anticonvulsant drugs.

Types	Commonly used drugs	Mechanism of action	Dose and route	Side effects
Barbiturate	Phenobarbitone	Barbiturates enhance the inhibitory neurotransmission in the CNS by enhancing the activation of GABASRS and thus facilitating the GABA- mediated opening of chloride ion channels	Gardenal 30, 60 mg tablets 20 mg/5 mL 5 years Luminal 30 mg tablet Phenobarbitone sodium 200 mg/mL Injection	Behavioral abnormality, impairment of learning and memory, rashes and megaloblastic anemia
Deoxybarbiturate	Primidone	Primidone is a GABA receptor agonist. The mechanism of primidone's antiepileptic action is not known	250–500 mg bd, children 10–20 mg/kg/day	
Hydantoin	Phenytoin, fosphenytoin	Phenytoin causes blockade of the voltage-dependent sodium channels and stabilizes the neuronal membrane	100 mg bid, maximum 400 mg/day; children 5–8 mg/kg/day Fosolin 50 mg/mL in 2 mL, 10 mL injection	Gum hypertrophy, hypersensitivity reactions, megaloblastic anemia
Iminostilbene	Carbamazepine, oxcarbamazepine	Its mechanism of action and antiepileptic actions are similar to phenytoin, i.e., it blocks sodium channels	200–400 mg tds; children 15–30 mg/kg/day	Sedation, dizziness, vertigo, diplopia and hypersensitivity reaction
Succinimide	Ethosuximide	Ethosuximide reduces the low threshold calcium(CA^{2+}) currents (T-currents) in the thalamic neurons. These T-currents are thought to be responsible for absence seizures	20–30 mg/kg/day	GI intolerance, tiredness, mood changes, agitation, headache, drowsiness

Contd...

Contd...

Types	Commonly used drugs	Mechanism of action	Dose and route	Side effects
Aliphatic carboxylic acid	Valproic acid (sodium valporoate)	It enhances the level of GABA by decreasing the metabolism of GABA. Like phenytoin, valproic acid blocks the sodium channels. Like ethosuximide valproate decreases low threshold Ca^{++} T-currents in the thalamus	Adults—start with 200 mg tds, maximum 800 mg tds; children—15–30 mg/kg/day	Anorexia, vomiting, loose motions, heartburn, drowsiness, ataxia and tremors
Benzodiazepines	Clonazepam, Diazepam, Lorazepam Clobazam	It enhances the effect of GABA by increasing GABA affinity for the GABA receptor. Binding of GABA to site opens the chloride channel, resulting in hyperpolarized cell membrane that prevents further excitation of cell	Adults 0.5–5 mg tds, children 0.02–0.2 mg/kg/day 0.2–0.5 mg/kg slow IV; maximum 100 mg/day 0.1 mg/kg IV at the rate of 2 mg/min Start with 10–20 mg at bd, up to 60 mg/day	Sedation, dullness, lack of concentration, irritability, behavioral abnormalities
Phenyltriazine	Lamotrigine	Inhibits the sodium channels and also inhibits the release of the excitatory amino acids like glutamate	50 mg/day initially, increase up to 300 mg/day as needed	Sleepiness, dizziness, diplopia, ataxia and vomiting
Cyclic GABA analogues	Gabapentin, Pregabalin	Exact mechanism of action is not known, but it does not act on GABA receptors	Start with 300 mg od, increase to 300–600 mg tds 75–150 mg bd, maximum 600 mg/day	Mild sedation, tiredness, dizziness and unsteadiness
Newer drugs	Topiramate, Zonisamide, Lavertiracetam, Vigabatrin Tiagabine, locasamide	It blocks the sodium channels, and also enhances GABASRS receptor currents	Initially 25 mg od, increase weekly up to 100–200 mg bd 25–100 mg bd 0.5 g bd, increase up to 1.0 G bd (maximum 3 g/day), children 4–15 year 10–30 mg/kg/day Initially 50 mg bd, increase up to 200 mg bd	Impairment of attention, sedation, ataxia, word finding difficulties, poor memory, weight loss, paresthesias and renal stones

(CNS, central nervous system; GABA, Gamma-aminobutyric acid, type-A-γ-aminobutyric acid receptors; bd, bedtime; tds, thrice a day; GI, gastrointestinal; IV, intravenous; od, orally daily)

Phenobarbitone

Phenobarbitone has specific anticonvulsant activity, which is not entirely dependent on general CNS depression. It has slow oral absorption and a long plasma t½ (80-120 hours). It has sedation effects also and can cause side effects like behavioral abnormalities, diminution of intelligence, impairment of learning and memory, hyperactivity in children and mental confusion in older people. On prolonged use it can cause rashes, megaloblastic anemia and osteomalacia. It has good efficacy in generalized tonic-clonic (GTC), simple partial (SP) and complex seizures (CS). It can be injected IV or IM. It is not effective in absence seizures. It is given in a dose of 60 mg one to three times a day in adults and in children 3-5 mg/kg/day.

Indications
- Infantile sperms
- Generalized tonic-clonic seizures
- Generalized myoclonic jerks
- Complex absences within autonomic manifestation
- Status epilepticus.

Contraindications
- Latent or manifest porphyria
- Respiratory obstructions.

Adverse Effects
- Nausea, vomiting, diarrhea, skin rash (2% patients)
- Muscle and joint pain
- Respiratory depression
- Paradoxical excitation (in children and elderly)
- Megaloblastic anemia.

Nursing Responsibilities
- Recognize that drugs may need vitamin D requirements by stepping up its metabolism, occasionally leads to rickets or osteomalacia within prolonged use.
- Be aware that prolonged use, even in rather low doses, can lead to tolerance and habituation watch for signs of tolerance and if necessary, withdraw drug slowly to avoid possibility of delirium and convulsions.
- Carefully weighs benefit versus risk in pregnant women; although a small incidence of fetal damage has been reported with their drugs, discontinuing them may result in increased seizure activity and fetal anoxia.

Phenytoin

Phenytoin is a major antiepileptic drug. It is not CNS depressant, but some sedation occur at therapeutic doses. Phenytoin causes blockade of the voltage-dependent sodium channels and stabilizes the neuronal membrane.

Indications
- Grand mal seizures
- Psychomotor seizures
- Alcohol withdrawn syndrome
- Cardiac arrhythmias
- Status epilepticus seizures during neurosurgery.

Contraindications
- Hematologic disorders
- Hepatic dysfunction
- In complete heart block
- Sinoatrial block
- Second third degree atrioventricular (AV) block.

Adverse Effects
- GI—nausea, vomiting, diarrhea, abdominal pain and dysphagia
- CNS—headache, depression, tremors, behavioral, disturbances
- Dermatologic—skin rashes, urticaria
- Other—gingival hyperplasia, hyperglycemia, osteomalacia and numbness.

Nursing Responsibilities
- Advise patient that excessive use of alcohol or other CNS depressant may reduce the efficacy of Phenytoin
- Counsel patient on the important of the maintenance of prescribed dosage regimen for good seizures control.
- Individualize dosage schedule in each patient to minimize toxicity (e.g. ataxia, confusion).
- Use parenteral solutions immediately after mixing and do not add to any IV infusion solubility may be altered by pH differences shape suspension thoroughly to obtain correct dosage. Avoid continuous infusion of Phenytoin solutions.
- Administer slowly IV do not gave IM in status epilepticus because sufficient plasma levels cannot be attained in most cases.
- Inform patient that Phenytoin may harmlessly turn color of urine from pink to reddish brown.
- Give oral drugs with meal if possible to minimize gastric irritation, because drug is strongly alkaline.
- Provide emotional support to the patient, instruct family member and close associates in the proper methods for dealing with seizure episode.
- Ask patient to carry an identification card with pertinent medical information.

Primidone

Primidone antiepileptic efficacy is similar to phenobarbitone. Its adverse effects are also similar to phenobarbitone, in addition it also causes anemia, leukopenia and psychotic reaction. It is given in dose of 250–500 mg bd in adults and 10–20 mg/kg/day in children.

Carbamazepine

Carbamazepine is the first-line antiepileptic drug and closely resembles phenytoin. Its mechanism of action and antiepileptic actions are similar to phenytoin, i.e., it blocks sodium channels. It is given in doses of 200–400 mg tds in adults and in children 15–30 mg/kg/day.

Indications

- Psychomotor seizures
- Mixed seizures
- Relief of pain associated trigeminal neuralgia
- Termination of intractable hiccoups (experimental use).

Contraindications

- History of bone marrow depression
- Concomitant use of monoamine oxidase inhibitors (MAOIs).

Adverse Effects

- CNS—confusion in coordination, speech disturbances, involuntary movements, dysphasia, visual Illusion, depression, peripheral neuritis and paresthesia
- Dermatologic—Rash, sweating, photosensitivity reactions and abnormal pigmentation
- Hematologic—blood dyscrasias.

Nursing Responsibilities

- Note that confusion, agitation and behavioral disturbance occur commonly in the elderly, supervised ambulation may be necessary.
- Advise periodic ophthalmologic examinations, because drug can produce ocular damage
- Counsel patient to observe for early signs of sore throat, mucosal ulceration, bruising, malaise and advise physician immediately.
- Use cautiously in patients within level, hepatic or cardiac disease, human immunodeficiency virus (HIV), glaucoma and in elderly, pregnant or nursing patients.
- Withdraw drug or make dosage adjustments slowly. Abrupt changes may produce seizures or status epilepsies.

Valproic Acid

Valproic acid is effective in partial seizures, GTC seizure and absence seizure. It enhances the level of GABA by decreasing the metabolism of GABA. Like phenytoin, valproic acid blocks the sodium channels. Like ethosuximide valproate decreases low threshold Ca^{2+} (T-currents) current in the thalamus. In adults start with 200 mg tds, maximum 800 mg tds and in children 15–30 mg/kg/day.

Indications

- Absence seizures (simple and complex)
- Adjunct in treatment of multiple seizure types
- Investigational uses include grand mal seizures, myoclonic seizures and prevention of recurrent febrile seizure and it is contraindicated in hepatic disease.

Warning
- Fatal hepatic failure has occurred in patients receiving valproic acid, usually during the first 6 months of treatment.
- Frequent liver function test are required, especially during initial months of therapy.

Adverse Effects
Diarrhea, abdominal cramps, visual disturbances, diplopia, dizziness, in coordination, tremor, dysarthria, skin rash, alopecia, depression, aggression, hyperactivity, behavioral disturbances, altered bleeding time, muscle weakness and hepatotoxicity.

Nursing Responsibilities
- Advise periodic blood counts during drug therapy because reports of platelet dysfunction and blood dyscrasias have appeared.
- Instruct patient to swallow capsule whole to avoid at level mouth and throat irritation
- Administer with food to minimize irritation.
- Note that drug is excreted in part as a ketone-containing metabolite, which can interfere with urine tests for ketone bodies.
- Instruct patient to report any visual disturbances immediately, because ocular toxicity has been noted.

Diazepam
Diazepam is a first line drug for emergency control of convulsions, e.g., status epilepticus, tetanus, eclampsia, convulsant drug poisoning, etc., hypotension and respiratory depression can occur so resuscitative measures should be kept ready before giving injection. Rectal instillation is preferred therapy for febrile convulsions in children. It is started with 0.2 –0.5 mg/ kg slow IV and can be extended maximum up to 100 mg/day.

Indications
- Adjunctive treatment of convulsive disorders, especially minor motor recurs
- Control of status epilepticus and other acute convulsive seizures
- Treatment of convulsions.

Contraindications
- Respiratory depression
- Acute pulmonary insufficiency
- Hypersensitivity.

Adverse Effects
Sedation and dullness, impaired alertness, ataxia, vertigo, dizziness, fatigue, nausea, vomiting, anemia, leucopenia, dry mounth and decreased appetite.

Nursing Responsibilities
- Be prepared to readminister diazepam IV as necessary to control acute seizures episodes effects.

- Do not administer IV to patient because status epilepticus can be precipitated in these patients.
- IV diazepam may cause venous thrombosis or phlebitis to protect this inject very slowly.

DRUGS FOR NEURODEGENERATIVE DISORDERS AND MISCELLANEOUS DRUGS

Antiparkinsonian Drugs

Parkinsonism

Parkinsonism is a chronic, progressive, extrapyramidal motor disorder characterized by rigidity, tremors and hypokinesia. With these manifestations defective posture and gait, mask like face, excessive salivation and dementia may occur. If it is not cured then it may progress into end stage disease in which the symptoms become worsen and includes inability to walk and breathing difficulty.

Classification (Fig. 3.24)

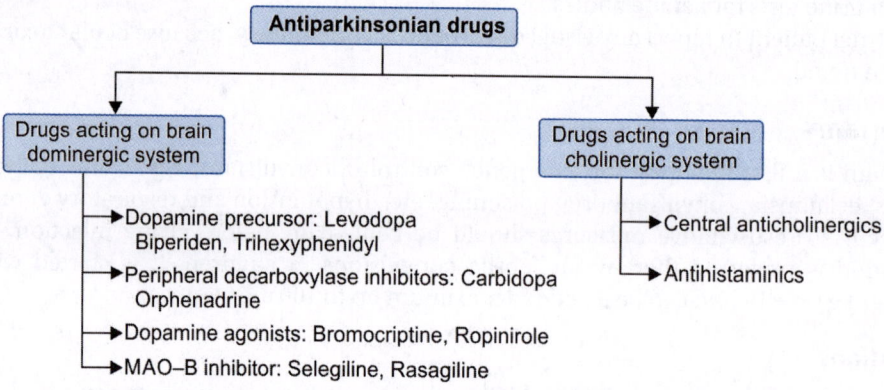

Fig. 3.24: Classification of antiparkinsonian drugs.

Notes on Individual Drugs

Dopamine Precursor

Levodopa

Levodopa is drug of choice for patients having Parkinsonism, as it crosses the blood-brain barrier (BBB) and is taken up by the surviving nigrostriatal neurons. It is converted to dopamine (DA) in the dopaminergic neurons in the striatum.

Mechanism of actions
- *CNS:* On administration of levodopa, symptoms resolves rapidly in individuals; hypokinesia and rigidity resolves first followed by tremors as well.
- *CVS:* It can lead to tachycardia, postural hypotension.
- *Endocrine:* They inhibit prolactin release.

Pharmacokinetics

Pharmacokinetic absorbed from small intestine and excreted in urine.

CHAPTER 3: Drugs Acting on Nervous System

Adverse effects
- *At initiation of therapy:* Nausea, vomiting, postural hypotension, cardiac arrhythmias and alteration in taste sensation.
- *After prolonged therapy:* Dyskinesias, anxiety, depression, mania and mental confusion.

Dose
- Start with 0.25 g bd after meals, gradually increase till adequate response is obtained usual dose is 2–3 g/day.
- It should be cautiously used in patients with ischemic heart disease, cardiovascular disease, peptic ulcer, hepatic or renal disorders, gout and glaucoma.

Peripheral Decarboxylase Inhibitors

Carbidopa
Carbidopa do not penetrate blood brain barrier and do not inhibit conversion of levodopa to DA in brain. Nausea, vomiting and cardiac complications are less prominent with its use. They are extracerebral dopa decarboxylase inhibitors. It causes postural hypotension, involuntary movements and behavioral abnormalities. The usual daily dose of levodopa is 0.4–0.8 g along with 75–100 mg carbidopa, given in three to four divided doses.

Dopaminergic Agonists

Bromocriptine
Bromocriptine are ergot derivatives having dopamine agonistic activity at D2 receptors. Bromocriptine is also a partial agonist, while pergolide is an agonist at D1 receptors. Symptoms resolve within ½–1 hour of oral dose and lasts for 6–10 hours. It causes vomiting, hallucinations, hypotension and conjunctival infection. It is used in dose of 1.25 mg once at night and increase up to 5 mg tds.

MAO–B Inhibitor

Selegiline
Selegiline has mild anti-parkinsonian action, but when combined with levodopa its action prolongs. It causes postural hypotension, nausea, confusion, psychosis; and is contraindicated in patients with convulsive disorders. It is given 5 mg with breakfast and with lunch, either alone or with levodopa. After 2–3 days, levodopa dose is reduced to one-fourth.

It is metabolized by liver into amphetamine.

Rasagiline
Rasagiline is five times more potent, longer acting and not metabolized to amphetamine. It is given as 1 mg od in the morning.

COMT Inhibitors

Entacapone
Entacapone is a catechol O-methyltransferase (COMT) inhibitors, which acts as adjuvant to levodopa/carbidopa, so they enhances and prolongs its therapeutic effects for advanced Parkinson disorder. It is given in 200 mg with each dose of levodopa/carbidopa, maximum 1,600 mg/day. Nausea, vomiting, dyskinesia, postural hypotension, hallucination, etc., are its adverse effects.

Glutamate Antagonist

Amantadine

Amantadine is an antiviral drug used for prophylaxis of influenza A2. It enhances the release of DA in the brain and diminishes the reuptake of DA. About 100 mg bd is used in patients and effect of single dose lasts for 8–12 hours. Classic side effect of drug includes bluish discoloration and edema of ankles; along with this some non-serious side effects, such as insomnia, restlessness, confusion and nightmares also occurs.

Central Anticholinergics

Central anticholinergics is drug of choice for drug-induced Parkinsonism. It helps to relieve tremor, sialorrhea. Hypokinesia and rigidity are affected the least. Its efficacy is lower than levodopa, but is cheaper and produces less side effects than levodopa. Impairment of memory, organic confusional states, blurred vision and urinary retention are its common side effects.

STIMULANTS, ETHYL ALCOHOL AND TREATMENT OF METHYL ALCOHOL POISONING

STIMULANTS

Stimulants are an agents that stimulate the functioning of the body's organs that are not function properly due to some reasons, such as depressants, lack of hormones, impaired nerve transmission. They are of different types. Every organ has their own stimulants.

Definition

The stimulants are defined as the substances that enhance the activity of organs of the body.

Classification

- Cardiac stimulants
- CNS stimulants
- Respiratory stimulants
- Laxative stimulants
- Uterine stimulants
- Immunostimulants

Cardiac Stimulants

Adrenergic drugs comes under this category.

Introduction

Adrenergic drugs are compounds, either natural or synthetic; these produce the activation of the sympathetic nervous system or resulting from adrenal medullary discharge. For this reason, these agents may also be termed as sympathomimetic (agents) drugs, i.e., drugs that mimic sympathetic nerve stimulation.

Definition

These are the drugs that produce affects that imitate or mimic those of sympathetic neurotransmitter norepinephrine, i.e., released by the postganglionic adrenergic nerve endings.

Classification of Sympathomimetic Drugs (Fig. 3.25)

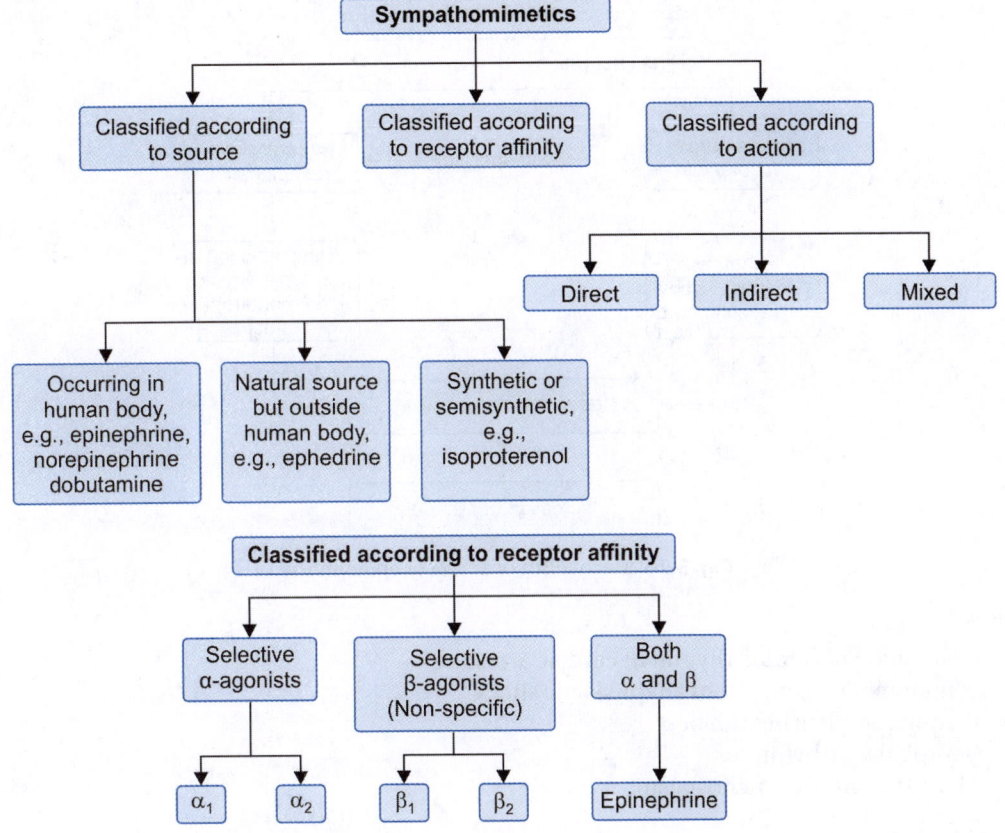

Fig. 3.25: Classification of sympathomimetic drugs.

Epinephrine
- It stimulates a receptors of sympathetic nervous system.
- It is used in cardiac arrest.
- It is used with local anesthesia for its vasoconstrictor properties, which decreases the rate of absorption of the anesthetic agent.

Dosage
- **Parenteral route**
- **Adrenaline:**
    - In cardiac arrest 0.5–1 mg
    - In adults 0.1–0.25 mg
    - In neonates 0.01– mg/kg

Mechanism of Action (Fig. 3.26)

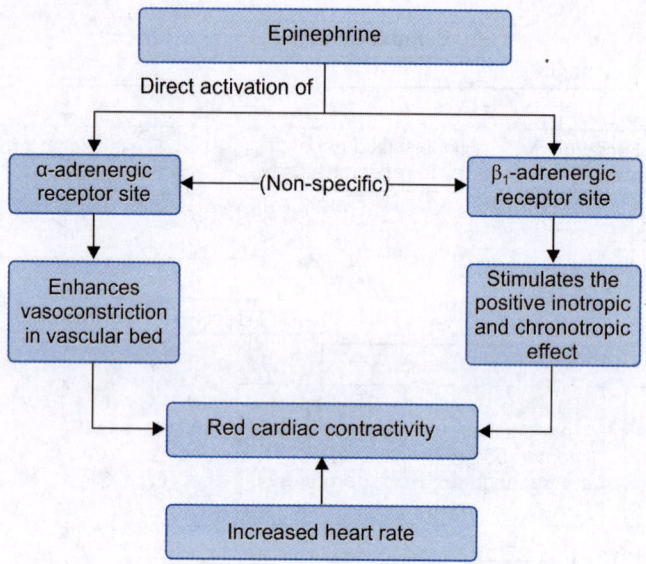

Fig. 3.26: Mechanism of action of epinephrine.

Indications
- Restoration of cardiac rhythm in cardiac arrest
- Symptomatic treatment of anaphylactic shock
- During complete heart block
- Ventricular arrhythmias
- Management of bronchospasm

Contraindications
- Severe hypertension
- Tachycardia caused by digitalis intoxication
- Organic brain damage
- In combination with general anesthesia

Adverse Effects
- **Systemic:**
  - Weakness
  - Dizziness
  - Hypertension
  - Tachycardia
  - Pulmonary edema
  - Dyspnea
  - Urinary retention
  - Cerebral hemorrhage
  - Lactic acidosis

- **Ophthalmic effects**
  - Conjunctival irritation
  - Pigmentation of eyelids and cornea
  - Shedding of eyelashes

Norepinephrine

- It is naturally occurring catecholamine with stimulating effects
- It increases blood pressure by stimulating peripheral vasoconstriction and myocardial contractility
- It increases myocardial oxygen consumption, but to a lesser degree
- Affinity for β2 receptors is very poor

Dosage
- **Route:** IV infusion
- Add 4 mL of the solution to 1,000 mL of 5% dextrose solution
- Observe response to an initial dose of 2–3 mL/min
- Average maintenance dose:-0.5–1 mL/min
- Slow infusion is given to maintain blood pressure

Mechanism of action (Fig. 3.27)

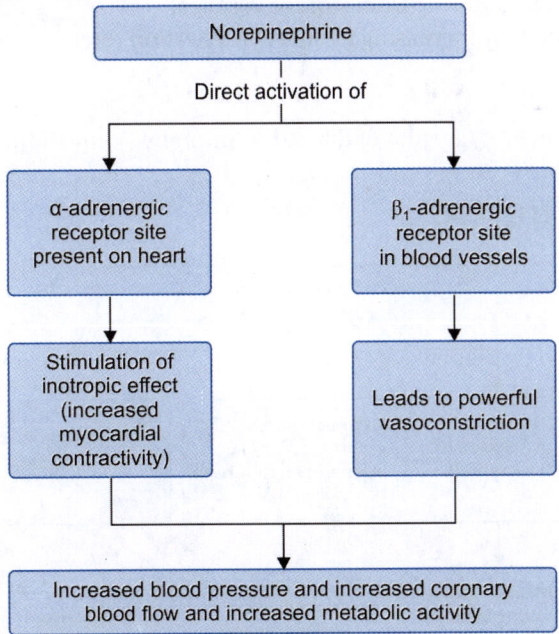

Fig. 3.27: Mechanism of action of norepinephrine.

Indications
- Restoration of blood pressure in certain hypotensive states (e.g., in myocardial infection, septicemia and blood transfusion).
- Treatment of cardiac arrest and profound hypotension.

Contraindications

- Hypovolemic shock
- Vascular thrombosis
- Extreme hypoxia during general anesthesia

Adverse Effects

- Hypertension (in combination with oxytocic drugs)
- Respiratory distress
- Arrhythmias in the presence of certain anesthesia
- Photophobia
- Chest pain in large dose
- Hyperglycemia
- Vomiting
- Cerebral hemorrhage and convulsions

Dopamine

- It is naturally occurring catecholamine and immediate precursor of norepinephrine.
- It acts on α, β1 and specific dopamine receptors.
- It also releases norepinephrine from storage vesicles.
- It increases urine flow by increasing glomerular filtration rate.

Dosage

Initially, 2 µg/kg/min to 5 µg/kg/min of diluted solution by IV infusion. It may increase up to 50 µg/kg/min.

Mechanism of action (Fig. 3.28)

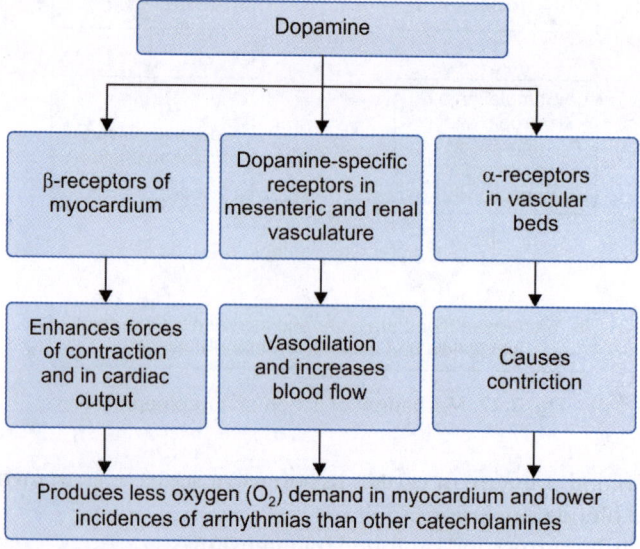

Fig. 3.28: Mechanism of action of dopamine.

Indications
- Shock due to hypovolemia
- Myocardial infection
- Septicemia
- Renal failure
- Heart surgery

Contraindications
- Ventricular arrhythmias
- Pheochromocytoma (it is a tumor that originates from chromaffin cells of the adrenal medulla)
- Hyperthyroidism

Adverse Effects
- Hypertension
- Nausea
- Vomiting
- Tachycardia
- Respiratory difficulty
- Headache

Isoproterenol
- It is similar to adrenaline.
- It is powerful cardiac stimulant (increases heart rate and increase force of contraction).
- It activates the β-adrenergic receptors.

Dosage
- **Cardiac arrest:** IV (injection) 1–3 mL of a 1:50,000 dilutions (0.02–0.06 mg)
- **Heart block-sublingual:** 10 mg initially (range 5–50 mg)

Mechanism of Action (Fig. 3.29)

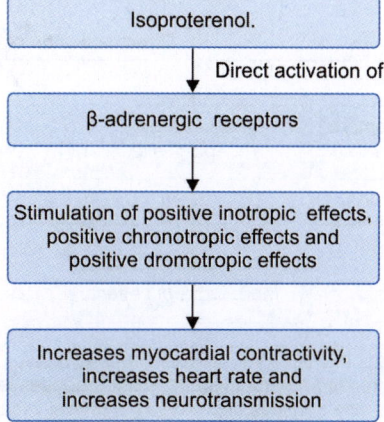

Fig. 3.29: Mechanism of action of isoproterenol.

Indications
- In management of shock
- Cardiac arrest
- AV block
- Carotid sinus
- Hypersensitivity
- Ventricular arrhythmias

Contradictions
- Arrhythmias associated with tachycardia
- Hypertension
- Tachycardia caused by digitalis toxicity
- Coronary artery diseases

Adverse Effects
- Buccal ulceration (sublingual)
- Bronchial irritation and edema
- Cardiac arrest
- Dry mouth
- Chest pain
- Tachycardia

Dobutamine
- It structurally resembles dopamine.
- Dobutamine has been recently introduced into clinical medicine as a seductive cardiac β1–adrenoceptor stimulant.
- It increases the force of contraction without increasing the heart rate.

Dosage
- µg/kg/min to 10 µg/kg/min IV infusion
- Infusion rates up to 40 µg/kg/min as required

Mechanism of Action (Fig. 3.30)

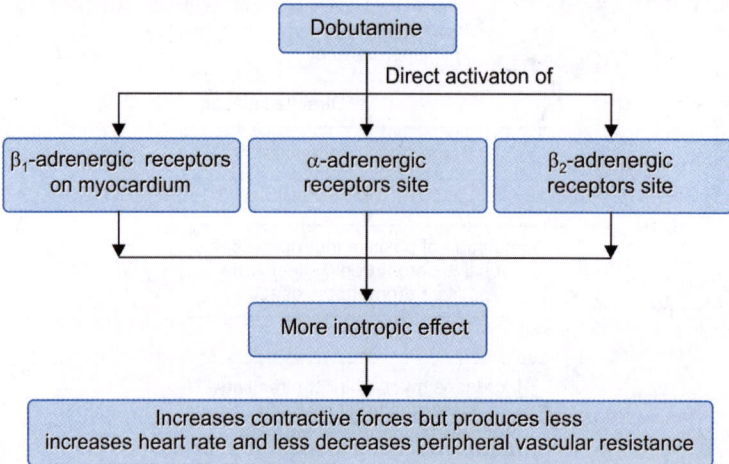

Fig. 3.30: Mechanism of action of dobutamine.

Indications
- Short-term treatment of acute heart failure due to depressed contractility
- For inotropic support in bacteremic shock

Contraindications
- Acute myocardial infection
- Subaortic stenosis

Adverse Effects
- Tachycardia (5–15 beats/min increases)
- Hypertension (10–20 mm Hg increases)

Nursing Responsibilities
- Before administration of the drug, the physical assessment of the patient should be done.
- The blood pressure, temperature, pulse and respiration (TPR) ECG and complete blood count, etc., should be done to obtain base line data future reference.
- Always observe basic principle of administration of drugs, such as:
    - Right patient
    - Right medicine
    - Right dose
    - Right time
    - Right route of administration
- Before administration of the drug check its label carefully; does not take oral orders; certain drugs may be pronounced similarly.
- Powerful drugs are given in small dose; it necessitates accuracy in the measurement of the drug.
- No drug should be mixed unless it is told; when it is to be administered as IV drip, each drug should be taken separately and IV sets should be connected with three way stopcocks.
- The drugs that have antagonizing effects should not be given to the patient at the same time.
- The nurse should be familiar with the toxic and side effects of the drug, so that the nurse should stop the drug temporarily and inform the physician immediately.
- The nurse should observe patient's clinical response to the drugs administered; the dose should be adjusted according to the condition of the patient.
- The patient should be reassured to relieve his anxiety.
- When administering drug, all care should be taken to reduce the side effects of the drugs, e.g., reduce the gastric irritation.
- Always study the manufacturer's instructions regarding the administration of the drug.
- Every drug given should be recorded in the patient's chart.

Patient Education
Patient's teaching is very important especially when the patient is discharged from the hospital and is going to the home with maintenance dose. Teach the patient about:
- Name of the drug and its action.
- Why he/she has to take and how has to take it for the best results.
- What is the dosage that he/she has to take, if any change in dosage is to be brought, how it can be done.
- What are the signs and symptoms that he/she has to report.

- The drug should be kept away from the light as instructed by the manufacturer.
- The drug should discard, if it has changed its original color and taste.
- The patient should be instructed to come for regular checkup.
- The patient should be told not to take any medication other than what is prescribed by the physician.

Central Nervous System Stimulants

Introduction
Central nervous system stimulants are used for the excitement and euphoria, decreased feeling of fatigue increased motor activity. They are having few clinical uses also, but mostly they are used for drug abuse.

Definition
They are the agents, which increase the energy or functional activity of the CNS by acting on neurons.

Classification (Fig. 3.31)

Classification of CNS stimulants CNS
- Caffeine
- Amphetamines
- pemoline
- Anorexiants
- Methylphenidate

Fig. 3.31: Classification of central nervous system (CNS) stimulants.

Caffeine
- Caffeine is most widely used CNS stimulant.
- In small amounts, it is a stimulant.
- Caffeine is a xanthine derivative possessing relatively very weak stimulant.

Dosage
- **Oral:** 100–250 mg every 3–4 hours
- **IM:** 50 mg
- **IV:** 500 mg in respiratory failure

Mechanism of action (Fig. 3.32)

Indications
- Relieves pain-associated spinal punctured.
- To relieve fatigue and increase awareness.

Contraindications
Peptic ulcer patients

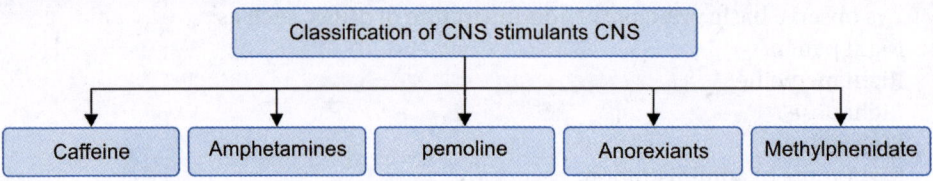

Fig. 3.32: Mechanism of action of caffeine.

Adverse Actions

- Nausea
- Vomiting
- Restlessness
- Irritability
- Hypotension

Amphetamine, Anorexiants and Methylphenidate

- **Interfere with** monoamine oxidase (MAO), an enzyme responsible for intracellular breakdown of monoamines, such as norepinephrine, dopamine, serotonin stimulant effects thought to be caused by an action on the cortex and possibly reticular formation
- **Anorexiant action:** May be caused by an inhibitory effect on hypothalamic feeding centers as well as elevation in mood.

Mechanism of Action (Fig. 3.33)

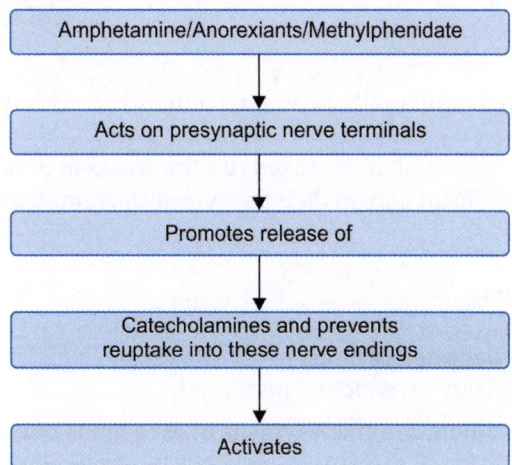

Fig. 3.33: Mechanism of action of amphetamine, anorexiants and methylphenidate.

Amphetamine

- They are synthetic sympathomimetic amines with marked CNS stimulatory action.
- They increase alertness and concentration, temporarily elevates the mood and stimulates motor activity.

Dosage: For example, Amphetamine Sulfate

- In narcolepsy—5–60 mg/day in divided doses
- **In minimal brain dysfunction:**
  - 3–5 years—2.5 mg/day
  - Over 6 years—5 mg one to two times/day
  - Obesity—5–30 mg/day.

Indications

- Treatment for narcolepsy
- Treatment of minimal brain dysfunction
- Short-term adjunct in the treatment of obesity

Contraindications:

- Cardiovascular diseases
- Hypertension
- Hyperthyroidism
- Pregnancy
- Under 3 years of age
- Arteriosclerosis
- Glaucoma
- Severe endogenous depression

Adverse Effects

- **CNS:** Nausea, euphoria, tremors, headache, chills, confusion, hallucinations, etc.
- **GI:** Nausea, vomiting, diarrhea, anorexia and weight loss.
- **Others:** urticaria, delayed or difficult urination, dyspnea, anginal pain, syncope, convulsions and coma.

Anorexiants

- Group of drugs-related structurally to amphetamines has been used in the treatment of exogenous obesity.
- Since their therapeutics benefit is restricted to a few weeks at best, because of developing tolerance, there is significant danger their prolonged consumption.

Dosage

- For example, Mazindol
- 1 mg three times/day
- Before meals or 2 mg daily before lunch
- Take with food if necessary to reduce GI discomfort

Indications: Short-term adjunctive management of exogenous obesity in conjunction with caloric restriction.

Adverse Effects

- **CNS:** Dizziness, euphoria, tremors, headache and confusion
- **CVS:** Tachycardia, hypertension, arrhythmias and precordial pain
- **GI:** Nausea, vomiting, anorexia, unpleasant taste, glossitis
- **Others:** Urticaria, dyspnea, anginal pain, syncope, convulsions, cramps and chills
- **Genitourinary tract:** Dysuria, polyuria, diuresis, cystitis, impotence, menstrual and change in libido

Contraindications

- Cardiovascular diseases
- Hypertension
- Hyperthyroidism
- Glaucoma
- Severe endogenous depression
- Pregnancy
- Under 3 years of age

Methylphenidate

A CNS stimulant with an action similar to that of amphetamines. It does not elevate blood pressure, heart rate and respiratory rate.

Dosage
As follows:
- **Adults:** Initially 10 mg, two to three times/day
- **Children (over 6 years):** Initially 5 mg, two times/day increases by 5–10 mg/week to optional dose
- Maximum dose 60 mg/day

Indications
As follows:
- Adjunctive therapy of minimal brain dysfunction syndrome in children
- Treatment for narcolepsy
- Relief of mild depression and apathetic or withdrawn senile behavior

Contraindications
- Tension
- Anxiety
- Glaucoma
- Seizure disorder
- Depression

Adverse Effects
- **CNS:** Nausea, dizziness, drowsiness and headache
- **CVS:** Blood pressure changes, tachycardia, anginal attacks and arrhythmias
- **Allergic:** Skin rashes, fever, urticaria, erythema, dermatitis, etc.
- **Others:** Anemia, abdominal pain, etc.

Nursing Responsibilities
- Before administration of drug, the physical assessment is required and the blood pressure, TPR, EEG should be done for base line.
- Advise the heavy caffeine users that headache, dizziness and nervousness can occur either during use or upon abrupt withdrawals.
- Use of amphetamine for weight control, only after other weight control programs have failed.
- Caution the patient that the ability to dine may be impaired.
- Administer last dose at least 6 hours before bedtime to minimize insomnia.
- Inform diabetic patients that insulin or dietary requirements may be altered by amphetamines.
- Attempt to determine the lowest effective dose for each patient to minimize danger.
- During treatment of minimal brain dysfunction in children, provide appropriate education, psychological and social intervention along with drug therapy.
- Watch for signs of excessive stimulation and notify physician immediately.
- Advise the patient that nervousness and insomnia may occur early in therapy but generally lessen with time, however dosage reduction may be required.
- Do not administer the last dose later than 4–5 hours prior to bedtime to minimize insomnia.

Respiratory Stimulants

Introduction
- Drugs having the ability to enhance depressed respiratory function are termed as respiratory stimulants or analeptics.
- Such agents act both at the level of respiratory centers in the brain stem as well as on the peripheral carotid chemoreceptor to increase the depth and also rate of respiration.
- They are antagonists to respiratory depressants and do not specifically block the effects of narcotics, barbiturates, muscle relaxants or other drugs.

Definition
- These are the agents stimulating the functions of respiratory system.
- They have the ability to enhance depressed respiratory functions.
- Caffeine and sodium benzoate also act as respiratory stimulants.

Classification (Fig. 3.34)

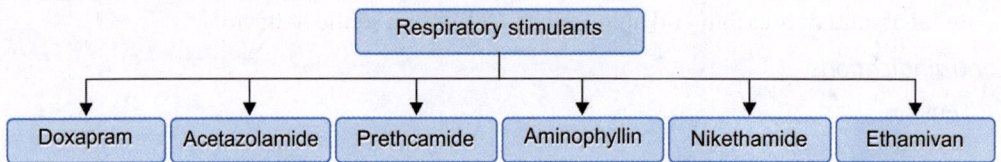

Fig. 3.34: Classification of respiratory stimulants.

Doxapram and Prethcamide
- Doxapram has a large margin between therapeutic and toxic doses.
- Continuous IV infusion of doxapram has been found to abolish episodes of apnea in the premature infant.
- Prethcamide is respiratory stimulant, such as doxapram.

Dosage
- **Doxapram:**
  - 40–80 mg—IM or IV
  - 0.5–2 mg/kg/hr—IV infusion
- **Prethcamide:**
  - 100–250 mg—oral, IM or IV

Mechanism of Action (Fig. 3.35)

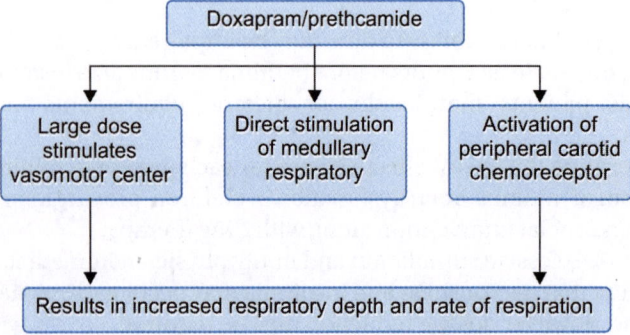

Fig. 3.35: Mechanism of action of doxapram and prethcamide.

Nikethamide, Ethamivan, Acetazolamide Nikethamide

Nikethamide cause increase in the salt and depth of respiration by stimulating the medullar respiratory centers.

Dosage

As follows—
- **Anesthetic dose:** 2–5 mL IV
- 5–15 mL to overcome respiratory distress

Ethamivan

Ethamivan is similar to nikethamide

Acetazolamide

Acetazolamide promotes bicarbonates diuresis and metabolic acidosis, which may be a useful stimulus to respiratory system.

Mechanism of Action of Nikethamide and Ethamivan (Fig. 3.36)

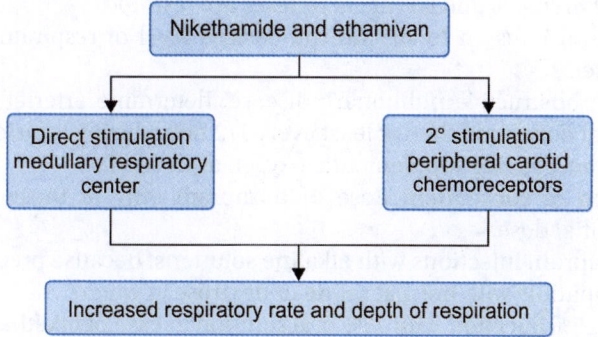

Fig. 3.36: Mechanism of action of nikethamide and ethamivan.

Indications

- As an expedient measure in hypnotic drug poisoning until mechanical ventilation is instituted; they are not dependable for long-term support
- Suffocation on drowning, acute respiratory insufficiency
- Apnea in premature infants
- Respiratory failure due to removal of hypoxic drive as a result of giving too high oxygen concentration to the patient with chronic lung disease
- Failure to ventilate spontaneously after general anesthesia.

Contraindications

- Ischemic asthmaticus
- Severe hypertension
- Thyrotoxicosis
- Epilepsy
- Pneumothorax
- Acute bronchial asthma

- Pulmonary embolism
- Respiratory failure due to neuromuscular disorder
- Uncompensated heart failure

Adverse Effects

- **CNS:** Flushing, sweating, pruritus, paresthesias, headache, dizziness, disorientation, mydriasis, tremors and involuntary movements.
- **Respiratory:** Cough, dyspnea, bronchospasm, hiccup (spasmodic contraction of diaphragm causing an abrupt aspiratory sounds.
- **Cardiovascular:** Chest pain, phlebitis (inflammation of vein, usually in legs) depressed T-wave arrhythmias.
- **GIT:** Nausea, vomiting and diarrhea
- **Others:** Urinary retention incontinence

Nursing Responsibilities

- Assess the patient by monitoring blood pressure, pulse and deep tendon reflexes during administration to prevent overdose.
- Maintain close observation of patient for at least 1 hour after injection or until patient is fully alert and pharyngeal and laryngeal reflexes are restored.
- Adjust flow rate of infusion to sustain the desired level of respiratory stimulation with minimal side effects.
- In patients with obstructive pulmonary disease, determine arterial blood gases before administration of doxapram then at least every 1/2 hour during infusion. Do not infuse for more than 2 hours. Provide supplemental oxygen as needed.
- Readministration of subsequent dose of doxapram only to those persons who have responded to initial dose.
- Do not mix doxapram injections with alkaline solutions, because precipitation will result. Injection is compatible with normal saline or dextrose in water.
- Do not confuse 25% injection with 25% oral solution in case of nikethamide.
- Note the drug is most effective and most hazardous when given by IV route.
- Record all the drugs given to the patient in nurse's record.

Ethyl Alcohol and Treatment of Methyl Alcohol Poisoning

Ethyl alcohol or ethanol is primarily ethane. It is an antiseptic drug, central nervous system depressant, a teratogenic acid. It is a clear, colorless liquid with pungent taste and vinous odor. Further *see* in **Chapter 6**

Drug Class

Antiseptics

Formulation

Local/Topical/Solution

Indications

- Neurolysis of nerve or ganglia
- Relied of chronic pain, such as trigeminal neuralgia
- Treatment of congenital venous malformation

- Treatment of uncontrolled primary hypertension
- Prevention and treatment of central line-associated bloodstream infection (CLABSI)
- Methyl alcohol poisoning

Contraindicated
- Alcoholic liver diseases
- Breastfeeding or lactating mothers

Adverse Effects
- Nausea
- Vomiting
- CNS depression
- Acute respiratory failure
- Death

Treatment of Methyl Alcohol Poisoning

Methyl alcohol or methanol poisoning is rate and acute condition which require emergency management and triaging. This methanol poisoning occur due to ingestion of gasoline additives, canned cooking fuels and other substance used in home like wind shield washers. Sometime, it is ingested accidently for attempting suicide. The ill effects of methanol poisoning are metabolic acidosis, blindness, kidney failure and death. Its treatment includes inhibition of alcohol dehydrogenase.

Clinical Features
- Decreased LOC
- Hypothermia
- Vomiting
- Abdominal pain
- Diminished vision
- Confusion
- Dizziness

Treatment

Treatment includes:
- Stabilizing the patient
- Give antidote fomepizole with ethanol, it reduce the action of alcohol dehydrogenase by competitive inhibition
- Hemodialysis in case of acidosis
- Mange the patient with folate, sodium bicarbonate and thiamine

MULTIPLE CHOICE QUESTIONS

1. **Gingival hyperplasia is an adverse effect of which drug?**
   a. Phenytoin sodium
   b. Valproic acid
   c. Barbiturate
   d. Carbamazepine
2. **Which of the following is considered as lethal for salicylate overdose?**
   a. 5–10 g
   b. 10–30 g
   c. 1–5 g
   d. 20–35 g

3. Which of the following drug is not an example of benzodiazepines?
   a. Alprazolam
   b. Chlordiazepoxide
   c. Clorazepate
   d. Phenytoin
4. Paracetamol is belonging to which class?
   a. Antipyretic
   b. Antihistamine
   c. Antiemetic
   d. Antifungal
5. Which of the following local anesthetic agent has shorter duration of action?
   a. Lidocaine
   b. Procaine
   c. Bupivacaine
   d. Ropivacaine

Answer Key

1. a   2. b   3. d   4. a   5. b

FURTHER READING

1. Aizenman CD et al. Use-dependent changes in synaptic strength at the purkinje cell to deep nuclear synapse. Prog brain Res. 2000;124:257.
2. Allain H et al. Disease-modifying drugs and Parkinson's disease. Prog Neurobiol. 2008;84:25.
3. Aminoff MJ. Treatment should not be initiated too soon in Parkinson's disease. Ann Neurol 2006:59:562.
4. Angot E, et al. Are synucleinopathies prion-like disorders? Lancer neurol. 2010;9:1128.
5. Antonini A. et al. Role of pramipexole in the management of Parkinson's disease. CNS Drugs. 2010;24:829.
6. Arroyo S. Rufinamide. Neurotherapeutics. 2007;4:155.
7. Avorn J. Drug warnings that can cause fits—communicating risks in a data-poor environment. N Engl J Med. 2008;359:991.
8. Baldwin CM, Keating GM. Rotigotine transdermal patch: a review of its use in the management of Parkinson's disease. CNS Drugs. 2007;21:1039.
9. Bhattacharjee J, El-Sayeh HG. Aripiprazole versus typical antipsychotic drugs for schizophrenia. Cochrane database Syst Rev. 2008;16(3)CD006617.
10. Bialer M. Progress report on new antiepileptic drugs: A summary of the tenth EILAT conference (EILAT X). Epilepsy Res. 2010;92:89.
11. Bredt DS, Nicoll RA. AMPA receptor trafficking at excitatory synapses. Neuron. 2003;40:361.
12. Breier A, Berg PH. The psychosis of schizophrenia: Prevalence, response to atypical antipsychotics, and prediction of outcome. Biol Psychiatry. 1999;46:361.
13. Brodie MJ, et al. Rufinamide for the adjunctive treatment of partial seizures in adults and adolescents: A randomized placebo-controlled trial. Epilepsia. 2009;50:1899.
14. Carlsson A, Waters N, Carlsson ML. Neurotransmitter interactions in schizophrenia-therapeutic implications. Biol Psychiatry. 1999;46:1388.
15. Catteral DE. et al. Compendium of voltage-gate ion channels: transient receptor potential channels, pharmacol Rev. 2003;55:591.
16. Catterall WA. et al. Compendium of voltage-gated ion channels: calcium channels. Pharmacol Rev. 2003;55:579.
17. Coyle JT. Glutamate and schizophrenia: beyond the dopamine hypothesis. Cell Mol Neurobiol. 2006;26:365.
18. Cross SA, Curran MP. Lacosamide in partial onset seizures. Drugs. 2009;69:449.
19. Eger EI II. The effect of inspired concentration on the rate of rise of alveolar concentration. Anesthesiology. 1963;89:774.
20. Eger EI II. Uptake and distribution. In: miller RD (Ed): anesthesia. 7th edition, Churchill livingstone; 2010.
21. Ertugral A, Meltzer HY. Antipsychotic drugs in bipolar disorder. Int J Neuropsychopharmacol. 2003;6:277.
22. Fragen RJ. Drug infusions in anesthesiology. Lippincott Williams & Wilkins; 2005.

23. Fremeau RT Jr, et al. VGLUTs define subsets of excitatory neurons and suggest novel roles for glutamate. Trends neruosci. 2004;27:98.
24. Hemming HC, et al. Emerging molecular mechanisms of general anesthetic action. Trends pharmacol sci. 2005;26:503.
25. Lugli AK, Yost CS, Kindler C. Anesthetic mechanisms: update on the challenge of unraveling the mystery of anaesthesia. Eur J Anaesth. 2009;26:807.
26. National Center for Biotechnology Information (2022). PubChem Compound Summary for CID 145068, Nitric oxide. Retrieved June 7, 2022 from https://pubchem.ncbi.nlm.nih.gov/compound/Nitric-oxide.
27. National Center for Biotechnology Information (2022). PubChem Compound Summary for CID 280, Carbon dioxide. Retrieved June 7, 2022 from https://pubchem.ncbi.nlm.nih.gov/compound/Carbon-dioxide
28. National Center for Biotechnology Information (2022). PubChem Compound Summary for CID 702, Ethanol. Retrieved June 7, 2022 from https://pubchem.ncbi.nlm.nih.gov/compound/Ethanol.
29. National Center for Biotechnology Information (2022). PubChem Compound Summary for CID 977, Oxygen. Retrieved June 7, 2022 from https://pubchem.ncbi.nlm.nih.gov/compound/Oxygen.
30. Weekley MS, Bland LE. Oxygen Administration. In: StatPearls. Treasure Island (FL): StatPearls Publishing; 2022.

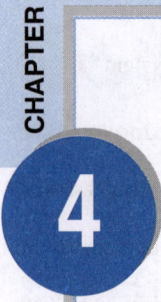

Drugs Used for Hormonal Disorders and Supplementation, Contraception and Medical Termination of Pregnancy

Prasuna Jelly, Hemlata, Suresh Sharma

ESTROGEN AND PROGESTERONE

Hypothalamus releases gonadotropin-releasing hormone (GnRH). This stimulates the anterior pituitary to release FSH and LH. FSH stimulates maturation of primary oocyte in an immature follicle. Follicle produces estrogen. Estrogen builds the uterine wall (the endometrium) and inhibits secretion of FSH. High levels of estrogen further stimulate secretion of LH by anterior pituitary. This plus FSH also causes ovulation of the secondary oocyte—leaving follicle without egg (the corpus luteum).

Corpus luteum secretes estrogen and progesterone. This maintains the endometrium for 15-16 days and inhibits LH (if oocyte is not fertilized and implanted in the uterine wall). The corpus degenerates (to corpus albicans) and stops producing estrogen and progesterone. Without estrogen and progesterone, endometrium breaks down—menstruation occurs. Menstruation is the sloughing off of the enlarged endometrial wall along with blood and mucus. This decrease in progesterone and LH. Low LH causes secretion of FSH by pituitary again. The cycle repeats.

Estrogen

A group of steroid hormones/female sex hormone that readily diffuse across the cell membrane. Inside the cell, they interact with estrogen receptors.

Natural Estrogens

Estradiol is the major estrogen secreted by ovary. It is synthesized in Graafian follicle, corpus luteum and placenta from cholesterol. Oxidized in the liver to weak estrogens like estrone, estriol.

Synthetic Estrogens

- To overcome the shortcomings of natural estrogens
- Steroidal—ethinyl estradiol, mestranol, tibolone
- Nonsteroidal—diethylstilbestrol, hexestrol, dienestrol

Estrogen Synthesis (Fig. 4.1)

- Estrogen is produced primarily by developing follicles in the ovaries, the corpus luteum, and the placenta
- The most abundant estrogen secreted by ovaries is estradiol
- The FSH and LH stimulate the production of estrogen in the ovaries
- Some estrogens are also produced in smaller amounts by other tissues such as the liver, adrenal glands and the breasts.

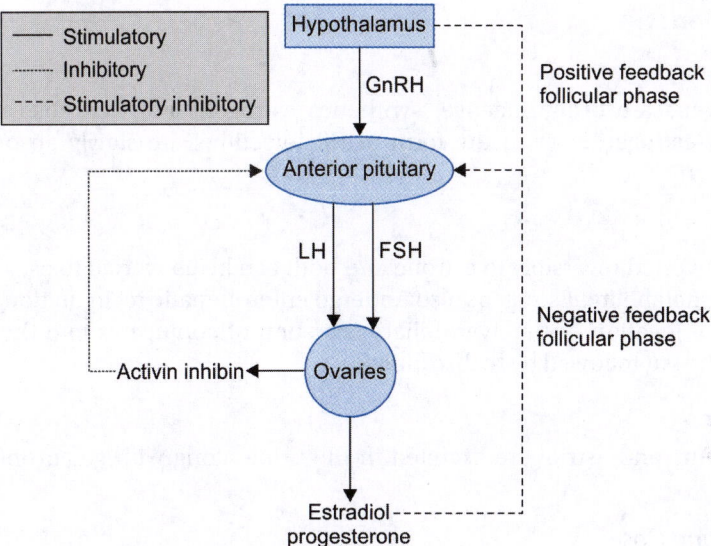

Fig. 4.1: Synthesis of estrogen and progesterone.

Effects of estrogen at various sites in the body

- Female reproductive system:
  - Fallopian tubes, uterus, vagina—pubertal growth and development. Thickening of vaginal epithelium
  - Mammary glands—proliferations of ducts and stroma
  - Uterine endometrium—proliferation
  - Cervix—watery secretion to facilitate sperm penetration
- CNS:
  - FSH/LH secretion—feedback control
  - Nausea and vomiting
- Blood:
  - Coagulation factors—decreased antithrombin III. Increasing circulating levels of factors II, VII, IX and X
  - Lipid profile—increase in HDL, decrease in LDL, increase in triglycerides
- Metabolic effects:
  - Anabolic effects
  - Glucose intolerance
  - Sodium and water retention
  - Maintain bone mass and decrease in bone resorption.
- Other effects:
  - Growth of hair, fat deposition, pigmentation on nipples
  - Gallbladder stones, cholestatic jaundice
  - Increased circulating level of proteins, hepatic adenoma on prolonged use.

Pharmacokinetics

Absorption
Natural estrogens are orally inactive; synthetics estrogens are well absorbed orally and transdermally, estrogen ester in the form of IM injections are slowly absorbed and have prolonged effect.

Metabolism
Estradiol is converted reversibly to estrone and both can be converted to estriol, which is the major urinary metabolite. Estrogens also undergo enterohepatic recirculation via sulfate and glucuronide conjugation in the liver, biliary secretion of conjugates into the intestine, and hydrolysis in the gut followed by reabsorption.

Excretion
Estradiol, estrone and estriol are excreted in the urine along with glucuronide and sulfate conjugates.

Preparations and Doses
The preparations and doses of estrogen along with their routes of administration has been presented in **Table 4.1**.

Indications

- **Hormonal replacement therapy:** It includes administrations of estrogen and progesterone combinations. Due to cessation of ovarian function at menopause women suffer a number of physical, psychological and emotional consequences..
- Acne and hirsutism—estrogen benefits by suppressing ovarian production of androgen by inhibiting gonadotropins released from pituitary.

Table 4.1: Estrogen preparations with doses and routes of administration.

Drug	Dose	Route
Natural steroidal estrogen: Estradiol benzoate, cypionate, enanthate	2.5–10 mg	IM
Conjugated estrogen	0.625–1.25 mg/day	Oral
Ethinylestradiol	0.02–0.2 mg/day	Oral
Mestranol	0.1–0.2 mg/day	Oral
Estriol succinate	4–8 mg/tds	Oral, cream tds
Dienestrol	0.01%	Topically in vagina
Transdermal estradiol: Estraderm-MX	25, 50,100 µg/24 h for 3–4 day	Apply to non-hairy skin below the waist, oral progestin is added
Gel formulations: Oestrogel	3 mg/5 g in 80 g tube	Applied over the arms once daily for hormonal replacement therapy (HRT)

- Dysmenorrhea—estrogen therapy benefits by inhibiting ovulation (anovulatory cycles) and decreasing prostaglandins secretions in endometrium.
- Carcinoma prostate—acts by suppressing the androgen production through pituitary.
- Senile vaginitis—effective in preventing as well as treating atrophic vaginitis that occurs in elderly women. An antibacterial may be combine.
- Delayed puberty in girls—Turner's syndrome or hypopituitarism.
- Dysfunctional uterine bleeding—this type of bleeding can result from the following three reasons:
  i. Estrogen withdrawal bleeding occurs when the estrogen given to postmenopausal women
  ii. Estrogen break through bleeding that occurs when there is a continuous stimulation of endometrium not interrupted by progesterone secretion, e.g. polycystic ovarian syndrome
  iii. Progesterone break through bleeding that occurs in presence of abnormally high progesterone, e.g. in women using low dose oral contraceptives.

Contraindications
- Pregnancy
- Thromboembolic disorders
- Diabetes
- Hepatic failure
- Estrogen dependent carcinoma of breast
- Endometrial carcinoma
- Endometriosis and undiagnosed genital bleeding.

Side Effects
- In males— gynecomastia, feminisation and decreased libido
- In females—breast tenderness, migraine, nausea, withdrawal bleeding, amenorrhea, endometrial hyperplasia, increased risk of vaginal and cervical adenocarcinoma
- In both sexes—gallstones and gallbladder, hepatic dysfunction, predisposition to thromboembolic disorders, precipitation of diabetes and fluid retention
- Fusion of epiphyses and reduction of adult stature when given to children.

Drug Interactions
- Need to increase the dose of warfarin, oral hypoglycemic or insulin
- Barbiturates, phenytoin, carbamazepine and rifampicin may decrease the effectiveness of estrogen
- Most antibiotics reduce the microbial flora of GIT, which retards the enterohepatic circulation of estrogens.

Nursing Responsibilities
- Assess BP prior to and periodically during use
- Monthly breast self-exam and annual mammograms are recommended
- In clients with breast cancer and bone metastasis, severe hypercalcemia may be caused by this therapy
- Nausea frequently occurs in morning, but disappears after 1–2 weeks of treatment.

Patient Education

- Teach client the correct dosage and amount and route of administration
- Advise client to take medicine with food, if nausea occurs
- Inform client that cigarette smoking can increase the risk of thrombus formation
- Advise client to report the signs of fluid retention
- Inform client that when cyclically taken vaginal bleeding will occur during the week each month when estrogen is withheld
- Instruct client to remain in lying down position for 30 minutes after administration of vaginal creams
- Instruct client to report positive Homan's sign
- Instruct client to take medication exactly as prescribed.

Antiestrogens and Selective Estrogen Receptor Modulators (SERM)

- **Antiestrogens:**
  - Pure antagonists
  - Clomiphene is for treatment of infertility in anovulatory women 50 mg OD for 5 days starting from 5th day of menstrual cycle.
  - Systemic inquiry (S/E) ovarian tumor, polycystic ovaries and gastric upset
  - Fulvestrant is used for the treatment of breast cancer
- **Selective estrogen receptor modulators (SERMs):**
  - Compounds with tissue-selective actions
  - The goal of these drugs is to produce beneficial estrogenic actions in certain tissues (e.g. brain, bone, liver) during postmenopausal hormone therapy
  - Antiestrogenic action is due to inhibition of human breast cancer cells
  - Tamoxifen(10–20 mg bd), raloxifene, toremifene.

Progesterone

- Progesterone is one of the steroid hormones
- It is secreted by the corpus luteum and by the placenta, and is responsible for preparing the body for pregnancy and, if pregnancy occurs, maintaining it until birth
- C21 steroid hormone—involved in the female menstrual cycle, pregnancy and embryogenesis
- Progesterone belongs to a class of hormones called progestogens and is the major naturally occurring human progestogen
- Progesterone should not be confused with progestins, which are synthetically produced progestogens
- **Synthetic progestogens:** Two classes of progestins are derivatives of either C21 or C19 steroid compounds:
  - **The C21 derivatives** are almost pure progestins, have weaker antiovulatory action and are used primarily as an adjuvant to estrogens for HRT, e.g. **medroxyprogesterone, dydrogesterone**
  - **The C19 nortestosterone derivatives** are having most potent antiovulatory action and more androgenic activity used in combined contraceptive pills, e.g. **norethisterone, levonorgestrel, desogestrel**

Synthesis
- Synthesized from pregnenolone, a derivative of cholesterol
- The precursor of the mineralocorticoid aldosterone
- Conversion to 17-hydroxyprogesterone of cortisol and androstenedione
- Androstenedione can be converted to testosterone, estrone and estradiol.

Sources
- Progesterone is produced in the adrenal glands, gonads, brain, and during pregnancy, in the placenta
- Increasing amounts are produced during pregnancy:
  - Initially, the source is the corpus luteum
  - After the 8th week production of progesterone shifts over to the placenta
  - The placenta utilizes maternal cholesterol as the initial substrate
  - Most of the produced progesterone enters the maternal circulation
  - Some is picked up by the fetal circulation and is used as substrate for fetal corticosteroids
  - At term the placenta produces about 250 mg progesterone per day

Mechanism of Action
- The progesterone receptor (PR) has a limited distribution in the body; confined mainly to female genital tract, breast, CNS and pituitary
- Since the ligand-binding domains of the two PR isoforms are identical, there is no difference in ligand binding
- However, the biological activities of PR-A and PR-B are distinct, and depend on the target gene in question:
  - PR-B mediates the stimulatory activities of progesterone
  - PR-A strongly inhibits this action of PR-B.
- Upon binding progesterone, the heat shock proteins dissociate, and the receptors are phosphorylated and that bind with high selectivity to progesterone response elements located on target genes and regulates transcription.

Pharmacokinetics
- **Absorption:** Progesterone undergoes high first pass metabolism. Therefore synthetic preparations are more commonly used
- Progesterone esters in oily solution for IM administration
- t½ is 5–7 minutes
- t½ of synthetic progestins is 8–24 hours
- **Metabolism:** By liver enzymes
- Excretion by urine after conjugation.

Effects of Progesterone

Reproductive System
- Fallopian tubes—growth and development, inhibition of uterine contraction during pregnancy and of immunologic rejection of fetus
- Uterine endometrium—induction of secretory phase in estrogen primed endometrium
- Mammary glands—development of secretory system for lactation

- Cervix—viscous, scanty mucus secretion as barrier to sperm penetration.
- **CNS**—body temperature increases, depressant effect and feedback control.
- **Metabolic effects**—increases basal insulin levels, increased appetite, fat deposition increases, decrease in HDL and catabolic action.

Preparations and Doses

The preparations and doses of progesterone along with their routes of administration has been presented in **Table 4.2**.

Indications

- As contraceptive
- Hormone replacement therapy
- Dysfunctional uterine bleeding
- To treat endometriosis—long-term therapy with progestins may be used as the progestin can inhibit estrogen-dependent growth of ectopic endometrial tissue
- Premenstrual syndrome/tension
- Threatened abortion—occurs in progesterone deficiency; pure progestins are used
- Endometrial carcinoma—repress the metastatic endometrial mass.

Contraindications

- In patients with hepatic disease or dysfunction
- Incomplete abortion, suspected pregnancy or undiagnosed vaginal bleeding
- Relatively contraindicated in patients with hyperlipidemia, thromboembolic disease (especially in smokers)
- Caution is appropriate in patients with heart disease due to increased fluid retention and edema.

Side Effects

- Breast engorgement, headache, rise in body temperature, edema, acne and mood swings may occur
- Irregular bleeding and amenorrhea can occur

Table 4.2: Preparation and doses of progesterone.

Drug	Dose	Route
Progesterone	10–100 mg, 100–400 mg	IM, oral
Hydroxyprogesterone	250–500 mg	IM
Medroxyprogesterone acetate	5–20 mg, 50–150 mg	Oral, IM
Dihydrogesterone	5–10 mg	Oral
Norethisterone	5–10 mg	Oral
Levonorgestrel	0.1–0.5 mg/day	Oral
Lynestrenol	5–10 mg	Oral
Allylestrenol	10–40 mg/day	Oral
Desogestrel	150 µg	Oral

- The 19-nortestosterone derivatives can lower plasma HDL levels—may promote atherogenesis
- Long-term use may increase the risk of breast cancer
- Blood sugar may rise and diabetes can be precipitated.

Nursing Responsibilities

- Prior to administration in clients with current H/o depression, make a plan to deal with worsening or recurrent depressive symptoms
- A thorough physical examination should be done with special attention to pelvic organs, breasts and hepatic function
- A Papanicolaou (Pap) test should be done prior to initiation of therapy and every 6–12 months while client is taking medicines
- Monitor vital signs including BP
- Monitor I/O

Patient Education

- Instruct client about dosing and timing of the medication
- Warn client about possible side effects
- Inform postmenopausal women of possibility of resumption of cyclical vaginal bleeding
- Instruct client to monitor BP and I/O
- Caution client to exposure to UV lights
- Instruct client to monitor the glucose level closely
- Instruct client to take medication with food

Antiprogestins

- Antiprogestin, first discovered in 1981, is mifepristone, used to terminate pregnancy
- In the presence of progesterone, mifepristone acts as a competitive receptor antagonist for both progesterone receptors
- When administered in the early stages of pregnancy, mifepristone causes decidual breakdown by blocking uterine progesterone receptors, which leads to detachment of the blastocyst, decreasing hCG production.

ORAL CONTRACEPTIVE AND HORMONE REPLACEMENT THERAPY

Hormonal Contraceptives

These are hormonal preparations used for suppression of fertility. The word 'contraception' means interception in the birth process at any stage ranging from ovulations to ovum implantation.

Definition

These are the birth control methods that act on the endocrine system. Hormonal contraceptives when properly used are the most effective spacing method contraception. Hormonal contraceptive may be estrogen, progesterone or testosterone.

Classification (Fig. 4.2)

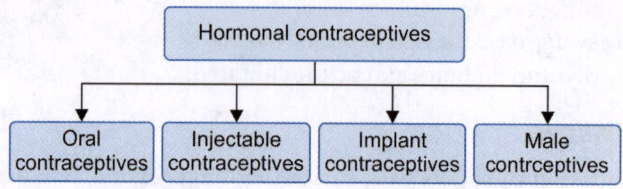

Fig. 4.2: Types of hormonal contraceptives.

Oral Contraceptives

Types of Oral Contraceptive

- Combined pills
- Mini pill (progesterone only pill)
- Post coital pill (emergency contraceptive)
- Centchroman (non-hormonal estrogen receptor antagonists)

Combined Pills

It contains estrogens and progestin. It is the most effective and popular method for contraception with 99%–99.5% success rate.

Combined pills can be:

Monophasic: No phasic increase or decrease in the estrogen, progestin content during 21 days of pill administration.

Biphasic/Triphasic: Level of estrogen remains same, but progestin level are altered.

The goal of these therapies are to minimize the occurrence of irregular bleeding while maintaining the efficacy. One tablet is taken daily for 21 days, starting on 5th day of menstruation. The next course is started after a gap of 7 days in which bleeding occur. Thus a cycle of 28 days is maintained.

Mini Pill (Progestin only Pill/Ezy Pill)

- It has been devised to eliminate the estrogen, because of many long-term risks associated with estrogen
- The efficacy is 96%–98%
- The menstrual cycle tends to become irregular and ovulation occurs in 20%–30% women, but other mechanisms contribute to contraceptive action
- Not associated with deep vein thrombosis (DVT) or heart disease.

Candidate for mini pill

- Cigarette smokers over age 35
- Women with H/O blood clots
- Women with H/O high BP
- Women who experience extreme migraine.

Postcoital Contraceptive (Morning after Pill)

- They are recommended within 48 hours of an unprotected intercourse
- High dose estrogen/progestins are quite effective in emergency contraception, when given immediately after unprotected coitus

- Acts by preventing ovulation and post-fertilization and implantation of blastocyst
- Delay in maturation of endometrium.

The following are the three regimens available:
- Levonorgestrel 0.5 mg + ethinyl estradiol 0.1 mg—taken as early as within 75 hours of unprotected intercourse and repeated after 12 hours. Women usually experience nausea and vomiting
- Levonorgestrel 0.75 mg taken twice with 12 hours:
    - Gap within 72 hours of intercourse. Effective mainly as post-ovulatory methods of fertility control
- Mifepristone 600 mg single dose taken within 72 hours of intercourse have high success rate and fewer side effects:
    Have high failure rate and side effects than oral combined pills.

Centchroman (Ormeloxifene/ Chhaya)

- It is a non-steroidal estrogen antagonist or selective estrogen receptor modulator (SERM) introduced in national family welfare program to be distributed as an oral contraceptive under the brand name Saheli
- Available as a tablet containing 30 mg of centchroman taken twice a week for first 3 months and then once a week subsequently to be continued irrespective of the following menstrual cycle, as long as contraceptive is desired
- The missed tablet should be taken as soon as possible, if the dose is missed for more than 7 days then reinitiate the therapy
- Contraceptive effects usually reversible within 6 months
- Has long plasma t½ about 1 week
- Acts as an anti-implantation agent by inducing embryo-uterine asynchrony, accelerated tubal transport and suppression of deciduation.

Preparation and Doses

Preparations and doses of oral contraceptives is presented in **Table 4.3**.

Advantages

- One of the most effective reversible method for birth control
- Simple and easy to use
- Regulate menstrual cycle
- Decrease acne
- Reduces the risk of ovarian and endometrial cancer
- May reduce perimenopausal symptoms

Disadvantages

- May be taken everyday
- May cause irregular bleeding
- Effectiveness may be reduced by other medication
- Not be used by women over age 35
- Does not protect against sexually transmitted infections (STIs)
- May increase the number of headaches
- May not be suitable for breastfeeding women

Table 4.3: Oral contraceptives with their doses.

Drug	Dose	
Combined pills		
Norgestrel, ethinyl estradiol	0.3 mg, 30 µg	Mala-D (21 tabs+ 7 ferrous sulfate 60 mg tablet
Levonorgestrel, ethinyl estradiol	0.25 mg, 50 µg	Ovral
Desogestrel, ethinyl estradiol	0.15 mg, 30 µg	Novelon
Desogestrel, ethinyl estradiol	0.15 mg, 20 µg	Femilon
Phased pills		
Levonorgestrel, ethinyl estradiol	50–75–125 mg, 30 µg	Triqular
Norethindrone, ethinyl estradiol	0.5–0.75–1.0 mg, 35 µg	Orthonovum
Postcoital pills		
Levonorgestrel, ethinyl estradiol	0.25 mg, 50 µg	Ovral (2+2)
Levonorgestrel	0.75 mg	Norlevo
Mini pills		
Norethindrone	0.35 mg	Nor-qd
Norgestrel	75 µg	Ovrette

Hormone Replacement Therapy

Hormone replacement therapy is a system of medical treatment for surgical menopausal, perimenopausal and to a lesser extends postmenopausal women. It includes administrations of estrogen and progesterone combinations. Due to cessation of ovarian function at menopause women suffer a number of physical, psychological and emotional consequences. Also aid in prolong life and may reduce incidence of dementia.

The benefits and risks of HRT are considered below:
- Reduction of vasomotor menopausal symptoms and vaginal atrophic changes
- Reduction in risk of osteoporosis and fractures
- Cardiovascular events—improves HDL/LDL RATIO, retard atherogenesis, risk of stroke increase
- Neuroprotective and CNS effects—insomnia and fatigue are reduced, improvement in cognitive abilities
- Cancers—predisposes to endometrial cancer and cause breast cancer. Protective effect on colorectal carcinoma
- Increase the risk of developing gall stones
- Trigger the migraine
- Improvement in quality of life
- Newer benefits:
  - Decreased risk of colorectal cancer by 37%
  - Decreased age-related tooth loss

CHAPTER 4: Drugs Used for Hormonal Disorders and Supplementation...

- Decreased age-related macular degeneration
- Delay of onset and progression of Alzheimer's disease when started early postmenopausal

Indications

- Relief of menopausal symptoms
- Prevention of osteoporosis
- To maintain the quality of life in menopausal years
- **Special group of women to whom HRT should be prescribed:** Premature ovarian failure, Gonadal dysgenesis, Surgical or radiation menopause

Dosage, Route and Indication of HRT (Table 4.4)

Low dose oral conjugated estrogen 0.3 mg daily is effective and has got minimal side effects. Dose interval may be modified as daily for initial 2-3 months then it may be changed to every other day for another 2-3 months and then every third day for the next 2-3 months. It may be stopped thereafter if symptoms are controlled.

Table 4.4: Dosage, route and indication of HRT.

Forms	Indication	Dosage	Route
Oral estrogen regime	Hysterectomy	Estrogen: Conjugated equine estrogen 0.3 mg or 0.625 mg	Orally
Estrogen and cyclic progestin	Intact uterus	Estrogen for 25 days and progesterone is added for last 12-14 days	Orally
Continuous estrogen and progestin therapy	Endometrial hyperplasia Hysterectomy	17 beta estradiol implants 25 mg, 50 mg or 100 mg (for 6 months)	Subdermal implants
	Endometrial hyperplasia	1 g applicator of gel, delivering 1 mg of estradiol daily	Percutaneous estrogen gel over skin and anterior wall of thigh
	Endometrial hyperplasia	3.2 mg of 17 betaestradiol, releasing about 50 ug of estradiol in 24 hours	Transdermal patch applied below the waistline
	Atrophic Vaginitis Urogenital atrophy Contraindicated to systemic HRT	Conjugated equine vaginal estrogen cream 1.25 mg daily	Vaginal cream
	Breast carcinoma Endometrial carcinoma Progestins	Medroxyprogesterone acetate 2.5 – 5 mg/day	Orally

Contraindication

- Known or suspected pregnancy or breast cancer
- Undiagnosed genital tract bleeding
- Presence estrogen dependent neoplasm in the body
- History of venous thromboembolism
- Active liver disease
- Gallbladder disease

Side Effects

- Fluid retention
- Bloating
- Breast tenderness or swelling
- Headaches
- Indigestion
- Depression
- Acne
- Backache
- Endometrial cancer
- Breast cancer
- Venous thromboembolic (VTE) disease
- Coronary heart disease (CHD)
- Lipid metabolism—increase the cholesterol level
- Dementia, Alzheimer's disease

Nursing Responsibilities (Table 4.5)

Table 4.5: Nursing responsibilities in process of hormone replacement therapy.

Prior to administration	• Obtain a complete history including personal or familial history of breast cancer, gallbladder disease, diabetes mellitus, liver or kidney disease. • Obtain a drug history to determine possible drug interactions and allergies. • Assess cardiovascular status including hypertension, history of MI, cerebrovascular accident, or thromboembolic disease.
During HRT	• Monitor for thromboembolic disease. (Estrogen increase risk for thromboembolism). • Monitor for abnormal uterine bleeding. (If undiagnosed tumor is present, these drugs can increase its size and cause uterine bleeding). • Monitor breast health. (Estrogen promote the growth of certain breast cancer). • Monitor for vision changes. (These drugs may worsen myopia or astigmatism and cause intolerance of contact lenses). • Encourage client not to smoke. (Smoking increases risk of cardiovascular disease) • Encourage client to avoid caffeine. (Estrogens and caffeine may lead to increased CNS stimulation). • Monitor glucose levels. (Estrogens may increase blood glucose levels) • Monitor for seizure activity. (Estrogen- induced fluid retention may increases risk of seizures). • Monitor client's understanding and proper self- administration. (Improper administration may incidence of adverse effects).
Evaluation phase	• The client verbalizes relief of unpleasant symptoms of menopause. • The client demonstrates an understanding of the drug's actions by accurately describing drug side effects and precautions. • The client accurately states signs and symptoms to be reported to the healthcare provider.

VAGINAL CONTRACEPTIVES (FIGS. 4.3A TO D)

Vaginal Rings
Vaginal rings containing levonorgestrel have been found to be effective. The hormone is slowly absorbed through vaginal mucosa. The ring is worn in the vagina for 3 weeks and removed for the fourth weeks **(Fig. 4.3A)**.

Female Condom
Female condom (FEMIDOM) is also a sheath made up of thin, transparent, soft plastic, closed at smaller end and opened at the wider end. It is of single time usage **(Fig. 4.3B)**.

Diaphragm (Vaginal Diaphragm and Dough Diaphragm)
Dough cap named after a German physician Dutch Neo Mathusians, 1882. It is a shallow, soft rubber cup, with a stiff but flexible rim, made up of coiled spring, which helps in retention. Size varies from 5 to 10 cm in diameter **(Fig. 4.3C)**.

Cervical Cap
It is thimble-shaped like diaphragm but smaller. It covers the vaginal portion of the cervix, thus acting as a barrier. The woman inserts the cervical cap with spermicidal, in the proper position in the vagina before having sexual intercourse **(Fig. 4.3D)**.

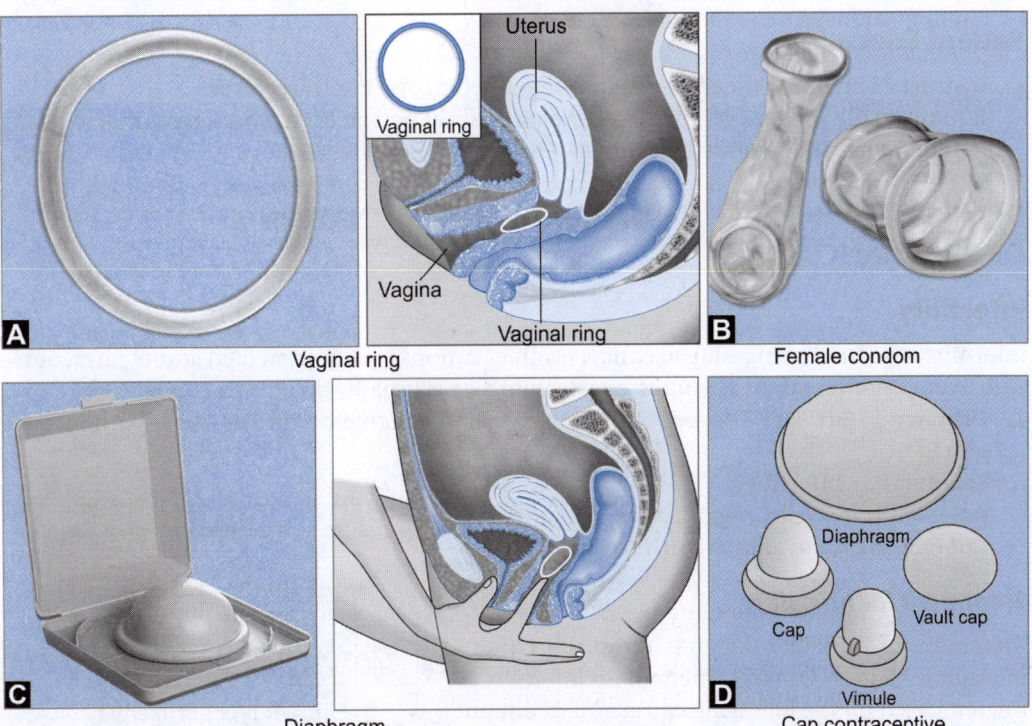

Figs. 4.3A to D: Types of vaginal contraceptives: A: Vaginal ring; B: Female condom; C: Diaphragm; D: Cap contraceptive.

Vault Cap (Dumas cap)

It fits into the vault of the vagina and occludes the cervix. Indicated when neither diaphragm nor cervical cap is suited to the women **(Fig. 4.3D)**.

Vimule Cap

It is a small, deep, cup like device with a flanged base, because of which it fits firmly on the cervix. It can be used by a woman, whose vaginal walls are lax and cannot use diaphragm **(Fig. 4.3D)**.

Merits

- Controlled by women, prevents both pregnancy and STDs, including AIDS
- No apparent side effects, no allergy and no contraindications
- It can be used even during menstruation
- More comfortable to men
- Offer greater protection as it covers both internal and external genitalia.

Demerits

- Expensive, not impressive, women must touch her genitals
- It is now available in India, but widely available in Europe and USA
- Costly, improvements are being worked out for universal acceptability

Patient Education

- Instruct client about the methods of using different oral contraceptives
- It requires the services of a medical or paramedical person for the demonstration of using it. It may tear while removing, if not careful

DRUGS FOR INFERTILITY AND MEDICAL TERMINATION OF PREGNANCY

Infertility

Infertility is defined as inability to conceive after 12 months of unprotected sexual intercourse with average frequency of 2-3 times/ week. Infertility is broadly divided into **(Fig. 4.4)**:

1. **Primary infertility:** The couple has never had pregnancy or has never produced a gestation.
2. **Secondary infertility:** Women have been pregnant previously, regardless of the outcome. But now she is not able to conceive again.

Treatment for Infertility

Treatment of infertility depends upon the type of infertility: Male or Female. The female infertility is treated based on the following cause and treatment modalities **(Tables 4.7 and 4.8)**.

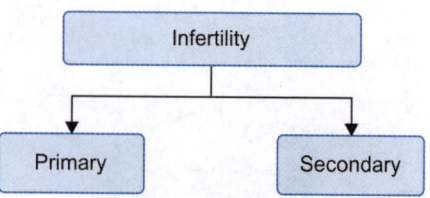

Fig. 4.4: Types of infertility.

Table 4.6: Cause and treatment modalities for infertility.

Cause of female infertility	Treatment modalities	Method/ Procedure of treatment
Ovulation disorders	Ovulation inducing drugs	Ovulation induction
Uterine and tubal abnormalities	Surgical procedures and assisted reproductive technology	• Laser vaporization • Tubo-tubal anastomosis • Gamete in-vitro fertilization Technique (GIFT) • Zygote in-vitro fertilization technique (ZIFT) • Intracytoplasmic sperm injection (ICSI)
Cervical mucus problem	Intrauterine insemination	Artificial insemination of donor, artificial insemination of husband
Endometriosis	Hormone suppressant or surgical procedure	Laparoscopy: Ablation and adhesiolysis or laparoscopic uterosacral nerve ablation (LUNA)
Hyperprolactinemia	Prolactin suppressing agents	Bromocriptine or cabergoline

Table 4.7: Drugs, mechanism of action, dose and side effect of the medical treatment for infertility.

Treatment of infertility	Drugs	Mechanism of action	Dosage	Side effect
Ovulation induction	Clomiphene citrate (CC)	It is anti-estrogenic which block the estrogen receptor in hypothalamus. It releases the gonadotrophins	50 mg maxim upto 250 mg Maximum 6 cycle	Hot flushes Nausea Vomiting Headache Visual symptoms
	Gonadotrophin releasing hormone analogs and dopamin agonists	Similar action of GnRH. It provokes the massive release of GnRH into circulation. It inhibits the secretion of estrogen	Buserelin 50-500 mcg SC/day or 300-1200 mcg IM/day	Hot flush Dizziness Diarrhea Constipation
	Gonadotrophins	Stimulates ovulation	Human menopausal gonadotrophin (HMG) 75 IU IM/day	Pain at the site of injection Fatigue Depression Irritation
Prolactin suppressing agents	Bromocriptine or cabergoline	It suppress the production of prolactin	0.25-0.5 mg once or twice weekly	Nausea Dizziness Headache Exhaustion

Table 4.8: Dose, composition and side effect of MTP kit.

Drug name	Composition and dosage	Storage	Side effect	Special consideration
MTP kit	Mifepristone (200 mg) + Misoprostol (200 mcg)	Store below 30°C	Nausea, vomiting, stomache, diarrhea, uterine contraction, menstrual bleeding (heavy)	Only recommended by medical professional Must be taken under the supervision as per dose

Nursing Responsibilities in Treatment of Infertility

- She must provide education regarding the treatment for alleviating her and couples fear
- Ensure counseling is done before imitating the treatment, as it is related to many ethical issues
- Teach the patient regarding the benefits of nutritious diet during the treatment
- Provide psychological support to the couple, to remain thoughtful.

Medical Termination of Pregnancy (MTP, 1971)

In India, the abortion was legalized by "Medical Termination of Pregnancy Act" of 1971, and has been enforced in the year April 1972. The Medical Termination of Pregnancy (Amendment) Act is launched in year 2021. It is deliberation of abortion by a registered medical practitioner in the interest of mother's health and life is protected by the MTP.

Indication

- Cardiac disease
- Chronic glomerulonephritis
- Malignant hypertension
- Intractable hyperemesis gravidarum
- Cervical or breast malignancy
- Diabetes mellitus with retinopathy
- Epilepsy or psychiatric illness with the advice of a psychiatrist

Recommendations

In the revised rule, a registered medical practitioner is qualified to perform an MTP provided:
- One has assisted in at least 25 MTP in an authorized center and having a certificate.
- One has got six months house surgeon training in obstetrics and gynecology.
- One has got diploma or degree in obstetrics and gynecology.
    - Termination can only be performed in hospitals, established or maintained by the government or places approved by the government.
    - Pregnancy can only be terminated on the written consent of the women. Husband's consent is not required.
    - Pregnancy in a minor girl (below the age of 18 years) or launatic cannot be terminated without written consent of the parents or legal guardian.
    - Termination is permitted upto 20 weeks of pregnancy. When the pregnancy exceeds 121 weeks, opinion of two medical practitioners is required.
    - The abortion has to be performed confidentially and the state in the prescribed form.

UTERINE STIMULANTS AND RELAXANTS

Uterine Stimulants

Introduction

The motility of uterus is important during pregnancy. Sedate uterus is needed during pregnancy, but at the time of delivery increases in uterus bone and motility are desired. These are various drugs and hormones, which act on uterus like uterine stimulants.

Definition

Uterine stimulants are those which stimulate the uterine contraction. One of the stimulants is oxytocin. They are the drugs that have the power to execute the contractions of the uterine muscles.

Classification (Fig. 4.5)

Oxytocin

Oxytocin is an octapeptide synthesized in hypothalamus and stored in posterior pituitary from where it is released in response to stimuli.

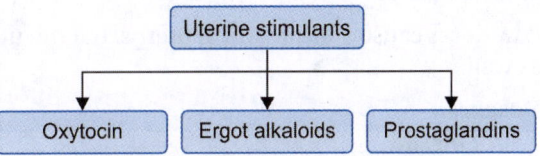

Fig. 4.5: Classification of uterine stimulants.

Dosage

- By IV infusion—10 units in 5% of dextrose 5% or ringer lactate.
- Oxytocin nasal solution—40 units/mL.

Mechanism of action (Fig. 4.6)

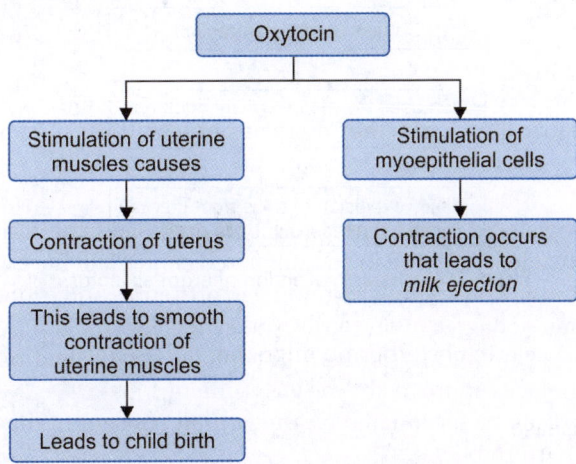

Fig. 4.6: Mechanism of action of oxytocin.

Indications

- **Pregnancy:** To induce abortion, oxytocin has been used for mid-trimester abortion
- To stop bleeding
- To induce labor

- **For oxytocin challenge test:** It is performed to determine uteroplacental adequacy in high risk pregnancy.

Contradictions
- Grand multipara
- Contracted pelvis
- Obstructed labor
- Cardiac disease

Adverse effects
- **GI:** Neonatal jaundice
- **CNS:** Hypotension
- **Reproductive system:** Hypertonic uterine activity:
  - Fetal distress and fetal death
  - Uterine ruptures

Ergot Alkaloids

Low doses cause contraction of uterus, but the uterus following each contraction relaxes fully as well.

Dosages
- *0.2 mg:* IM
- *1–2 mg:* Sublingually
- *0.2 mg:* Orally

Mechanism of action (Fig. 4.7)

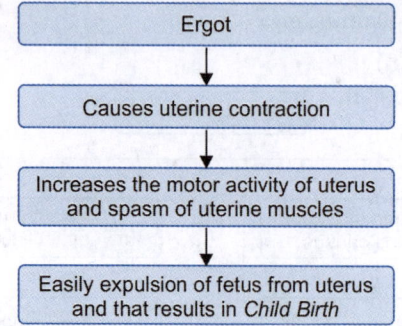

Fig. 4.7: Mechanism of action of ergot alkaloids.

Indication

The major therapeutic use is in obstetric and migraine.

Contraindications
- Organic cardiac disease
- Rh–ve mother
- Severe preeclampsia (in this convulsions may occur as a result of an acute toxemia of pregnancy)

Adverse effects
- Hypertension
- Interference in lactation by decreasing concentration of prolactin

Nursing responsibilities
- Assess the condition of patient having labor contractility
- Assess for H_2O intoxication
- Monitor BP temperature, pulse and respiration
- Identify length and duration of contraction
- Check any type of allergic reaction
- Do not mix two drugs
- Monitor the level of calcium and prolactin, and for decreased breast milk production

Patient Education
- Advise the patient to blow nose before administration
- Teach the patient to report the increased blood loss
- Advice patient that contraction will be similar to menstrual cramps
- To reported blood loss, headache, sweating, nausea, vomiting, etc

UTERINE RELAXANTS (TOCOLYTICS)

These are the drugs, which decrease uterine motility. These agent either act directly to suppressing myometrial smooth muscle contractions; or indirectly by inhibiting synthesis, release, receptor action of prostaglandin. Common drugs categories are beta- adrenergic agonists (terbutaline, ritodrine), calcium channel blockers (nifedipine), NSAIDs (indomethacin). Others are like oxytocin receptor antagonists (atosiban), nitrates, general anesthetics are drugs, which can depress uterine contractions.

Classification

- **Adrenergic antagonist:** Ritodrine
- **Calcium channel blocker:** Nifedipine
- **Oxytocin antagonist:** Atosiban
- Magnesium sulfate
- **Miscellaneous drugs:** Ethyl alcohol, nitrates, progesterone, general anesthetics, halothane and indomethacin.

The drugs commonly used for uterine relaxation are presented in **Table 4.9.**

Table 4.9: Commonly drugs used for uterine relaxation.

Trade name	Category	Dose
Terbutaline	β blockers	SC: 0.25 mg q 20 min up to 3 dose IV: 10–80 µg/min PO: 2.5 mg q 4–6 h
Ritodrine	β blockers	IV: Initially 50 µg/min, increase by 50 µg/min q 10 min to maximum 350 µg/min PO:10 mg q 2 h for 24 h
Nifedipine	CCB*	PO: 10 mg q 20 min for 2–3 dose; maximum 40 mg in 1 h
Indomethacin	NSAIDs†	50 mg loading dose rectally, followed by 25 mg PO q 6 h for 2–3 day
Atosiban	Oxytocin antagonist	Not yet approved

*CCB, calcium-channel blockers; †NSAIDs, non-steroidal anti-inflammatory drugs.

Mechanism of Action (MOA) Selective β₂ Agonists
- Known to relax uterine myometrium
- Ritodrine is β-2 adrenergic agonist. It binds to β-2 adrenergic receptors on outer membrane of myometrial cell, activates adenyl cyclase to increase the level of cAMP, which decreases intracellular calcium and leads to a decrease of uterine contractions
- Drugs in this category are terbutaline and ritodrine.

MOA Calcium Channel Blockers
- Nifedipine is the drug under this category
- It acts by impairing the calcium entry into myometrial cells via voltage dependent channels to inhibit uterine contractility

Indications
- Delay or postpone preterm labor
- Arrest threatened abortion
- In dysmenorrhea
- Prevent uterine hyperstimulation.

Contraindications
- Known fetal anomaly incompatible with life
- β adrenergics contraindicated in presence of pulmonary edema
- Severe hypertension and CAD
- Caution use, if cervix is dilated greater than 5 cm or if gestational age is less than 20 weeks.

Side Effects
- Beta adrenergics—maternal and fetal tachycardia, palpitations, tremors and anxiety
- May cause or exacerbate constipation
- Nausea and vomiting.

Adverse Effects
- Beta adrenergics—pulmonary edema
- Nifedipine and indomethacin can cause oligohydramnios
- Indomethacin can cause premature closure of ductus arteriosus leading to fetal death.

Drug Interactions
Increased incidence of pulmonary edema, when used concurrently with corticosteroids for fetal lung maturity.

Patient Education
- Educate client as to possible side effects and coping strategies
- Instruct client about use and dose of oral medications and importance of taking them on time
- *Nifedipine*—encourage client change position slowly due to possible orthostatic hypotension
- Advise client to consult physician prior to taking over-the-counter (OTC) medications.

Nursing Responsibilities

- **β-adrenergics:** If client continues on to deliver after receiving uterine relaxant medications, be prepared with oxytocic for treatment of PPH
- Monitor vital signs and I/O
- **Nifedipine:** Avoid grapefruit juice during administration
- Use indomethacin for short period of time
- If mother is using terbutaline during pregnancy, monitor the neonate for hypoglycemia.

MULTIPLE CHOICE QUESTIONS

1. Which of the following is a non-steroidal form of estrogen?
   a. Diethylstilbestrol
   b. Ethinylestradiol
   c. Mestranol
   d. Tibolone
2. What is the effect of estrogen on cervix?
   a. Proliferation
   b. Thickening
   c. Watery secretion
   d. Both a and c
3. Preferred route of administration of estradiol.
   a. Topical
   b. Oral
   c. IM
   d. IV
4. Clomiphene is used in treatment of:
   a. Dysmenorrhea
   b. Infertility
   c. Gynecomastia
   d. Delayed puberty
5. Route of administration of progesterone esters.
   a. Oral
   b. Topical
   c. IM
   d. IV

Answer Key

1. a   2. c   3. c   4. b   5. c

FURTHER READING

1. Acconcia F, et al. Palmitoylation-dependent estrogen receptor alpha membrane localization: regulation by 17 beta-estradiol. Mol Biol Cell. 2005;16:231.
2. Action to control cardiovascular risks in Diabetes study group: effects of intensive glucose lowering in type 2 diabetes. N Engl J Med. 2008;358:2545.
3. Adler AL, et al. Association of systolic blood pressure with macrovascular and microvascular complications of type 2 diabetes (UKPDS 36): prospective observational study. By Med J. 2000;321:412.
4. Advance collaborative group: Intensive blood glucose control and vascular outcomes in patients with type 2 diabetes. N Engl J Med. 2008;358:2560.
5. Alesci S, et al. Glucocorticoid-induced osteoporosis: from basic mechanisms to clinical aspects. Neuroimmunomodulation. 2005;12:1.
6. American thyroid association (http://www.thyroid.org).
7. Anderson GL. et al. Women's Health Initiative Steering Committee: effects of conjugated equine estrogen in postmenopausal women with hysterectomy. JAMA. 2004;291:1701.
8. Bacopoulou F, Greydanus DE, Chrousos GP. Reproductive and contraceptive issues in chronically ill adolescents. Eur J Contracept Reprod Health Care. 2010;15:389.
9. Baggio LA, et al. Biology of incretins: GLP-1 and GIP. Gastroenterology. 2007;132:2131.
10. Bamberger CM, Schulte HM, Chrousos GP. Molecular determinants of glucocorticoid receptor function and tissue sensitivity. Endocr Rev. 1996;17:221.

11. Bamberger CM, Schulte HM, Chrousos GP. Molecular determinants of glucocorticoid receptor function and tissue sensitivity to glucocorticoids. Endocr Rev. 1996;17:245.
12. Barlier A, Jaquet P. Quinagolide-a valuable treatment option for hyperprolactinaemia. Eur J Endocrinol 2006;154:187.
13. Basaria S, et al. Adverse events associated with testosterone administration. N Engl J Med. 2010;363:109.
14. Becker DJ, Kilgore ML, Morrisey MA. The societal burden of osteoporosis. Curr Rheumatol Rep. 2010;12:186.
15. Bikkle DD. Nonclassic actions of vitamin D. J Clin Endocirnol Metabol. 2009;94:26.
16. Biondi B Cooper DS. The clinical significance of subclinical thyroid dysfunction. Endocr Rev. 2008;29:76.
17. Black DM. et al. One year of alendronate after one year of parathyroid hormone (1-84) for osteoporosis. N Engl J Med. 2005;353:555.
18. Bloomgarden ZT. Gut-dervied incretin hormones and new therapeutic approaches. Diabetes care. 2004;27:2554.
19. Carel JC, et al. Consensus statement on the use of gonadotropin-releasing hormone analogs in children. Pediatrics. 2009;123:752.
20. Carter-Su C, Schwartz J, Smit LS. Molecular mechanism of growth hormone action. Annu Rev Physiol. 1996;58:187.
21. Chandraharan E, Arulkumaran S. Acute tocolysis. Curr Opin Obster Gynecol. 2005;17:151.
22. Charmandari E, Kino T. Chrousos syndrome: A seminal report, a phylogenetic enigma and the clinical implications of glucocorticoid signaling changes. Eur J Clin Invest. 2010;40:932.
23. Charmandari E, Tsigos C, Chrousos GP. Neuroendocrinology of stress. Ann Rev Physiol. 2005;67:259.
24. Chrousos GP. Stress and disorders of the stress system. Nat Endocrinol Rev. 2009;5:374.
25. Clines GA, Guise TA. Mechanisms and treatment for bone metastases. Clin Adv Hematol Oncol. 2004;2:295.
26. Colaro A. The prolactinoma. Best Pract Res Clin Endocrinol Metab. 2009;23:575.
27. Cooper DS, et al. The thyroid gland. In: Gardner DG, Shoback D (Eds): Greenspan's Basic Clinical Endocrinology, 9th edn. McGraw-Hill, 2011.
28. Cummings SR, et al. Denosumab for prevention of fractures in postmenopausal women with osteoporosis. N Engl J Med, 2009;361:756.
29. Dutta DC. Textbook of Gynecology. Infertility 6th edn New Delhi. Jaypee Brothers Medical Publishers, pp.230-324.
30. Fitzpatrick DL, Russell MA. Diagnosis and management of thyroid disease in pregnancy. Obstet Gynecol Clin N Am. 2010;37:173.
31. Galli E, Pingitore A, Iervasi G. The role of thyroid hormone in the pathophysiology of heart failure: clinical evidence. Heart fail Rev 2010;15:155.
32. Laurberg P, et al. Iodine intake as a determinant of thyroid disorders in populations. Best Pract Res Clin Endocrinol Metab. 2010;24:13.

CHAPTER 5

Drugs Used for Pregnant Women During Antenatal, Labor and Postnatal Period

Hemlata, Suresh Sharma

TETANUS PROPHYLAXIS

The tetanus toxoid vaccine program for pregnant women was launched in year 1983. The disease tetanus is caused by *Clostridium tetani* bacteria. These bacteria present everywhere including soil and dust which enters to the host via cut or wounds. The toxin release by this bacteria cause muscle spasm and even death. This tetanus is more common among the newborn and pregnant women due to unsterile home deliveries. Tetanus can only be prevented by the vaccination. To prevent this transmission; the tetanus prophylaxis is given to pregnant women.

Mechanism of Action (Fig. 5.1)

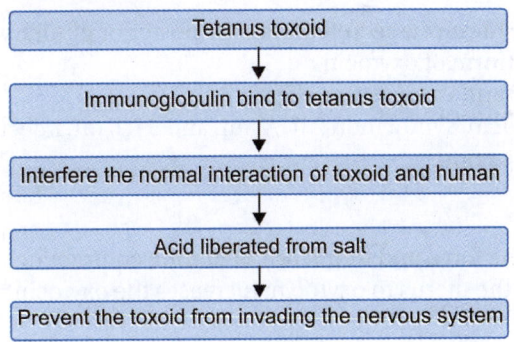

Fig. 5.1: Mechanism of tetanus toxoid vaccine.

Tetanus Prophylaxis

The tetanus prophylaxis among pregnant women provide the protection from tetanus. It is recommended to give 2 doses of TT in pregnant women. Dosage, route and site of tetanus prophylaxis is shown in **Table 5.1**.

Table 5.1: Dosage, route and site of tetanus toxoid.

Vaccine dose	Due age	Dose	Route	Site
Tetanus toxoid-1	Early in pregnancy	0.5 mL	Intramuscular	Upper arm
Tetanus toxoid-2	After 4 weeks of TT-1	0.5 mL	Intramuscular	Upper arm
Tetanus Toxoid-booster	If not received 2 TT doses in pregnancy within the last 3 years	0.5 mL	Intramuscular	Upper arm

Tetanus toxoid vaccine is safe no contraindication and no side effects reported.

IRON AND VITAMIN K1 SUPPLEMENTATION

Anemia is the most common hematological abnormality which occurs during pregnancy. Anemia is the defined as reduction in the erythrocytes concentration or hemoglobin less than 10 g/dL. This occurs due to acute loss of blood, iron deficiency and increase requirement of iron in pregnancy. This iron deficiency fails to maintain the normal and result in maternal and fetal complications. The recommended daily dietary allowance (RDA) of iron during pregnancy is 27 mg. This requirement is fulfilled by giving the iron supplementation during pregnancy. The Centers for Disease Control and Prevention (CDC) recommends providing the low-dose iron supplement to all pregnant women at the first prenatal visit. The deficiency of folic acid is prevented by giving folic acid tablets with iron supplement **(Table 5.2)**.

Vitamin K1 (Phytonadione)

Vitamin K1 is a fat-soluble vitamin help in coagulation. This immunization is recommended in the newborn at birth. Newborn are at risk of bleeding die to immature liver cell which need supplement to prevent the risk of bleeding **(Table 5.3)**.

OXYTOCIN, MISOPROSTOL

Oxytocin

- Oxytocin is a peptide hormone secreted from the posterior pituitary along with vasopressin
- Pitocin is a synthetic form of oxytocin
- Also has antidiuretic and vasopressor effect
- **Formulations:** Oxytocin/syntocinon 2 IU/2 mL and 5 IU/mL injection **(Table 5.4)**.
- Pitocin 5 IU/1 mL injection

Action

- Oxytocin increases the force and frequency of uterine contractions
- Estrogens sensitizes the uterus to oxytocin; increases the oxytocin receptors

Table 5.2: Recommended iron and folic acid supplementation in pregnant mother and lactating women.

Supplement	Composition/dose	Frequency	Duration	Side effects
Iron and folic acid	Iron—100 mg elemental iron Folic acid—500 µg (0.5 mg)	1 tab daily OD	For first 100 days and at 14–16 week Followed by 100 days of postpartum	Constipation Diarrhea Bloating Dry mouth

Table 5.3: Dose, route, frequency and site of vitamin K1 supplement.

Vitamin K	dose	Route	Frequency	Site
Vitamin K1 (Phytonadione)	Birth weight 1000 g or more : 1 mg less than 1000 g : 0.5 mg	Intramuscular	Soon after delivering by ensuring skin-to-skin contact with mother Not less than 24 hours of birth	Antero-lateral aspect of thigh

Table 5.4: Oxytocin with doses and routes of administration.

Trade name	Action	Dose and route
Oxytocin (Pitocin)	Tonic contractions	*Induction of labor:* 10–20 units in 1 L of IV fluids *Postpartum:* 10–20 units in IV bag or IM *Intranasal:* to promote milk ejection reflex
Desamino-oxytocin	Buccal formulation	*Induction of labor:* 50 IU buccal tb repeated 30 minutes maximum dose is 10 tb (500 IU) *Uterine inertia:* 25 IU every 30 minutes *Lactation:* 25–50 IU before feeding

- Non-pregnant uterus and that during early pregnancy is rather resistant to oxytocin; sensitivity increases in third trimester; there is sharp increase near term and quick fall during puerperium.
- The increased contractility is restricted to the fundus and body; lower segment is not contracted, may even relax at term.

Mechanism of Action

- Oxytocin receptors acts on specific G-protein coupled oxytocin receptors, which mediate the response mainly by depolarization of muscle fiber and influx of Ca^{2+} ions as well as through phosphoinositide hydrolysis and IP mediated intracellular release of Ca^{2+} ion
- **(A comprehensive review may be obtained from the Chapter 4 Page No. 129)**
- Oxytocin also increase prostaglandin synthesis and release by the endometrium, which may contribute to contractile response.

Pharmacokinetics

- Inactive orally
- **Onset of action:** Uterine contractions
  - IM 3–5 minutes
  - IV 1 minute.
- **Duration:** IM—2–3 hour; IV: 1 hour
- **Metabolism:** Rapidly hepatic and via plasma (by oxytocinase) and to a smaller degree, the mammary gland
- **Half-life elimination:** 1–5 minutes
- **Excretion:** Urine.

Indications (Fig. 5.2)

Therapeutic Indication

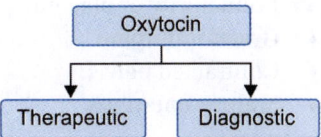

Fig. 5.2: Types of indication of oxytocin.

1. Induction and augmentation of labor

It increases both amplitude and frequency of uterine contractions. Labor needs to be induced in case of postmaturity or prematurely in toxemia of pregnancy, diabetic mother, ruptured membranes or placental insufficiency.

2. Active management of third Stage labor (AMTSL)

It is used during the third stage of labor (Placenta expulsion stage). It is recommended to administer 10 IU (2 mL) oxytocin intramuscularly for the management of third stage. It helps in the separation of placenta from uterine wall.

3. Early pregnancy abortion
For accelerating the abortion, oxytocin is used while performing dilatation and curettage procedure

4. Uterine inertia
When uterine contractions are feeble and labor is not progressing.

5. Postpartum hemorrhage/Cesarean section
Acts forcefully by contracting uterine muscles which further compresses the blood vessels to arrest hemorrhage. Also it help in promotion of involution of uterus in postpartum period.

6. Breast engorgement
It may occur due to insufficient milk ejection reflex—intranasal may be given few minutes before suckling. It causes induction of smooth muscle contractions in lactating breast, leading to let down reflex. Induce abortion and or facilitate removal of uterine contents after miscarriage.

Diagnostic Indication

Contraction stress test (CST)
This test is performed to assess whether the fetus can sustain the stress of the labor. In this oxytocin infusion (1 mIU/mL) is started and monitor the fetal heart rate (FHR). If there is an alteration of FHR, it suggest of fetal hypoxia.

Oxytocin sensitivity test (OST)
This test is used to assess the responsiveness of injection oxytocin. The initial dose is 0.01 units/min given intravenously to induce uterine contraction. If no contraction begins after 4 attempts, it suggest of irresponsive uterus.

Contraindications
- Hypersensitivity
- Unfavorable fetal position or presentation that are undeliverable
- Fetal distress
- Uterine scar (previous surgery of uterus or cervix including CS)
- Hypertonic or hyperactive uterus
- Prematurity or placenta previa
- Grand multipara
- Contracted pelvis
- Malpresentations

Side effects
- **CV**: Tachycardia, hypotension, dysrhythmias
- **CNS**: Maternal seizures, feeling faint or lightheadedness fetal (ICH), hypoxia, trauma, bradycardia and dysrhythmias
- **F and E**: Hyponatremia
- **GI**: Nausea and vomiting
- **Other**: Hypersensitivity
- **Genitourinary**: Impaired uterine blood flow, pelvic hematoma, tetanic uterine contractions, uterine rupture, postpartum hemorrhage

Adverse effects
- Uterine tetany leading to fetal demise
- Uterine rupture has been documented with over dosage, i.e., hyperstimulation
- Newborns exposed to oxytocin in utero have higher incidence of hyperbilirubinemia
- Prolonged use can cause water intoxication due to antidiuresis

Nursing responsibilities
- Assess character, frequency and duration of contractions frequently throughout administration and postpartum
- Monitor maternal vital signs frequently throughout administration
- Use fetal monitoring and assess FHR continuously throughout administration
- Monitor maternal electrolytes
- Monitor Intake/output chart
- Monitor for symptoms of water intoxication, such as anuria, headache, drowsiness and confusion
- Have Mg sulfate available, if needed to treat severe contractions
- Notify healthcare provider, if symptoms of fetal disstress occur
- Massage the injection site after deep injection of oxytocin into deltoid muscle to assist quick absorption
- Do not increase rate of oxytocin once the desired contraction pattern is achieved (contraction frequency of 2-3 minutes lasting 60 second)

Patient education
- Explain to client the indication for administration
- Prepare client for the route of administration and possible side effects
- Instruct client to report sudden headache

Misoprostol

Misoprostol is a methyl ester of prostaglandin E1. It is synthetic prostaglandin used in the induction of labor and abortion as it is rapidly absorbed. It is more effective than oxytocin and prostaglandin E2. It is also used as NSAIDs (details are discussed in Chapter 3, Volume 2).

Indications and Dosage (Table 5.5)

Risk

- Tachysystole (hyperstimulation of uterus)
- Fetal heart increase and meconium can be passed by fetus
- Rupture of uterus but, rare

Table 5.5: Indications and dosage of misoprostol.

Indication	Dosage
Cervical repining	25–50 µg vaginally every 3–4 hourly
Induction of labor	25–50 µg orally (Buccal)
Second trimester medical termination of pregnancy (MTP)	400 µg vaginally 3–4 hourly
Prevention and management of PPH	600–800 µg per rectal

ERGOMETRINE

Ergot Derivatives

These alkaloids are produced by fungus, which affects the cereal crops:
- **Ergotoxine**—has an alpha adrenergic blocking activity and an antihypertensive, and cerebral vasodilator
- **Ergotamine, dihydroergotamine**—used in acute attack of migraine
- **Methysergide**—it is mainly anti 5-HT; used for migraine prophylaxis
- **Bromocriptine**—is a dopaminergic agonists, used for Parkinsonism
- **Ergometrine**—is an oxytocic, used to prevent postpartum hemorrhage

Ergometrine and its Analogue (Table 5.6)

- Ergometrine and its derivatives are more potent and has a selective action on uterus
- **Small doses:** Rhythmic uterine contraction and relaxation
- **Larger doses:** Substantial, prolonged contractions

Mechanism of Action

- Ergot alkaloids significantly increase the motor activity of the uterus
- It affects primarily uterine smooth muscles producing sustained contractions and thereby shortens the third stage of labor.
- **Stimulant action:** Involves serotonergic, alpha-adrenergic receptor
- Uterine sensitivity changes during pregnancy (possibly due to progressively increasing numbers of $a1$ receptors
- After small doses contractions are increased in force or frequency, or both, but are followed by a normal degree of relaxation.

As the dose is increased, contractions become more forceful and prolonged, resting tonus is markedly increased, and sustained contracture can result.

For more details *see* **Chapter 4, Page No. 130.**

Indications

Therapeutic	Prophylactic
• Atonic postpartum hemorrhage • Inevitable abortion • Expulsion of hydatidiform mole pregnancy • Medical termination of pregnancy	• AMTSL (Active Management of Third Stage Labor) in case of excessive bleeding

Table 5.6: Ergot derivative preparations along with doses.

Drug	Dose
Ergometrine	0.25, 0.5 mg tablet 0.5 mg/mL injection
Methylergometrine Methergin, metherone, ergomet	0.125 mg tablet 0.2 mg/mL injection

Contraindications
- Hypersensitivity
- Heart disease
- Severe pre-eclampsia and eclampsia
- Caution in patients with hypertension, vascular disease, presence of sepsis—may cause gangrene, liver and kidney disease

Side Effects
- Increase in BP
- Hour glass contraction of uterus
- Nausea and vomiting
- Uterine cramping
- Decreased milk production

Adverse Effects
- Weakness
- Muscle pain
- Insensitivity to cold
- Paresthesia of extremities

Pharmacokinetics
- Rapidly and completely absorbed orally
- Onset of action—oral (15 minutes), IV (almost immediate)
- Metabolized in liver
- Excreted in urine
- Plasma t½ is 1–2 hours
- Duration of action—3–4 hours

Nursing Responsibilities and Patient Education
- Closely monitor lochia and BP after administration
- Explain indication for administration to client
- Prepare clients for route of administration and possible side effects, such as cramping
- Instruct client to report excessive blood loss
- Instruct client not to smoke because of increased/additive vasoconstrictor with ergonovine use

METHYL PROSTAGLANDIN E2 ALPHA

Prostaglandins
Prostaglandins are biologically active derivatives of 20 carbon atom polyunsaturated fatty acids that are released from cell membrane phospholipids:
- PGE2—its synthetic analogue dinoprostone
- PGF2—its synthetic analogue carboprost
- The PGF2 released from decidua (endometrium during pregnancy), PGE_2 from fetal membrane (Amnion) and PGI_2 from myometrium of uterus

- These are used as uterine stimulants especially in latter part of pregnancy and to cause ripening of cervix.

Types

The following is a comparison of different types of prostaglandin **(Table 5.7)**, prostacyclin I_2 (PGI_2), prostaglandin E_2 (PGE_2), and prostaglandin F_{2a} (PGF_{2b}).

Classification

The classification of prostaglandin E_2 has been given in **Table 5.8** along with its doses, routes of administration and indications.

Mechanism of Action

- The PGs uniformly contract human uterus, pregnant as well as non-pregnant
- Sensitivity is higher during pregnancy and also increase with progress of pregnancy

Table 5.7: Types of prostaglandins.

Type	Receptor	Receptor type	Function
PGI_2	IP	G_s	• Vasodilation • Inhibit platelet aggregation • Bronchodilation
PGe_2	EP_1	G_q	• Bronchoconstriction • GI tract smooth muscle contraction
	EP_2	G_s	• Bronchodilation • GI tract smooth muscle relaxation • Vasodilation
	EP_3	G_i	• Decrease gastric acid secretion • Increased gastric mucus secretion • Uterus contraction (when pregnant) • GI tract smooth muscle contraction • Lipolysis inhibition • Increased autonomic neurotransmitters • Increased platelet response to their agonists and • Increased atherothrombosis in vivo
	Unspecified		• Hyperalgesia • Pyrogenic
$PGF_{2\alpha}$	FP	G_q	• Uterus contraction • Bronchoconstriction

Table 5.8: Classification of prostaglandins.

Category	Generic name	Dose and route	Indications
Prostaglandin E2	Dinoprostone Prepidil, Cervidil	Intracervical gel—0.5 mg vaginal insert—10 mg	Ripening of cervix
Prostaglandin F2	Carboprost Hemabate	250 µg IM may repeat at 50–90 min intervals as needed up to 2 mg	Postpartum hemorrhage (PPH)

- The PGs increase tone as well as amplitude of uterine contractions
- At term, PGs at low doses soften the cervix and make it more compliant

Indications

- Abortion—uterine contractions are provoked and the conceptus is expelled within next few hours
- Induction and augmentation of labor
- Cervical ripening—good results in case of unfavorable cervix
- PPH

Contraindications

- Use with caution in HTN and with the history of asthma
- Acute pelvic inflammatory disease
- History of pelvic surgery

Clinical Uses

- Synthetic prostaglandins are used
- To induce childbirth or abortion (PGE2 or PGF2, with/without mifepristone, a progesterone antagonist)
- To prevent closure of patent ductus arteriosus in newborns with particular cyanotic heart defects (PGE1)
- To prevent and treat peptic ulcers (PGE)
- As a vasodilator in severe Raynaud's phenomenon or ischemia of a limb in pulmonary hypertension
- In treatment of glaucoma (as in bimatoprost ophthalmic solution, a synthetic prostamide analog with ocular hypotensive activity)
- To treat erectile dysfunction or in penile rehabilitation following surgery (PGE1 as alprostadil)
- As an ingredient in eyelash and eyebrow growth beauty products due to side effects associated with increased hair growth

Side Effects

- Diarrhea, nausea, vomiting
- Uterine cramping
- Tension headache
- Flushing, cardiac dysrhythmias
- Fever and malaise
- Chest pain

Adverse Effects

- HTN
- Uterine tetany
- Uterine rupture

Nursing Responsibilities

- **Prenatal:** Follow manufacturer's instructions for placement of medication; client must remain recumbent for up to 20–30 minutes after administration, and have fetal monitoring during this time.
- **Postpartum:** Monitor lochia and BP, be prepared for clients to develop diarrhea.

Patient Education

- **Prenatal:** Client should report long or continuous contractions, as uterine tetany may develop; client should count fetal movements as an indicator of fetal well-being
- **Postpartum:** Prepare client for route of administration and possible side effects.

MAGNESIUM SULFATE

- It is neither a specific antihypertensive nor an anticonvulsant, controls convulsions and reduce BP in patients of preeclampsia.
- The $MgSO_4$ is usually preferred over B2 agonists inpatients having cardiac problems, diabetes, hypertension and hyperthyroidism
- When given parentally, it acts as CNS depressant and also depresses smooth, skeletal and cardiac muscle function
- Used to arrest preterm labor and to prevent or treat seizures with pre-eclampsia and eclampsia
- It is used in conjunction with B-adrenergics, which increases risk of pulmonary edema.
- It is used in the case of eclampsia during pregnancy.

Indication

- Severe pre-eclampsia
- Management of eclampsia

Available form

Each ampule of 2 mL contains 1 g of $MgSo_4$. It is available in 50% w/v strength.

Dose and Regimen (Table 5.9)

Table 5.9: Dose and regimen of magnesium sulfate.

Regimen	Dosage
Pritchard method	*Loading dose:* 4 g (20% Solution) IV over 5 min and 5 g IM (50%) buttock *Maintenance dose:* 5 g every 4 hourly into alternate buttock
Dhaka method	*Loading dose:* 4 g slow IV over 15 min 3 g IM (50%) in each buttock *Maintenance dose:* 2.5 g IM in alternate buttock till 24 hours of first dose
Zuspan method	*Loading dose:* 4 g (20% solution) IV over 5–10 min *Maintenance dose:* 1 g per hour IV infusion
Sibai method	*Loading dose:* 4–6 g over 15–20 min in 100 mL NS *Maintenance dose:* 2 g per hour IV infusion

Contraindication

Myasthenia gravis

Side Effects

- Flushed warm feeling
- Drowsiness
- Decreased deep tendon reflexes
- Decreased hand grasp strength
- Fluid and electrolyte imbalance
- Hyponatremia
- Nausea and vomiting

Toxicity

- Depression of patellar reflex
- Respiratory depression in neonate and mother
- **Antidot:** Calcium gluconate
- In case of toxicity, injection calcium gluconate 10% 10 mL IV is recommended.

Nursing Responsibilities

- Check patellar reflex prior to dose
- Monitor hand grasp, deep tendon reflexes, and serum levels
- Monitor IV site closely to avoid extravasation
- Monitor vital signs (Blood pressure) and take accurate daily weight

Patient Education

- Educate client about side effects of medication
- Advise client to report side effects of preeclampsia including headache, epigastric pain and visual disturbance
- Instruct family to report any signs of confusion

CALCIUM GLUCONATE

Calcium gluconate is a calcium salt, used as a medicine to manage hypocalcemia, cardiotoxicity due to hyperkalemia and hypermagnesemia. In pregnancy, it is used as a antidote of magnesium sulfate. In case of hypermagnesemia, which occur as a toxicity of magnesium sulfate given during the prevention and treatment of eclampsia. It work as a antagonism of magnesium site of action.

Indication

- Toxicity of magnesium sulfate
- Hypocalcemia
- Hyperkalemia
- Hypermagnesemia

Available Form

- Each ampule contain 100 mg/mL of calcium of Calcium gluconate
- 1 mL of 10% calcium gluconate contains 9.3 mg of elemental calcium
- Available in 1 mL ampule and 10 mL vial

Dosage

- In case of cardiac arrest, calcium gluconate 10% 15–30 mL IV over 2–3 min
- In case of toxicity of $MgSO_4$ (treatment of eclampsia), calcium gluconate 10% 10 mL IV over 2–3 min
- In case of hypermagnesemia due to renal impairment, calcium gluconate 1–2 g (10–20 mL) over 5–10 min

Contraindications

- Hypercalcemia
- Hypersensitivity
- Sarcoidosis
- Hypophosphatemia

Side Effects

- Syncope
- Bradycardia
- Paresthesia
- Extravasation
- Necrosis

Toxicity

- Extravasation injury can cause necrosis
- Fatigue
- ECG changes with short QT interval
- Muscle weakness
- Polydipsia

Nursing Responsibilities

- Check for hypersensitivity and other contraindication
- Monitor serum calcium level before administering and during infusion every 1–4 hourly
- Monitor IV site closely to avoid extravasation
- Check the ECG for any changes

MULTIPLE CHOICE QUESTIONS

1. What is the recommended dose of tetanus toxoid in pregnancy?
   a. 0.1 mL
   b. 0.5 mL
   c. 1 mL
   d. 0.25 mL

2. **Recommended dose of iron and folic acid in pregnancy:**
   a. Iron 100 mg elemental iron and folic acid 500 µg
   b. Iron 500 mg elemental iron and folic acid 50 µg
   c. Iron 250 mg elemental iron and folic acid 100 µg
   d. Iron 100 mg elemental iron and folic acid 250 µg
3. **Oxytocin is contraindicated in:**
   a. Induction of labor
   b. Uterine inertia
   c. Postpartum hemorrhage
   d. Placenta previa
4. **Action of ergot derivates:**
   a. Induces tonic contractions
   b. Depolarize muscle fibers
   c. Increases motor activity of uterus
   d. Induce abortion
5. **Antidote of magnesium sulphate:**
   a. Calcium gluconate
   b. Protamine sulfate
   c. Potassium hydrochloride
   d. N-acetylcysteine

Answer Key

1. b   2. a   3. d   4. c   5. a

FURTHER READING

1. American Academy of Pediatrics Committee on Nutrition. Vitamin K compounds and the water soluble analogues. Pediatrics. 1961;28:7.
2. Bellad A, Kapil R, Gupta A. National Guidelines for Prevention and Control of Iron Deficiency Anemia in India. Indian J Comm Health. 2017;30,1:89-94.
3. Chakraborty A, Can AS. Calcium gluconate. Treasure Island (FL): StatPearls Publishing;2022.
4. National Health Mission. Ministry of Health and Family Welfare GoI. Operational Guidelines for Injection Vitamin K prophylaxis at birth (in Facilities). 2014; Pg 3-4.
5. Park K. Epidemiology of communicable diseases. In: Park JE (Ed). Park's Textbook of Preventive and Social medicine. Jabalpur, India: Banarsidas Bhanot Publishers. 2014;21:154-5.
6. Pritchard IA, et al. The Parkland Memorial Hospital Protocol for Treatment of Eclampsia: Evaluation of 245 cases. American Journal of Obstetrics and Gynecology. 1984;48:95.
7. Tandon R, Jain A, Malhotra P. Management of Iron Deficiency Anemia in Pregnancy in India. Indian journal of hematology & blood transfusion: an official journal of Indian Society of Hematology and Blood Transfusion. 2018;34(2),204–15. https://doi.org/10.1007/s12288-018-0949-6
8. World Health organization (WHO) Expanded Programme on Immunization. Tetanus Neonatal Tetanus (NT): 2015. Available from: http://www.wpro.who.int/immunization/factsheets/tetanus_nt/en/.

CHAPTER 6

Miscellaneous Drugs

Vasantha Kalyani, Hemlata, Suresh Sharma

DRUGS USED FOR DEADDICTION

Many drugs are habit forming or addictive. A person has control over his/her choice to start using drugs, but once started, the pleasurable effect of drugs makes one want to keep reusing. Drug addiction is a condition characterized by compulsiveness for drug, abuse of drug, and long-lasting chemical changes in the brain. The addict is dependent on a substance, which is harmful or dangerous for physical and/or mental health, social and economic well- being. De-addiction includes assessment, pharmacological treatment, individual and family counseling, psychotherapy, follow up and rehabilitation. Medications are used to control withdrawal, detoxification, and relief of symptoms, reduce craving for drug and produce aversion.

Disulfiram Aversion Therapy

Disulfiram (Trade Name: Antabuse) inhibits the enzyme aldehyde dehydrogenase or alcohol antagonist drug. If alcohol is taken after disulfiram, acetaldehyde concentration in the body increases producing symptoms like, headache, burning sensation, flushing, perspiration, heaviness in the chest, dizziness, vomiting, confusion, hypotension, circulatory collapse, severe anxiety, etc. So this therapy is given only for patients who are well motivated to leave the habit of alcoholism.

The effect lasts for 7–14 days after stopping disulfiram. The reactions can sometimes be very severe and therefore treatment should be given in a hospital. Sensitization to alcohol develops after 2–3 hours after first dose and lasts for 2 weeks after stopping the drug. It is contraindicated in patients with liver disease, cardiac failure, coronary artery disease and history of cerebrovascular accident, hypertension, psychoses, pregnancy and breastfeeding and patients physically dependent on alcohol. Disulfiram has psychotic reaction with metronidazole and inhibit the metabolism of tricyclic antidepressants, phenytoin and benzodiazepines.

Available form: Tablet of dose 200 mg/500 mg.

Note: Disulfram should be given after assuring that person has not consumed alcohol in past 12 hours. Common drugs used in de-addiction are given in **Table 6.1**.

DRUGS USED IN CPR AND EMERGENCY

Drugs Used in Emergencies

The term emergency care refers to management of patients with urgent and critical needs. But in reality emergencies include all the conditions the patient and the family consider as emergency. Emergency department is a challenging environment for patients, families and medical personnel. Large number of people seeks emergency care every day. The common emergencies include acute coronary syndrome, other cardiac conditions, trauma, anaphylaxis,

Table 6.1: Common drugs used in de-addiction.

Drug	Indications	Dose	Action
Diazepam	• Sedation in alcohol and benzodiazepine withdrawal • Detoxification for other drugs such as amphetamines, cocaine and benzodiazepines	5–10 mg	• Long acting benzodiazepine • Anti-anxiety and produce sedation and amnesia • Muscle relaxant
Lorazepam	Alcohol detoxification with suspected liver dysfunction	1–2 mg	• Short acting benzodiazepine • Causes sedation and amnesia • Anti-anxiety
Buprenorphine	• Opioid withdrawal and detoxification • Long lasting pain—cancer pain	4–16 mg daily	• Suppress some withdrawal symptoms • Opioid—antagonist
Clonidine	• Opioid withdrawal and detoxification • Facilitate in smoking cessation	0.1–0.2 mg every 4 hours, for 10 days; the dose is tapered	• Alpha-2 agonist; reduces symptoms of sympathetic overactivity like tremors and tachycardia • Central sympatholytics • Suppress some of the autonomic withdrawal symptoms like anxiety, nausea, vomiting and diarrhea
Methadone	• Adjunct in treatment of opioid dependence • Analgesic as morphine	10–40 mg daily, increased by up to 10 mg daily (maximum 30 mg weekly); usual dose 60–120 mg daily	• Synthetic opioid • Methadone is effective orally and by this route no 'kick' is experienced • More potent, long-acting and prevents withdrawal symptoms because it is slowly released from the tissues
Thiamine	Alcoholism (thiamine deficiency occurs with alcoholism)	100–150 mg/day	Water soluble—vitamin B_1
Nicotine chewing gums	Severe tobacco withdrawal symptoms	–	Similar to nicotine in tobacco, but less effect
Disulfiram	Adjunct in the treatment of chronic alcohol dependence	Tablet 250 mg 0.75–0.25 g daily	Aldehyde dehydrogenase inhibitor

shock, hypoglycemia, poisoning, etc. For prompt management of the emergency condition Crash Cart is used. The purpose of the Crash cart is to provide all emergency drug at one place. The drugs commonly used in emergency and critical care is presented in **Table 6.2**.

Table 6.2: Common emergency/critical care drugs.

Classification	Drugs	Indications	Dose and administration
Cardiac stimulant	Adrenaline (Epinephrine)	Ventricular fibrillation; pulseless ventricular tachycardia	*Available form:* 1 mg/1 mL (1:1,000) is given every 3 minutes intravenously *Adult dosage:* 1 mg in 9 mL normal saline (1 mg/10 mL) *Pediatric dosage:* 0.01 mg/kg (10 μg/kg) in normal saline (up to 5 mL)
		Anaphylaxis	Adrenaline is given every 5 minutes intramuscularly (IM) until clinical features have improved. Up to 10 doses may be given *Adult dosage:* 0.5 mg *Pediatric dosage:* 0.01 mg/kg (10 μg/kg) in adults, if there is a poor response, consider glucagon 1–2 mg intravenously (IV) over 5 minutes IV adrenaline if shock persists after two IM doses
Injectable anesthetic	Lignocaine	Ventricular fibrillation; pulseless ventricular tachycardia	1 mg/kg
Anticholinergics	Atropine	Asystole or severe bradycardia	1.2–3.0 mg (adult); 20 μg/kg (child)
Oxygen	Oxygen	Asthma and bronchospasm	8 L/min (controlled oxygen therapy in cases of acute exacerbations of chronic obstructive pulmonary disease—oxygen at 2 L/min via nasal prongs)
		Acute coronary syndrome (coronary artery disease, myocardial infarction, angina)	8 L/min
		Acute pulmonary edema	8 L/min
		Status epilepticus	8 L/min
Adrenergic	Inj. Dopamine	Shock—cardiogenic, hypovolemic and septic shock	Dose—5 mL–200 mg 2–10 μg/kg body weight
Opioid antagonist	Pentazocine (Fortwin)	Postoperative and chronic pain	Dose–1mL–30 mg 50–100 mg oral; 30–60 mg IM

Contd...

Contd...

Classification	Drugs	Indications	Dose and administration
Calcium channel blocker	Verapamil	Supraventricular tachycardia, atrial flutter, fibrillation, hypertrophic cardiomyopathy	*Dose:* 2 mL–5mg 120–240 mg daily in divided doses or sustained release form intravenous dosage. 2.5–5 mg. Slow IV bolus up to 10 mg
	Nifedipine	Angina pectoris, systemic hypertension, Raynaud's phenomenon	*Dose:* 5 mg, 10 mg, 20 mg tablets 30 mg once daily
Anti-hypertensive and anti-convulsant	$MgSO_4$	Prevention of seizures in preeclampsia and management of eclampsia	4 g over 5–15 minutes IV, followed by IV infusion, 1 g/ hour for at least 24 hours after the last seizure or delivery (whichever occurs later) or by deep intramuscular injection 5 g into each buttock then 5 g every 4 hours into alternate buttocks for at least 24 hours after the last seizure or delivery (whichever occurs later)
Anti-anginal	Nitroglycerin	Acute myocardial infarction, unstable angina, refractory angina, coronary artery spasm, pulmonary edema following LVF, infarct limitation, intraoperative hypertension	The drug is diluted in normal saline (5 mg/500 mL) and administered as a constant infusion; started at a small dose at 5 µg/kg/min and increased gradually
	Sorbitrate	Chronic angina pectoris, prevention of acute episodes of angina	10–30 mg three times a day
Benzodiazepines	Lorazepam	Status epilepticus, anxiety or insomnia	*Status epilepticus:* 0.1 mg/kg Anxiety 1–6 mg od in divided doses; Elderly start at 1–2 mg/day in divided doses; insomnia associated with anxiety 1–2 mg HS (Bedtime) parenteral; IM or IV injection into a large vein
	Diazepam	Status epilepticus rectally in febrile convulsions	*Adult dosage:* 5–10 mg IV or 10–20 mg per rectum (dilute with 5 mL of saline) *Pediatric:* Diazepam IV 10 mg/2 mL, 0.04 mL/kg Diazepam per rectum 10 mg/2 mL, 0.10 mL/kg
	Midazolam	IV anesthesia, sedation of intubated and mechanically ventilated patients Epilepsy	*Adult dosage:* 5–10 mg IM or 2.5–5.0 mg IV *Pediatric dosage:* 0.2 mg/kg IM or 0.1 mg/kg IV (dose can be repeated after 15 minutes if there is persistent or recurrent convulsion)

Contd...

Contd...

Classification	Drugs	Indications	Dose and administration
Rehydration therapy	Dextrose	Hypoglycemia, maintenance fluid in newborn, fluid replacement without significant electrolyte deficit, management of hyperkalemia	*Dose:* 5%; 10% isotonic solutions of 500 mL bottles. 10% and 20% solutions 1,000 mL for parenteral nutrition, 25%, 50% hypertonic solutions as 25 mL ampules 25% dextrose 2 mL/kg with insulin for correction of hyperkalemia
	Normal saline	Anaphylactic shock, hypovolemia	20 mL/kg
Antacid	Inj. sodium bicarbonate	Alkalinize the urine in poisoning	1–2 mg/kg/h IV infusion needed to maintain urine pH between 7.5 and 8.5
		Metabolic acidosis	*Dose:* 7.5% Conc-25 mL or 1–2 mg/kg/hr IV infusion
Corticosteroids	Hydrocortisone	Anaphylaxis	250 mg (4 mg/kg), single dose IV
		Asthma and bronchospasm	*Adult:* 250 mg (4 mg/kg) IV *Pediatric:* 4 mg/kg IV
Bronchodilators	Salbutamol nebulization	Asthma and bronchospasm	*Adult:* 10 mg by oxygen, 8 L/min every 15 minutes *Pediatric:* 5 mg/2.5 mL by oxygen, 8 L/min
	Ipratropium	Asthma and bronchospasm	*Adult:* Nebulization 500 µg 2 hourly *Pediatric:* 20 µg/dose metered dose inhaler (MDI) via spacer, 2–4 puffs every 20 minutes in 1st hour
NSAIDs—salicylates	Aspirin	Acute coronary syndrome (coronary artery disease, myocardial infarction, angina)	300 mg orally
Vasodilators	Glyceryl trinitrate (GTN) spray	Acute coronary syndrome (coronary artery disease, myocardial infarction, angina) Acute pulmonary edema	1 dose repeated after 5 minutes if no improvement
Opioids	Morphine	Acute coronary syndrome (coronary artery disease, myocardial infarction, angina)	2.5 mg IV every 5 minutes as required, maximum of 15 mg
		Acute pulmonary edema	2.5 mg IV
Loop diuretics	Frusemide	Acute pulmonary edema	20 – 40 mg IV

LASA drugs: Look alike and sound like:
- Dopamine and dobutamine
- Adenosine and adrenaline
- Morphine and pethidine
- Adrenaline and atropine

Nursing Responsibilities
- Rapid response of the emergency situation with full awareness of LASA Drugs.
- Always ensure safety of patient, must follow 6 rights of medication administration, i.e. calling out loudly while administering.
- Must ensure the Crash Cart is fully equipped with the drugs and other inventory.

IV FLUIDS AND ELECTROLYTE REPLACEMENT

Intravenous fluid and electrolyte imbalance occur due to many conditions like diarrhea, vomiting, wasting, trauma or bleeding, accidents, etc. The IV fluid replacement aims to restore the circulatory volume and correct electrolyte imbalance. The replacement therapy occurs due to different means of fluid transport: Diffusion, osmosis, filteration and active transport. The fluid and electrolyte is already discussed in details in Vol. 1.

These fluid replacement therapies include three different types of IV fluids:
1. Crystalloids
2. Colloids
3. Blood and blood products

Crystalloids (Table 6.3)

The crystalloids are discussed in Chapter 3 (Volume1). Based on the osmolality it is broadly divided as:
1. Isotonic solution like ringer lactate, dextrose 5 % in water (D5W) and normal saline
2. Hypotonic solution like 0.45% normal saline
3. Hypertonic solution like dextrose 5 % in normal saline

Colloids (Table 6.4)

The colloids contain solute in the protein form. It cannot cross the wall of capillaries and remain in the blood vessel for longer time. This mechanism increases the intravascular volume. These includes albumin, dextran, hetastarch and mannitol.

Blood and Blood Products

Blood transfusion of blood and blood products help in the replacement of the fluid and electrolytes. These blood and its products includes transfusion of plasma, red blood cells, white blood cells and platelets.

COMMON POISONS, DRUGS USED FOR TREATMENT OF POISONING

Management of Common Poisoning

A poison may be defined as any substance, which if administered or comes in contact with a living being produces ill-health, disease or death. Every drug in a high dose can cause

Table 6.3: Types of crystalloids and its usage.

Types of crystalloid	IV solution	Usage	Nursing responsibilities
Isotonic	Normal saline (0.9% sodium chloride)	• Shock • Blood transfusion • Diabetic ketoacidosis (DKA) • Resuscitation • Hyponatremia	• Monitor the fluid flow rate to prevent overload • Use with caution among patients with edema and heart failure
	Ringer lactate (Hartmann's)	• Burns • Acute blood loss • Hypovolemia • Dehydration • Lower GI fluid loss	• Check the contraindication of RL, as it should be avoided among patients with renal failure, liver disease • Check the lab values of serum potassium before administering
	Dextrose 5% in water (D5W)	Fluid loss Dehydration Hypernatremia	• Check for the sign of hyperglycemia or osmotic diuresis • Monitor the fluid flow to prevent overload
Hypotonic	½ Normal saline (0.45% sodium chloride)	• Water replacement in case of vomiting • Diabetic ketoacidosis (DKA)	• Monitor the fluid flow to prevent overload • Check the contraindication, as it should be avoided among patients with, liver disease • Use with cause, as it can raise Intracranial pressure
Hypertonic	Dextrose 5% in NS	Diabetic ketoacidosis (DKA)	Administer when blood sugar is less than 250 mg/dL
	Dextrose 5% in ½ NS	Temporary treatment in case of shock	Check the contraindication, as it should be avoided among patients with cardiac and renal disease.
	Dextrose 10% in water	Fluid replacement	Monitor the blood sugar levels

poisoning. Poisoning could be accidental, suicidal or homicidal. Millions of poisoning cases are seen every year with several hundred dying, but several more are unreported. Mortality rate varies from country to country. In India, it is around 35%, while in America, it is 2%. When treated on time with appropriate drugs, treatment of poisoning can be successful. Drugs causing poisoning, their signs/symptoms and their management are given in **Table 6.5**.

Treatment of Snake Bite

There are more than 3,000 species of snakes in the world of which about 216 are found in India and out of them about 52 types of the snakes in India are poisonous. Vipers, cobras and kraits are the common poisonous snakes.

In all cases of snake bite, the patient is in great fear and is in a stage of neurogenic shock. The patient is in a semiconscious state with cold, clammy skin, feeble pulse, rapid and shallow

Table 6.4: Types of colloids and its usage.

Type of colloid	Mechanism of action	Indications	Nursing responsibilities
Albumin	It is a plasma protein, keep fluid in blood vessel and maintain blood volume	• Protein replacement in case of nephritic syndrome • Treatment of shock • Therapeutic plasma exchange	• Monitor the fluid flow to prevent overload • Monitor the patient for sign of anaphylaxis
Dextran	It is polysaccharides which shift the fluid into vessel and cause vascular expansion.	• Hypovolemia results from trauma, burn • Pulmonary embolism	• Monitor the fluid flow to prevent overload • Check for hypersensitivity • Rule out the contraindication before administering, i.e., bleeding disorder, renal failure and CHF
Hetastarch (HES)	It is a synthetic starch which shift the fluid into vessel and cause vascular expansion	• Hypovolemia • Leukapheresis	• Check for hypersensitivity • It increases the risk of bleeding
Mannitol	It is alcohol sugar cause oliguric diuresis.	• Eliminate toxins • Cerebral edema • Acute renal failure	• Monitor the fluid flow to prevent overload • Must perform neurologic assessment

breathing. Other symptoms vary according to the type of snake. The signs and symptoms of systemic toxicity appear in about half an hour.
- **Elapid bite (cobra, krait, etc.—neurotoxic):** Local reactions are pain, burning, swelling, discoloration of the site, oozing of blood stained fluid are seen in 1–3 hours. Blisters and local necrosis may occur. Systemic effects include vomiting, headache, loss of consciousness, ptosis, ophthalmoplegia (eyes become fixed in central position) convulsions followed by flaccid paralysis.
- **Viper bite—hemotoxic:** Local reactions are prominent with swelling, discoloration, blister formation and bleeding from the site. Bleeding from the gums, hematuria, disseminated intravascular coagulation are seen.
- **Sea snakes (hydrophids):** Local reactions are mild swelling and pain. Systemic myotoxic effects include muscle pain, stiffness, renal and hepatic necrosis.

Treatment

First Aid
- Ensure safe place
- Calm and reassurance
- Immobilize the bitten part
- Clean the wound, monitor for swelling

Table 6.5: Drugs causing poisoning, their signs/symptoms and their management.

Type of poisoning	Signs and symptoms	Management
Paracetamol poisoning 10–15 g in adults can cause serious toxicity	First 24 hours—nausea, vomiting, anorexia and abdominal pain; within 2–4 days—increased serum transaminases, jaundice, liver tenderness and prolonged prothrombin time, which may progress to liver failure in some patients nephrotoxicity may result in acute renal failure	Stomach wash is given; activated charcoal prevents further absorption *Antidote is N-acetylcysteine* (150 mg/kg IV infusion over 15 minutes repeated as required; oral loading dose—140 mg/kg followed by 70 mg/kg every 4 hours—17 doses) more effective when given early
Salicylates poisoning	Dehydration, hyperpyrexia, gastrointestinal irritation, vomiting, sometimes hematemesis, acid-base imbalance, restlessness, tremors, delirium, hallucinations, metabolic acidosis, convulsions, coma and death due to respiratory failure and cardiovascular collapse (CVC)	*Treatment is symptomatic:* Gastric lavage correct acid-base imbalance and dehydration—IV fluids, Na^+, K^+, HCO_3^- and glucose Blood pH should be monitored Temperature is brought down by external cooling with alcohol or cold water sponges if hemorrhagic complications are seen, blood transfusion and vitamin K are needed. Forced alkaline diuresis with sodium bicarbonate and a diuretic like frusemide is given along with IV fluids
Morphine and other opioids poisoning (lethal dose of morphine in nonaddicts is about 250 mg, but addicts can tolerate gram)	Respiratory depression with shallow breathing, pinpoint pupils, hypotension, shock, cyanosis, flaccidity, stupor, hypothermia, coma and death due to respiratory failure and pulmonary edema	Positive pressure respiration Maintenance of blood pressure (BP) Gastric lavage with potassium permanganate to remove unabsorbed drug *Specific antidote is naloxone*—0.4–0.8 mg IV repeated every 10–15 minutes
Organophosphorous poisoning	Symptoms result from muscarinic, nicotinic and central effects—vomiting, abdominal cramps, diarrhea, miosis, sweating, increased salivary, tracheobronchial and gastric secretions and bronchospasm; hypotension, muscular twitchings, weakness, convulsions and coma. Death is due to respiratory paralysis	Maintain BP and patent airway; if poisoning is through skin—remove clothing and wash the skin with soap and water; If the poison is consumed by oral route, gastric lavage is given. Drug of choice is atropine IV 2 mg every 10 minutes till pupil dilates; maximum dose can be anything from 50 to 100 mg or more depending on the severity of the poisoning. Cholinesterase reactivators—pralidoxime, obidoxime and diacetylmonoxime; thus, they reactivate the cholinesterase enzyme. They should be given within minutes after poisoning. In severe poisoning, 1–2 g of IV pralidoxime given within 5 minutes of poisoning gives best results. *Antidote is atropine sulfate*—2–5 mg IV

Contd...

Contd...

Type of poisoning	Signs and symptoms	Management
Atropine poisoning	Dry skin, fever, dry mouth, dysphagia, dilated pupils, muttering delirium, palpitation, restlessness, excitement, hallucinations, hypotension, difficulty in passing urine and passing stools, convulsions and coma may result in death Scopolamine causes central nervous system (CNS) depression instead of CNS stimulation	Gastric lavage with tannic acid—if the poisoning is by oral route Saline purgatives to prevent absorption of the poison Tepid sponging to reduce temperature. Small sips of water to moisten the mouth. Sterile saline to be instilled into the eye to prevent drying. *Physostigmine 1–2 mg IV is the antidote*; it is an anticholinesterase drug. Physostigmine 1% eye drops to overcome mydriasis, catheterization of the bladder
Barbiturates	Manifestations include respiratory depression with slow and shallow breathing, hypotension, skin eruptions, cardiovascular collapse and renal failure	Gastric lavage followed by administration of *activated charcoal* to prevent further absorption of barbiturates. Maintenance of patent airway, adequate ventilation and oxygen administration. General supportive measures like maintenance of BP and fluid balance. Forced alkaline diuresis with sodium bicarbonate, a diuretic (frusemide) and IV fluids will hasten the excretion of long-acting barbiturates through the kidneys since they are acidic drugs. Hemodialysis should be done especially if there is renal failure
Digitalis	*Extracardiac:* Anorexia, nausea, vomiting and diarrhea are the first symptoms to appear; weakness, confusion, hallucinations, blurred vision	Stop digitalis Oral or parenteral K$^+$ supplements are given Ventricular arrhythmias are treated with IV phenytoin
	Cardiac toxicity: Arrhythmias of any type including extrasystoles, bradycardia, pulses bigeminy and AV block (ventricular tachycardia and fibrillation) can be caused by cardiac glycosides; hypokalemia enhances digitalis toxicity	Bradycardia is treated with atropine and supraventricular arrhythmias with propranolol *Antidigoxin immunotherapy* is now available; it is life-saving in severe poisoning
Methanol	Manifestations of toxicity are vomiting, headache, vertigo, severe abdominal pain, hypotension, delirium, acidosis and coma. Formic acid has affinity for optic nerve and causes retinal damage resulting in blindness. There are reports of even 15 mL of methanol causing blindness. Death is due to respiratory failure	*Correction of acidosis:* As retinal damage occurs faster in presence of acidosis, immediate correction of acidosis with IV sodium bicarbonate infusion helps in preventing blindness. *Protect eyes:* Patient should be kept in a dark room to protect the eyes. Gastric lavage should be given.

Contd...

Contd...

Type of poisoning	Signs and symptoms	Management
		BP and ventilation should be maintained. Ethyl alcohol is given immediately. It competes with methanol for alcohol dehydrogenase A loading dose of 0.6 g/kg is followed by an infusion of 10 g/hour *Antidote: Fomepizole* inhibits the enzyme alcohol dehydrogenase Hemodialysis to enhance the elimination of methanol
Acute alcohol Intoxication	Signs of intoxication are prominent when blood alcohol concentration exceeds 200 mg% Fatal alcohol concentration varies between 500 and 800 mg % The symptoms are of CNS depression, dilated pupils, slurred speech, nausea, vomiting, tachycardia, loss of reflexes, hypotension, circulatory collapse, hypothermia, stupor and coma	Stomach wash using normal saline Maintenance of circulation and respiration 50 mL of 50% glucose given IV to treat hypoglycemia 100 mg thiamine IV to prevent Wernicke's encephalopathy Maintenance of fluid and electrolyte balance Hemodialysis—clearance of ethanol can be enhanced by hemodialysis
Heparin	In heparin overdosage, bleeding can occur	Mild heparin over dosage can be treated by just stopping heparin because heparin is short acting *Protamine sulfate* is a protein obtained from the sperm of certain fish. Given intravenously, it neutralizes heparin (1 mg for every 100 units of heparin) In the absence of heparin, protamine sulfate can itself act as a weak anticoagulant; hence, protamine overdose should be avoided
Warfarin	In warfarin overdosage, hemorrhage is the main hazard Bleeding in the intestines or brain can be troublesome. Minor episodes of epistaxis and bleeding gums are common	Depends on the severity Stop the anticoagulant Fresh blood transfusion is given to supply clotting factors Antidote—the specific *antidote is vitamin K^1 oxide;* it allows the synthesis of clotting factors. But even on IV administration, the response to vitamin K^1 oxide needs several hours. Hence, in emergency, fresh whole blood is necessary to counter the effects of oral anticoagulants
Insulin	Hypoglycemia is the most common complication of excess insulin. Symptoms include sweating, palpitation, tremors,	Oral glucose or fruit juice like orange juice or in severe cases, IV glucose promptly reverse the symptoms

Contd...

Contd...

Type of poisoning	Signs and symptoms	Management
	blurred vision, weakness, hunger, confusion, difficulty in concentration and drowsiness. Severe hypoglycemia may result in convulsions, coma and death	50 mL of 50% glucose is given intravenous- ly followed by dextrose infusion depending on the requirement
Iron	Manifestations include vomiting, abdominal pain, hematemesis, bloody diarrhea, shock, drowsiness, cyanosis, acidosis, dehydration, cardiovascular collapse and coma. Immediate diagnosis and treatment are important as death may occur in 6–12 hours	Gastric lavage is given with 2% sodium bicarbonate solution *Desferrioxamine* is the antidote 5–10 g is instilled into the stomach at the end of the stomach wash, to prevent iron absorption; It is injected intramuscularly 2 g every 12 hours or IV 10–15 mg/kg/hr correction of acidosis and shock Hemodialysis or exchange transfusion help in severe cases
Cyanide	Cyanide rapidly binds to cytochrome oxidase and other vital enzymes; this results in inhibition of cellular respiration and blocks the utilization of oxygen; cyanide poisoning can be rapidly fatal; it requires immediate treatment	Amylnitrite is given by inhalation and sodium nitrite by IV injection (10 mL of 3% solution). *Sodium thiosulfate* is given IV (50 mL of 25% solution) It reacts with cyanmethemoglobin to form thiocyanate, which is easily excreted by the kidneys, nitrates convert hemoglobin to methemoglobin, which has a high affinity for cyanide and binds to cyanide forming cyanmethemoglobin. It thus, protects the important enzymes from binding to cyanide
Iodine overdosage	Acute toxicity with iodine can be fatal (3–4 g fatal dose). Nausea, vomiting, diarrhea and an unpleasant metallic taste, vesication, desquamation and corrosion of skin and mucous membrane with brownish-yellow stains, corrosion and perforation of mouth, throat and gastrointestinal mucosa, nephritis and renal failure, delirium, stupor Inhalation produces edema of glottis and pulmonary edema. Anaphylactic reactions can occur Iodism is a term used to denote chronic poisoning with iodide salts and is characterized by ery- thema, urticaria, acne, stomatitis, conjunctivitis, rhinorrhea, parotid swelling, lymphadenopathy, anorexia and insomnia	Administer starch or flour solution (30 g per liter of water) Milk is also helpful *Sodium thiosulfate is the antidote* A solution of 1%–5% sodium thiosulphate is given orally. This will convert iodine to iodide, which is relatively harmless Skin lesions can be treated with 20% alcohol. Supportive therapy treatment involves liberal intake of sodi- um chloride, which promotes excretion of iodides Induction of vomiting or stomach wash are contraindicated

- Identify the snake if possible
- Rapid evacuation to emergency
- Measures like local incision, suction, application of ice, and giving alcoholic beverages are all found to be harmful and no more recommended.

Supportive Therapy

Blood pressure, respiration and urine output are to be monitored. ECG and blood gas analysis are needed. Fresh blood transfusion may be needed to correct coagulation parameters. Initiate intravenous fluid, analgesics like paracetamol for pain, prophylactic antibiotics as required and tetanus toxoid injection are to be given in all cases. Aseptic cleaning of the bitten area, Antisnake venom (ASV) is indicated in presence of signs of systemic envenomation or grade as depicted in **Table 6.6**.

Infusion should be done after test dose. Watch for reactions to ASV. Hypersensitivity reactions including anaphylaxis can occur. Clean the bite site with providone iodine.

Food Poisoning

Food poisoning can occur on consumption of food that is contaminated with microorganisms, toxins or chemicals.

Nausea, vomiting, abdominal pain, fever, weakness and diarrhea are the common symptoms of food poisoning. Other symptoms depend on the causative agent.

Causes for Food Poisoning

- **Microorganisms:**
    - Bacteria
    - Protozoa
    - Viruses.
- **Toxins:** Present in certain fish, plants and mushrooms.
- **Chemicals.**

Food Poisoning due to Microorganisms

Consumption of food contaminated with microorganisms is the most common cause of food poisoning. The incubation period varies from a few (1–2) hours to a few days.

Microorganisms: Bacteria including *Staphylococcus aureus, Salmonella typhi, Shigella, Vibrio cholerae, Vibrio parahaemolyticus, Bacillus cereus, Clostridium botulinum, (Clostridium perfringens), Streptococcus, Campylobacter* and *Escherichia coli* can cause food poisoning. Viral gastroenteritis may be caused by rotavirus, parvovirus and adenovirus. Treatment is symptomatic.

Table 6.6: Recommended dose ASV based on level of envenomation.

Grade and level of envenomation	Dose of antivenom
Grade –I (No envenomation)	None
Grade –II (Mild envenomation)	4–5 vials
Grade –III (Moderate envenomation)	5–10 vials
Grade –IV (Severe envenomation)	10–15 vials
Grade –V (Very severe envenomation)	15–20 vials

Fungi: The spores of moulds grow on food and can release mycotoxin. These mycotoxins are heat stable. *Aspergillus flavus* can produce aflatoxins, *Penicillium islandicum* can produce islanditoxin.

Others: Protozoa like *Entamoeba histolytica* (amebiasis) and *Giardia lamblia* (giardiasis) are common causes of food poisoning. *Metronidazole* is the drug of choice in both.

Mushrooms are available in large variety, out of which only about 5% are poisonous. Consumption of such mushrooms can cause a variety of toxic effects depending on the toxin—they can cause cellular destruction, affect central or autonomic nervous system, gastrointestinal system or the kidney.

Treatment however, is symptomatic in all these cases except when autonomic nervous system is involved. *Inocybe, Clitocybe* and some species of amanita contain muscarine which stimulates the cholinergic muscarinic receptors. Symptoms include salivation, sweating, diarrhea, constricted pupils, dyspnea, bradycardia and hypotension. The specific *antidote is atropine* (1 mg IV repeated as required).

Chemicals: Contamination of food with chemicals like arsenic, mercury, antimony or insecticides in fruits and vegetables can cause poisoning. Monosodium glutamate is a food additive commonly used in chinese food. Dose more than 1 g can cause troublesome symptoms including burning and numbness of face and neck, chest pain, headache, vomiting and vertigo. In children, convulsions can sometimes occur. Treatment is supportive and symptomatic.

VITAMINS AND MINERALS SUPPLEMENTATIONS

Vitamins

Vitamins are organic compounds required for normal metabolism in the body. They are required by the body in very small amounts. They are supplied by the diet. A balanced diet supplies adequate amounts of vitamins to fulfill the daily requirement. Vitamins are classified into fat-soluble and water-soluble vitamins **(Fig. 6.1)**.

Types of vitamin B-complex
- Vitamin B1 (thiamine)
- Vitamin B2 (riboflavin)
- Vitamin B3 (nicotinic acid, niacin)
- Vitamin B_5 (pantothenic acid)

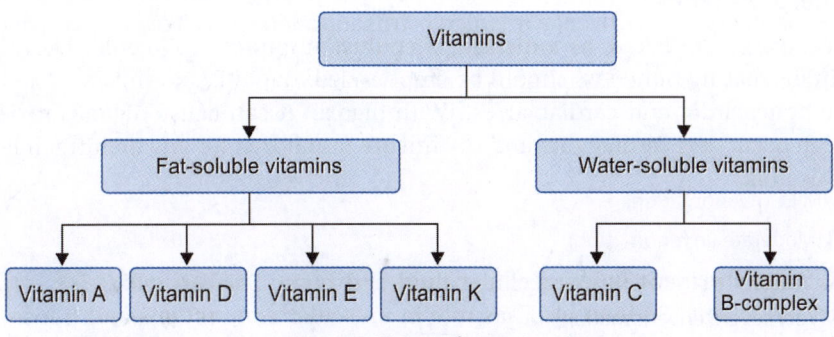

Fig. 6.1: Types of vitamin.

- Vitamin B6 (pyridoxine)
- Vitamin B7 (niotin)
- Vitamin B_9 (folic acid)
- Vitamin B_{12} (cyanocobalamin)

The requirement of vitamins is increased during periods of rapid growth, pregnancy and lactation and in disease conditions. Vitamin deficiencies result in characteristic signs and symptoms. The **Table 6.7** describes the important vitamins, their functions in the body, dietary sources, daily requirements, deficiency diseases caused by them and the prophylaxis and treatment of deficiency.

Minerals

Minerals are natural elements found in the human body, which are required for growth, repair and other vital functions. Some minerals are needed in large quantities, while others are in small quantities.

Minerals needed in large quantities (major minerals are calcium, sodium, potassium, magnesium, phosphorus, chloride, sulfur. Minerals needed in small quantities (trace minerals) are iron, zinc, manganese, copper, iodine, fluoride, cobalt.

Calcium

Calcium is essential for formation of bones and teeth, tissue excitability, muscular contraction, myocardial contractility, normal blood coagulation and secretion from glands. The normal plasma calcium level is 9–11 mg/dL. Daily requirement—400–600 mg/day. The main source of calcium are milk and dairy products, green leafy vegetables like kale (curly), lady finger, soya drink and fish.

Available Forms

- 10% in 10 mL ampule. 1 mL 9 mg
- Oral—tablet calcium phosphate and calcium carbonate—500–1,000 mg.

Indications

Hypocalcemia, hypocalcemic tetany/seizures, osteoporosis and vitamin D deficiency rickets

Adverse effects: Oral calcium can produce constipation.

Nursing Responsibilities

Safety precautions are taken, as indicated, if confusion is present. Regular weight-bearing exercise in decreasing bone loss should be emphasized. Rapid IV administration of calcium can cause bradycardia and cardiac arrest. With digoxin it can cause digitalis toxicity. ECG changes can occur and cardiac rate and rhythm are monitored for any abnormalities in case of hypercalcemia.

Sodium

Sodium is mainly present in extracellular fluid and bone. Sodium maintains extracellular fluid (ECF) osmolality. Sodium also has role in muscular contractions and transmission of nerve impulses. The normal plasma level of sodium is 135–145 mEq/L. Daily requirement of

Table 6.7: Description of fat soluble and water soluble vitamins.

Vitamins	Functions	Dietary sources	Daily allowance	Deficiency	Prophylaxis and treatment of deficiency
Vitamin A	Synthesis of rhodopsin, the pigment in retina of the eye; maintenance of the integrity of epithelial cells, for growth and cell-mediated immunity	Green leafy vegetables carrots, mango, papaya, eggs, butter, cheese, milk, liver, fish liver oils	3,000–4,000 IU	Night blindness, xerophthalmia, Bitot's spots; keratomalacia, perforation of the cornea, necrosis and blindness	*Prophylaxis:* 3,000–5,000 IU/day when there is an increased requirement. Treatment — 50,000–1,00,000 IU intramuscularly or orally for 1–3 days followed by oral supplementation in vitamin A deficiency
Vitamin D	Calcium and phosphate absorption in the intestine and Ca^{++} reabsorption from the kidney; promotes osteoclastic activity	Liver, egg yolk, fish liver oils, milk, butter	200–400 IU	Rickets and osteomalacia	*Prophylaxis:* 400 IU daily or 300,000 IU every 3–6 months IM; 6,00,000 units IM repeated after 4–6 weeks is needed in rickets and osteomalacia with calcium supplements
Vitamin E	Antioxidant; it is essential for normal structure and function of the nervous system and integrity of the biological membranes	Wheat germ, nuts like almonds, sunflower, seeds, cerals, egg, yolk green leafy vegetables	10–15 mg	Deficiency is not common; deficiency can lead to sterility and hemolysis of red blood cells	
Vitamin K	Vitamin K is essential for the biosynthesis of clotting factors—prothrombin bin and factors VII, IX and X by the liver	Vitamin K_1—from plant source green leafy vegetables, liver, meat, cheese, egg yolk and tomatoes. Vitamin K_2 is produced in the gut by bacteria	50–100 mg	Prolonged clotting time, hemorrhagic disease in newborn	Administration of vitamin K, 1 mg IM to the newborn baby prevents hemorrhagic diseases of the newborn

Contd...

Contd...

Vitamins	Functions	Dietary sources	Daily allowance	Deficiency	Prophylaxis and treatment of deficiency
Thiamine (B_1)	Converted to thiamine pyrophosphate, which acts as a coenzyme in carbohydrate metabolism	Cereals, rice polishing, liver, egg yolk	1.2–1.4 mg	Beriberi: Dry beriberi and wet beriberi; Wernicke's encephalopathy and Korsakoff's psychosis	Prophylactically in increased demand as in pregnancy, lactation and infants; beriberi—50 mg daily parenterally. Once the patient recovers, maintenance dose of 10 mg/day is given orally; chronic alcoholics—50 mg daily
Riboflavin (B_2)	Flavin mononucleotide (FMN) and flavin adenine dinucleotide (FAD) containing the active form of riboflavin are coenzymes in various oxidition-reduction reactions	Milk, cereals, pulses, leafy vegetables, eggs and meat	1.5–2 mg	Angular stomatitis, glossitis, seborrheic keratosis of the nose, mouth ulcers, dry skin, burning sensation in the plantar surface of the feet	Prevention and treatment of deficiency (2–10 mg)
Nicotinic acid (niacin B_3)	Involved in several oxidation reduction reactions; a lipid-lowering agent	Rice polishings, cereals, fish, pulses, groundnut, liver, meat	20 mg	Pellagra characterized by dermatitis, diarrhea and dementia	Prophylaxis and treatment of pellagra (50–500 mg); nicotinic acid is used in hyperlipoproteinemia because it can lower plasma lipid levels
Pantothenic acid (B_5)		Rice polishings, whole grains, meat, egg yolk	4–7 mg	Pantothenic acid deficiency in human beings is not known	Calcium pantothenate is one of the components of multivitamin preparations
Pyridoxine (B_6)	Pyridoxal phosphate is a coenzyme involved in the synthesis of several amino acids and other compounds like GABA	Whole grains, pulses, green vegetables, milk, liver, egg yolk	2 mg	Glossitis, peripheral neuritis, anemia, dermatitis and risk of convulsions due to decreased GABA levels in the brain	Prophylaxis and treatment of pyridoxine deficiency; the antitubercular drug INH can cause peripheral neuritis—pyridoxine is used both for the prophylaxis and treatment of this peripheral neuritis; convulsions due to pyridoxine deficiency in infants

Contd...

Contd...

Vitamins	Functions	Dietary sources	Daily allowance	Deficiency	Prophylaxis and treatment of deficiency
Biotin (B_7)	Biotin is a coenzyme in several metabolic reactions	Liver, nuts, egg yolk	0.1–0.2 mg	Biotin deficiency in humans is not known	Present in many multivitamin preparations
Folic acid (B_9)	Essential for normal DNA synthesis	Leafy vegetables, milk, liver, meat, cereals, Orange	100–200 mg	Megaloblastic anemia, glossitis, diarrhea and weakness	*Megaloblastic anemia:* Folic acid 2–5 mg/day is given orally along with vitamin B_{12}. In folic acid deficiency due to malabsorption syndromes, it is given IM. Prophylaxis: in pregnancy, lactation, infancy and other situations with increased requirement —500 mg daily orally
Vitamin (B_{12})	Essential for normal DNA synthesis	Milk, egg yolk, liver, meat, fish	1–2 µg	*Pernicious anemia:* Deficiency of intrinsic factor resulting in failure of B^{12} absorption; causes are gastrectomy, chronic gastritis, malabsorption and fish tapeworm infestation	Prophylaxis and treatment of megaloblastic anemia due to B_{12} deficiency of any cause; if B_{12} deficiency is due to lack of intrinsic factor, it is given IM or SC Preparations: Cyanocobalamin—100 µg/mL injection; hydroxocobalamin—100, 500, 1,000 µg/mL injection
Vitamin C	Ascorbic acid is involved in several metabolic reactions; it is essential for the integrity of connective tissue, for the development of cartilage, bone and teeth and for wound healing	Goose berry (amla), citrus fruits, green vegetables and tomatoes	50 mg	*Scurvy:* Characterized by connective tissue defects resulting in hemorrhages, impaired wound healing, tender bleeding gums, deformed teeth, brittle bones, anemia and growth retardation	*For prevention of vitamin C deficiency:* 50–100 mg daily *Scurvy:* 500–1,000 mg daily

sodium varies from 5 to 15 g. The main source of sodium is table salt, sunflower seed, beet root, spinach, coriander, and egg.

Available Forms

Sodium chloride Injectable solution—0.9% isotonic, 0.45% saline, 3% and 5% hypertonic, glucose with sodium chloride injectable solution—5% glucose, 0.9% sodium chloride, 5% glucose, 0.45% sodium chloride.

Indications

Hyponatremia, fluid and electrolyte replacement, diabetes ketoacidosis.

Nursing Responsibilities

Hypertonic saline solutions should be administered under close observation. Monitor fluid intake and output as well as daily body weights. Serum sodium level and renal function should be monitored.

Potassium

Potassium is mainly present inside the cells. Potassium has an important role in regulating muscular activity, maintaining water and electrolyte balance and acid-base balance; potassium is also essential for neuronal activity.
Daily requirement: 3–5 g in adults.
The main source of potassium are banana, dry fruits, lentils, spinach, broccoli, coconut water, tomatoes, chicken and fish

Available Forms

Potassium chloride oral solution: 15 mEq in 20 mL solution
- *Injectable solution:* 15% in 20 mL ampule, 10% in 10 mL ampule
- *Sources:* Coconut water, vegetables, fruits, nuts, meat and liver.

Nursing Responsibilities

Patients receiving digitalis, who are at risk for potassium deficiency should be monitored closely for signs of digitalis toxicity. Monitor cardiac function and renal function for patients on oral or intravenous potassium. Oral potassium supplements can lead to gastrointestinal (GI) lesions; and the patients should be cautiously monitored for abdominal distention, pain or GI bleeding.

Magnesium

Magnesium is the most abundant intracellular cation after potassium. It acts as an activator for many intracellular enzyme systems and plays a role in both carbohydrate and protein metabolism. Magnesium balance is important in neuromuscular function. Sources of magnesium are vegetables, grains, nuts, cocoa, fish, meat. Daily requirement is 300 mg in adults. Plasma magnesium levels 1.8–2.4 mg/dL.

Therapeutic Uses

- **Magnesium deficiency:** Magnesium hydroxide is given orally in mild cases and magnesium sulfate slow IV in severe deficiency—5 mL of 50% magnesium is given slow IV.

- **As antacids:** Magnesium hydroxide and magnesium trisilicate are used as antacids.
- **Osmotic purgative:** Magnesium sulfate is used as an osmotic purgative.
- **As anticonvulsant:** Magnesium sulfate is used IV (or IM) to control seizures in toxemia of pregnancy.
- **Tocolytic:** Intravenous magnesium sulfate may be used as an alternative to relax the uterus in preterm labor.
- **Cardiac arrhythmias:** Magnesium chloride may be used in the treatment of arrhythmias that may follow myocardial infarction.
- **In raised intracranial tension:** Rectal administration of magnesium sulfate solution may help to reduce intracranial tension.
- **Topical:** 25%–50% magnesium sulfate in glycerin (Mag sulf poultice) is used topically to relieve local edema. $MgSO_4$ exerts osmotic effect, while glycerin is hygroscopic and together they reduce local inflammation.

Phosphorus

Phosphorus is necessary for the formation of bones and teeth. Phosphorus is essential for phosphorylation reactions. Phosphorus is important in maintaining the acid-base balance in the plasma and the cells —phosphates are buffers. Phosphorus is present in many food items including milk, cereals, fish, meat, pulses and nuts. Daily requirement of phosphorus is about 900–1,000 mg in adults.

Uses of Phosphorus

- Phosphorus deficiency.
- Chronic hypercalcemia (without hyperphosphatemia).

VACCINES AND SERA (UNIVERSAL IMMUNIZATION PROGRAM SCHEDULE)

Vaccines and Sera

Substances, which provide immunity either actively or passively are called immunizing agents. They can be classified as vaccines, immunoglobulin and antisera. Immunity can be active or passive. Commonly used vaccines and seras are presented in **Tables 6.8 and 6.9**.

Active Immunity

Active immunization occurs when the natural immune system of the body develops immunity on exposure to an antigen. Vaccines are used for active immunization. Vaccines are suspensions of specific antigens. They are of three types:

1. **Live attenuated vaccine:** These are made from live organisms, which does not have the capacity to cause the disease but retain immunogenicity. Two live vaccine must be administered after a gap of 4 weeks(1 month)
   For example, Bacille Calmette-Guerin, oral polio vaccine
2. **Inactivated or killed vaccine:** These are prepared from killed microorganisms, which on entering the body induce immunity.
   For example, Cholera, Salk's polio vaccine.
3. **Toxoids:** Certain microorganisms produce exotoxins, which when chemically treated loss their toxicity but retain antigenicity called toxoids. Toxoids can be used to in immunization.
   For example, Tetanus toxoid, diphtheria toxoid.

Table 6.8: Commonly used vaccines.

Vaccine	Type of agent	Route of administration	Primary immunization	Booster	Indication
Bacille Calmette-Guerin (BCG)	Live attenuated	ID*/SC†	At birth	7 and 14 year	In all children
Cholera	Inactivated	SC/IM‡	*Adults:* Two doses 1 month apart	Every 6 month endemic areas	People living in endemic area
Diphtheria	Toxoid	IM	6, 10, 14 week of age	18 month and at 4–6 year	For all children
Pertussis	Inactivated	IM	6, 10, 14 week of age	18 month and at 4–6 year	For all children
Tetanus	Toxoid	IM	6, 10, 14 week of age	18 month and at 4–6 year	*For all children; adults:* Postexposure prophylaxis if > 5 years has passed since last dose
Typhoid/paratyphoid	Inactivated	SC	After 3 year at any age: Two doses 4 week apart	Every 3 year	Risk of exposure to typhoid fever
Typhoid (Typhoral)	Live inactivated	Oral (capsules)	Above 6 year at any age: 3 doses on alternate days 1 hour before food	Every 3 year	Risk of exposure to typhoid fever
Meningococcal vaccine	Bacterial polysaccharides	SC	One dose	–	Travelers to areas with Meningococcal epidemics control of outbreak in closed population
Pneumococcal vaccine	Bacterial polysaccharides	SC	One dose	Every 3–5 years if there is high risk of exposure	Travelers to areas with epidemics, close contacts, military recruits
Plague	Inactivated	IM	One dose	–	In an epidemic
Haemophilus Influenzae (type B)	Polysaccharide	IM	One dose	–	For all children, patients at risk

Contd...

Contd...

Vaccine	Type of agent	Route of administration	Primary immunization	Booster	Indication
Poliomyelitis (OPV)	Live virus	Oral	6, 10 and 14 week of age	18 month; again at 4–6 year	For all children
Measles, mumps, rubella (MMR)	Live virus	SC	12–15 month	11–12 year	For all children
Hepatitis A	Inactivated virus	IM	1 dose (2–4 week)	After 6–12 month	Travelers to endemic areas, homosexual men persons at occupational risk
Hepatitis B	Inactive viral	IM	At birth, 1 month, 6–18 month	After 5 years but not routinely recommended	For all children, persons at occupational risk, hemophiliacs, post-exposure prophylaxis
Influenza	Inactivated virus	IM	One dose	Yearly	High-risk people like elderly, asthmatics
Rabies (Rabipur)	Inactivated virus	IM/ID	Pre-exposure: 3 doses at days 0, 7 and 21. Post-exposure: 6 doses IM 0, 3, 7, 14, 30 and 90	After 1 year then at 2–5 year	Post-exposure treatment pre-exposure prophylaxis in persons at risk for contact with rabies virus
Varicella	Live virus	SC	2 doses 4–8 week apart at 18 month	–	All children from 18 months to 13 years with no history of varicella infection
Yellow fever	Live virus	SC	1 dose	Every 10 year	Travelers to areas where yellow fever is seen, laboratory personnel at-risk of exposure
Japanese encephalitis	Killed	SC	2 doses 7–14 day apart	Before 12 month	Population at risk

*ID, intradermal; †SC, subcutaneous; ‡IM, intramuscular.

Table 6.9: Commonly used immunoglobulins and sera.

Preparation with source	Dose and route	Indications
Diphtheria antitoxin (horse)	IV or IM 20,000–120,000 units	Diphtheria clinical diphtheria—to be given immediately
Tetanus immunoglobulin (human)	IM *Prophylaxis:* 2,500 units *Treatment:* 3,000–6,000 units	Tetanus Treatment and post-exposure prophylaxis, of unclean wounds in inadequately immunized persons
Tetanus antitoxin [anti-tetanus serum (ATS) (horse)] (If tetanus Ig is not available)	IM/SC *Prophylaxis:* 1,500–3,000 IU *Treatment:* 50,000–100,000 IU	Tetanus Treatment and post-exposure prophylaxis of unclean wounds in inadequately immunized persons
Rabies immunoglobulin (human)	20 IU/kg; half the dose infiltrated around the wound; remaining IM	Rabies Postexposure prophylaxis combined with rabies vaccine
Botulinum antitoxin	IM/IV 10,000 IU	Treatment and post-exposure prophylaxis botulism
Antirabies serum (ARS) (horse)	IM 40 IU/kg	Used if rabies Ig is not available, but is inferior to it
Gas gangrene antitoxin (AGS) (horse)	IM/SC/IV *Prophylaxis:* 10,000 IU *Treatment:* 30,000–75,000 IU	Gas gangrene Post-exposure prophylaxis and treatment
Hepatitis B immunoglobulin (HBIG)	IM 0.06 mL/kg	Post-exposure prophylaxis in nonimmune persons
Antisnake venom polyvalent (horse)	IV 20–30 mL to be given within 4 hour after the bite; additional doses may be required	Snake bite–cobra, vipers, krait
Human gamma globulin		Gamma globulin deficiency; prophylaxis of hepatitis A, measles, mumps, rubella
Anti-Rh D Ig	Less than 12 weeks—50 µg IM More than 12 weeks—300 µg IM Postpartum period—300 µg IM	To the Rh-negative mother after the birth of Rh-positive baby or after uncompleted pregnancy with Rh-positive fetus

Passive Immunization

Passive immunization is the administration of antibodies or serum containing antibodies to provide immunity against specific organisms. Newborns receive natural passive immunity from the maternal antibodies that is transferred transplacentally. Passive immunization provides rapid, but temporary protection. Antibodies are immunoglobulins (Ig) like normal human gamma globulin, tetanus Ig, rabies Ig, anti-diphtheria Ig and hepatitis B Ig. Antisera like tetanus antitoxin, gas gangrene antitoxin, diphtheria and antirabies serum are obtained from sera of horses, which are actively immunized against the specific organism. Sensitivity tests should be done before giving antisera. Allergic reactions including serum sickness and anaphylaxis can occur with antisera, while it is uncommon with immunoglobulins.

Immunoglobulins

Immunoglobulins are human gamma globulins that carry the antibodies—like normal human gamma globulins, tetanus Ig, rabies Ig, anti-diphtheria Ig and hepatitis B Ig. Allergic reactions including serum sickness and anaphylaxis can occur with antisera, while it is uncommon with Igs.

Immunization and Universal Immunization Program

Vaccines and antisera are used for immunization against bacterial and viral infections. Vaccines stimulate the host immune system while antisera supplement and support the immune system with readymade antibodies. In 1978, the expanded program was launched in urban areas. Later on, in year 1985, the Universal Immunization Program was launched by Government of India. Immunization is an important tool for eliminating and controlling the life threatening infectious disease. The current immunization program schedule is given in **Table 6.10**.

ANTICANCER DRUGS: CHEMOTHERAPEUTIC DRUGS COMMONLY USED

Chemotherapy uses the chemicals for the treatment of infectious diseases caused by bacteria and the other pathologic microorganisms, parasites and tumor cells.

Anticancer drugs, which inhibit the growth of cancer cells by killing them or modifying their growth. These drugs are also used in conjunction with surgery and radiotherapy.

Classification

Classification of anticancer drug is given in **Table 6.11**.

NOTES ON INDIVIDUAL DRUGS

Alkylating Agents

Mechlorethamine: It has cytotoxic and radiomimetic action (like ionizing radiations). It is highly reactive and given in dosage of 0.1 mg/kg IV daily for 4 days. It is mainly used in case of Hodgkin's and non-Hodgkin's lymphomas. Nausea, vomiting and hemodynamic changes are its common side effects.

Cyclophosphamide: It has immunosuppressant properties and is popularly used in many solid tumors. It can be given as 2–3 mg/kg/day orally or 10–15 mg/kg IV every 7–10 days IM. Alopecia and cystitis are its common side effects.

Ifosfamide: It is useful in case of bronchogenic, breast, testicular, bladder, head and neck carcinomas, osteogenic sarcoma and some lymphomas. It causes less alopecia and is less emetogenic than cyclophosphamide.

Chlorambucil: It is slow-acting agent and is mainly active on lymphoid tissue. It is drug of choice in case of chronic lymphatic leukemia, non-Hodgkin's lymphoma and some other solid tumors. It is used in dosage of 4–10 mg (0.1–0.2 mg/kg) daily for 3–6 weeks, then 2 mg daily for maintenance.

SECTION 1: Pharmacology-II

Table 6.10: Universal immunization program schedule.

Vaccine	Due age	Dose	Route	Site
BCG	At birth till 1 year	(0.05 mL until 1 month) 0.1 mL beyond age 1 month	Intradermal	Upper arm—left
Hepatitis B - Birth dose	At birth or within 24 hours	0.5 mL	Intramuscular	Anterolateral side of mid-thigh—left
OPV-0	At birth or within the first 15 days	2 drops	Oral	Oral
OPV 1, 2 and 3	At 6 weeks, 10 weeks and 14 weeks till 5 years of age	2 drops	Oral	Oral
Pentavalent 1, 2 and 3 (Diphtheria + Pertussis + Tetanus + Hepatitis B + Hib)	At 6 weeks, 10 weeks and 14 weeks Or upto 1 year of age	0.5 mL	Intramuscular	Anterolateral side of mid-thigh—left
Fractional IPV (inactivated polio vaccine	At 6 and 14 weeks or upto 1 year of age	0.1 mL	Intradermal	Upper arm
Rotavirus (where applicable)	At 6 weeks, 10 weeks and 14 weeks	5 drops	Oral	Oral
Pneumococcal conjugate vaccine (PCV) (where applicable)	At 6 weeks and 14 weeks At 9 completed months—booster 1 year of age	0.5 mL	Intramuscular	Anterolateral side of mid-thigh—right
Measles/rubella 1st dose	At 9 completed months to 12 months. 5 years of age	0.5 mL	Subcutaneous	Upper arm—right
Japanese encephalitis – 1 (where applicable)	At 9 months to 12 months upto 15 years of age	0.5 mL	Subcutaneous	Upper arm—left
Vitamin A (1st dose)	At 9 months upto 5 years of age (1 lakh IU)	1 mL	Oral	Oral

Melphalan: It is used in advanced ovarian cancer and is effective in multiple myeloma. It is given in dosage of 10 mg daily for 7 days or 6 mg/day for 2–3 weeks. Bone marrow depression, infections, pancreatitis and diarrhea are its common complications.

Busulfan: It is mainly used in case of chronic myeloid leukemia in dosage of 2–6 mg/day orally. Hyperuricemia, pulmonary fibrosis, skin pigmentation and sterility are its side effects.

CHAPTER 6: Miscellaneous Drugs

Table 6.11: Classification of anticancer drugs.

Group	Drugs
Cytotoxic drugs	
• Alkylating agents	Mechlorethamine, cyclophosphamide, ifosfamide, chlorambucil, melphalan, busulfan, dacarbazine, procarbazine
• Platinum coordination complexes	Cisplatin, carboplatin, oxaliplatin
• Antimetabolites	Methotrexate, 6-mercaptopurine, 5-fluorouracil, capecitabine, cytarabine
• Microtubule damaging agents	Vincristine, vinblastine, paclitaxel, estramustine
• Topoisomerase–II inhibitors	Etoposide
• Topoisomerase-I inhibitors	Topotecan, irinotecan
• Antibiotics	Actinomycin-D, doxorubicin, epirubicin, mitomycin C
• Miscellaneous	Hydroxyurea, tretinoin
Targeted drugs	Imatinib, gefitinib, erlotinib, cetuximab, bevacizumab, sunitinib
Hormonal drugs	Glucocorticoids, estrogens, antiandrogens, gonadotropin-releasing hormone (GnRH) agonists, progestins

Dacarbazine: It is drug of choice in case of malignant melanoma and also used in case of Hodgkin's lymphoma. It is given in dosage of 3.5 mg/kg/day IV for 10 days, repeated after 4 weeks. Nausea, vomiting, flu-like symptoms, neuropathy and myelosuppression are its adverse effects.

Platinum Coordination Complexes

Cisplatin: It is drug of choice in case of metastatic testicular and ovarian carcinoma and can also be used in other solid tumors like lung, bladder, esophageal, gastric, hepatic, head and neck carcinomas. It is administered as slow IV infusion in dosage of 50-100 mg/m^2. It has highly emetic action, so antiemetics are routinely administered before infusing it. It can also cause renal toxicity, tinnitus, deafness, sensory neuropathy and hyperuricemia.

Carboplatin: It is better tolerated drug than cisplatin as nephrotoxicity, ototoxicity and neurotoxicity are low. It is used in case of ovarian carcinoma of epithelial origin and squamous cell carcinoma of head and neck, small cell lung cancer, breast cancer and seminoma.

Oxaliplatin: It is choice of drug in case of colorectal cancer; and is also helpful in gastroesophageal and pancreatic cancers. It is used in dosage of 85 mg/m^2 IV every 2 weeks. Diarrhea, acute allergic reactions and sensory paresthesias are reported.

Antimetabolites

Methotrexate: It is highly efficacious antineoplastic drug and is widely used in non-Hodgkin's lymphoma, breast, bladder, head and neck cancers and osteogenic sarcoma. It can also have immunosuppressant action, so useful in rheumatoid arthritis, psorasis and many other autoimmune disorders. In dosage of 15–30 mg/day for 5 days orally or 20–40 mg/m^2 body surface area (BSA) IM or IV it can be used in choriocarcinoma. It can cause megaloblastic anemia in lower doses and in higher doses pancytopenia can occur. Mucositis, diarrhea and GI bleed can also occur.

Mercaptopurine: It is highly effective antineoplastic agent. It is used in childhood acute leukemia, choriocarcinoma and in some solid tumors. It is given as 2.5 mg/kg/day, half dose for maintenance. Its toxic effects are bone marrow depression, nausea, vomiting, reversible jaundice and hyperuricemia.

5-Fluorouracil (5-FU): It is commonly used drug for colon, rectum, stomach, pancreas, liver, urinary, bladder, head and neck malignancies. It is given in dosage of 500 mg/m^2 IV. Infusion over 1–3 hours weekly for 6-8 weeks or 12 mg/kg/day IV for 4 days followed by 6 mg/kg Iv on alternate days. Myelosuppresion, mucositis, diarrhea, nausea and vomiting are its common side effects.

Cytarabine: It is mainly used for leukemias and lymphomas not for solid tumors. It is administered IV 100 mg/m^2 once or twice for 5–10 days or by continuous infusion over 5–7 days. Leukopenia, thrombocytopenia, anemia, mucositis and diarrhea are its major toxic effects.

Microtubule Damaging Agents

Vincristine: It is used for myeloid leukemia, Hodgkin's disease, Wilms' tumor, Ewing's sarcoma, neuroblastoma and carcinoma lung. It is administered as 1.5–2 mg/m^2 BSA IV weekly. Peripheral neuropathy, alopecia, ataxia, nerve palsies, postural hypotension, paralytic ileus, urinary retension and seizures are its adverse effects.

Vinblastine: It is used for Hodgkin's disease, Kaposi sarcoma, neuroblastoma, non-Hodgkin's lymphoma, breast and testicular carcinoma in dosage of 0.1–0.15 mg/kg IV weekly 3 doses. Bone marrow toxicity, neurotoxicity and alopecia are its adverse effects.

Paclitaxel: It is used in metastatic ovarian and breast carcinoma after failure of first-line chemotherapy and relapse cases. It is also useful in advanced cases of head and neck cancer, small cell lung cancer, esophageal adenocarcinoma, urinary and hormone refractory prostate cancer. It is administered in dosage of 135–175 mg/m^2 by infusion over 3 hour and repeated every 3 weeks. Nausea, chest pain, arthralgia, myalgia, mucositis and edema are its adverse effects.

Estramustine: It is drug of choice in case of advanced and metastatic prostate cancer. It is used in dosage of 4–5 mg/kg orally three times daily. Gynecomastia, impotence, fluid retention, increased risk of thromboembolism and impaired glucose tolerance are its adverse effects.

Topoisomerase-II Inhibitors

Etoposide: It is used in testicular tumors, lung cancer, Hodgkin's lymphoma, carcinoma of bladder and stomach. It is administered in dosage of 50–100 mg/m^2/day IV for 5 days or 100–200 mg/day orally. Alopecia, leukopenia and GIT disturbances are its adverse effects.

Topoisomerase-II inhibitors

Topotecan: It is used in combination with cisplatin for cervical cancer. It can also be used for metastatic carcinoma of ovary and small cell lung cancer after primary chemotherapy has failed. It is administered in dosage of 1.5 mg/m^2 IV over 30 min daily for 5 days every 3 weeks, 4 or more cycles. Bone marrow depression pain in abdomen, vomiting, anorexia and diarrhea are its adverse effects.

Irinotecan: It is used for metastatic/advanced colorectal carcinoma and also in cancer of lung, cervix, ovary and stomach. It is given in dosage of 125 mg/m^2 IV over 90 min, weekly for 4 weeks. Its side effects are neutropenia, thrombocytopenia, hemorrhage, bodyache and weakness.

Antibioitics

Actinomycin D: It is drug choice for Wilms' tumor and childhood rhabdomyosarcoma and can also be used for Ewing's sarcoma and metastatic testicular carcinoma. Its dosage is 15 µ/kg IV daily for 5 days. Vomiting, stomatitis, diarrhea, erythema and desquamation of skin, alopecia and bone marrow depression are its adverse effects.

Doxorubicin: It is used for acute myeloid, lymphoblastic leukemia and in many solid tumors like breast, thyroid, ovary, bladder and lung cancer, sarcomas and neuroblastoma. They act by blocking DNA as well as RNA synthesis. It is administered in dosage of 30–50 mg/m^2 BSA IV for 3 days then repeated every 3–4 weeks. Cardiotoxicity, bone marrow depression, alopecia, stomatitis, vomiting and local tissue damage are its adverse effects.

Epirubicin: It is used for breast cancer, gastroesophageal, pancreatic, hepatic and bladder carcinoma. Its dosage is 60–90 mg/m^2 IV over 5 min, repeated at 3 weeks, total dose 900 mg/m2 is to be given to avoid cardiotoxicity. Its common adverse effects are alopecia, hyperpigmentation of skin and oral mucosa, painful oral ulcers, fever and GI symtoms.

Mitomycin C: This drug is usually combined with 5-Flu and radiation to treat resistant cancers of stomach, cervix, colon, rectum, breast, etc. It generates free radicals to damage DNA. It is administered in dosage of 10 mg/m^2 BSA, infused IV in one day or divided in 5 doses and infused over 5 days. Injections are repeated only after 6 weeks or more. It mainly affects bone marrow and GIT for its toxic effects.

Miscellaneous Cytotoxic Drugs

Hydroxyurea: It is first-line drug for sickle cell anemia in adults and can also be used for myeloid leukemia, psoriasis and polycythemia vera. It is administered in dosage of 20–30 mg/kg daily or 80 mg/kg twice weekly. Myelosuppression, GI disturbances and cutaneous reactions are its common toxic effects.

Tretinoin: It is used for acute myelocytic leukemia. About 45 mg/m^2/day is administered till one after remission occurs. Dryness of skin, eye, nose, mouth, priritus, epiataxis, rise in serum lipids, hepatic transaminases and intracranial pressure are its adverse effects. It can also cause retinoic acid syndrome comprising of breathlessness, fever, pleural/pericardial effusion and pulmonary infiltrates.

Targeted Drugs

Imatinib: It is first drug to be introduced as targeted drug for the treatment of malignancy. It is effective drug for treatment of chronic myeloid leukemia. It is administered 400 mg/day with meals and in accelerated phase of chronic myeloid leukemia (CML) dose is increased to 600–800 mg/day. Abdominal pain, vomiting, fluid retention, periorbital edema, pleural effusion, myalgia, liver damage and chronic heart failure (CHF) are its adverse effects.

Gefitinib: It is used in patients of non-small cell lung cancer. Its dosage is 250 mg/day orally. Skin rashes, diarrhea, nausea, anorexia and itching are its common side effects.

Erlotinib: It can be combined with gefitinib for advanced metastatic pancreatic cancer. Rest of its indications and adverse effects are similar to gefitinib. It is administered in dosage of 100–150 mg od to be taken 1 hour before or 2 hours after meals.

Bevacizumab: In combination with 5-Fu it is used for metastatic colorectal cancer. It also improves the survival in metastatic non-small cell lung cancer, breast cancer and glioblastoma. It is administered IV every 2–3 weeks. Rise in BP, arterial thromboembolism leading to heart attack and stroke, hemorrhage, heart failure, proteinuria, GI perforation and healing defects are its adverse effects.

Sunitinib: It is used in metastatic renal cell carcinoma and resistant GI stromal tumor. It is administered orally daily in 4 weeks cycle. Hypertension, rashes, diarrhea, weakness, bleeding, proteinurea, hypothyroidism and neutropenia are its adverse effects.

Hormonal Drugs

Glucocorticoids: It is primarily used for acute childhood leukemia and lymphomas. It can also be used for controlling malignancy/chemotherapy associated complications like hypercalcemia, hemolysis, bleeding due to thrombocytopenia, retinoic acid syndrome, increased intracranial tension and mediastinal edema. Amongst all prednisolone/dexamethasone are most commonly used drugs.

Estrogens: They help to reduce symptoms in carcinoma prostate—Fosfestrol 600–1,200 mg IV initially and for maintenance 120–240 mg orally can be used.

Gonadotropin-releasing hormone (GnRH) agonists: They are generally used in combination with antiandrogens. They have palliative effect in advanced estrogen/androgen-dependent carcinoma breast/prostate.

Progestins: They are used in palliative treatment of metastatic carcinoma of breast.

NURSING RESPONSIBILITIES

- Weekly assess complete blood count (CBC) and platelet count, withhold drug if WBC is < 4,000/mm^3 or platelet count is < 75,000/mm^3.
- Strict asepsis and protective isolation is to be maintained if WBC levels are low.
- Assess intake-output ratio and inform the physician if urine output falls below 30 mL/h.
- Monitor body temperature q4h as it may indicate beginning infection.
- Assess for liver function tests before and during therapy as per the need.
- Assess for bleeding, yellowing skin, sclera, dark urine, edema in feet, pain in joints and stomach as well as the inflammation of mucosa and breaks in skin.
- Regularly check the IV site for irritation and phlebitis.
- Provide comprehensive oral hygiene, using careful techniques and soft bristle brush.

PATIENT EDUCATION

- Teach the client and family members to report the signs of infection and anemia.
- Teach them to report if any bleeding occurs.
- Teach them to avoid use of razor.
- Teach them to use the commercial mouthwash.

CAUSES FOR FAILURE OF CHEMOTHERAPY

- Delay in diagnosis or therapy.
- Wrong or incomplete diagnosis:
  - No infection; other causes of fever like collagen diseases or malignancy
  - Non-bacterial infection
  - Polymicrobial infection.
- Errors in antimicrobial susceptibility testing
- Inadequate concentration of antibiotic at the site of infection:
  - Improper dose
  - Decreased absorption from food or drug interaction
  - Increased elimination of agent
  - High protein binding
  - Poor delivery (e.g. vascular disease).
- Decreased activity at the site:
  - Chemical factors (pH and others)
  - Antibiotic antagonism
- Other factors at the site of infection:
  - Collection requiring drainage
  - Necrotic tissue
  - Foreign body
- Other host factors:
  - Impaired immune defenses
  - Infection in a protected site requiring bactericidal drug or combination (infecting organism present behind barriers such as vegetation on heart valves, inside the eyeball, blood-brain barrier).
- Development of resistance to antimicrobial agents such as presence of dormant or altered organisms, which later give rise to relapse.
- Superinfection.

SUPERINFECTION

Superinfection is the appearance of bacteriological and clinical evidence of new infection during the chemotherapy of a primary one. Superinfections mostly occur in broad spectrums. Due to antimicrobial therapy there is removal of the inhibitory influence of the drug-sensitive flora that is normally inhibited in the nasopharynx and other body orifices. Many of these floras produce antibacterial substance called bacteriocin. As a result of alteration of normal microbial flora of the host, there is establishment of growth of exogenous microorganism and endogenous proliferation of microorganism, which are relatively not sensitive to that particular antibiotic. So, secondary infection is superimposed on the original infection.

Common Causative Organism of Superinfection

- *Candida* or fungal infection commonly
- Enterobacteriaceae *(Shigella, Salmonella, Escherichia, Klebsiella)*
- *Pseudomonas*
- *Staphylococcus.*

CHEMOPROPHYLAXIS

Chemoprophylaxis is the use of antimicrobial agents to prevent infection. This is recommended in the following situations:
- **In healthy persons:**
  - Penicillin G is given for prevention of gonorrhea or syphilis in patients after contact with infected persons called post-exposure prophylaxis.
  - *Malaria:* In healthy individuals visiting an endemic area—chemoprophylaxis with chloroquine is given.
- **To prevent infection in high-risk patients:**
  - In neutropenic patients receiving anticancer drugs, immunosuppressive agents and patients with acquired immunodeficiency syndrome (AIDS), antibacterials like penicillin or fluoroquinolones or cotrimoxazole may reduce the incidence of bacterial infection.
  - In patients with contaminated or exposed wounds as in road traffic accidents.
  - Catheterization of urinary tract—norfloxacin is used.
  - In burns, to prevent colonization by bacteria.
- **Surgical prophylaxis:** Prior to surgery chemoprophylaxis is recommended. Adequate antibacterial activity should be present during surgery. Hence, the drug is started parenterally 30–60 minutes before surgery. A drug which is effective against all organisms that are likely to contaminate the wound is usually selected.
- **In close contacts:** Chemoprophylaxis is recommended particularly in children, when infectious (open) cases of leprosy or tuberculosis (TB) are in close contact.

IMMUNOSUPPRESSANTS AND IMMUNOSTIMULANTS

Immunosuppressants

Immunosuppressants are drugs, which inhibits cellular/humoral or both type of immune responses. These drugs are used to prevent graft rejection in organ transplantation and in autoimmune diseases.

Common Immunosuppressant Drugs

For common immunosuppressant drugs *see* **Table 6.12**.

Immunestimulants

Immunostimulating and immunomodulating agents are drugs that modulate the immune response and can be used to increase the immune responsiveness.

Thalidomide: It is a teratogenic drug. It enhances cell-mediated immunity by action on T cells. Thalidomide is used in multiple myeloma, lepra reactions and in lupus erythematosus.

Interferons are cytokines with antiviral and immunomodulatory properties. Recombinant interferons α, β and γ bind to specific receptors and bring about immune activation and increase host defenses leading to an increase in the number and activity of cytotoxic and helper T cells and killer cells. Interferons α and β are mainly used for antiviral effects, while interferon γ for its immunomodulating actions. Interferons are indicated in several tumors including malignant melanoma, hairy cell leukemia lymphomas, Kaposi's sarcoma, condylomata acuminata and in viral infections.

Table 6.12: Classification, uses, and nursing considerations of common immunosuppressants.

Group	Name of the drug	Uses	Nursing action
Calcineurin inhibitor	*Cyclosporine:* Oral/IV 10–15 mg/kg/day	Most effective for prevention and treatment for graft rejection in renal, hepatic, cardiac, bone marrow and other transplantations It is the second line drug in autoimmune diseases like rheumatoid arthritis, uveitis, bronchial asthma, inflammatory bowel diseases, dermatomyositis, psoriasis, etc	Initial dose till 1–2 weeks after transplantation. Maintenance dose 2–6 mg/kg/day. Medicine administer with milk or fruit juice; patient should be monitored for infection and regular blood drug level. Monitor vital signs regularly Strict aseptic technique to be followed, while taking care of patient
	Tacrolimus: Oral/IV 0.05–0.1 mg/kg for renal transplant 0.1–0.2 mg/kg for liver transplant	Useful in patients with rejection is not suppressed by cyclosporine and suitable for acute rejection; it is very much useful for liver transplantation and fistulating Crohn's disease	Regular blood level monitoring Monitor vital signs regularly Follow strict aseptic techniques
	Mycophenolate mofetil 1 g, 250 mg, 500 mg tablet/capsule	It is the add on drug with the cyclosporine to reduce the dose and its toxicity in graft transplantations	Monitor the patient for GI bleeding Check vital signs periodically Follow strict aseptic techniques
MTOR inhibitors	*Sirolimus and evorolimus:* Tablet 1 mg	Useful for prevention and treatment of graft rejection by alone or with combination of cyclosporine or tacrolimus; it is useful for stem cell replacement	Monitor vital signs regularly; strict aseptic technique to be followed, while taking care of patient
Cytotoxic drugs/antiproliferative drugs	*Azathioprine:* 1–5 mg/kg	It is used in combination with cyclosporine in prevention of graft rejection; it is also useful for progressive rheumatoid arthritis, inflammatory bowel diseases and alternative to long-term steroids in autoimmune diseases	Check for hypertensive reactions
	Methotrexate: 10–25 mg oral; if, IM/IV will be a single dose	Useful as first line drugs in autoimmune disease such as rheumatoid arthritis, severe psoriasis, pemphigus, myasthenia gravis, uveitis, chronic active hepatitis	Regularly check for renal functions, any signs of bleeding, presence of blood in urine and hematological monitoring

Contd...

Contd...

Group	Name of the drug	Uses	Nursing action
	Cyclophosphamide	It is very much useful in bone marrow transplantation and as a maintenance therapy in pemphigus, systemic lupus exythematosus, thrombocytopenic purpura	Regularly monitor vital signs, blood pressure, blood sugar, blood level drug and provide hygienic care and infection prevention precautions
	Chlorambucil: 0.1–0.3 mg/kg/day	It is a weak immunosuppressant used in autoimmune diseases	
Glucocort-icoids	Corticosteroids	These are companion drugs to cyclosporine; it is useful in graft rejection and autoimmune diseases	Provide hygienic care. Check blood sugar periodically
Antibody reagents	TNFα inhibitors	Mainly used in autoimmune disease	Check for cytokine release syndrome, continuous monitor of vital signs Provide side rails Follow institute protocol while administering drug
	Anti-cD3 antibody	It is useful in acute transplant rejection; mainly in steroid resistant cases; it is also used to deplete T cells from the donor bone marrow before transplantation	Check for cytokine release syndrome, continuous monitor of vital signs; provide side rails Follow institute protocol while administering drug
	Antithymocyte globulin (ATG)/polyclonal antibodies: Lyphoglobulin 100 mg Thymoglobulin 1.5 mg/kg/day	It is used to suppress acute allograft rejection episodes among steroid resistant cases	Check for cytokine release syndrome, continuous monitor of vital signs Provide side rails Follow institute protocol while administering drug

Hypothalamus releases gonadotropin-releasing hormone (GnRH). This stimulates the anterior pituitary to release FSH and LH. FSH stimulates maturation of primary oocyte in an immature follicle. Follicle produces estrogen. Estrogen builds the uterine wall (the endometrium) and inhibits secretion of FSH. High levels of estrogen further stimulate secretion of LH by anterior pituitary. This plus FSH also causes ovulation of the secondary oocyte—leaving follicle without egg (the corpus luteum).

Corpus luteum secretes estrogen and progesterone. This maintains the endometrium for 15–16 days and inhibits LH (if oocyte is not fertilized and implanted in the uterine wall) corpus degenerates (to corpus albicans) and stops producing estrogen and progesterone. Without estrogen and progesterone, endometrium breaks down—menstruation occurs. Menstruation is the sloughing off of the enlarged endometrial wall along with blood and mucus. Decrease in progesterone and LH. Low LH causes secretion of FSH by pituitary again. The cycle repeats.

MULTIPLE CHOICE QUESTIONS

1. **Drug for opioid withdrawal and detoxification:**
   a. Clonidine
   b. Methadone
   c. Thiamine
   d. Nicotine
2. **Disulfiram aversion therapy should be initiated, patient has not consumed alcohol in past: _____ hours.**
   a. 2 hours
   b. 12 hours
   c. 24 hours
   d. 48 hours
3. **Availability of adrenaline:**
   a. 1 mg/1 mL
   b. 5 mg/1 mL
   c. 10 mg/mL
   d. 5 mg/2 mL
4. **Indication of atropine in emergency:**
   a. Ventricular fibrillation
   b. Bronchospasm
   c. Pulseless VT
   d. Severe bradycardia
5. **0.45% NS is considered as:**
   a. Isotonic
   b. Hypotonic
   c. Hypertonic
   d. Colloid

Answer Key

1. a
2. b
3. a
4. d
5. b

FURTHER READING

1. Ada G. Vaccines and vaccination. N Engl J Med. 2001;345:1042.
2. Advice for travelers. Treat Guidel Med Lett. 2009;7:83.
3. Avery RK. Immunizations in adults immunocompromised patients: which to use and which to avoid. Cleve clin J Med. 2001;68:337.
4. CDC Website: http://www.cdc.gov/vaccines/
5. Dennehy PH. Active immunization in the united states: developments over the past decade. Clin Micro Rev. 2001;14;872.
6. Gardner P, Peter G. Vaccine recommendations: challenges adncontroversies. Infect Dis Clin North Am. 2001;15:1.
7. Gardner P, et al. Guidelines for quality standards for immunization. Clin Infect Dis. 2002;35:503.
8. General recommendations on immunization. Recommendations of the Advisory Committee on Immunization Practices (ACIP). MMWR Morb Mortal Wkly Rep. 2011;60(2):1.

9. Hill DR, et al. The practice of travel medicine: guidelines by the infectious diseases society of America. Clin infect Dis. 2006;43:1499.
10. Huether SE. Fluids and electrolytes, acids and bases. In: Huether SE, McCance KL. Understanding Pathophysiology, 5th edn. Mosby. St. Louis. 2012: 105-26.
11. Keller MA, Stiehm ER. Passive immunity in prevention and treatment of infectious disease. Clin microbiol Rev. 2000;13:602.
12. Ministry of Health and Family Welfare-GOI. Immunization Handbook for Health Workres. National Health Mission. 2018:33-34
13. Pickering LK, et al. Immunization programs for infants, children, adolescents, and adults: clinical practice guidelines by the infectious diseases society of America. Clin infect Dis. 2009;49:817.
14. Recommended adult immunization schedules-United States, 2010. MMWR Morb Mortal Wkly Rep. 2010;59:1.
15. Recommended immunization schedules for persons aged 0 through 18 years-United States, 2010. MMWR Morb Mortal Wkly Rep. 2007;58(51 and 52).

CHAPTER 7

Introduction to Drugs Used in Alternative Systems of Medicine

Raj Kumar, Hemlata, Suresh Sharma

Endless varieties of traditional health practices exist in the world. Alternative systems of medicine (ASM) use elements from the domain of traditional medicine. A number of traditional systems of medicine exist in India among which Ayurveda and Siddha are of fully originated and developed in India. **Figure 7.1** depicts the AYUSH—alternative system of medicine.

AYURVEDA, HOMEOPATHY, UNANI, AND SIDDHA, ETC.

Ayurveda

- The term 'Ayurveda' meaning knowledge of life has derived from the Sanskrit words 'ayu' (life) and 'veda' (knowledge). The origin of Ayurveda dates back to the early Vedic period 3000–1000 BC. Rigveda (2000 BC) describes the use of plants as medicine in India and Atharvaveda (1500–1000 BC), which described more plants and introduced further more basic concepts of Ayurveda.
- In Hindu mythology, the origin of ayurvedic medicine is attributed to Dhanvantari, the physician of the Gods. Hinduism and Buddhism have been an influence on the development

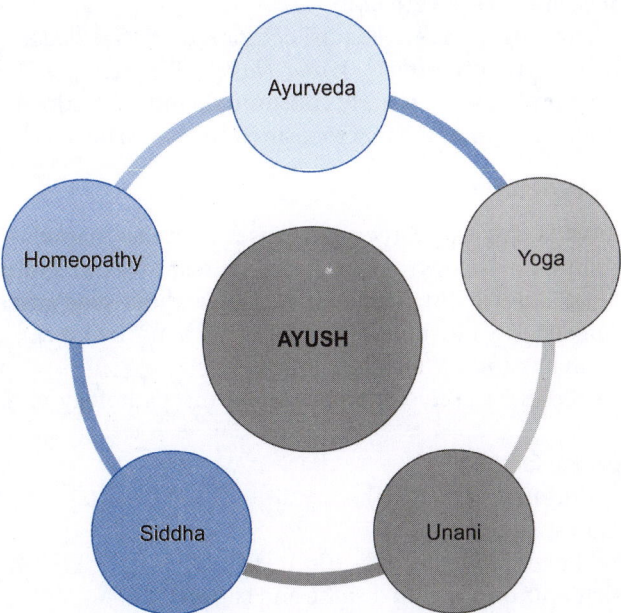

Fig. 7.1: AYUSH—alternative system of medicine.

of many of Ayurveda's central ideas. Ayurveda had tremendous development during the Buddhist period. During this period, there were institutions to teach and practice this system of medicine.
- Charaka and Sushruta are the two celebrated pioneers in Ayurvedic medicine. Charaka compiled Charaka Samhita, which is the basic textbook of Ayurveda in which he mentioned the use of many drugs. Sushruta, who is considered as the father of Indian surgery, compiled Sushruta Samhita, which describes early surgical knowledge.
- In Ayurveda, treatment involves two different types of experts—practitioners and dispensers.
- Among the category of practitioners, there is a subcategory for Ayurveda therapists, which is of two types; those who practice as panchakarma therapists and those who practice as Ayurveda dietitians.
- Panchakarma is a therapeutic way of eliminating toxic elements from the body.
- Health is defined as the state of equilibrium of:
  - *Dosha:* The humors
  - *Agni:* Digestive juices, enzymes and hormones involved in metabolism (biofire)
  - *Dhatu:* Tissues
  - *Mala:* Waste materials

Along with a happy state of atma (soul), indriya (sensory and motor organs), and manas (mind). Thus, Ayurveda aims to maintain equilibrium of dosha, dhatu and mala, patency of srotas (channels) and a healthy state of the agni.

Basic Concepts and Fundamental Principles of Ayurveda

- Ayurveda is based on the principle that the entire universe and the human body are one, and that the same principles govern both.
- The Universe, according to Ayurveda is composed of five basic elements—Pancha Mahabhutas, such as *Earth (Prithvi), Water (Jala), Fire (Agni), Air (Vayu) and Space/Ether (Akash)*. Human body is similarly constituted, and a healthy balance between the microcosm (human being) and the macrocosm (universe) is the basis of health.

Concept of Disease in Ayurveda

- According to Ayurveda, there are three main causes of disease, namely—Asatmendriyartha samyoga (indiscriminate use of senses organs and their objects), Prajnaparadha (error of intellect resulting in a loss of discrimination between wholesome and unwholesome with subsequent indulgence in unwholesome diets and behavior) and Parinama (seasonal variation, cosmic effects and the effects of time).
- Pancha lakshana nidana, the five components of the pathology of a disease, assists in diagnosis. They are:
  1. Nidana (causative factors)
  2. Purvarupa (prodromal symptoms)
  3. Rupa (signs and symptoms)
  4. Samprapti (pathogenesis)
  5. Upashaya (elements opposite to disease and causes)
- The concept of shat kriyakala (six stages of pathogenesis) is vital for an understanding of the pathological states of the doshas that result in disease. These are chaya (accumulation),

prakopa (aggravation), prasara (overflowing), sthanasamsraya (localization), vyakti (manifestation) and bheda (classification or dissolution) of doshas.
- The Charaka Samhita recommends a ten-fold examination of the patient—constitution, abnormality, essence, stability, body measurements, diet suitability, psychic strength, digestive capacity, physical fitness and age.

Treatment Principles in Ayurveda

In Ayurveda, the equilibrium of the dhatus in healthy individuals is preserved, so that disease is prevented. In diseased people, treatment eliminates the disequilibrium between the doshas, and the body is restored to normality. From this point of view, a wholesome substance is said to be one of two types, either one that maintains health or one that disequilibrium between the doshas thereby alleviating the disorders. The latter is used for treatment of the diseased and the former is used for healthy people to maintain and promote health. In addition, vajikarana (aphrodisiac) and rasayana (rejuvenative/promotive) measures are also prescribed for removing toxins accumulated in the body, maintaining equilibrium and preventing senility and related problems.

Ayurveda also focuses on diet, hygiene, exercise, yoga and meditation. This focus on offering a healthy sytem rather than fighting with disease.

Types of Treatment

Ayurveda considered as one of the oldest medicinal and healing system. This ayurvedic treatment foucs on balance of mind, body and spirit. Following are the type of ayurvedic treatment:
- **Shodhana therapy:** Purification of body by detoxing include emesis induction, oil enema, etc.
- **Shamana therapy:** Treating body imbalances or stabilizing the dosha by herbal medicines includes sunbathing. Use of digestives and appetizers
- **Pathya vyavastha:** Modification of several diet and activities plan include intermittent fasting, stimulation of *Jathr Agni* (Fire).
- **Rasayana therapy:** Improving immune system of the patient

Drugs in Ayurveda

In Ayurveda, substances of natural origin including whole plants or their parts, animal parts and minerals are used as medicines, either alone or usually in combination. Hundreds of plant- based medicines are employed including cardamom and cinnamon. Some animal products may also be used, e.g., milk, bones, and gallstones. In addition, fats are used both for consumption and for external use. Minerals, including sulfur, arsenic, lead, copper sulfate and gold are also consumed as prescribed. This practice of adding minerals to herbal medicine is known as rasa shastra. Alcohol or opium was used as a narcotic. Both oil and tar were used to stop bleeding. Traumatic bleeding was said to be stopped by four different methods of ligation of the blood vessel; cauterization by heat; using different herbal or animal preparations locally, which could facilitate clotting; and different medical preparations, which could constrict the bleeding or oozing vessels. Various oils could be used in a number of ways including regular consumption as a part of food, anointing, smearing, head massage and prescribed application to infected areas.

Siddha System

- The Siddha medicine is believed to be more than 10,000 years old. This system of medicine originated as a system of medicine in the Tamil speaking regions. This system was very popular in Ancient India and was well flourished during the Indus Valley civilization.
- The system is believed to be developed by the 18 siddhars, who possessed the Ashta Siddhis, or the eight supernatural powers. Sage Agastya is considered the guru of all siddhars. Palm leaf manuscripts say that Siddha System was first described by Lord Shiva to his wife Parvati who passed on this knowledge to her son Lord Muruga and he taught his disciple Sage Agastya, who in turn taught 18 siddhars and they spread this knowledge to human beings. The siddhars contributed thousands of texts on Siddha in palm leaf manuscripts, fragments of which were found in different parts of South India.
- Siddhars were of the concept that a healthy soul can only be developed through a healthy body. So they developed methods and medication that are believed to strengthen their physical body and thereby their souls. 'Siddha medicine' means medicine that is perfect. Siddha medicine maintains the ratio of vata, pitta and kapha, and revitalize and rejuvenate dysfunctional organs that cause the disease.
- Generally the basic concepts of the Siddha medicine are almost similar to ayurveda. But siddha medicine recognizes the predominance of vata, pitta and kapha in childhood, adulthood and old age, respectively whereas in Ayurveda, kapha is dominant in childhood, vata in old age and pitta in adults.
- National Institute of Siddha, Chennai, Tamil Nadu, India was the first institute which focuses on growth and development of Sidhha by promoting research and healthcare in Siddha. This institute was established on 3rd May 2005.

According to the Siddha medicine, various psychological and physiological functions of the body are related to the combination of seven elements:
- Plasma (saram) responsible for growth, development and nourishment
- Blood (cheneer) responsible for nourishing muscles, imparting color and improving intellect
- Muscle (ooun) responsible for shape of the body
- Fatty tissue (kollzuppu) responsible for oil balance and lubricating joint
- Bone (elumbu) responsible for body structure and posture and movement
- Brain (moolai) responsible for strength
- Semen (sukila) responsible for reproduction

It is assumed that when the normal equilibrium of the three humors (vata, pitta and kapha) is disturbed, disease is caused. The factors, which affect this equilibrium are environment, climatic conditions, diet, physical activities and stress. Under normal conditions, the ratio between these three humors (vata, pitta and kapha) is 4:2:1, respectively.

According to the siddha system, diet and lifestyle play a major role, not only in health but also in curing diseases. This concept is termed 'pathyam and apathya', which is essentially a list of 'do's and don'ts'.

In diagnosis, examination of eight items is required:
1. **Tongue (na):** Black in vatha, yellow or red in pitta, white in kapha, ulcerated in anemia.
2. **Color (varna):** Dark in vatha, yellow or red in pitta, pale in kapha.
3. **Voice (svara):** Normal in vatha, high-pitched in pitta, low-pitched in kapha, slurred in alcoholism.

4. **Eyes (kan):** Muddy conjunctiva in vatha, yellowish or red in pitta, pale in kapha.
5. **Touch (sparisam):** Dry in vatha, warm in pitta, chill in kapha, sweating in different parts of the body.
6. **Stool (mala):** Black stools indicate vatha, yellow pitta, pale in kapha, dark red in ulcer and shiny in terminal illness.
7. **Urine (neer):** Early morning urine is examined; straw color indicates indigestion, reddish-yellow color in excessive heat, rose in blood pressure, saffron color in jaundice, and looks like meat washed water in renal disease.
8. **Pulse (nadi):** The confirmatory method recorded on the radial artery.

Siddha system focus on treating the disease, such as skin problems (psoriasis) and sexually transmitted disease) but not emergency cases. It is also effective for diarrhea, postpartum anemia and arthritis.

Drugs in Siddha

- The drugs used by the siddhars could be classified into three groups—*thavara (herbal product), dhathu (inorganic substances)* and *jangamam (animal products)*.
- The drugs used in siddha medicine were classified on the basis of five properties—*suvai (taste), guna (character), veerya (potency), pirivu (class)* and *mahimai (action)*.
- According to their mode of application, the siddha medicines could be categorized into two classes; internal medicine was used through the oral route and further classified into 32 categories based on their form, methods of preparation, shelf-life, etc. External medicine includes drugs, certain applications (such as nasal, eye and ear drops), and certain procedures (such as leech application) further classified into 32 categories based on their form, methods of preparation, shelf-life, etc.
- The siddha medicine includes leaves, flowers, fruits, various roots and even some metals in a mixed basis.
- The treatment in siddha medicine is thus aimed at keeping the three humors in equilibrium and maintenance of seven elements. Hence, proper diet, medicine and a disciplined regimen of life are advised for a healthy living and to restore equilibrium of humors in diseased condition.

Homeopathy

Homeopathy has its own unique philosophy and therapeutics. The credit of deriving an entire system of therapeutics from this principle, goes to the German physician Samuel Hahnemann. Drugs are living, vibrating personalities, each, full of specific energy and capable of influencing life in all the three planes, viz. physical, mental and spiritual. Each drug performs a specific type of work of a specific degree. 'Materia Medica' contains the description of drugs used in homeopathy. The first National Institute of Homeopathy was established on 10th December, 1975 in Kolkata, West Bengal.

Fundamental Principles of Homeopathy

There are a few fundamental principles, which form the basis of this science—seven cardinal principles in homeopathy. They are as follows:
1. Law of similia
2. Law of simplex
3. Law of minimum dose

4. Doctrine of drug proving
5. Theory of chronic diseases
6. Theory of vital force
7. Doctrine of drug dynamization

Law of Similia

The word 'homoeos' means 'like' or 'similar' and 'pathos' means 'suffering' and so homeopathy is a 'medicine of likes'. It is a method of curing the sufferings in a diseased individual by administration of remedies that have the capacity to produce similar sufferings in a relatively healthy individual. This is the law that governs Homeopathy and forms the most fundamental basis of this science. This law is also called **Similia Similibus Curantur**, which means 'Let likes be treated by likes'.

Law of Simplex

- Hahnemann states 'only one, single, simple remedy should be administered to the patient at one time'.
- This is the law of simplex. At any given time, only one remedy can be the exactly similar to the presenting condition of the patient. If the physician administers more than one remedy at a time, he/she will be unable to ascertain the curative action of the remedy. Administration of more than one drug can lead to symptoms, which can be harmful to the patient.

Law of Minimum Dose

Homeopathic medicines act at a dynamic level and only a minute quantity of the medicine is enough to stimulate the dynamically deranged vital force to bring about the necessary curative change in a patient. The minuteness of drug avoids the unwanted medicinal aggravation caused by crude substances, and prevents chances of any organ damage.

Doctrine of Drug Proving

Drug proving is a systematic investigation and evaluation of the disease producing power of a substance on healthy human beings of both sexes, different age groups and people from different places. Healthy individuals should be chosen for conducting a drug proving, because if a diseased person is chosen, the actions of the drug to be proved and the disease symptoms will merge with each other and an accurate picture of the drug may not emerge.

Theory of Chronic Diseases

Hahnemann after 12 years of experiment and observations, concluded that the chronic miasms are the main cause of chronic diseases. Miasm is an obnoxious disease-producing agent, dynamic in nature and inimical to life. He founded the theory of miasms and named the miasms as—Psora, Sycosis, Syphilis.

Theory of Vital Force

Vital force is the invisible vital energy that animates each organism and is the essence of the individual. In health, it is this spirit-like force that governs the life and maintains all the bodily sensations and functions in equilibrium. In disease, there is dynamic derangement of the vital force, which leads to disharmony and alteration of all the bodily functions and sensations.

Doctrine of Drug Dynamization

Drug dynamization is a process by which all the medicinal properties, which are latent in a substance, are extracted from their crude form for the curative purpose by diluting drug on a specific scale and this process is called 'potentization'. By potentization, there is a quantitative reduction and a qualitative enhancement of the medicinal substance, hence medicinal aggravation is minimized. Toxic materials and venoms of certain animals, when potentized are rendered harmless for therapeutic purpose.

Unani System

- The word Unani or Yunani has its origins in the Greek word—ωνία (Iōnía), the name of a place in Greek populated coastal region of Anatolia. In Hindi, Urdu and Persian, it means 'Greek Medicine' and is a form of traditional medicine widely practiced in South Asia. It is a tradition of Greco-Arabic medicine, which is based on the teachings of Greek physician Hippocrates and Roman physician Galen, and developed into an elaborate medical system by Arab and Persian physicians such as Rhazes, Avicenna (Ibn Sena), Al-Zahrawi and Ibn Nafis.

  Unani medicine is based on the concept of the four humors:
  1. Phlegm (Balgham)
  2. Blood (Dam)
  3. Yellow bile (Safrā')
  4. Black bile (Saudā')

  The basic knowledge of Unani medicine as a healing system was developed by Hakim Ibn Sina (known as Avicenna in the West) in his medical encyclopedia 'The Canon of Medicine'.

- Any cause and/or factor is countered by Quwwat-e-Mudabbira-e-Badan (the power of body responsible to maintain health), the failing of which may lead to derangement of the normal equilibrium of akhlat (humors) of the body, which contribute to the disease. The abnormal humor leads to pathological changes in the tissues and exhibits the clinical manifestations. After diagnosing the disease, Usool-e-Ilaj (principle of management) of disease is determined on the basis of etiology on the following pattern:
  - Izala E Sabab (elimination of cause)
  - Tadeele Akhlat (normalization of humors)
  - Tadeele Aza (normalization of tissues/organs)
  - *Ilaj-Bil-Advia (pharmacotherapy):* For this purpose, mamulat e matlab nuskha (prescription) is formulated which contain the single and/or compound Unani drugs having desired actions as per requirements.
  - Ilaj-Bil-Yad (surgery)

- Unani practitioners can practice as qualified doctors in India, as the government approves their practice. Unani medicine is very close to Ayurveda. Both are based on theory of the presence of the elements (in Unani, they are considered to be fire, water, earth and air) in the human body. According to followers of Unani medicine, these elements are present in different fluids and their balance leads to health and their imbalance leads to illness.

- National Institute of Unani Medicine was established on 19th November 1984 in Bengaluru. The vision of institute is to propagate and develop Unani system of Medicine.

DEPARTMENT OF AYUSH UNDER THE MINISTRY OF HEALTH AND FAMILY WELFARE

A department for Indian Systems of Medicine and Homeopathy was established under the Ministry of Health and Family Welfare and later renamed as Department of AYUSH (Ayurveda, Yoga & Naturopathy, Unani, Siddha and Homeopathy). The department works for improving the quality and standards of drugs, education, research and development and awareness generation in the fields of these systems of medicine. The Drug Control Cell in the Department of AYUSH has reviewed the essential drug lists of Ayurveda, Siddha, Unani and Homeopathy and published a new list to guide the procurement and stocking of these medicines in the health facilities. Ayurvedic, Siddha and Unani Drug Technical Advisory Board (ASUDTAB) have recommended shelf-life/expiry date for Ayurvedic, Siddha and Unani (ASU) drugs.

Pharmacopoeia Commission

The safety concerns tend to get more and more stringent regarding the ASU drugs. To establish Pharmacopoeia Standards for Ayurvedic, Siddha and Unani drugs, Government of India has three Pharmacopoeia Committee for Ayurveda, Siddha and Unani. It is an independent body, which conducts ongoing exercises and regularly upgrades the standards.

Role of Nurses ASM

- Mainstreaming alternative and Indian Systems of Medicine provides a wide variety of challenges and opportunities for nurses. Several ayurvedic institutions are already running degree and diploma courses in Ayurvedic Nursing and Panchakarma. Indira Gandhi National Open University (IGNOU) also started certificate in AYUSH nursing (Ayurveda) for Auxiliary Nurse Midwives. Many people are using traditional medicines in addition to Allopathic system. It should be immediately reported to the physician and if possible consult with an AYUSH practitioner.
- The dilution and mode of administration of AYUSH medicines are different from the allopathic system. Certain drugs are mixed and diluted with different substances, such as honey, milk, water, palm jaggery, ginger juice, etc. The time of administration of drugs is also sensitive. So, it is necessary to read the instructions given with these medicines and check the date of expiry also.
- Certain drugs are contraindicated in certain conditions such as pregnancy, and certain disease conditions. Many drugs of traditional medicine system contain metals and compounds, which in large doses can be poisonous. According to the traditional medicine system these compounds are purified and do not have any poisonous effects. So, it is necessary to establish pharmacopoeia standards for alternative systems of medicine. Nurses should have basic awareness on these and the basic nursing curriculum should be updated according to these needs.

DRUGS USED IN COMMON AILMENTS

The alternative system of medicine is used for many common ailments. These ailments are treated with drugs used in Ayush, Homeopathy, Unani and Siddha. The rational usage of these drugs requires supervision and prescription. **Table 7.1** illustrated the drugs used in common ailments.

CHAPTER 7: Introduction to Drugs Used in Alternative Systems of Medicine

Table 7.1: Usage of AYUSH drugs for managing common ailments.

System	Common ailments	Drugs used for managing ailments
Circulatory system	Iron deficiency disorder	*Ayurveda:* Buttermilk, dry grapes, spinach, jaggery with tepid water, rice water with mandura bhasma 0.5 g twice daily *Homeopathy:* Arsenic album, ferrum phosphoricum, natrum muriaticum
	Weakness	*Homeopathy:* Ferrum metallicum
	Palpitation/tachycardia	*Homeopathy:* Arsenic album, calcarea carbonicum
Digestive system	Abdominal pain	*Ayurveda:* Hinguvachadi churna, lashunadi vati two tablet twice a day with warm water, hing churan with mustard oil for massaging near umbilicus or mix I warm water *Homeopathy:* Cyn-D. every 2 hours, coloc. 30 every half an hour
	Constipation	*Ayurveda:* Triphala 5 g with tepid water, 8–10 dried grapes in boiled 250 mL milk
	Peptic ulcer, acidity and burning sensation, indigestion	*Ayurveda:* Kushmanda or petha 7–14 mL with 3 g of yashtimadu powder twice daily, nimbu Juice *Unani:* Qurs-e-Tankar 1 tab/bd. Qurs-e-Kabid 1 tab/bd *Naturopathy:* Hydrotherapy, massage and mud therapy *Yoga:* Asana, kriya, cleansing process
	Worm infestation	*Ayurveda:* Hing Churanin luke warm water
	Vomiting	*Ayurveda:* Hing churan, jatiphala with tulsi, kali mirch, nimbu juice *Homeopathy:* Phosphorus
	Hemorrhoids	*Ayurveda:* Kulattha or horse gram dal soup trice daily
	Diarrhea and dysentery	*Ayurveda:* Tirakatuor panchakola powder 2 g bd, lavang water *Homeopathy:* Cyn-D. every 2 hours *Naturopathy:* Hydrotherapy, massage and mud therapy
Urinary system	Urinary calculi	*Ayurveda:* Kulattha or horse gram 1–2 g in water, musli root 5–10 g
	Edema	*Homeopathy:* Ferrum metallicum
	Dysuria	*Ayurveda:* Kushmanda or petha 60 mL with yavakshara 5 g and sugar 25 g bd
Musculoskeletal system	Rheumatoid arthritis	*Ayurveda:* Kulattha or horse gram dal soup trice daily *Naturopathy:* Massage with mustard oil
Respiratory system	Allergic rhinitis	*Ayurveda:* Haridra khanda
	Cough	*Ayurveda:* Lavang or laung with honey, mircha or kali mirch
Reproductive system	Leukorrhea or vaginal disorder	*Ayurveda:* Pushyanuga churna 3 g with honey *Homeopathy:* Kali carbonicum
	Menstrual disordrs	*Ayurveda:* Kulattha or horse gram decoction of seed in 30 mL water *Homeopathy:* Kali carbonicum, natrum muriaticum, pulsatilla
	Pregnancy	*Unani:* Sharbat-e-faulad 15 mL bd *Ayurveda:* Hyperemesis gravidarum lavang with sugar syrup
	Oligospermia	*Ayurveda:* Musli 3–6 g with sugar candy and milk
Integumentary system	Skin disorders, such as rash	*Ayurveda:* Haridra Khanda
Nervous system	Epilepsy or fits	*Ayurveda:* Kushmanda or petha 7–14 mL with 3 g of yashtimadhu powder twice daily

SECTION 1: Pharmacology-II

MULTIPLE CHOICE QUESTIONS

1. **The term 'Ayurveda' means:**
   a. Science of life
   b. Knowledge of life
   c. Life of human
   d. Science of medicine
2. **Pancha Mahabhutas is related to which system of Indian medicine:**
   a. Ayurveda
   b. Siddha
   c. Unani
   d. Naturopathy
3. **Rasayana therapy is the treatment that:**
   a. Modifies diet
   b. Treating body imbalances
   c. Body purification
   d. Improving immune system
4. **Vata, pitha and kapha are related to which system of Indian medicine:**
   a. Ayurveda
   b. Siddha
   c. Unani
   d. Naturopathy

Answer Key

1. b   2. a   3. d   4. b

FURTHER READING

1. Cherukara JM. Medical Tourism in Kerala—Challenges and Scope, paper presented at the Conference on Tourism in India—Challenges ahead, 15–17 May, Indian Institute of Management, Kozhikode; (2008).
2. Mehta R. Integrating AYUSH systems in healthcare perspective, in Technopak Perspective, 4; 2010.
3. Ministry of Health and Family Welfare, Government of India. National Health Programmes, AYUSH and Management of Minor Ailments. Book 4.2006;1–33.
4. Priya R, AS Shewtha. Status and role of AYUSH and local health care traditions under the National Rural Health Mission. Government of India; 2010;73–116.
5. The Ayurvedic Pharmacopoeia of India. Part-I, Volume-III. New Delhi: Ministry of Health and Family Welfare, Government of India; 2001.

CHAPTER 8

Fundamental Principles of Prescribing

Suresh Sharma

PRESCRIPTIVE ROLE OF NURSE PRACTITIONERS: INTRODUCTION

Nursing practice has become multifaceted with the development of innovative extended roles and levels of practice in nursing worldwide. Prescriptive authority is one among these advancements and should be sensitive to the country's environment and necessity. As a result, the method to describe and implement nurse prescribing varies from country to country. The variances between countries replicate differences in "healthcare systems", the development in nursing, and administrative authority that impacts decision-making and policy.

Approaches to implementing and developing nurse prescribing need vigorous leadership and positive action to promote this essential service for international healthcare provision. Prescriptive authority for nurses has originate as a reply to the altering landscape of "healthcare demands and concerns regarding access to care, the evolution of healthcare systems, and the professionals who provide care". It is significant to remember that the roles and responsibilities of all healthcare professionals evolve in response to the demands and needs of individuals and communities. The prescriptive authority has been a positive and practical example of this type of change. Prescribing is included as a component of undergraduate nursing program in the US.

Nursing roles are changing, and with the introduction of nurse practitioner programs in critical care, midwifery, and primary care, there is a need to move towards empowering these nurses in terms of quality, standards, monitoring, and evaluation. Their clinical expertise is also highly valued by patients. The professions, their education and professional progress, credentialing, and models of prescribing differs within and between countries. Though there is narrow standardization, the precise aims of prescriptive authorization for healthcare professionals to prescribe are generally related to:
- Improving access to treatment for the patient
- Enlightening patient outcomes without compromising patient safety
- Optimal utilization of possible skills and proficiency of health professionals
- Supportive legal protection for the prescriber and others with delegated responsibilities

The role and responsibilities of nurses are developing and altering universally. Nursing practice has become additional multifaceted and varied as nurses are a progressively observable and essential part of multidisciplinary teams with their knowledge and expertise in managing patient care. Nurses are emerging with up-to-date developments in the provision of healthcare services; prescriptive authority is one aspect of these advances in the nursing profession. The motivation for nurse prescribing is subtle to the country's context and the healthcare culture in which this possibility develops. Consequently, the method of significant and implementation nurse prescribing follows a distinctive pattern in different countries.

Standards of Proficiency (Nursing and Midwifery Council—NMC, UK)

Nurse prescribers must have sufficient knowledge and competence to:
- Assess a patient's clinical condition
- Undertake a thorough health history that includes medication history
- Diagnose and decide on management of the presenting condition and whether or not to prescribe where necessary
- Identify appropriate products, if medication is required
- Advise the patient on the effects and risks
- Prescribe if the patient agrees and as per legal provision
- Monitor response to medication and lifestyle advice

Prescribing became a part of nursing practice in a few countries from decades. The level of education and credentialing for nurse prescribing differs among authorities and ranges from diploma-prepared generalist nurses to advanced practice nurses with master's or doctoral degrees. The various perspectives on the prescriptive role of nurse practitioners are described below:
- The various models of prescriptive authority serves as a foundation for safe and effective prescribing tool for the nurses.
- Prescriptive authority for nurses can advance effective and effective healthcare service provision and enable more integrated patient care, rise professional satisfaction, and increase the complete quality of the health service.
- Nurses' prescribing practice comes under three different categories: "Independent prescribing, supplementary prescribing, and prescribing via a structured prescribing arrangement (or protocol)".
- Authorities need a set period of clinical experience before starting recommending practice.
- Nurse prescribing is progressively becoming an essential role within nursing practice and improves job satisfaction and self-empowerment.

LEGAL AND ETHICAL ISSUES RELATED TO PRESCRIBING

Prescribing is a multifaceted task that needs the application of comprehensive judgment, precise knowledge, skills, and attitudes to an individual at a given point in time. An increasing number of medicines available to the prescriber, many people receiving multiple drugs, and a variety of treatments and therapies increased the complexity to a complicated state.

Understanding about legal and ethical aspects involved in drug prescribing is essential for safe practice by the nurses. Nurse practitioners must work under the professional code of conduct and legislative limitations. The framework of safe and competent prescription contains five core components which are described in **Figure 8.1**. The necessities under each of the components may differ based on the needs of the selected nurse prescribing model.

Completion of An Accredited Education Program

The healthcare worker looking for prescriptive authority should undergo an accredited education program that is reliable with their scope of practice and validates competence. The education should be certified by "the appropriate nursing board or accreditation council". Accreditation guarantees that the course has the relevant content and that the curricula meet or exceed the standards that experts have developed to protect the nursing profession and the public. An education program should be developed that can adequately assess the performance of the nurse seeking prescriptive authority to a set standard. The following are the core components of the education program related to safe and competent prescriptions.

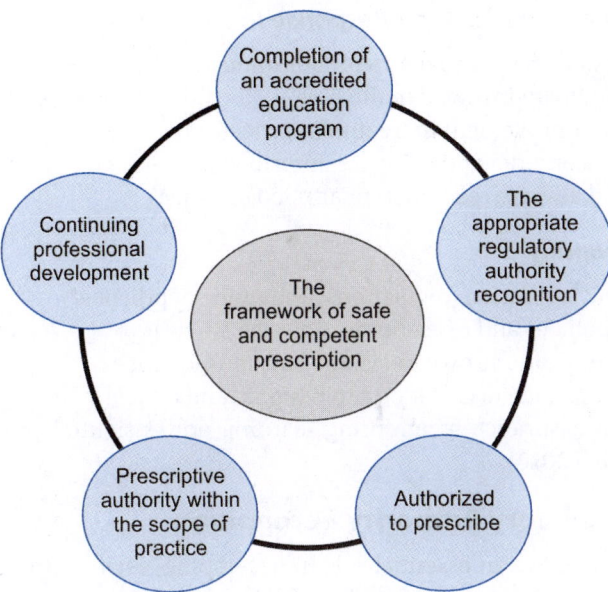

Fig. 8.1: The framework of safe and competent prescription.

People Centeredness in Care
- Place individuals at the center of all practice
- Promote individual and public agency
- Provide culturally sensitive, respectful, and empathetic care
- Incorporate a systems approach to health
- Demonstrate clinical reasoning and decision-making capacities

Evidenced-based and Informed Practice
- Identify the utmost suitable treatment based on the person's needs
- Avoid the overdoing or mistreatment
- Maintain present knowledge of prescribing procedures or algorithms

Communication and Collaboration
- Adapt good communication skills to goal oriented and compassionate communication
- Listen keenly and thoughtfully
- Convey information purposefully
- Manage information sharing, consider patient in decision making
- Engage in collaborative practice
- Build and maintain believing partnerships

Pharmacological Essentials
- Demonstrate knowledge of human anatomy and physiology
- Apply to the understanding of pharmacodynamics
- Maintain up to date knowledge
- Prepare prescriptions reliable according to laws and policies

Monitors and Reviews the Person's Response to Treatment
- Monitor the person's response to drugs continuously
- Share details with team involved in the care
- Work for quality improvement in treatment procedures
- Enabling person-centered and evidence-informed practice
- Report suspected adverse reactions (pharmacovigilance)

Practices Professionally
- Practicing under "legislation, regulations, and scope of practice"
- Faithfulness to policies and procedures
- Take accountability for one own decisions and consequences
- Practice as per "the code of conduct, professional and ethical standards"
- Demonstrate an assurance to enduring learning and insightful practice (Nursing and Midwifery Council 2018)

Appropriate Regulatory Authority Recognition

Regulatory authorities hold an essential role in developing, establishing, implementing, and regulating nursing roles. An essential function of the body is to guard the community by making sure that only "nurses who are appropriately educated, qualified, competent and ethical in practice are credentialed". The regulatory authority must be able to identify nurses who are authorized to prescribe. The establishment of a governing regulatory authority is beneficial in the following aspects.
- Helps in the authentication of the proficiency of the employee
- Continuing validation of the persons who provide care
- Research and development in prescriptive authority for nurses

Authorized to Prescribe

The relevant legislation permits authorization to prescribe, related regulations and professional standards within countries, states, regions, or territories, and the policies and procedures of health service providers in which the nurse works.

Prescriptive Authority within the Scope of Practice

The scope of nursing practice is defined "within a legislative and regulatory framework and describes the competencies (knowledge, skills, attitudes, and judgment), professional accountabilities, and responsibilities of the nurse prescriber". It provides the foundation for beginning a standard for nursing practice, nursing education, nursing roles, and responsibilities (ICN 2013). Prescriptive authority is most usually related to the increasing emergence of Advanced Practice Nursing (APN) and relevant scopes of practice for the APN roles/advanced levels of nursing. The scope of practice for the prescriptive authority is mediated by certain factors within the professional and individual domains **(Fig. 8.2)**. The legislation, regulations and standards set by professional organizations will determine the scope of practice to the prescriptive authority of the professionals. In addition, the scope of practice may vary with certain individual domains, such as competency and skills, knowledge, experience, ethics, accountability.

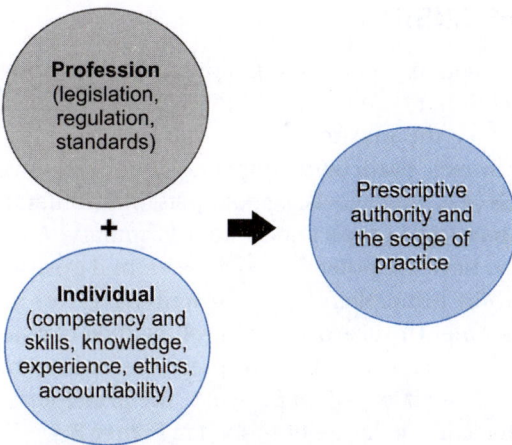

Fig. 8.2: Factors affecting the prescriptive authority and the scope of practice.

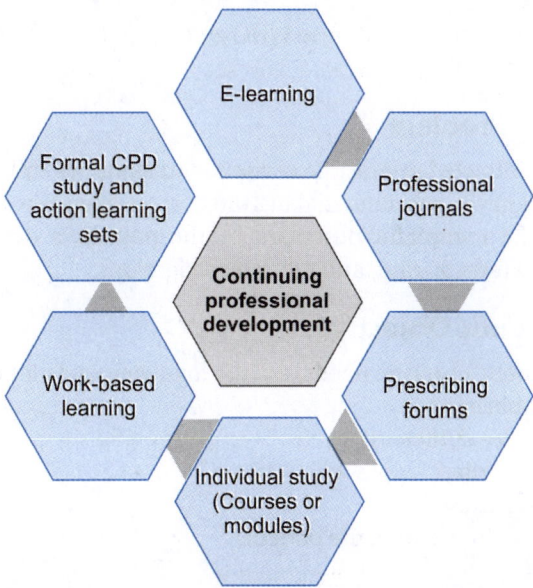

Fig. 8.3: Measures to achieve continuing professional development.

Continuing Professional Development to Uphold the Capability to Prescribe

Continuing professional development (CPD) is recognized as maintaining up-to-date knowledge and skills that influence prescribing competence to ensure quality healthcare and patient safety. Maintaining professional competence for nursing practice and the nurse prescriber is a continuous process. In some countries, mandatory demonstration of CPD is required for ongoing licensure and credentialing. Credentialing bodies or authorities usually determine the requirements and timeline for verification of competence maintenance. The measures to achieve continuing professional development is illustrated in **Figure 8.3**.

PRINCIPLES OF PRESCRIBING

Prescribing is one of the main approaches to treating and preventing diseases. Currently, in India, only medical practitioners are involved in it. However, it is extended to other health professionals in the west for the maximum utilization of resources. Thus, the prescription practices is extended to nurses, particularly nurse practitioners in developed countries, and other health professionals (e.g., pharmacists, podiatrists, physiotherapists) who are permitted to prescribe within the restricted scope and limited formulary. All medicines can enhance health; however, they also have the potential to cause harm if misused. For these reasons, all prescribers should follow the principles of good prescribing. Errors in prescribing can lead to ineffective and unsafe treatment, exacerbation or prolongation of illness, distress, harm to the patient, and higher costs. They can also make the prescriber vulnerable to influences that can cause irrational prescribing, such as patient pressure. The principles of prescribing according to the British Pharmacological Society are described in **Figure 8.4**.

STEPS OF PRESCRIBING

The steps of prescribing process according to WHO guide to good prescribing (1994) is depicted in **Figure 8.5**.

Define the Patient's Problem

The health assessment knowledge must be revised, and skills are utilized when defining the patient's situation. Whenever possible, making the correct diagnosis is based on integrating information, such as the complaint described by the patient, a detailed history, physical examination, laboratory tests, X-rays, and other investigations.

Specify the Therapeutic Objective

After examining the patient's holistic needs, ask the following questions:
- Is the diagnosis established?
- Is information or advice sufficient?
- Is there a need to prescribe?
- What does the patient expect?
- What is your objective for treating the patient?

Select the Therapeutic Strategies

Making a choice involves the consideration of appropriateness, effectiveness, safety, cost, and acceptability of the drug. Select the method based on the knowledge of pathophysiology and the findings from history, examination, lab tests, and other investigations. Medication or drug history and allergies are vital in the past that including the following:
- List of medications the patient is on with the repeat prescription of the medication
- Record from the history the name, dose, frequency, and route of medication
- Prescribed or not
- Inquiry about OTC (over-the-counter) drugs or any other herbal preparations
- Any allergies reaction to the medication, foods, or environmental factors and treatment given

CHAPTER 8: Fundamental Principles of Prescribing

1. Be clear about the reasons for prescribing	• Make an accurate diagnosis whenever possible • Be clear in what the patient is likely to gain from the prescribed medicines
2. Take into account the patient's medication history before prescribing	• Obtain an accurate list of current and recent medications (including over-the-counter and alternative medicines), prior adverse drug reactions, and drug allergies from the patient, their carers, or colleagues
3. Take into account other factors that might alter the benefits and risks of treatment	• Consider other individual factors that might influence the prescription (e.g., physiological changes with age and pregnancy, or impaired kidney, liver or heart function)
4. Take into account the patient's ideas, concerns, and expectations	• Seek to form a partnership with the patient when selecting treatments, making sure that they understand and agree with the reasons for talking the medicine
5. Select effective, safe and cost effective medicines individualized for the patient	• The likely beneficial effect of the medicine should outweigh the extent of any potential harms • Prescribe medicines that are unlicensed, off-lable or outside standard practice only if satisfied • Choose the best formulation, dose, frequency, route of administration, and duration of treatment
6. Adhere to national guidelines and local formularies where appropriate	• Be aware of guidance produced by respected bodies, but always consider the individual needs of the patient • Select medicines with regard to costs and needs of other patients • Be able to identify, access, and use reliable and validate sources of information, and evaluate potentially less reliable information critically
7. Write unambiguous legal prescription using the correct documentation	• Be aware of common factors that cause medication errors and know how to avoid them
8. Monitor the beneficial and adverse effects of medicines	• Identify how the beneficial and adverse effects of treatment can be assessed • Understand how to alter the prescription as a result of this information • Know how to report adverse drug reactions
9. Communicate and document prescribing decisions and the reasons for them	• Communicate clearly with patients, their carers, and colleagues • Give patients important information about how to take the medicine, what benefits might arise, adverse effects, and any monitoring that is required • Use the health record and other means to document prescribing decisions accurately
10. Prescribe within the limitations of your knowledge, skill and experience	• Always seek to keep the knowledge and skills that are relevant to your practice up to date • Be prepared to seek the advice and support of suitably qualified professional colleagues • Make sure that, where appropriate prescriptions are checked (e.g., calculations of intravenous doses)

Fig. 8.4: Principles of prescribing.

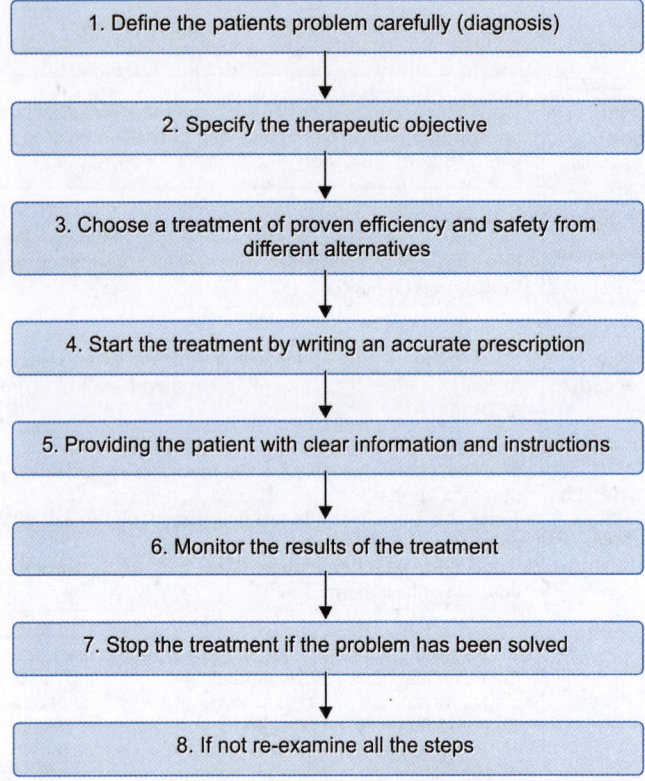

Fig. 8.5: Steps of prescribing.

- Recording the observations. Collect history related to age, sex, hereditary factors, lifestyle factors, social and community networks, living and working conditions, socio-economic, cultural, and environmental conditions. The selected strategy should be agreed upon with the patient (concordance)

Pharmacological Treatment

Pharmacological treatment involves selecting the correct group of drugs, selecting the medicine from the chosen group, and verifying the suitability of the selected drug for each patient. These drugs cause adverse reaction. The measures to avoid these drugs adverse reaction are presented in **Table 8.1.**

Knowledge about the pathophysiology of the clinical condition, pharmacokinetics, and pharmacodynamics of the chosen drug are fundamental principles for rational therapeutics.

Start the Treatment

A prescription is an instruction from a prescriber to a pharmacist/dispenser. The prescriber is not always a doctor; it could be a nurse, medical assistant, etc. The dispenser is not always the pharmacist, it could be an assistant nurse. Every country has its standards, laws, and regulations as to who should prescribe, dispense, and the required information in a prescription form, drugs that require a prescription or not, special laws regarding narcotics, etc.

Table 8.1: Measures to avoid adverse drug reaction.

The selection process of any drug must consider the efficacy and safety of the drug; For safety, the potential benefits of the treatment must always be balanced against known safety concerns. The following are the measures to avoid adverse drug reaction:
• Use as few concurrent drugs as possible
• Use the lowest effective dose
• Check if patient is pregnant or breastfeeding
• Is the patient at extremes of life?
• Do you know all the drugs that the patient is taking?
• Check for over-the-counter medicines
• Drug allergies or previous reaction to medications

Information Regarding Prescription

A prescription should contain the name and address of the prescriber with telephone no (if possible), date of medication, name (generic name) and strength of the drug, dosage form (only use standard abbreviations) (tablet paracetamol 500 mg (10 tablets) BD x 5 days), label: how much, how often, special instruction, name, address, age of the patient, and prescriber's initials signature, license number. Every prescription serve as a legal document. Therefore, clarity, precision and legibility are essential the prerequisites of every prescription.

Give Information, Instruction and Warnings

Accurate information on the prescription would increase drug compliance. Giving adequate instruction are essential to ensure patient compliance. Compliance to drug treatment can be improved by the following ways:
- Selecting the best drug for serving the best purpose
- Maintaining a therapeutic relationship
- Providing adequate amount of time to give necessary information, instructions, and warnings
- Usage of certain compliance tools, such as patient leaflets, pictorials, day calendars, drug passports, and dosage boxes

Monitor the Treatment (Stop or Continue)

Monitoring enables to determine whether the treatment has been successful or additional action is required. This allows stopping or reformulating, if necessary, or continuation of therapy. It may be passive monitoring (self-monitoring) and active monitoring (future appointment and consultation). The guideline for evaluating treatment outcomes are mentioned in **Table 8.2**.

There are certain techniques through which the prescriber can effectively monitor the treatment outcomes which are listed below:
- Make an inventory of available sources of information
    - Reference books and medical journals
    - Drug compendia—handbooks for desk reference national formulary
    - National lists of essential drugs and treatment guidelines

Table 8.2: The decision algorithm regarding monitoring the treatment outcomes.

Was the treatment effective?
• Yes, disease cured, stop the treatment
• Yes, but not yet completed—any side effects ▪ No, treatment can be continued ▪ Yes, reconsider dosage or drug choice
• No, disease not cured—verify all steps: ▪ Diagnosis correct ▪ Therapeutic objective correct ▪ Drug prescribed correctly ▪ Effect monitored correctly

- Drug formularies
- Drug bulletins, drug information centers
- Verbal information
- Drug industry sources of information
- Choose between sources of information that are credible and accessible, e.g., medical journals, drug bulletins, pharmacology or clinical reference books, national formulary revisions
- **Effective reading:** Awareness about the recent updates helps in the formulation of decision during conflicting situations

PRESCRIBING COMPETENCIES

A competency is a quality or characteristic of a person that is related to effective performance. Competencies can be described as a combination of knowledge, skills, motives and personal traits. A competency framework is a collection of competencies thought to be central to effective performance. The prescribing competency framework provides an outline of common competencies to maintain the uniformity in the in the area of practice. It can also be used by regulators, education providers, professional organisations and specialist groups to inform standards, the development of education, and to inform guidance and advice. The competency framework sets out the good prescribing competencies while rendering service (**Fig. 8.6**).

According to this framework, there are two domains, each containing some dimensions of competency which describe the activity or outcomes relevant to all prescribers taking into account their scope of practice.

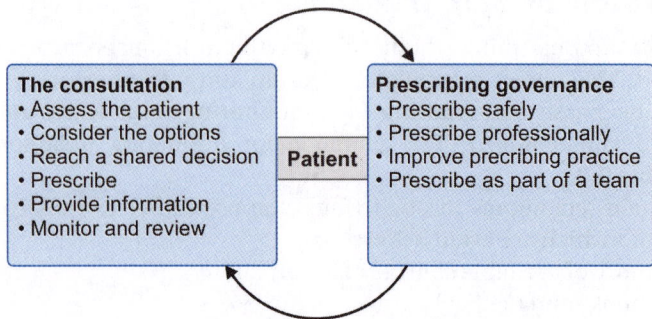

Fig. 8.6: Prescribing competency framework.

Domain 1: The Consultation

1. Assess the Patient

The points to be kept in mind while assessing the patient are to undertake the consultation in an appropriate setting by considering patient dignity, capacity, consent, and confidentiality. Introduce self and prescribing role to the patient/carer and confirms patient/carer identity with good communication skills to build good consultation skills and build rapport with the patient/carer. Collect an appropriate medical, psychosocial, and medication history, including allergies and intolerances, and record. Identifies and addresses possible susceptibilities that may be causing the patient to seek treatment. Accesses and interprets all available and relevant patient records to ensure knowledge of the patient's management to date and relevant investigations for appropriate treatment.

2. Identify Evidence-based Treatment Options Available for Clinical Decision Making

Consider both non-pharmacological and pharmacological treatment approaches and assess the risks and benefits to the patient of taking or not taking medicine or treatment. Understand the pharmacokinetics and pharmacodynamics of drugs and how individual patient factors may alter these. Additionally, assess how comorbidities, existing medication, allergies, intolerances, contraindications, and quality of life impact management options.

3. Present Options and Reach a Shared Decision

Actively involve and work with the patient to make informed choices and agree on a plan that respects the patient's preferences by considering patient diversity, background, personal values, and beliefs about their health, treatment, and medicines, supporting the importance of equality and inclusivity and developing cultural competence. Explain the material risks and benefits and the rationale behind management options in a way the patient understands to make an informed choice.

4. Prescribe

Prescribe a medicine with up-to-date awareness of its actions, indications, dose, contraindications, interactions, cautions, and adverse effects. Understand the potential for adverse effects and take steps to recognize and manage them while minimizing risk and understanding and using relevant national, regional and local frameworks for the use of medicines. Prescribe generic medications where practical and safe for the patient, and knows when treatments should be prescribed by branded product.

5. Provide Information

Assess the patient's health literacy and adapts appropriately to provide clear, understandable, and accessible information, and guide the patient/carer on how to identify reliable sources of information about their condition, medicines, and treatment. Ensure the patient knows what to do if there are any concerns about managing their condition, if the situation deteriorates or if there is no improvement in a specific timeframe.

6. Monitor and Review

Establish and maintain a plan for reviewing the patient's treatment and establish and maintain a program to monitor the effectiveness of treatment and potential unwanted effects. Adapt the management plan in response to ongoing monitoring and review of the patient's condition and preferences.

Domain 2: Prescribing Governance

7. Prescribe Safely

Prescribe within own scope of practice, recognize the limits of own knowledge and skill, know about common types and causes of medication and prescribing errors, and know-how to minimize their risk. Identify and mitigate potential risks associated with prescribing via remote methods. Report near misses, critical incidents, and medication and specify errors using appropriate reporting systems while regularly reviewing practice to prevent a recurrence.

8. Prescribe Professionally

Ensure confidence and competence to prescribe are maintained by accepting personal responsibility and accountability for defining clinical decisions and understanding legal and ethical implications. Work within legal and regulatory frameworks affecting prescribing practice. Make prescribing decisions based on the needs of patients and not the prescriber's personal views. Work within the organizational, regulatory, and other codes of conduct when interacting with the pharmaceutical industry.

9. Improve Prescribing Practice

Improve by reflecting on own and others' prescribing practices, acting upon feedback and discussion, and acting upon inappropriate or unsafe prescribing practices using appropriate processes. Understand and use available tools to improve prescribing practice and take responsibility for own learning and continuing professional development relevant to the prescribing role. Use networks for support and education and encourage and support others with their prescribing practice and continuing professional development.

10. Prescribe as Part of a Team

Work collaboratively as part of a multidisciplinary team to ensure that the transfer and continuity of care (within and across all care settings) are developed and not compromised. Establish relationships with other professionals based on understanding, trust, and respect for each other's roles concerning the patient's care. Agree on the appropriate level of support and supervision for their role as a prescriber.

MULTIPLE CHOICE QUESTIONS

1. Which of the following include in the standards of proficiency?
    a. Assessment of patient's condition
    b. Advise the patient about effects and risks
    c. Monitor response to medication
    d. All of the above

CHAPTER 8: Fundamental Principles of Prescribing

2. In which year World Health Organization issue guidelines to good prescribing?
   a. 1990
   b. 1992
   c. 1994
   d. 1999

Answer Key

1. d
2. c

FURTHER READING

1. Australian Nursing and Midwifery Federation (2018). Registered nurse and midwife prescribing. ANMF Position Statement Retrieved from http://www.anmf.org.au/documents/policies/P_Registered_Nurse_and_Midwife_Prescribing.pdf
2. American Nurses Association (2010). Credentialing Definitions [online]. Retrieved from https://www.nursingworld.org/education-events/faculty-resources/research-grants/styles-credentialing-research-grants/credentialing-definitions/
3. Abuzour AS, Lewis PJ, Tully MP (2018). Practice makes perfect: A systematic review of the expertise development of pharmacist and nurse independent prescribers in the United Kingdom. Res Social Adm Pharm, 14(1), 6–17. doi:10.1016/j.sapharm. 2017.02.002
4. Canadian Nurses Association (2015). Framework for the Practice of Registered Nurses in Canada. Retrieved from https://www.cna-aiic.ca/~/media/cna/page-content/pdf-en/framework-forthe-pracice-of-registered-nurses-in-canada.pdf
5. Indian Nursing Council (2016). Nurse practitioner in critical care (post graduate-residency program). Retrieved from https://main.mohfw.gov.in/sites/default/files/57996154451447054846_0.pdf
6. Indian Nursing Council (2018). Integration of mid-level health provider in basic BSc Nursing and post basic BSc nursing curriculum. Retrieved from file:///Users/elissaladd/Documents/Nurse%20Prescribing/India%20Mid%20level%20provider.pdf
7. International Council of Nurses (2021). Guidelines on prescriptive authority for nurses.
8. International Council of Nurses (2006). Fact Sheet: Credentialing.
9. International Council of Nurses (2009). Implementing Nurse Prescribing: An Updated Review of Current Practice Internationally. Trends and issues in nursing. Developed by Ball, J for the International Council of Nurses.
10. International Council of Nurses (2013). ICN Position Statement: Scope of nursing practice. Retrieved from http://www.icn.ch/images/stories/documents/publications/position_statements/B07_Scope_Nsg_Practice.pdf
11. International Council of Nurses (2019). Core Competencies in Disaster Nursing. Retrieved from https://www.icn.ch/publications?page=1
12. World Health Organization (2016). Medicines in Healthcare Delivery: Thailand. Retrieved from https://www.who.int/docs/default-source/searo/hsd/edm/csa-thailand-situational-assessment-2015.pdf?sfvrsn = 5b7590c4_2
13. World Health Organization (2017). WHO Global Patient Safety Challenge: Medication without Harm. Retrieved from: http://apps.who.int/iris/bitstream/10665/255263/1/WHO-HIS-SDS-2017.6-eng.pdf?ua=1&ua=1
14. World Health Organization (2018). The third WHO Global Patient Safety Challenge: Medication without Harm. Retrieved from https://www.who.int/initiatives/medication-without-harm
15. World Health Organization (2019). WHO Medicines, Vaccines and Pharmaceutical Annual Report 2018. Promoting access to safe, effective, quality and affordable essential medical products for all. Retrieved from https://apps.who.int/iris/handle/10665/324765
16. World Health Organization (DAP/94.11) Guide to Good Prescribing: A practical Manual
17. Aronson JK. Balanced prescribing. Br J Clin Pharmacol. 2006;62:629–32.doi:10.1111/j.1365-2125. 2006. 02825.x

18. Aronson JK. Changing beta-blockers in heart failure: When is a class not a class? Br J Gen Pract. 2008;58:387–9.doi:10.3399/bjgp08X299317
19. Royal Pharmaceutical Society, A Competency Framework for all prescribers; 2016.
20. Ten Principles of Good Prescribing, British Pharmacological Society, retrieved from www.bps.ac.uk
21. A Single Competency Framework for all prescribers, National Prescribing Centre-NPC (Provided by NICE), 2012, NPC is part of NICE (National Institute for Health and Clinical Excellence, NICE) Ref. NICE (2012) A Single Competency Framework for all Prescribers NPC.

SECTION 2

PATHOLOGY-II

CHAPTERS

- Kidney and Urinary System
- Male Genital System
- Female Genital System
- Breast
- Central Nervous System

CHAPTER 9

Kidney and Urinary System

Aminder Singh, Nancy Kurien, Suresh Sharma

GLOMERULONEPHRITIS

- Glomerulonephritis (GN) is the inflammation and subsequent damage to the nephrons present in the kidney. GN or Bright's disease is the term used that primarily involves the renal glomeruli. It is the bilateral inflammation of the glomeruli.
- **Glomerulonephritis is broadly classified into two groups**:
  1. *Primary:* In this, the glomeruli are the predominant site of involvement. GN has occurred without any other systemic disease.
  2. *Secondary:* GN has occurred secondary to any other disease. In this certain systemic or hereditary diseases affect the glomeruli, e.g., infections, diabetes.
- These categories are further divided into many forms as tabulated in **Table 9.1**.

Etiopathogenesis

Figure 9.1 shows the etiopathogenesis of glomerulonephritis.

Clinical Manifestations

- Decreased urination or oliguria due to decreased glomerular filtration rate (GFR)
- Smoky or coffee-colored urine due to hematuria
- Dyspnea or orthopnea due to pulmonary edema secondary to hypervolemia
- Periorbital edema

Table 9.1: Categories of primary and secondary glomerulonephritis.

Primary	Secondary
Acute GN • Post-streptococcal • Non-streptococcal	Lupus nephritis
Rapidly progressive GN	Diabetic nephropathy
Minimal change disease	Systemic infectious diseases
Membranous GN	
Membranoproliferative GN	
Focal proliferative GN	
Focal segmental glomerulosclerosis	
IgA nephropathy	
Chronic GN	

(GN: glomerulonephritis)

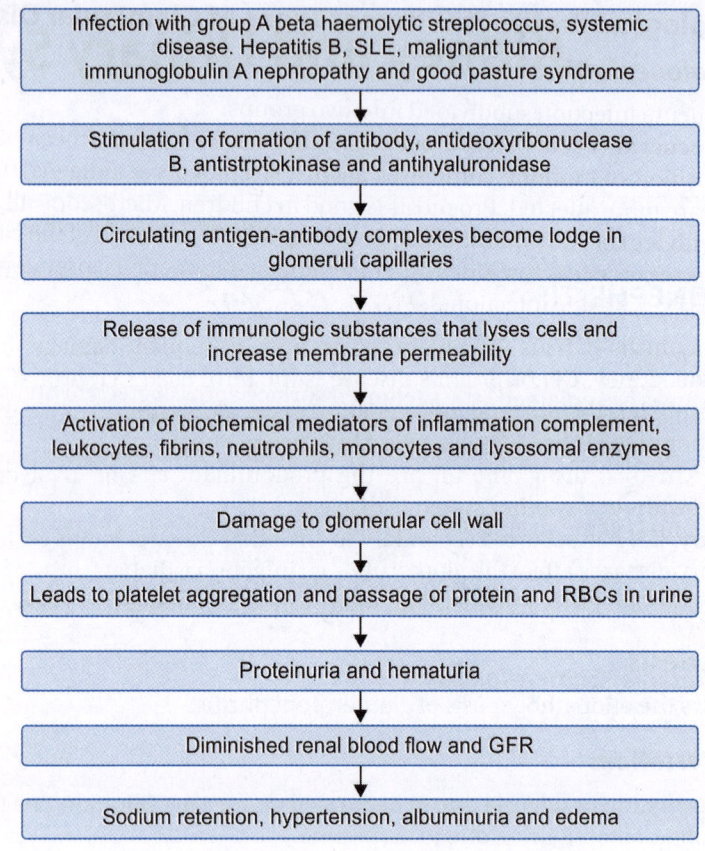

Fig. 9.1: Etiopathogenesis of glomerulonephritis.
(GFR: glomerular filtration rate; RBC: red blood cell; SLE: systemic lupus erythematosus)

- Mild-to-severe hypertension
- Proteinuria

Diagnostic Tests

Blood Analysis

- Elevated electrolyte, BUN, and creatinine levels
- Decreased serum protein level
- Decreased hemoglobin (Hb) level
- Elevated antistreptolysin O titers

Urine Analysis

- RBC, WBC, mixed cell casts, and protein indicating renal failure
- Fibrin degradation products and C protein
- Throat culture for group A β-hemolytic *Streptococcus*
- X-ray of the kidney
- Renal biopsy

Histomorphological Profile of Different Types of Glomerular Diseases

Acute Glomerulonephritis

Acute GN is an acute infection subdivided into two groups:
1. **Post-streptococcal** (occurs after a person is affected with streptococcal skin infections, due to deposition of immune complexes against streptococcal antigens). Children (6–10 year of age) are more affected. Prognosis is good in children. Microscopically hypercellular glomeruli with leukocytic infiltration and obliteration of the lumen of the capillary is seen.
2. **Acute non-streptococcal** (includes other bacteria like salmonella, pseudomonas, staphylococci, viruses, parasitic infections).

Pathological Changes

- **Grossly:** Kidneys are enlarged. The sectioned surface shows petechial hemorrhages giving a flea-bitten kidney **(Fig. 9.2A)**.
- **Microscopically:** Glomeruli are large and hypercellular. There is infiltration of leukocytes, polymorphs, and monocytes. There are fibrins within the capillary lumina. There may be swelling and hyaline droplets in tubular cells and may contain red cell casts. There is interstitial edema and leukocytic infiltration. Immunofluorescence microscopy reveals that there are irregular deposits along the GBM consisting principally of IgG and complement C3 **(Fig. 9.2B)**.

Rapidly Progressive Glomerulonephritis

Rapidly progressive GN is caused by immune-mediated glomerular damage leading to acute renal failure in a few weeks or months. There is a deposition of immune complexes, deposits of anti—GBM antibodies, and activation of neutrophilic cytoplasmic antibodies. Oliguria may progress within weeks.

Pathological Changes

- **Grossly:** The kidneys are enlarged and pale with a smooth outer surface. Cut surface shows congested medulla.

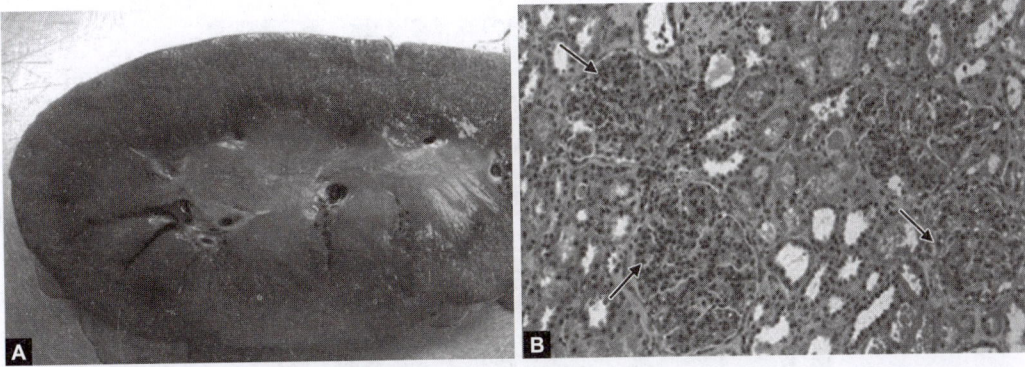

Figs. 9.2A and B: Acute glomerulonephritis: (A) Grossly; (B) Microscopically (post-infection glomerulonephritis—low power light micrograph showing diffuse, proliferative glomerulonephritis as may be seen in postinfectious glomerulonephritis. The glomeruli are so hypercellular (arrows) that open capillary lumens cannot be seen and the glomeruli may be hard to distinguish from the surrounding interstitium).

- **Microscopically:** Crescents are seen inside Bowman's capsule. Crescents are a collection of polygonal cells, which elongates. Fibrin and thrombi are also present in the glomerular tuft. The tubular epithelium shows hyalinization. The interstitium is edematous and may show fibrosis. Vascular changes associated with hypertension are also seen. Immunofluorescence shows granular IgG and C3 along a capillary wall **(Fig. 9.3)**.

Minimal Change Disease

Minimal change disease accounts for 80% of cases of nephrotic syndrome in children. There are fatty changes in tubules with no apparent change in glomeruli mainly the cause is idiopathic or it is associated with systemic diseases and drug therapy.

Pathological Changes

- **Grossly:** The kidneys are of normal size and shape.
- **Microscopically:** No abnormality is seen in glomeruli except an increase in the mesangial matrix. Hyaline droplets and lipid vacuolation are present in the cells of proximal convoluted tubules. There may be edema of the interstitium. There are minimal changes seen in blood vessels. There is foot process flattening of epithelial cells due to increased suppressor T-cell activity.

Membranous Glomerulonephritis

In membranous GN, there is a thickening of the glomerular capillary, which is secondary to certain conditions like systemic lupus erythematosus (SLE), malignancies, syphilis, and in the majority of cases it's idiopathic. It is an immune complex disease induced by antibodies formed against glomerular antigens.

Pathological Changes

- **Grossly:** Kidneys are enlarged, pale and smooth.
- **Microscopically:** There is a thickening of glomerular capillary walls. Immune complex deposits are incorporated in the thickened basement membrane, producing duplication of

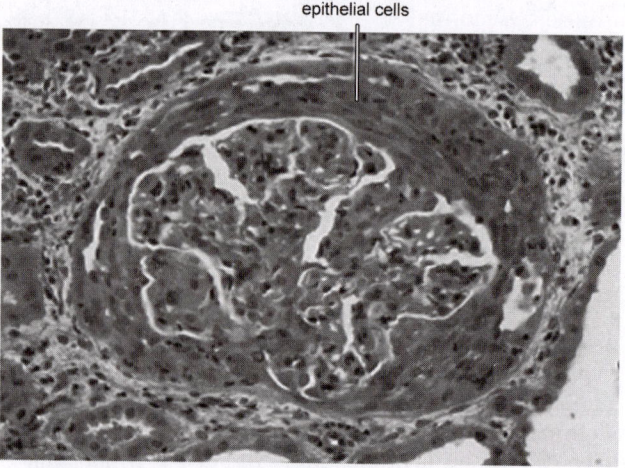

Fig. 9.3: Microscopy of rapidly progressive glomerulonephritis.

the membrane. Best seen under acid—Schiff stain. Lipid vacuolation seen. Shows fibrosis and scanty chronic inflammatory cells. Electron microscopy shows deposits in GBM, and the basement membrane protrudes between deposits as spikes.

Membranoproliferative Glomerulonephritis

It is an immune-mediated glomerular disease presented with hypercellular mesangium and thickening of the capillary wall as seen in nephritic syndrome.

Pathological Changes

- **Grossly:** Kidneys are pale and firm in consistency.
- **Microscopically:** Glomeruli are enlarged due to variable degrees of mesangial cell proliferation and increase in the mesangial matrix. GBM staining shows two basement membranes with a clear zone between them. This is referred as double contour or tram track appearance. Tubular cells may show vacuolation and hyaline droplets. The interstitium shows infiltration of inflammatory cells and some granular cells. Vascular changes are seen due to hypertension. Electron microscopy shows dense deposits in subendothelial locations.

Focal Glomerulonephritis

In this damage is confined to only one or two lobules or only a certain number of glomeruli. It occurs because of systemic diseases such as SLE, bacterial endocarditis, and Wegner's granulomatosis, as a component of known renal diseases in IgA nephropathy.

Pathological Changes

By light microscopy, the important feature seen is focal or segmental glomerular involvement. There is a cellular proliferation of mesangial cells and endothelial cells. By Immunofluorescence, mesangial deposits IgA, IgG, complement and, fibrin is seen.

Focal Segmental Glomerulosclerosis

In this again involvement is focal and segmental. It may be idiopathic or due to superimposed primary glomerular disease, secondary type as seen in certain diseases such as HIV, diabetes mellitus, and reflux nephropathy.

Pathological Changes

Under light microscopy, the affected glomeruli will show solidification or sclerosis of one or more lobules. Besides this, there is interstitial fibrosis and infiltration of mononuclear leukocytes and tubular epithelial cell atrophy and degeneration. Hyalinosis occurs in the capillary loop. Under an electron microscope, diffuse loss of foot processes is seen. Immune complexes deposits are also seen. Immune complex deposits are also seen. Immunofluorescence (IF) shows IgM and C3 **(Fig. 9.4)**.

IgA Nephropathy

It is characterized by the aggregation of IgA in the mesangium. Etiology remains unclear, under most circumstances idiopathic, as a part of Henoch-Schonlein purpura and also sometimes associated with chronic inflammation of the body system, e.g., trabecular bone density (TBD), leprosy, ankylosing spondylitis.

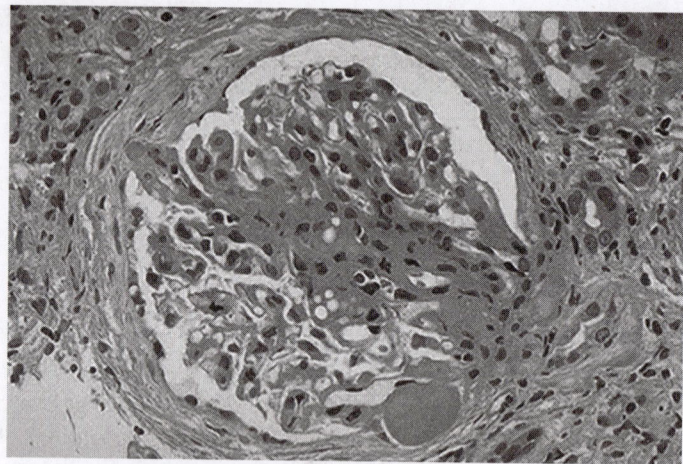

Fig. 9.4: Microscopy of focal segmental glomerulosclerosis.

Pathological Changes

Under light microscopy, there is a marked widening of mesangium proliferation of mesangial cells. IF shows deposition of IgA with or without IgG and C3. Electron microscopy shows dense deposits in the mesangium.

Chronic Glomerulonephritis

It is the final stage in which there is irreversible impairment of renal function. The most common causes include rapidly progressive GN (90%), membranous GN (50%), membranoproliferative GN (50%), focal segmental glomerulosclerosis (50%), IgA nephropathy (40%), acute post-streptococcal GN (1%).

Pathological Changes

- **Grossly:** Kidneys are usually small and contracted. The capsule is adherent to the cortex. The cortical surface is diffuse and granular.
- **Microscopically:** Glomeruli are reduced in number, showing hyalinized tufts giving an acellular, eosinophilic appearance. Tubules are completely disappearing atrophied. Tubular cells show hyaline droplets, degeneration, and tubular lumina contain eosinophilic, homogenous casts. There is delicate and fine fibrosis of interstitial tissue and a varying number of chronic inflammatory cells are also seen. It is characterized by hypertension, uremia, and progressive deterioration of renal function (**Fig. 9.5**).

Secondary Glomerular Disease

In this, glomerular involvement occurs secondary to systemic and hereditary diseases. The important examples are as follows.

Lupus Nephritis

It occurs secondary to SLE. The incidence of renal involvement in SLE ranges from 40 to 75%. The two important clinical features are proteinuria and hematuria.

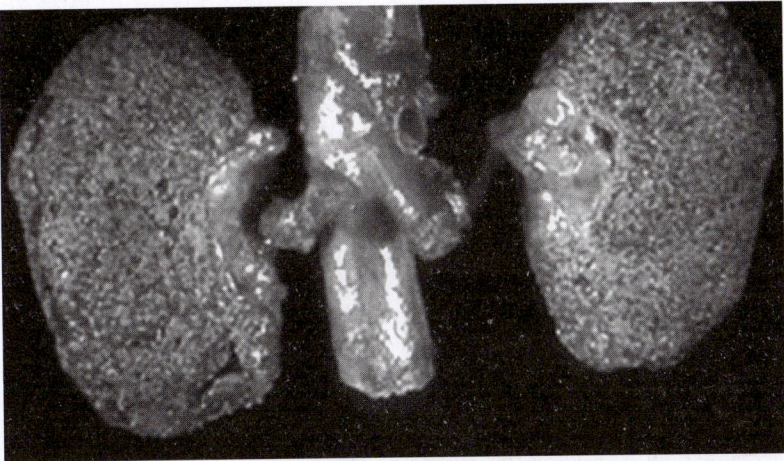

Fig. 9.5: Chronic glomerulonephritis.

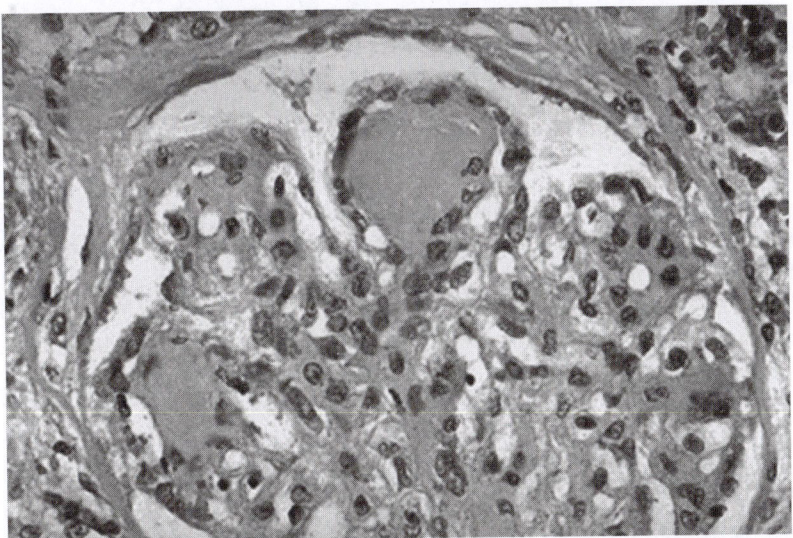

Fig. 9.6: Diabetic nephropathy.

Pathological Changes

Immunofluorescence shows deposits in the mesangium, which consists of IgG and C3. Sometimes there is a focal and segmental proliferation of endothelial and mesangial cells with infiltration of neutrophils and macrophages. Glomeruli are sclerosed and hyalinized and there are remains of lesions.

Diabetic Nephropathy

It is a chronic complication of diabetes mellitus. There are four types of renal lesions diabetic glomerulosclerosis, vascular lesion, diabetic pyelonephritis, and tubular lesions **(Fig. 9.6)**.

Pathological Changes

There is hypoperfusion, deposition of proteins in the mesangium. Cellular infiltration is seen in renal lesions. In regions of glomerular capillary loops, nodules are formed as a result of the increased mesangial matrix. This is known as Kimmelstiel-Wilson lesion which is related to diabetes mellitus. Hyaline arteriosclerosis affects both afferent and efferent arterioles of glomeruli further leading to renal ischemia that results in tubular atrophy and fibrosis. In tubules, epithelial cells of proximal convoluted tubules develop extensive glycogen deposits appearing as vacuoles. These are called Armanni—Ebstein lesions.

Hereditary Nephritis

In this, nephropathy occurs because of hereditary diseases like Alport syndrome, Fabry's disease, and Nail-patella syndrome.

Alport's syndrome: This is an X-linked dominant disorder having a mutation in the alpha-5 chain of type 4 collagen located on the X chromosome.

Pathological Changes

- Glomeruli show segmental proliferation of mesangial cells and increased mesangial matrix and segmental sclerosis.
- Presence of lipid-laden form cells in the interstitium.
- As a disease, progress increases sclerosis of glomeruli, tubular atrophy and interstitial fibrosis.
- Electron microscopy (EM) reveals characteristic basement membrane splitting or lamination in affected parts.
- Immunofluorescence microscopy (IM) shows deposits of Ig and complement:
  - *Fabry's disease:* It is characterized by the accumulation of neutral glycosphingolipids in lysosomes of glomerular, tubular, vascular, and interstitial cells.
  - *Nail-patella syndrome/osteo-onychodysplasia:* It is an abnormality in the alpha-1 chain of collagen 5 on the chromosome and is associated with multiple defects of elbows, knees, and nails dysplasia. About half of the cases develop nephropathy.

PYELONEPHRITIS

- Pyelonephritis is the inflammation of kidneys caused by pyogenic bacteria.
- It is mainly categorized into two types, i.e., acute and chronic pyelonephritis.

Acute Pyelonephritis

- Acute pyelonephritis is an acute suppurative inflammation of kidneys caused by pyogenic bacteria.
- The bacteria gain entry into the urinary tract and then into the kidney by two routes: **(1) Ascending infection and (2) hematogenous infection**.

Etiopathogenesis

In acute pyelonephritis, bacterial entry may happen through two different routes as discussed below **(Fig. 9.7)**.

1. **Ascending infection:** The route may be fecal contamination of the urethral orifice, urethral trauma, diabetes, pregnancy, urinary tract obstruction or instrumentation, vesicourethral

CHAPTER 9: Kidney and Urinary System

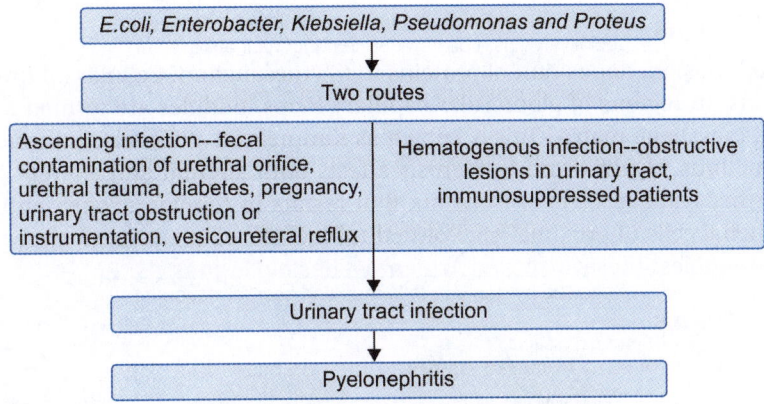

Fig. 9.7: Etiopathogenesis of acute pyelonephritis.

reflux. The common pathogenic organism causes contamination of the urethral orifice leading to urethritis and cystitis. The bacteria in small proportions ascend further up against the flow of urine, extending into the renal pelvis and then the renal cortex.
2. **Hematogenous infection:** It is caused by obstructive lesions in the urinary tract. The infection results from blood-borne spread.

Clinical Manifestations
- Pyuria
- Chills, fever
- Lumbar tenderness and back pain
- Dysuria, proteinuria, glycosuria and ketonuria
- Frequency of micturition
- Bacteriuria (urine will show bacteria in excess of 100,000/mL, pus cells and pus cell casts).

Complications
There are three major complications:
1. **Papillary necrosis:** It affects one or both kidneys. Grossly, the necrotic papillae are yellow to gray-white, sharply defined areas with congested borders and resemble infarction. The pelvis may be dilated. Microscopically, necrotic tissue is separated from the viable tissue by a dense zone of polymorphs.
2. **Pyonephrosis:** There is an abscess in the kidneys, usually occurs in case of obstruction which does not allow the abscess to drain, and kidneys are transfused into a multilocular sac filled with pus.
3. **Perinephric abscess:** The abscesses in the kidneys may extend through the capsule of the kidney into perinephric tissue forming an abscess.

Pathological Changes
- **Grossly:** Kidneys appear enlarged and swollen. Cut surface shows small, yellowish-white abscesses with hemorrhagic rim mainly situated in the cortex **(Fig. 9.8)**.
- **Microscopically:** A large number of neutrophils are seen in the interstitial tissue and in tubules. May form neutrophilic abscesses in renal parenchyma.

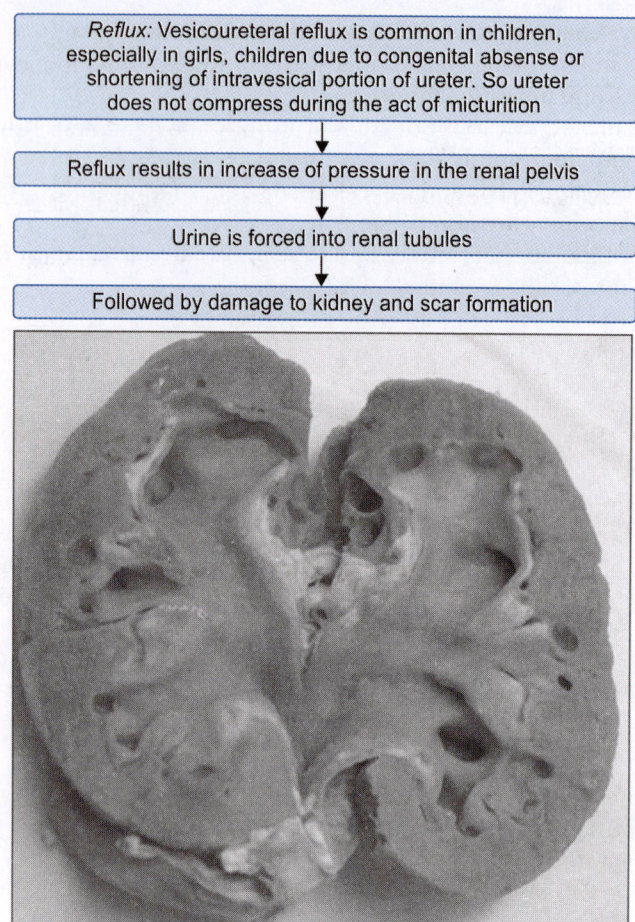

Fig. 9.8: Acute pyelonephritis.

Chronic Pyelonephritis

Chronic pyelonephritis condition results from separated attacks of inflammation and scarring. The two types of chronic pyelonephritis are reflux and obstructive.

Etiopathogenesis

Obstructive: Repeated attacks of urine obstruction and renal infection result in renal damage and scarring.

Clinical Features

Patients present with clinical signs and symptoms of hypertension.

Pathological Changes

- **Grossly:** Kidneys are small and contracted showing unequal reductions. The surface of the kidneys is irregularly scarred. The scares are of variable size and show U-shaped depression on the cortical surface. The pelvis is dilated and calyces are blunt.

- **Microscopically:** Changes occur in interstitium and tubules.
  - *Interstitium:* Inflammatory reaction is seen composed of lymphocytes, plasma cells, macrophages, and interstitial fibrosis.
  - *Tubules:* Tubules show varying degrees of atrophy and dilatation. Tubules may contain eosinophils and neutrophils.
  - *Pelvicalyceal system:* Pelvis and calyces are dilated, sharing fibrosis. Lymphoid follicles with germinal centers are also present.
  - *Blood vessels:* Blood vessels are scarred showing obliterative endarteritis.
  - *Glomeruli:* Fibrosis and hyalinization of glomeruli are seen.

Diagnostic Methods
- Culture of urine
- Intravenous pyelography
- Antibiotic sensitivity tests
- CT scan of kidney, ureter and, bladder

RENAL CALCULI

The formation of renal calculi at any level of the urinary tract from kidneys to ureters.

Etiopathogenesis (Fig. 9.9)

The main etiological factors of the urinary calculi are as follows:
- Idiopathic hypercalciuria without hypercalcemia
- Hyperparathyroidism associated with hypercalcemia
- Urinary tract infection
- Genetic defect in cystine transport
- Hyperuricosuria and hyperuricemia due to myeloproliferative disorders
- Patients on chemotherapeutic agents
- Urinary pH less than 6 (acidic)

Types of Urinary Calculi (Fig. 9.10)

- **Calcium stones:** It is a more common type comprising about 75% of all urinary calculi made up of calcium oxalate and calcium phosphate.
- **Mixed stones:** It contributes about 15% made up of magnesium-ammonium-calcium phosphate, often called struvite. Staghorn calculus (Coral calculi) is commonly formed in struvite stones.

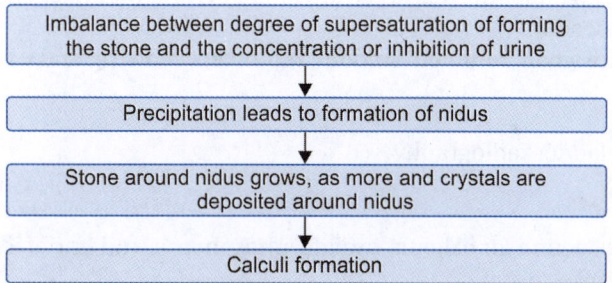

Fig. 9.9: Etiopathogenesis of the urinary calculi.

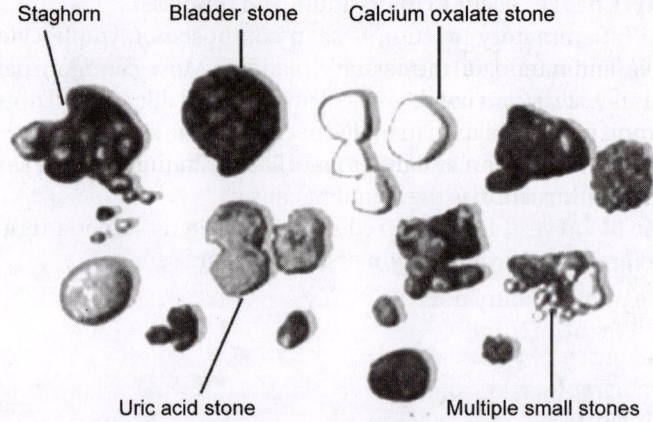

Fig. 9.10: Pathology and types of urinary calculi.

- **Uric acid stone:** It contributes about 6% made up of uric acid.
- **Cystine stones:** It contributes about 2% made due to defects in cystine transport associated with genetic defects resulting excessive in excretion of cysteine.
- **Xanthine:** It contributes less than 2%, and occurs mainly due to abnormal xanthine metabolism.

Clinical Manifestations
- Colicky pain resulting from obstruction
- Nausea and vomiting
- Fever and chills from infection
- Abnormal metabolism of xanthine
- Hematuria when calculi abrade a ureter
- Abdominal distension
- Anuria from bilateral obstruction

Pathological Changes
- Calcium stones are small, ovoid, hard, dark brown with a granular rough surface. They are dark brown due to old blood pigment deposition as a result of repeated trauma to the urinary tract by these sharp edges.
- Struvite stones are yellow-white or gray, soft, friable, and irregular in shape.
- Uric acid stones are smooth, yellowish-brown, hard, and multiple. They show laminated structure on cut section.
- Cystine stones are small, rounded, smooth, multiple, yellowish, and waxy.

Diagnostic Tests
- Kidney-ureter-bladder radiography
- Ultrasonography
- Urine culture
- 24-hour urine collection for calcium oxalate, phosphorus, and uric acid excretion
- Blood protein level

CYSTITIS

- Cystitis is the inflammation of the urinary bladder. Most common pathogenic microorganism in this is *Escherichia coli*.
- It is more common in females than in males because of the shortness of the urethra, which is prone to fecal contamination and due to mechanical trauma during sexual intercourse. In males, prostatic obstruction is the frequent cause.

Etiology

- Spread from the upper urinary tract
- Instrumentation in the urethra
- Radiation exposure
- Direct exposure to chemical irritant
- Foreign bodies and local trauma
- Bacterial (E. coli, Klebsiella, Enterobacter, Pseudomonas), Fungal (*Candida Albicans*), parasitic infestations (schistosoma hematoma)
- **Nephrotoxins:** Infectious chemical agents, antibiotics, heavy metals, poisons, drugs like cyclophosphamide and autoimmune responses

Etiopathogenesis

Figure 9.11 shows the etiopathogenesis of cystitis.

Clinical Manifestations

- Severe lower abdominal or pelvic pain
- Urgency
- Frequency
- Nocturia, dysuria
- Dyspareunia
- Fever, chills, malaise

Types of Cystitis

- Acute
- Chronic
- Interstitial
- Cystitis cystica

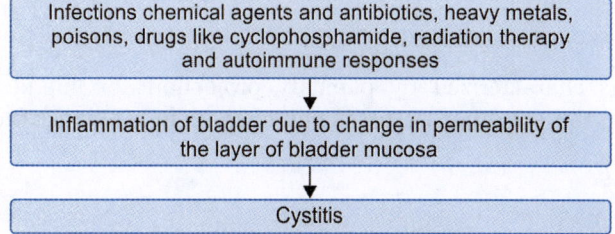

Fig. 9.11: Etiopathogenesis of cystitis.

- Malakoplakia
- Polyploid cystitis

Pathological Changes

Acute Cystitis
- **Grossly:** Mucosa is red, swollen, hemorrhages and suppurative exudates or ulcers on bladder mucosa.
- **Microscopically:** Infiltration with neutrophilic exudates mixed with lymphocytes and macrophages. Mucosa appears to be edematous and congested.

Chronic Cystitis
Repeated attacks lead to chronic cystitis:
- **Grossly**: Epithelium is thickened, red, granular with formation of polyploidy masses. There is thickened bladder wall and shrunken cavity.
- **Microscopically**: Patchy creation of mucosa with formation of granulation tissue.
- Fibrosis of muscular and submucosal layer with infiltration of inflammatory cells.
- Formation of lymphoid follicles in bladder mucosa is also seen (cystitis follicularis).

Interstitial Cystitis
Interstitial cystitis occurs usually in middle-aged women. Microscopically, the submucosal and muscular tissue is replaced with fibrotic tissues and infiltration of inflammatory cells appear (lymphocytes, plasma cells, eosinophils).

Cystitis Cystica
Due to chronic inflammation, there is a downward projection of epithelial nests known as Brunn's nests. These epithelial cells are small cystitic inclusions in the bladder wall and develop into columnar metaplasia with secretions in the lumen of cysts.

Malakoplakia
Malakoplakia occurs most frequently in immunosuppressed patients and recipients of transplants.
- **Grossly:** The lesions appear soft, flat, yellowish plaques on bladder mucosa.
- **Microscopically:** The plaques are composed of a massive accumulation of macrophages with multinucleated giant cells and some lymphocytes and macrophages contain concretions of calcium phosphate called Michaelis-Gutmann bodies. These bodies represent lysosomes filled with debris of bacteria phagocytosed by macrophages.

Polypoid Cystitis
Polypoid cystitis is characterized by papillary projections on bladder mucosa due to submucosal edema. This condition occurs in patients with indwelling catheters and infection.

Diagnostic Tests
- Urine culture
- Cystoscopy
- Urine flow study

RENAL CELL CARCINOMA

The two forms of tumors are benign and malignant **(Table 9.2)**. They generally arise from renal tubules, embryonic tissue, mesenchymal tissue, medullary interstitial, and the epithelium of the pelvis.

Etiology

- Tobacco, exposure to asbestos, heavy metals, petroleum products
- In women, obesity and estrogen therapy
- Hereditary and acquired cystic diseases
- Analgesic nephropathy
- Hypertension

Etiopathogenesis of Renal Tumor

Figure 9.12 shows the etiopathogenesis of renal tumors.

Histomorphological Profile of Different Tumors

Benign Tumors

- **Cortical adenomas:** They are the most common than other tumors and are multiple. Grossly, these tumors are in the form of tiny nodules encapsulated, usually in white or yellow color. Microscopically, they are composed of cords or papillary structures projecting into cystic space. Cells are usually uniform, cuboidal with no division.
- **Oncocytoma:** They are arising from the collecting duct. Grossly, the tumor is encapsulated and of variable size usually having tan color. Microscopically, tumor cells are plump with abundant, finely granular, acidophilic cytoplasm and round nuclei.

Table 9.2: Types of renal tumors.

Benign	Malignant
Epithelial tumors of renal parenchyma	
Adenoma oncocytoma	Adenocarcinoma renal cell carcinoma
Epithelial tumors of renal pelvis	
Transitional cell papilloma	Transitional cell carcinoma Squamous cell carcinoma
Embryonal tumors	
Mesoblastic nephroma multicystic nephroma	Wilms' tumor
Non-epithelial tumors	
Angiomyolipoma medullary interstitial tumor	Sarcomas
Miscellaneous	
Juxtaglomerular cell tumor	
Metastatic tumors	

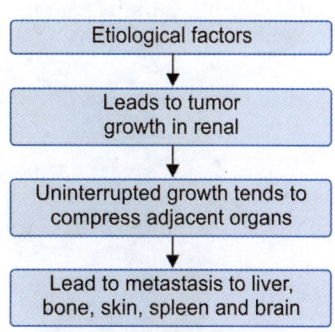

Fig. 9.12: Etiopathogenesis of renal tumors.

- **Juxtaglomerular tumor or reninoma:** It is a rare tumor.
- **Angiomyolipoma:** It is a hamartoma of the kidney derived from blood vessels, smooth muscles, and fat. Grossly, the tumor resembles a uterine leiomyoma having a whorled appearance. Microscopically, it shows the cellular growth of spindle cells derived from secondary mesenchyma.
- **Mesoblastic nephroma:** It is a congenital benign tumor usually characterized same as an angiomyolipoma.
- **Multicystic nephroma:** It occurs in early infancy. Grossly, it is a solitary, unilateral well-demarcated tumor of varying size showing multilocular appearance. Microscopically, the cysts are lined by tubular epithelium while the stroma between the cysts contains mesenchymal tissues.
- **Medullary interstitial cell tumor:** It is the tiny nodule arising from the medulla consists of fibroblasts like cells. Also called renal fibromas tumor of renal cortex consisting of sheets of epitheloid cells with many small blood vessels. These tumors secrete excessive quantity of renin, thus patient is hypertensive.

Malignant Tumors

- **Renal cell carcinoma:** Another name for this tumor is hypernephroma, adenocarcinoma comprises of 70–80% of all renal cancers. Mainly they are classified into six major types— (1) clear cell, (2) papillary, (3) granular, (4) chromophobe, (5) sarcomatoid, and (6) collecting duct. *Grossly*, the RCC commonly arises from the poles of the kidneys as a solitary and unilateral tumor. The tumor appears to be large, golden yellow usually multifocal, and bilateral. Cut surface shows ischemic necrosis, cystic change, and foci of hemorrhages **(Fig. 9.13A)**. *Microscopically*, the tumor appears to be a solid mass and acini of uniform appearing tumor cells. Clear cells predominate with some granular cells. The stroma is composed of fine and delicate fibrous tissue **(Fig. 9.13B)**.

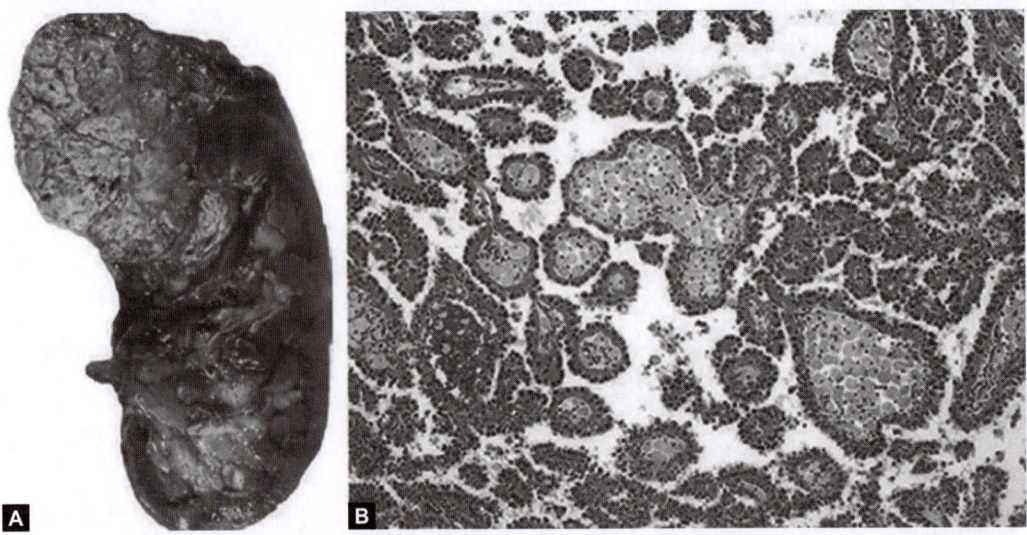

Figs. 9.13A and B: Renal cell carcinoma: (A) Grossly; (B) Microscopy.

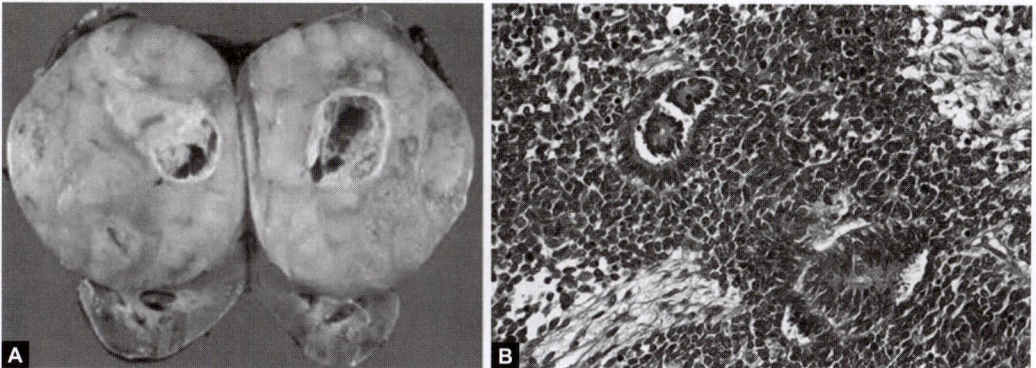

Figs. 9.14A and B: Wilms tumor: (A) Grossly; (B) Microscopy.

- **Wilms' tumor:** Also called nephroblastoma. It is an embryonic tumor derived from the renal epithelium and mesenchymal components and is seen most commonly in 1–6 age group with equal sex incidence. Grossly, it is quite large, spheroidal, replacing most of the kidney. It is usually solitary and unilateral, in 5–10% cases bilateral. Cut surface shows soft, fish-flesh-like gray-white to cream-yellow tumor of foci of necrosis and hemorrhages. Microscopically, it shows a mixture of epithelial and mesenchymal elements. Smooth muscle, cartilage, bone, fat cells, and fibrous tissue may be seen sometimes. Most of the tumor consists of small, round to spindled, anaplastic, sarcomatoid tumor cells **(Figs. 9.14 A and B)**.

Clinical Manifestations

- Pain resulting from tumor pressure and invasion
- Hematuria
- Smooth, firm, non-tender mass palpable over affected kidney
- Fever
- Hypertension (HTN) from compression of renal artery
- Urinary retention secondary to obstruction of urinary flow
- Pulmonary embolism

Diagnostic Tests

- CT scan
- Intravenous retrograde pyelography
- Ultrasound
- Cystoscopy
- Renal angiography
- Liver function tests (LFTs)
- Complete blood shows anemia, polycythemia

RENAL FAILURE

Regardless of the cause, renal failure has two major syndromes, i.e., acute renal failure and chronic renal failure:

- **Acute renal failure** is a syndrome characterized by rapid onset of dysfunction, caused by obstruction, poor circulation, or underlying kidney disease, usually reversible with treatment, but if not treated, may progress to end-stage renal disease and death.
- **Chronic renal failure** is a syndrome characterized by progressive destruction and irreversible deterioration of renal function, rapidly progressive destruction of nephrons, eventually terminating in death.

Etiopathogenesis

Figure 9.15 shows the etiopathogenesis of renal failure.

Clinical Manifestations

Respiratory System

- Tachypnea
- Kussmaul's breathing
- Tenacious sputum
- Pain with coughing
- Pulmonary edema

Gastrointestinal System

- Anorexia
- Abdominal distension
- Gastrointestinal bleeding
- Nausea and vomiting
- Diarrhea and constipation

Neurological System

- Lethargy, confusion
- Convulsions

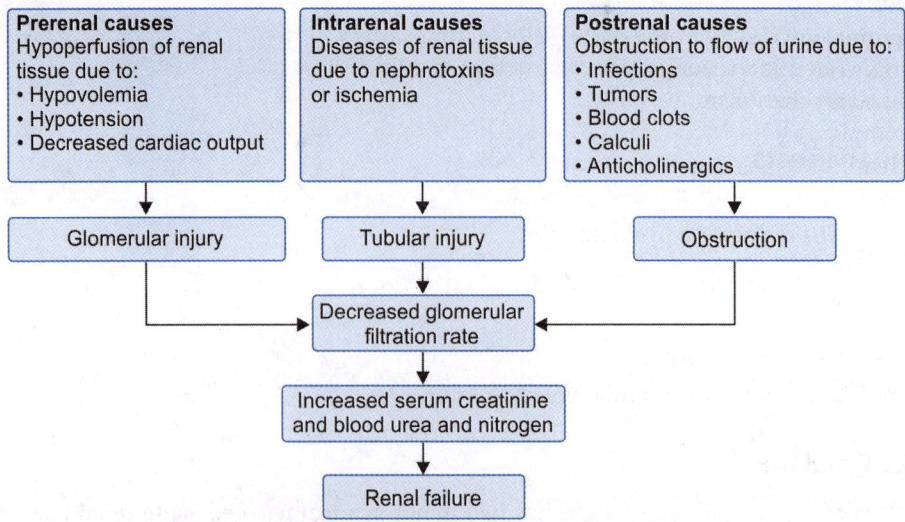

Fig. 9.15: Etiopathogenesis of renal failure.

- Unusual behavior
- Sleep disturbances

Skeletal System
- Bone resorption
- Osteoporosis
- Increased risk of bone fracture
- Ecchymosis

Genitourinary System
- Decreased urine output
- Proteinuria
- Casts and cells in urine
- Decreased urine sodium

Reproductive System
- Infertility
- Decreased libido
- Erectile dysfunction
- Amenorrhea

Pathological Changes
- Varying degrees of tubular necrosis with disrupted, necrotic, or regenerating tubular epithelium can be seen.
- Following direct nephrotoxic injury or uniform diffuse necrosis of proximal convoluted tubules is observed.
- Crescents are present inside the Bowman's capsule.

Diagnostic Methods
- Serum creatinine is elevated
- BUN values more than 100 mg/dL indicates severe kidney impairment
- Blood biochemistry, electrolyte imbalance
- Complete blood count (CBC) Hb, and hematocrit are decreased
- Creatinine clearance is decreased
- Serum uric acid is increased
- Renal biopsy to identify underlying disease
- Reduced kidney size on X-ray, renal scan

MULTIPLE CHOICE QUESTIONS

1. **Inflammation of mucosa of urinary bladder is called** _____
   - a. Urethritis
   - b. Cystitis
   - c. Pyruvitis
   - d. Renalitis
2. **Tumors that arise from collecting ducts are** _____
   - a. Oncocytoma
   - b. Malakoplakia
   - c. Polypoid cystitis
   - d. Wilms' tumor

3. **Common causative organism of cystitis is** _____
   a. Salmonella
   b. Escherichia coli
   c. Epstein Barr virus
   d. Streptococcus
4. **Pyelonephritis is** _____
   a. Inflammation of ureters
   b. Infection of urinary tract
   c. Inflammation of kidneys
   d. Inflammation of urethra
5. **Embryonic tumor which is derived from renal epithelium is** _____
   a. Reninoma
   b. Oncocytoma
   c. Angiomyolipoma
   d. Wilms' tumor

Answer Key

1. c   2. a   3. b   4. c   5. d

FURTHER READING

1. Bostwick DG, Eble JN. Urologic surgical pathology. St Louis, Mosby, 1997.
2. Cohen HT, McGovern FJ. Renal cell carcinoma. N Engl J Med. 2005;353:2477.
3. Epstein JI, et al. The WHO/International society of urologic pathologic consensus classification of urothelial (transitional cell) neoplasms of the urinary bladder. Am J Surg Pathol. 1998;22:1435.
4. Freedman BI, et al. The link between hypertension and nephrosclerosis. Am J Kidney Dis. 1995;25:207.
5. Heptinstall RH. Pathology of the kidney (3 volts). London, Little, Brown and Company, 1992.
6. Hrick DE, et al. Glomerulonephritis. N Engl J Med. 1998;339:888.
7. Joshi VV. Cystic lesions of the kidney. In proceedings of III International CME and Update in surgical pathology, Gupta RK (Ed). Lucknow SGPGI, 1998.
8. Lamm DL, Torti FM. Bladder cancer 1996. CA Cancer J Clin. 1996;46(2):93–112.
9. Mostofi FK, et al. WHO-Histological typing of kidney tumours, number 25. Geneva, WHO, 1981.
10. Phillips JL, et al. The genetic basis of renal epithelial tumours: Advances in research and its impact on prognosis and therapy. Curr Opin Urol. 2001;11:463.
11. Proceedings of international CME on Renal transplant pathology held at PGI, Chandigarh (20–22 February 2009).
12. Webb JN. Aspects of tumours of the urinary bladder and prostate gland. In recent advances in histopathology, number 15, Anthony PP, et al (Eds). Philadelphia, Churchill Livingstone. 1992. pp 157.

Male Genital System

Aminder Singh, Nancy Kurien, Suresh Sharma

CRYPTORCHIDISM

Cryptorchidism or undescended testis is a condition in which a testicle is arrested at some point in its descent. It is a congenital disorder in which one or both testis fails to descend into the scrotum remaining in the abdomen or inguinal canal **(Fig. 10.1)**. Cryptorchidism is a common birth anomaly of the male genital organ.

Etiopathogenesis

The mechanism by which the testes descend into the scrotum is still unexplained. The possible causes of cryptorchidism **(Fig. 10.2)**.

Clinical Manifestations

- Testis on the affected side not palpable in the scrotum
- Scrotum enlarged on the unaffected site due to compensatory hypertrophy
- Infertility after puberty due to prevention of spermatogenesis
- Inguinal hernia.

Pathological Changes

- **Grossly:** Testis is small in size, firm, and fibrotic.
- **Histologically:** There is a progressive loss of germ cell element, the tubular basement membrane is thickened, increase in the interstitial stroma, Leydig cells are seen as prominent **(Fig. 10.3)**.

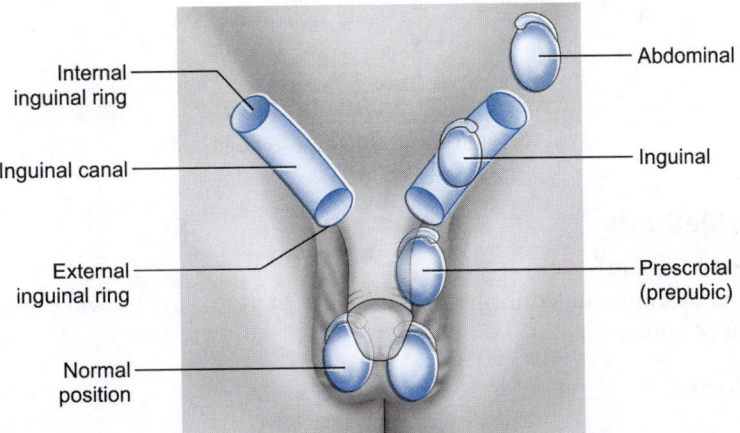

Fig. 10.1: Cryptorchidism/undescended testis.

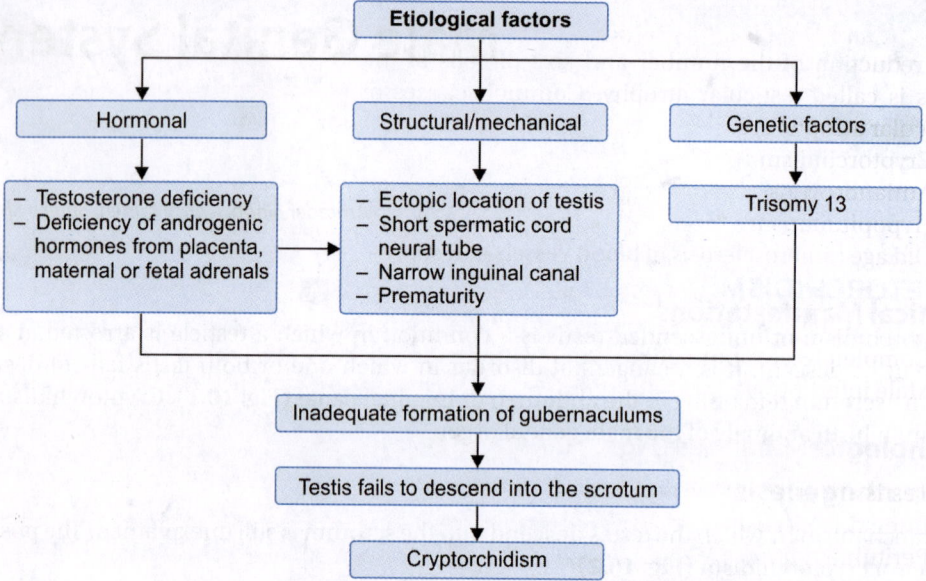

Fig. 10.2: Etiopathogenesis of cryptorchidism.

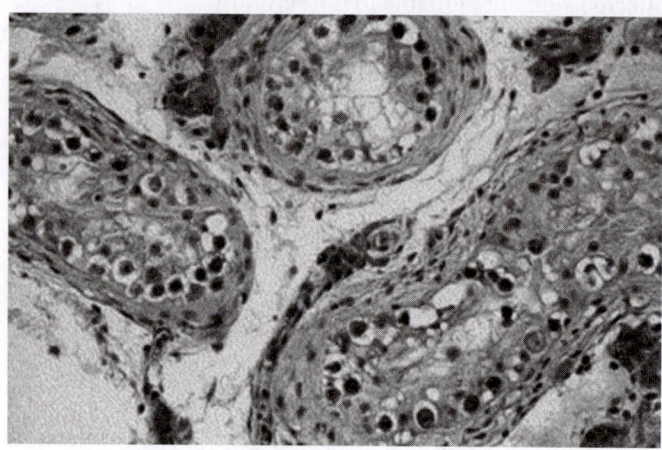

Fig. 10.3: Microscopy of undescended testis.

Diagnostic Methods
- Physical examination
- Serum gonadotropin to confirm the presence of testis by showing the presence of circulating hormone

Complications
- Sterility
- Increased risk of testicular cancer

TESTICULAR ATROPHY

The reduction of the number and size of cells of the testis is called testicular atrophy. Common causes of testicular atrophy are:
- Cryptorchidism
- Antiandrogens
- Hypopituitarism
- Old age (atherosclerosis of blood vessels of testis)

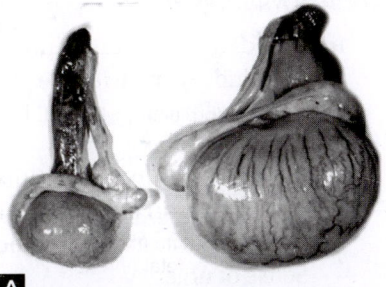
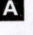

Clinical Manifestations
- Completely asymptomatic
- Male infertility

Pathological Changes (Figs. 10.4A and B)
- Testis are small in size and firm
- Interstitial fibrosis
- Peritubular fibrosis
- Reduced germ cells elements
- Increased Leydig cells

Diagnostic Methods
- Physical examination
- Doppler sonography

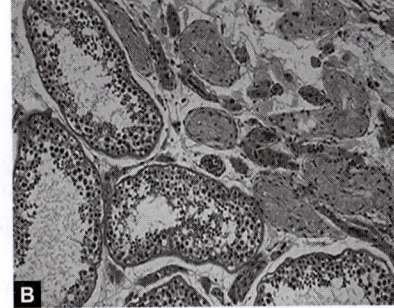

Figs. 10.4A and B: Testicular atrophy: (A) Grossly; (B) Microscopy.

PROSTATIC HYPERPLASIA

Enlargement of the prostate gland is called prostatic hypertrophy. It is a non-neoplastic condition and commonly called benign nodular hyperplasia.

Benign Prostate Hypertrophy
- Although most men aged 50 and older have some prostatic enlargement, also known as benign prostate hypertrophy (BPH). In benign prostatic hyperplasia, the prostate gland enlarges enough to compress the urethra and cause overt urinary obstruction.
- Depending on the size of the enlarged prostate, the age, the health of the patient, and the extent of the obstruction, BPH is treated symptomatically or surgically. BPH is common, affecting up to 50% of men over age 50 and older, and 75% of men over age 80 and older.

Causes
- The main cause of BPH may be age-associated changes in hormone activity. Androgenic hormone production decreases with age, causing an imbalance in androgen and estrogen levels and high levels of dihydrotestosterone, the main prostatic intracellular androgen.
- Other causes include:
  - Arteriosclerosis
  - Inflammation
  - Metabolic or nutritional disturbances

Clinical Manifestation

- It depends on the extent of prostatic enlargement and the lobes affected. Characteristically, the condition starts with the group of symptoms known as prostatism, which includes:
  - Reduced urinary stream, caliber, and force
  - Urinary hesitancy
  - Difficulty starting micturition
- As the obstruction increases, it causes:
  - Frequent urination with nocturia
  - Sense of urgency
  - Dribbling
  - Urine retention
  - Incontinence
  - Possible hematuria

Pathological Changes

- **Grossly:** Affected prostate is enlarged, nodular, smooth, and firm and weighs around 40–80 g. Cut surface contains many fairly well-circumscribed nodules, which may be glandular or fibromuscular. In glandular, the tissue is yellow—pink, soft, honeycombed, and milky fluid exude. In fibromuscular, the cut surface is firm and does not exude milky fluid. The hyperplastic glands are lined by tall, columnar epithelial cells and a peripheral layer of flattened basal cells **(Figs. 10.5A and B)**.
- **Histologically:** Glandular hyperplasia is more commonly characterized by increased intra-acinar papillary infoldings with fibrovascular cores. The epithelium is two-layered, the inner columnar and outer cuboidal. The fibromuscular hyperplasia appears as aggregates of spindle cells. Areas of infarction and squamous metaplasia are fairly common in advanced cases **(Fig. 10.6)**.

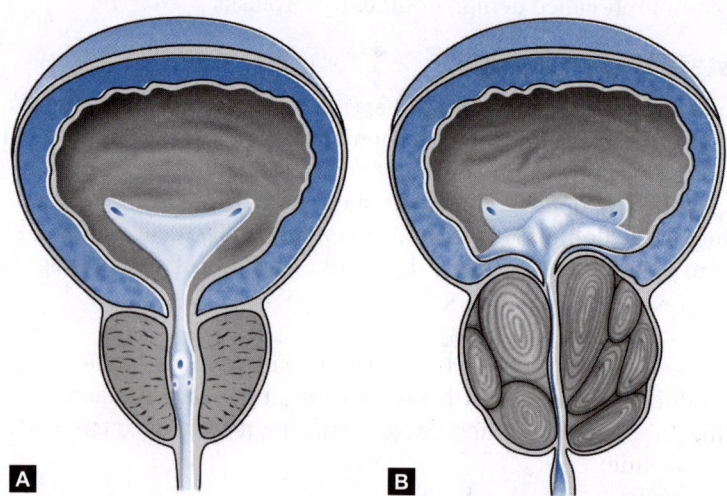

Figs. 10.5A and B: Illustration comparing normal prostate and prostatic hyperplasia: (A) Normal prostate; (B) Prostatic hypertrophy.

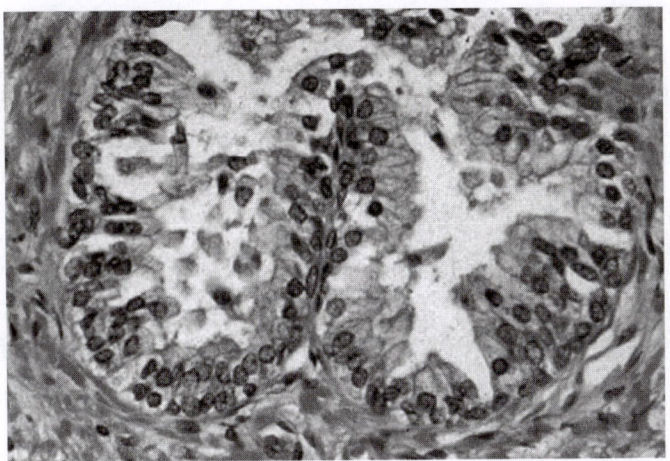

Fig. 10.6: Microscopy of prostatic hyperplasia.

Diagnostic Methods

- Visible midline mass above the symphysis pubis
- Enlarged prostate with rectal palpation
- Other findings that help confirm the diagnosis may include excretory urography to rule out urinary tract obstruction, hydronephrosis, calculi or tumors, and filling and emptying defects in the bladder
- Alternatively, if the patient is not cooperative, cystoscopy to rule out other causes of obstruction
- Elevated BUN and serum creatinine levels
- Elevated prostate-specific antigen (PSA)
- Urinalysis and urine cultures showing hematuria, pyuria, and with bacterial count more than 100,000/microliter, urinary tract infection
- Cystourethroscopy for severe symptoms showing prostate enlargement, bladder wall changes, and a raised bladder

CARCINOMA OF PENIS

- More than 95% of penile neoplasms originate from squamous epithelium
- In developing countries, however, penile carcinoma occurs at much higher rates
- Most cases occur in uncircumcised patients older than 40 years of age
- Several factors have been implicated in the pathogenesis of squamous cell carcinoma of the penis:
  - Poor hygiene
  - Smoking
  - Infection with human papillomavirus, particularly type 16 and 18

Pathological Changes (Figs. 10.7A and B)

- The penis appears as a gray, crusted, papular lesion, most commonly on the glans penis or prepuce

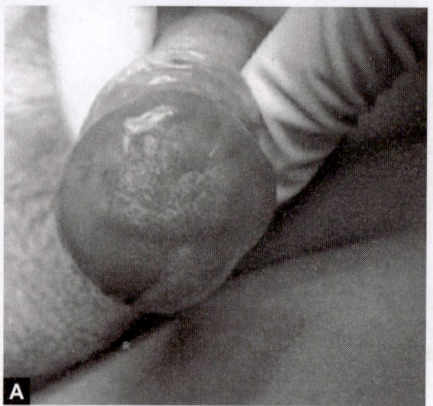 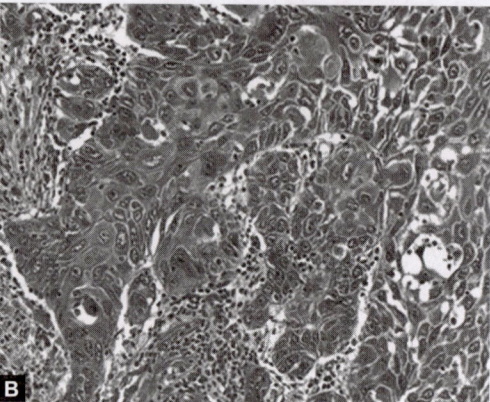

Figs. 10.7: Carcinoma of penis: (A) Gross; (B) Microscopy.

- Malignant cells throughout the epidermis with no invasion of the underlying stroma and central keratin pearls
- The tumor may be cauliflower-like and papillary
- Occurs on the shaft and glans of the penis as an ulcerated infiltrative lesion that may spread to inguinal nodes and infrequently to distant sites

CARCINOMA OF PROSTATE

Carcinoma of the prostate is one of the most common forms of malignant disease and is the second leading cause of male deaths from malignancy. The tumor is rare below 50 years of age, the peak incidence is between 60 and 85 years.

Clinicopathological Types

Two clinicopathological types of prostatic carcinoma are recognized by the difference in their behavior, i.e., clinical (symptomatic) carcinoma and latent (incidental) carcinoma.

Clinical Carcinoma

- Arise in the posterior subcapsular area of the gland
- Adenocarcinoma
- Invasion of stroma and perineural spaces
- Asymmetric firm enlargement of the prostate may be palpable per rectum
- Metastasis, especially to the bone

Latent Carcinoma

- Microscopic focus of tumor found incidentally
- Common incidence high in old age
- Dormant lesions, metastasis in 30% after 10 years

Clinical Findings

Generally, symptoms appear only in the late stage of carcinoma of the prostate. Some of the most common symptoms are given below:

- Difficulty initiating a urinary stream, dribbling, urine retention secondary to obstruction of the urinary tract from tumor growth
- Hematuria from infiltration of the bladder

Mode of Spread

The spread of prostatic carcinoma may be:
- **Direct:** Stromal invasion, prostatic capsule, urethra, bladder base, seminal vesicle
- Via lymphatics to sacral, iliac, and para-aortic nodes
- Via blood to bone, lungs, and liver

Diagnostic Test Results

- Biopsy confirms cell type
- Direct rectal examination reveals a small hard nodule
- Prostatic surface antigen is elevated
- Serum acid phosphatase levels are elevated
- Magnetic resonance imaging (MRI), CT scan and excretory urography identify tumor mass
- Elevated alkaline phosphatase levels and positive bone scan indicate bone metastasis

Confirmatory test for carcinoma of prostate is biopsy. Pathologists use Gleason score to grade the carcinoma.

Pathological Changes

- **Grossly:** The prostate is enlarged, normal in size, or smaller. The cut section shows an irregular yellowish area **(Fig. 10.8A)**.
- **Microscopically:** Four histologic types are described—adenocarcinoma, squamous cell carcinoma, transitional cell carcinoma, and undifferentiated carcinoma **(Fig. 10.8B)**.

Adenocarcinoma

Adenocarcinoma being more common is characterized by:
- Loss of intra-acinar papillary convolutions
- The tumor cells may penetrate and replace fibromuscular stroma

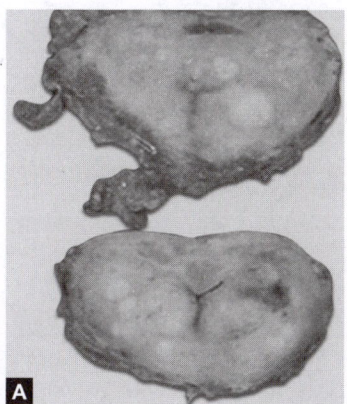
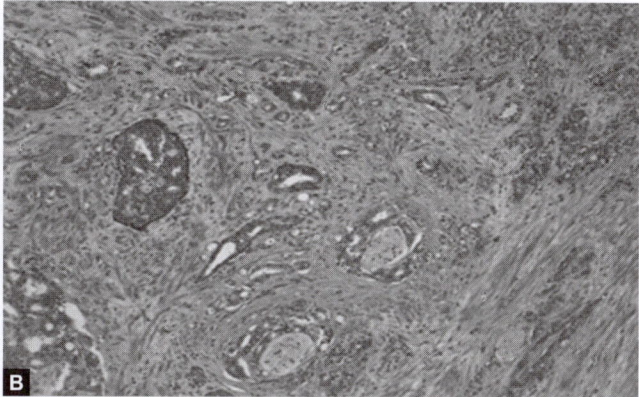

Figs. 10.8A and B: Carcinoma prostate: (A) Gross; (B) Microscopy.

- The glands are well-differentiated small and medium-sized, sometimes cribriform or fenestrated
- The tumor cell may be clear, dark, and eosinophilic
- Invasion of intraprostatic perineural spaces

MULTIPLE CHOICE QUESTIONS

1. **The causative organism for carcinoma of the penis is _____**
   a. Staphylococcus
   b. Papillomavirus
   c. Herpes simplex virus
   d. Streptococcus
2. **A medical condition in which testis are undescended is _____**
   a. Testicular agenesis
   b. Testicular degeneration
   c. Cryptorchidism
   d. Testicular atrophy
3. **Benign prostate hypertrophy is commonly seen in _____**
   a. Male aged 35–45
   b. Male aged 20–35
   c. Male aged 50 and above
   d. Male of any age group
4. **In BPH, hyperplastic glands are lined with _____**
   a. Tall columnar epithelial cells
   b. Squamous epithelial cells
   c. Simple cuboid cells
   d. Stratified epithelial cell
5. **Elevated prostate-specific antigen is seen in _____**
   a. Testicular agenesis
   b. Prostate agenesis
   c. Benign prostate hypertrophy
   d. Cancer of penis

Answer Key

1. b   2. c   3. c   4. a   5. c

FURTHER READING

1. Berney DM. A practical approach to the reporting of germ cell tumours of the testis. Curr Diagn Pathol. 2005;11:151.
2. Chevelle JC. Classification and pathology of testicular germ cell and sex cord stromal tumors. Urol Clin Am. 1999;26: 585.
3. Garnik MB, Fair WR. Prostate cancer: Emerging concepts. Part I. Ann Intern Med.1996;125:118.
4. Gleason DF. Atypical hyperplasia, benign hyperplasia and well differentiated adenocarcinoma of the prostate. Am J Surg Pathol. 1985;9:53.
5. Mostofi FK, et al. Pathology of carcinoma of the prostate. Cancer. 1992;70(suppl 1):235.
6. Mostofi FK, et al. WHO-histological typing of prostate tumours, number 22. Geneva, WHO, 1980.
7. Nelson WG, et al. Prostate cancer. N Engl J Med. 2003;349:366.
8. Stenman UH, et al. Prostate specific antigen. Semin Cancer Biol. 1996;9:83.

CHAPTER 11

Female Genital System

Neena Sood, Nancy Kurien, Suresh Sharma

CARCINOMA CERVIX

- Despite dramatic improvements in early diagnosis and treatment, cervical carcinoma continues to be one of the major causes of cancer-related deaths in women, particularly in the developing world
- There are cytologic changes in layers of squamous epithelium, the changes being progressive

Clinical Manifestations

- No symptoms or other clinically apparent changes in preinvasive cervical cancer
- Abnormal vaginal bleeding with persistent vaginal discharge and postcoital pain and bleeding related to cellular invasion and erosion of the cervical epithelium
- Pelvic pain secondary to pressure on surrounding tissues and nerves from cellular proliferation
- Vaginal leakage of urine and feces from fistulas due to erosion and necrosis of the cervix
- Anorexia, weight loss, and anemia are related to the hypermetabolic activity of cellular proliferation and increased tumor growth needs

Infection with human papillomavirus (HPV) for a long period of time highly increases the risk for carcinoma of the cervix. HPV strain 16 and HPV strain 18 are predominantly linked to carcinoma of the cervix.

Staging of Cervical Cancer

The staging of cervical cancer is based on clinical and pathological assessments, which are as follows:
- **Stage I:** Cervical cancer is strictly confined to the cervix.
- **Stage II:** Cancer extends beyond the cervix but has not extended onto the pelvic wall. It involves the vagina, but not the lower third.
- **Stage III:** Cancer may extend onto the pelvic wall and involves the lower third of the vagina.
- **Stage IV:** Implies extension outside the reproductive tract. Tumors may then involve the adjacent organs, e.g., the mucosa of the bladder or rectum.

Diagnostic Test Results

- Pap smear reveals malignant cellular changes
- Colposcopy identifies the presence and extent of early lesions
- Biopsy confirms cell type
- CT scan, nuclear imaging scan, and lymphangiography identify metastasis

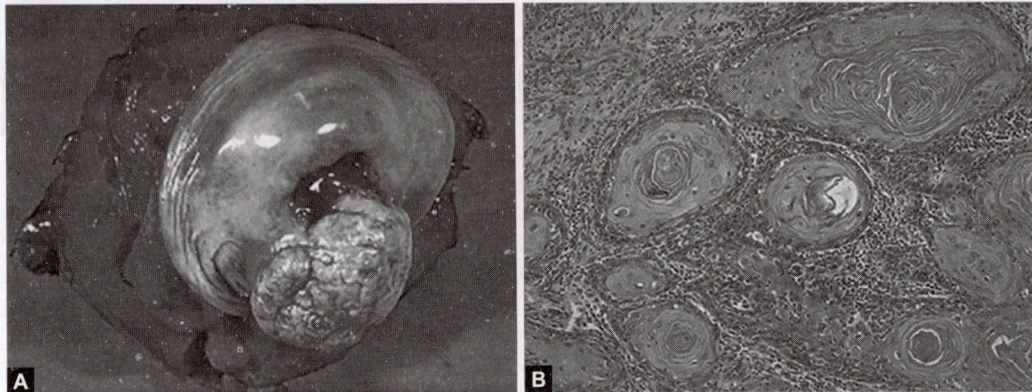

Figs. 11.1A and B: Carcinoma of the cervix: (A) Gross; (B) Microscopy.

Pathological Changes

- **Grossly:** Cervical carcinoma may present three types of the pattern **(Fig. 11.1A)**:
  1. Fungating (cauliflower-like growth infiltrating adjacent vaginal walls)
  2. Ulcerating
  3. Infiltrating
- **Histologically:** The following patterns are seen **(Fig. 11.1B)**:
  - *Epidermoid carcinoma:* It comprises around 80% of cervical carcinomas; the most common is moderately differentiated non-keratinizing large cell type with better prognosis (70%); then is well-differentiated keratinizing epidermoid carcinoma (25%) and at last, small cell undifferentiated carcinoma with poor prognosis (5%).
  - *Adenocarcinoma:* These are well-differentiated mucus-secreting adenocarcinomas, or clear cell types containing glycogen, but no mucin.
  - *Others:* The remaining cases are, such as adenosquamous carcinoma, verrucous carcinoma, and undifferentiated carcinoma.

Primary prevention of carcinoma of the cervix can be done by HPV vaccination of girls aged 9 to 14.

CARCINOMA ENDOMETRIUM

- The most common neoplasm of the body of the uterus are endometrial polyps, smooth muscle tumors, and endometrial carcinomas. All tend to produce bleeding from the uterus as the earliest manifestation.
- Endometrial carcinoma is the most frequent cancer occurring in the female genital tract and appears most frequently between the ages 55 and 65 years.

Risk Factors

- Obesity
- Increased synthesis of estrogen from adrenal and ovarian precursors
- Diabetes
- Hypertension

- Infertility
- Women tend to be nulliparous, often with nonovulatory cycles

Clinical Manifestation
- Uterine enlargement secondary to tumor growth
- Postmenopausal bleeding or persistent and unusual premenopausal bleeding from erosive effects of tumor growth
- Pain and weight loss related to progressive infiltration and invasion of tumor cells and continued cellular proliferation

Staging
- **Stage IA:** Tumor limited to the endometrium
- **Stage IB:** Invasion of less than one-half of the myometrium
- **Stage IC:** Invasion of more than one-half of the myometrium
- **Stage IIA:** Endocervical glandular involvement only
- **Stage IIB:** Cervical stromal invasion
- **Stage IIIA:** Tumor invades serosa and/or adnexa and/or positive peritoneal cytology
- **Stage IIIB:** Metastasis to pelvic and para-aortic lymph nodes
- **Stage IVA:** Tumor invasion of bladder and/or bowel mucosa
- **Stage IVB:** Distant metastasis include intra-abdominal and/or intrainguinal lymph nodes

Diagnostic Test Results
- Endometrial, cervical, and endocervical biopsies are positive for malignant cells, revealing cell type
- Dilatation and curettage identify malignancy in patients whose biopsies were negative
- Multiple cervical biopsies and endocervical curettage, pinpoint cervical involvement
- Schiller's test reveals cervix resistant to staining
- Chest X-ray and CT scan reveal metastasis; barium enema identifies possible bladder or rectal involvement

Pathological Changes
- **Grossly:** Endometrial carcinoma has two patterns localized polyploid tumor or diffuse tumor. The tumor protrudes into the endometrial cavity as an irregular, friable and gray-tan mass. The cut section shows the extension of growth in the myometrium **(Fig. 11.2A)**
- **Histologically:** Endometrial carcinomas are adenocarcinomas. These may be moderately differentiated, poorly differentiated, or well-differentiated **(Fig. 11.2B)**
  - **Well-differentiated adenocarcinoma** is characterized by an increase in the number of glands, which are closely packed. The glandular epithelium shows stratification, formation of tufting, and papillae.
  - **Moderately differentiated adenocarcinoma** shows all the above features along with the presence of some solid sheets of malignant cells.
  - **Poorly differentiated adenocarcinoma** is characterized by the presence of solid sheets and ribbons of malignant epithelial cells.

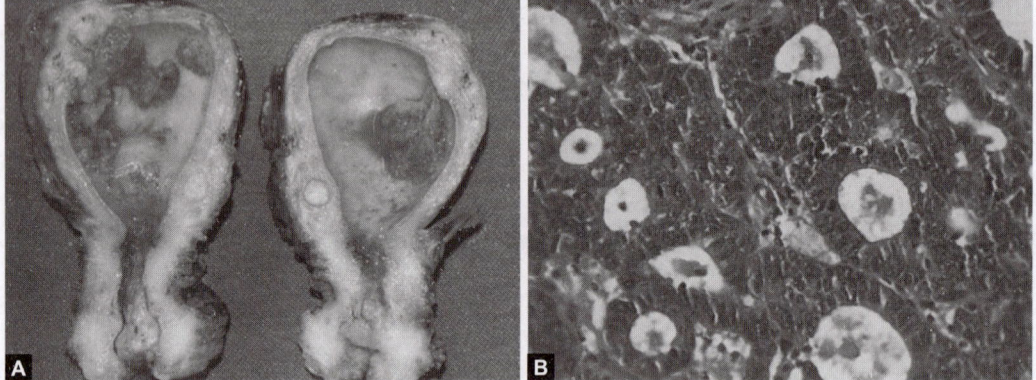

Figs. 11.2A and B: Endometrial carcinoma: (A) Gross; (B) Microscopy.

UTERINE FIBROIDS

Uterine fibroids, which are also known as uterine leiomyomas, the most common benign tumors in women, are also known as *myomas, fibromyomas or fibroids.* These tumors are composed of smooth muscle that usually occurs in the uterine corpus, although they may appear on the cervix, or on the round or broad ligament. Uterine leiomyomas occur in women of childbearing age.

Risk factors

- Obesity
- Family history of fibroids

Causes

The cause of uterine leiomyomas is unknown, but some factors implicated as regulators of leiomyoma growth include:
- Several growth factors, including epidermal growth factors
- Steroid hormones, including estrogen and progesterone (leiomyomas typically arise after menarche and regress after menopause, implicating estrogen as a promoter of leiomyoma growth).

Signs and Symptoms

Most leiomyomas are asymptomatic. Signs and symptoms of leiomyoma include:
- Abnormal bleeding, typical menorrhagia with disrupted submucosal vessels
- Pain only associated with torsion of pedunculated subserous tumor or leiomyomas undergoing degeneration. This can be artificially induced through myolysis, a laparoscopic procedure to shrink fibroids or uterine artery embolization
- Pelvic pressure and impingement on adjacent viscera resulting in mild hydronephrosis (this is not believed to be an indication for treatment because renal failure rarely if ever results)

Classification

Leiomyomas are classified according to the location:
- Within the uterine wall occur in the myometrium (intramural or interstitial)
- Protrude into the endometrial cavity (submucosal)
- Protrude from the serosa surface of the uterus (subserosal)

Pathological Changes

- **Grossly:** Fibroids are multiple, circumscribed, firm, nodular, gray-white masses of variable size. The cut surface shows a whorled appearance **(Fig. 11.3A)**
- **Microscopically:** It is composed of a whorled bundle of smooth muscle cells with connective tissue **(Fig. 11.3B)**
- The pathological characters may alter due to secondary changes, such as hyaline degeneration, cystic degeneration, infarction, calcification, infection and suppuration, necrosis, and fatty changes.

Complications

Various disorders have been attributed to uterine leiomyomas, including:
- Recurrent spontaneous abortion
- Preterm labor
- Malposition of the fetus
- Anemia secondary to excessive bleeding
- Bladder compression
- Infection (if tumor protrudes out of the vaginal opening)
- Secondary infertility
- Bowel obstruction

Diagnosis Methods

The diagnosis is based on:
- Clinical findings and patient history suggesting uterine leiomyomas
- Blood studies showing anemia from abnormal bleeding
- Bimanual examination showing enlarged, firm, non-tender, and irregularly contoured uterus

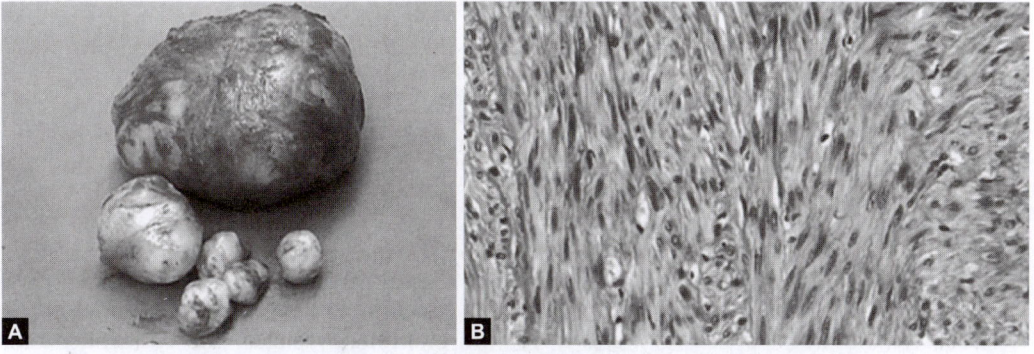

Figs. 11.3A and B: Uterine leiomyomas: (A) Gross; (B) Microscopy.

- Ultrasound for accurate assessment of the dimension, number, and location of tumors
- Magnetic resonance imaging

Other diagnostic procedures include:
- Hysterosalpingography
- Hysteroscopy
- Endometrial biopsy
- Laparoscopy

VESICULAR MOLE (HYDATIDIFORM MOLE)

- The typical vesicular or hydatidiform mole is the voluminous mass of swollen, dilated, chorionic villi, appearing grossly as a grape-like structure.
- It originates from hydatidiform means drop of water and mole means shapeless mass. Its incidence is high in teenagers and in older women. It may be invasive or noninvasive.
- The swollen villi are covered by varying amounts of normal to the highly atypical chorionic epithelium.
- Two distinctive subtypes of moles have been characterized as complete and partial moles:
  1. *The complete hydatidiform mole* does not permit embryogenesis and therefore never contains fetal parts. All of the chorionic villi are abnormal and the chorionic epithelial cells are diploid.
  2. *The partial hydatidiform mole* is compatible with early embryo formation and therefore contains fetal parts, has some normal chorionic villi, and is almost always triploid.

Two Patterns Result from Abnormal Fertilization

1. In a complete mole, an empty egg is fertilized by two spermatozoa, yielding a diploid karyotype composed of entirely paternal genes.
2. In a partial mole, a normal egg is fertilized by two spermatozoa, resulting in a triploid karyotype with a preponderance of paternal genes.

Clinical Manifestations

The condition usually arises in the 4th to 5th-month gestation characterized by:
- Increase in uterine size
- Vaginal bleeding
- Symptoms of toxemia
- History of the passage of grape-like masses per vagina

Diagnostic Tests

The only test, which confirms this is, elevated hCG level both in urine and blood as compared to normal levels in pregnancy. Removal of the mole is accompanied by a fall in hCG levels.

Pathological Changes (Figs. 11.4A and B)

Complete Mole
- **Grossly:** The uterus is enlarged and filled with grape-like vesicles. The vesicle contains clear watery fluid.

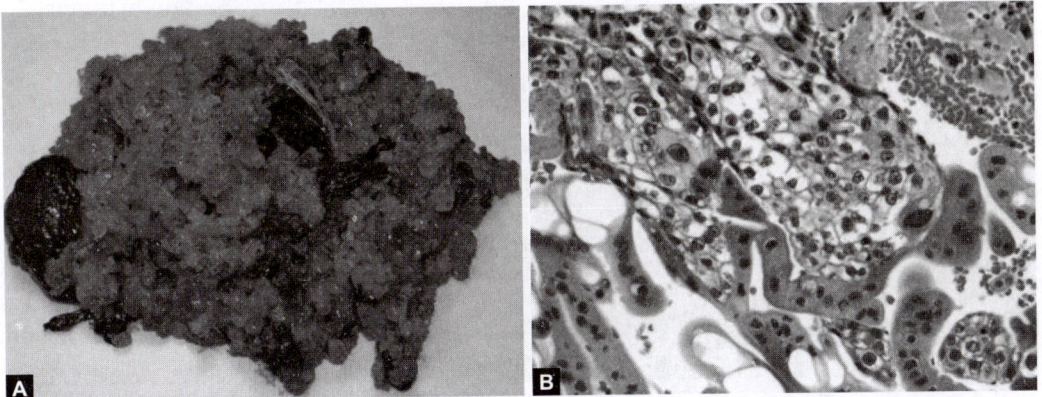

Figs. 11.4A and B: Hydatidiform mole: (A) Gross; (B) Microscopy.

- **Microscopically:** Mole appears as large, round edematous villi with hydropic degeneration and decreased vascularity of villous stroma. Trophoblastic proliferation is also seen.

Partial Mole
- **Grossly:** The uterus is smaller and contains cystic villi.
- **Microscopically:** Villi show edematous change. Trophoblastic proliferation is slight and focal.

CHORIOCARCINOMA

- Choriocarcinoma (CC) is an aggressive malignant tumor that arises either from gestational chorionic epithelium or less frequently, from totipotential cells within the gonads or elsewhere.
- Approximately 50% of choriocarcinomas arise in complete hydatidiform moles. About 25% arise after an abortion. Most of the remainder occur during what had been a normal pregnancy. The positive correlation between increasing maternal age and increasing frequency of this neoplasm suggests an origin from an abnormal ovum rather than from retained chorionic epithelium.
- Choriocarcinomas are basically two types, i.e., gestational (placental origin) and non-gestational (ovarian origin), as discussed below:
  - The non-gestational CC is found in young, under the age of 20 years and is more malignant and disseminated widely in the bloodstream to the lung, liver, bone, brain, and kidney.
  - Gestational CC is a highly malignant, metastasizing tumor of trophoblasts; the last 50% of the cases occur after a hydatidiform mole, 25% following spontaneous delivery, and 5% after ectopic pregnancy.

Clinical Manifestations
- Vaginal bleeding following a normal or abnormal pregnancy
- Metastasis in brain and lungs
- High level of hCG in plasma and urine

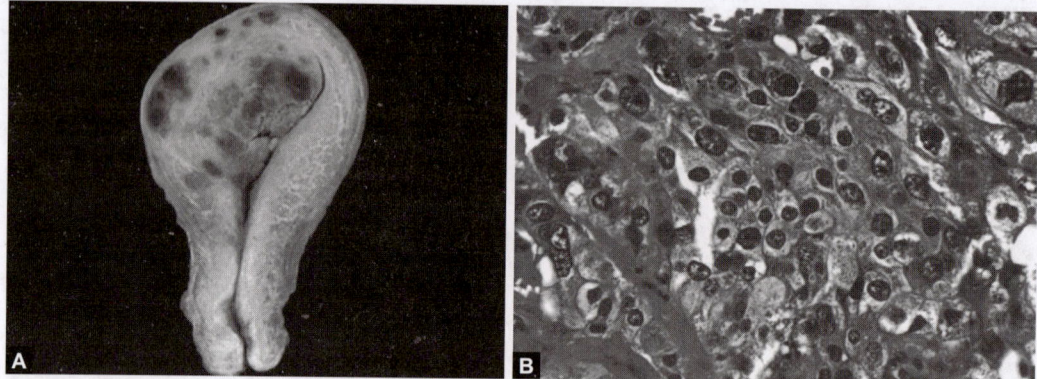

Figs. 11.5A and B: Choriocarcinomas: (A) Gross; (B) Microscopy.

Pathological Changes (Figs. 11.5A and B)

- **Grossly:** The tumor appears hemorrhagic, soft, and fleshy mass.
- **Microscopically:** There is—
  - Absence of villi
  - Masses of highly anaplastic and bizarre cytotrophoblast cells are mixed
  - Presence of hemorrhage and necrosis
  - Invasion of the myometrium and other structures like blood vessels and lymphatics.

OVARIAN CYSTS

The polycystic ovarian syndrome (PCOS) is a metabolic disorder characterized by multiple ovarian cysts.

Causes

The precise cause of the polycystic ovarian syndrome is unknown. Theories include:
- Abnormal enzyme activity triggering excess androgen secretion from the ovaries and adrenal glands.
- Endocrine abnormalities causing all of the signs and symptoms of polycystic ovarian disease, amenorrhea, polycystic ovaries on ultrasound, and hyperandrogenism.

Etiopathogenesis

- A general feature of all ovulation syndromes is a lack of pulsatile release of gonadotropin-releasing hormone.
- Initial ovarian follicle development is normal.
- Many small follicles begin to accumulate because there is no selection of a dominant follicle.
- These follicles may respond abnormally to the hormonal stimulation, causing an abnormal pattern of estrogen secretion during the menstrual cycle.
- Endocrine abnormalities may be the cause of the polycystic ovarian syndrome.

Clinical Manifestations

The signs and symptoms of the classic polycystic ovarian syndrome include:
- Mild pelvic discomfort
- Lower back pain
- Dyspareunia
- Abnormal uterine bleeding
- Hirsutism
- Male pattern hair loss
- Acne

Complications

Possible complications include:
- Malignancy due to sustained estrogenic stimulation of the endometrium
- Increased risk of cardiovascular disease and type 2 diabetes mellitus due to insulin resistance

The polycystic ovarian disease may produce:
- Secondary amenorrhea
- Oligomenorrhea
- Infertility

Diagnosis Tests

Diagnosis of polycystic ovarian disease includes:
- History and physical examination showing bilateral enlarged polycystic ovaries and menstrual disturbances, usually dating back to menarche
- Visualization of ovaries through ultrasound, laparoscopy, or surgery, often for another condition
- Slightly elevated urinary 17-ketosteroid levels and anovulation
- Elevated ratio of luteinizing hormone to follicle-stimulating hormone, and elevated levels of testosterone and androstenedione
- Unopposed estrogen action during the menstrual cycle due to anovulation
- Direct visualization by laparoscopy to rule out paraovarian cysts of the broad ligament, salpingitis, endometriosis, and neoplastic cysts.

Pathological Changes (Figs. 11.6A and B)

- **Grossly:** The ovaries are usually involved bilaterally and are sized twice the normal ovary. They are gray-white in color with small bluish cysts just beneath the cortex. The medullary stroma is abundant, solid, and gray.
- **Histologically:** The outer cortex is thick and fibrous. The subcortical cells are lined by prominent luteinized theca cells and represent follicles in various stages of maturation.

OVARIAN TUMORS

Ovarian cancer is the third most important cancer in women. It is also the fifth leading cause of death in women. Both benign and malignant tumors occur in the ovaries.

SECTION 2: Pathology-II

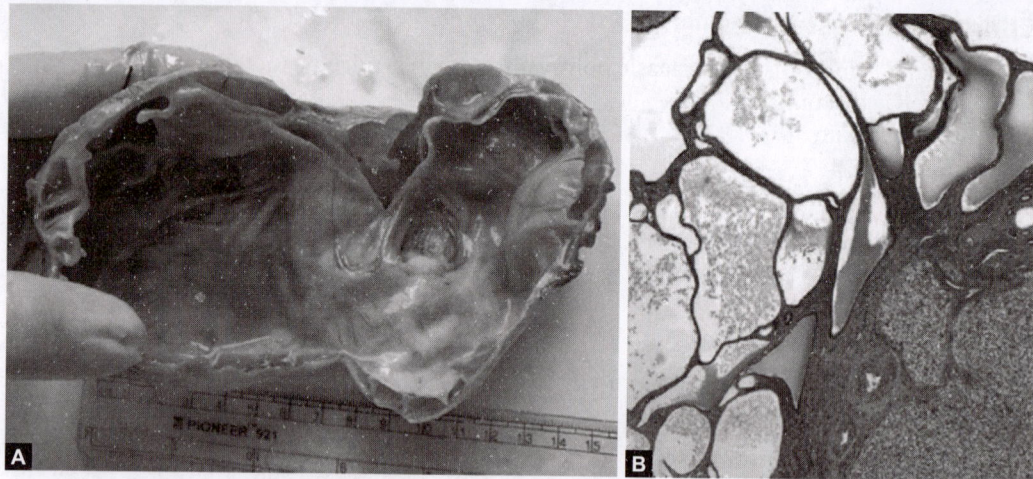

Figs. 11.6A and B: Polycystic ovarian disease: (A) Gross appearance; (B) Microscopy.

Etiology

Few risk factors are:
- **Nulliparity:** There is a higher incidence of ovarian cancer in unmarried women and married women with low or no parity.
- **Hereditary:** Women having a family history are more susceptible to a mutation in the *BRCA* gene and in the *TP53* tumor suppressor gene.
- **Complex genetic syndromes:** The syndrome associated with ovarian tumors are:
  - Peutz-Jeghers syndrome
  - Gonadal dysgenesis
  - Nevoid basal cell carcinoma.

Clinical Manifestations

- Vague abdominal discomfort, dyspepsia, and other mild gastrointestinal complaints from the increasing size of tumor-exerting pressure on nearby tissues
- Urinary frequency, constipation from obstruction resulting from increased tumor size
- Pain from tumor rupture, torsion, or infection
- Feminizing or masculinizing effects secondary to cellular type
- Ascites related to invasion and infiltration of the peritoneum
- Pleural effusion related to pulmonary metastasis

Simplified Clinical Staging of Ovarian Cancer

- **Stage I:** Tumor limited to ovaries
- **Stage II:** Involvement of other pelvic structure
- **Stage III:** Intra-abdominal spread beyond the pelvis
- **Stage IV:** Distant metastasis

Classification

According to WHO, ovarian tumors arise from normally occurring cellular components of the ovary:

- Tumors of surface epithelium
- Germ cell tumors
- Sex—cord-stromal tumors
- Miscellaneous tumors
- Metastatic tumors

Pathological Changes

Tumors of Surface Epithelium

This group constitutes about 60–70% of all ovarian neoplasms and 90% of malignant ovarian tumors. The common epithelial tumors are of three major types, i.e., serous, mucinous and endometrioid:

1. **Serous tumors:** It comprises the largest group; constitutes 20% of benign and 40% malignant. Grossly, the tumors are large and spherical masses, which are unilocular and multilocular. Microscopically, they are divided into:
   - *Serous cystadenoma:* It is characteristically lined by properly oriented low co- columnar epithelium, which is ciliated and resembles tubal epithelium.
   - *Borderline serous tumor:* It is characterized by stratification of benign serous type of epithelium.
   - *Serous cystadenocarcinoma:* It is characterized by multilayered malignant cells, which show loss of polarity, presence of solid sheets of anaplastic epithelial cells, and stromal invasion. Papillae formation is associated with psammoma bodies.

2. **Mucinous tumors:** It comprises about 20% of ovarian tumors and 10% of ovarian cancers. Grossly, these tumors are larger than serous tumors. They are smooth-surfaced cysts with characteristic multilocation containing thick and viscid gelatinous fluids. Benign tumors generally have thin walls and septa, and malignant tumors have thickened areas. Histologically, they are divided into:
   - *Mucinous cystadenoma:* It is characterized by a single layer of cells having basal nuclei and mucinous vacuoles.
   - *Borderline mucinous tumor:* It is characterized by the same histologic criteria as for borderline serous tumor, i.e., stratification of typical epithelium without stromal invasion.
   - *Mucinous cystadenocarcinoma:* It is characterized by pilling up of malignant epithelium at places forming solid sheets, papillary formation, and infiltration into stroma with/without pools of mucin.

3. **Endometrioid tumors:** It comprises about 5% of all ovarian tumors. Most of them are malignant having bilateral involvement. Grossly, these tumors are partly solid and partly cystic and may have foci of hemorrhages. Histologically, the endometrioid adenocarcinoma is distinguished from serous and mucinous carcinoma by a typical glandular pattern that closely resembles that of uterine endometrial adenocarcinoma.

4. **Clear cell tumor:** It comprises about 5% of all ovarian cancers. They are also called mesonephroma. Grossly, these tumors are large, usually unilateral, partly solid and partly cystic. Histologically, it is characterized by tubules, glands, papillae, cysts, and solid sheets of tumor cells resembling cells of renal adenocarcinoma.

5. **Brenner tumor:** It comprises about 2% of all ovarian tumors. Most tumors are benign. The borderline form is also seen, called proliferating Brenner tumor, and one with

carcinomatous change is termed as malignant Brenner tumor. Grossly, the Brenner tumor is typically solid, yellow, gray, and firm mass of different sizes. Histologically, this tumor consists of nests, masses, and columns of epithelial cells, dispersed in a fibrous stroma. These epithelial cells are ovoid in shape, having clear cytoplasm, vesicular nuclei having a coffee-bean shape.

Germ Cell Tumor

It comprises about 15–20% of all ovarian neoplasms. These tumors occur mainly in young females:
- **Teratomas:** These tumors arise from their germ cell layers—ectoderm, mesoderm, and endoderm. They are further divided into mature, immature, monodermal, or highly specialized teratomas:
    - *Mature teratoma:* It is also called a dermoid cyst. Grossly, they are unilocular, 10–15 cm in diameter, usually cystic filled with paste-like sebaceous secretions and desquamated keratin mixed with masses of hair. The cyst wall is thin and opaque gray-white. Microscopically, the cyst wall is lined by stratified squamous epithelium. Benign cystic teratoma produces kaleidoscopic patterns.
    - *Immature teratomas:* They account for 0.2% of all ovarian tumors. Grossly, it is a unilateral, solid mass, which shows a characteristic variegated appearance revealing areas of hemorrhages, necrosis, and tiny cysts. Microscopically, the tumor is having embryonic appearance.
    - *Monodermal teratoma:* They include two important examples—struma ovary and carcinoid tumor
        - *Struma ovary:* It is a teratoma composed of thyroid tissue. A tumor has the appearance of follicular adenoma.
        - *Carcinoid tumor:* This teratoma arises from argentaffin cells interstitial epithelium leading to carcinoid syndrome.
- **Dysgerminomas:** It comprises about 20% of all ovarian cancers. Grossly, it is a solid mass of variable size. The cut section shows gray-white to pink, lobular soft, and fleshy foci of hemorrhages and necrosis. Histologically, tumor cells are arranged in diffuse sheets, islands, and cords separated by scanty fibrous stroma. The tumor cells are uniform in appearance and large with vesicular nuclei and clear cytoplasm.
- **Yolk sac tumor:** It is the second most common germ cell tumor. The tumor is unilateral, highly aggressive, and grows rapidly. Grossly, the tumor is generally solid with areas of degeneration. Histologically, it is characterized by the presence of papillary projections having central blood vessels with perivascular layers of anaplastic embryonic germ cells.
- **Choriocarcinoma:** It is a highly malignant and metastasizing tumor of the trophoblast. Grossly, the tumors appear hemorrhagic, soft, and fleshy mass. Microscopically, there is the absence of villi, cytotrophoblast, and syncytiotrophoblast cells are intermixed with the invasion of underlying myometrium, other structures, blood vessels, and lymphatics.
- **Other germ cell tumors:** These are embryonal carcinoma, polyembryoma, and mixed germ cell tumors.

Sex Cord-stromal Tumors

It comprises 5–10% of all ovarian neoplasms. It includes tumors originating from granulose cells, theca cells, and Sertoli-Leydig cells:

- **Granulose theca cell tumor:** It comprises 5% of all ovarian tumors. It includes granulosa, thecoma and fibroma.
    - *Granulosa tumor* occurs at all ages and invades locally, aggressive, malignant behavior. Grossly, it is small, cystic, and usually unilateral. The cut section is yellowish-brown. Microscopically, granulose cells are arranged in a variety of patterns including micro-macro follicular, trabecular, bands, and diffuse sheets. There is the presence of rosette-like Exner bodies having a pink center and circular row of granulosa cells.
    - *Thecoma:* These are always benign and occur more frequently in postmenopausal-women. Grossly, the coma is solid and firm mass, 5–10 cm in diameter. The cut section is yellowish. Microscopically, thecoma consists of spindle-shaped theca cells of the ovary admixed with hyalinized collagen. The cytoplasm is lipid-rich and vacuolated, which reacts with lipid stain.
    - *Fibroma:* These tumors are associated with pleural effusion and benign as cites termed Meigs syndrome. Grossly, tumors are large, firm, and fibrous. Histologically, they are composed of spindle-shaped well-differentiated fibroblasts and collagen.
- **Sertoli-Leydig cell tumors:** These are called neuroblastomas. Grossly, they resemble granulose, theca cells. *Histologically,* these tumors are composed of Sertoli cells or Leydig cells forming well-defined tubules, having a biphasic pattern with the formation of solid sheets in tumors with intermediate differentiation.
- **Gynandroblastoma:** It is an extremely rare tumor in which there is a combination of pattern of both granulose theca cell tumor and Sertoli-Leydig cell tumor.

Miscellaneous Tumors

- **Lipid cell tumors:** This is a small group of ovarian tumors that appears as soft yellowish or yellow-brown nodules, which are composed of lipid-laden cells. Some examples are hilus cell tumors, adrenal rest tumors, and luteomas.
- **Gonadoblastoma:** This is a rare tumor occurring in dysgenetic gonads. Microscopically, it is composed of a mixture of germ cells and sex cord components.

Metastatic Tumors

- Metastasis occurs by lymphatics or hematogenous routes, but direct extension from adjacent organs. Most common sites where metastasis to ovaries are carcinoma of the breast, genital tract, gastrointestinal (GI) tract, and hematopoietic malignancies.
- *Krukenberg tumor* is one of the examples. It is a distinctive bilateral tumor metastatic to ovaries by trans coelomic spread characterized by the presence of mucus-filled signet ring cells accompanied by a sarcoma-like proliferation of ovarian stroma. In most of the cases, it arises from the gastrointestinal site.

Diagnostic Test Results

- Pap test may be normal
- Abdominal ultrasound, CT, or X-ray delineates tumor presence and size
- Complete blood count (CBC) may show anemia
- Excretory urography reveals abnormal renal function and urinary tract abnormalities and obstruction
- Chest X-ray reveals pleural effusion with distant metastasis
- Barium enema shows obstruction and size of the tumor

- Lymphangiography reveals lymph node involvement
- Mammography is normal to rule out breast cancer as the primary site
- Liver functions studies are abnormal with ascites
- Paracentesis fluid aspiration reveals malignant cells
- Tumor markers, such as CEA and hCG are positive.

MULTIPLE CHOICE QUESTIONS

1. Intraductal carcinoma of the breast occurs _____
   a. Within large mammary duct
   b. Within the lobule
   c. Outside the duct
   d. Within the stroma
2. Stage III of ovarian cancer indicates _____
   a. Distant metastasis
   b. Involvement of other pelvic organs
   c. Intra-abdominal spread beyond the pelvis
   d. Within ovaries
3. Highest incidence of ectopic pregnancy is in _____
   a. Ampulla
   b. Isthmus
   c. Ovary
   d. Fimbriae
4. The voluminous mass of swollen, dilated, chorionic villi, appearing grossly as a grape-like structure is _____
   a. Mole
   b. Ectopic pregnancy
   c. Ovarian cyst
   d. Hydatidiform mole
5. Prolonged infection with HPV-18 is linked with _____
   a. Ovarian cancer
   b. Carcinoma of the cervix
   c. Endometrial cancer
   d. Uterine polyp

Answer Key

1. a   2. c   3. a   4. d   5. b

FURTHER READING

1. Anderson TJ, Page DL. Risk assessment in breast cancer. In recent advances in histopathology, number 17, Anthony PP, et al. (Eds). London Churchill Livingstone, pp 69, 1997.
2. Arver B, et al. Hereditary breast cancer: A review. Semin cancer biol. 2000;10:271.
3. Ross JS. Predictive and prognostic molecular markers in breast cancer. In recent advance in histopathology, number 21, pignatelli M and underwood JCE (Eds). Philadelphia, Churchill Livingstone, pp 31–50, 2005.
4. Tavassoli FA. Pathology of the breast. Edinburgh, Churchill Livingstone, 1992.

CHAPTER 12

Breast

Aminder Singh, Joyce Joseph, Suresh Sharma

FIBROCYSTIC CHANGES

Fibrocystic changes or disease of breast are benign breast changes, mediated by hormones (increase in estrogen level), commonly seen in premenopausal women. Originate from terminal duct lobular unit of breast with or without fibrosis.

These changes are also associated with polycystic ovaries.

Clinical Manifestations
- Pain in breast
- Tender swellings bilateral and multifocal.

Morphology
- **Gross:** Grayish white, fibrous tissue with multiple cysts filled with semitranslucent fluid
- **Microscopic:** Cyst shows eosinophilic secretions and foamy macrophages. Mild epithelial hyperplasia may be present. Atypical hyperplasia is associated with increased risk of breast cancer development.

Types
- Non-proliferative
- Proliferative.

FIBROADENOMA

Fibroadenomas are solid, benign tumors of the female breast, common in young age, but can occur at any age. Originate from terminal duct lobular unit.

Clinical Manifestations
- Firm
- Well-circumscribed
- Painless
- Mobile breast lump.

Morphology

Gross
- Usually measures around 1–5 cm
- Grayish white, well-circumscribed rubbery in appearance
- Cut section appear gelatinous

Microscopy
- Proliferating epithelial and mesenchymal components are part of tumor
- Hyalinization and myxoid changes are noticed in tumor.

Management
Fibroadenomas seldom develop into breast carcinomas. The treatment modality used is surgical removal of the tumor.

BREAST CANCER
No cancer is more feared by women than carcinoma of the breast. The physiological and pathological changes in women's breasts vary during different phases of their life. This is due to variations in hormone levels that occur before, during, and after the period of reproductive life; hormones are important in the regulation of growth, development, and function of the breast.

Clinical Manifestations
- Lumps can vary in their nature depending on their cause
- Well-circumscribed or ill-defined
- Single or multiple small nodules
- Soft or firm
- Mobile or attached to skin or underlying muscle.

These features assist in clinical distinctions between benign breast lesions and breast carcinomas.

Risk Factors
Well-established Influences
- Age after 35 years
- First-degree relative with breast cancer
- Postmenopausal period
- Age at menarche <12 years
- Age at menopause >55 years
- First live birth after age 35 years
- Nulliparous
- Benign breast disease
- Lobular carcinoma in situ.

Less Well-established Influences
- Exogenous estrogens
- Oral contraceptives
- Obesity
- High-fat diet
- Alcohol consumption
- Cigarette smoking.

General Features and Classification
- Cancer of the breast occurs more frequently in the left breast than the right and is bilateral
- In 50% of cases, the upper quadrant is a most common anatomic site half of the cases, followed by the central portion and then the lower
- Carcinoma of the breast arises from ductal epithelium in 90% of cases, while the remaining 10% originate from the lobular epithelium
- For a variable period, tumor cells remain confined within ducts or lobules before they become invasive
- There are two patterns in non-invasive carcinoma—ductal and lobular, whereas there are varieties of histological patterns of invasive carcinoma breast.

Non-invasive Carcinoma
In this in situ form, tumor form cells are localized within ducts or lobules without evidence of invasion. Two forms are recognized, i.e., intraductal or lobular.

Intraductal Carcinoma
It is confined within larger mammary ducts. The tumor usually begins with atypical hyperplasia of ductal epithelium followed by filling of ducts with tumor cells.

Pathological changes are as follows:
- **Grossly:** The tumor may vary from a small poorly defined focus to a 3–5 cm diameter mass. Cut surface shows, cystically dilated ducts containing cheesy necrotic material or the intraductal tumor may be polypoid and friable resembling intraductal papilloma.
- **Histologically:** The proliferating tumor cells within the ductal lumina may have four types of patterns in different combinations, i.e., solid, comedo, papillary and cribriform:
  1. Solid pattern is characterized by filling and plugging of ductal lumina with tumor cells.
  2. Comedo pattern is centrally placed necrotic debris surrounded by neoplastic cells.
  3. Papillary pattern has the formation of intraductal papillary projections of tumor cells.
  4. Cribriform pattern is recognized by neat punched-out fenestrations in the intraductal tumor.

Lobular Carcinoma
It is not a palpable tumor.
- **Grossly:** No visible tumor is identified.
- **Histologically:** It is characterized by filling up terminal ducts and ductules or acini by uniform cells, which are small, rounded nuclei with cytoplasmic margins.

Invasive Carcinoma
Invasive breast cancer has various morphologic types.

Infiltrating Duct Carcinoma
It accounts for 70% of cases of breast cancer. They are found most commonly in the left breast.

Pathological changes are as follows:
- **Grossly:** The tumor is irregular, 1–5 cm in diameter, hard cartilage-like mass that cuts with a grating sound. The cut surface shows gray-white to yellowish chalky streaks.

- **Histologically:** There is infiltration of tumor cells into diffuse fibrous stroma and fat with invasion into perivascular and perineural spaces. There is the presence of poorly form glandular structures and intraductal foci.

Infiltrating Lobular Carcinoma

It accounts for 5% of cases of breast cancer and occurs more frequently bilateral having multicentric origin.

Pathological changes are as follows:
- **Grossly:** The appearance varies from well-defined scirrhous mass to poorly defined area of induration.
- **Histologically:** There is a linear arrangement of stromal infiltration by tumors cells. Infiltrating cells show concentric arrangements around ducts. Tumor cells are sound and regular with pleomorphism and infrequent mitosis.

Medullary Carcinoma

It accounts for 1% of all breast cancers. This tumor has better prognosis due to good host immune response:

Pathological changes are as follows:
- **Grossly:** The tumor is characterized by large, circumscribed well-circumscribed, rounded masses that is soft and fleshy, also called encephaloid carcinoma. Cut surface shows areas of hemorrhages, and necrosis.
- **Histologically:** Tumor cells appear as sheets of large, pleomorphic cells with abundant cytoplasm, and vesicular nuclei with atypical mitosis. The loose connective tissue stroma is scanty and prominent lymphoid infiltrate.

Colloid Carcinoma

It occurs more frequently in older women and is usually slow-growing.

Pathological changes are as follows:
- **Grossly:** The tumor is a soft and gelatinous mass with well-demarcated borders.
- **Histologically:** Colloid carcinoma contain large amount of extracellular mucin or acini filled with mucin. Cuboidal to tall columnar tumor cells are also seen floating in mucin.

Papillary Carcinoma

It is a rare variety of infiltrating duct carcinoma in which stromal invasion is in the form of papillary structures.

Tubular Carcinoma

This tumor is having most favorable prognosis.

Histologically, the tumor is highly well-differentiated and has an orderly pattern. The tumor cells are regular and form single well-defined tubules.

Adenoid Cystic Carcinoma

This tumor is having excellent prognosis. There is stromal invasion by islands of cells having a characteristic fenestrated appearance.

Secretory (Juvenile) Carcinoma

This pattern is found more frequently in children and has a better prognosis. The tumor is well-circumscribed, which on histologic examination shows intra/extra PAS (periodic acid-Schiff) positive clear spaces.

Inflammatory Carcinoma

It does not constitute any histologic type and it is associated with extensive invasion of dermal lymphatics.

Carcinoma with Metaplasia

Invasive ductal carcinomas may have various types of metaplastic alterations such as squamous metaplasia, cartilaginous and osseous metaplasia.

MULTIPLE CHOICE QUESTIONS

1. **Intraductal carcinoma of the breast occurs** _____
   a. Within large mammary duct
   b. Within the lobule
   c. Outside the duct
   d. Within the stroma
2. **Stage III of ovarian cancer indicates** _____
   a. Distant metastasis
   b. Involvement of other pelvic organs
   c. Intra-abdominal spread beyond the pelvis
   d. Within ovaries
3. **Highest incidence of ectopic pregnancy is in** _____
   a. Ampulla
   b. Isthmus
   c. Ovary
   d. Fimbriae
4. **The voluminous mass of swollen, dilated, chorionic villi, appearing grossly as a grape-like structure is** _____
   a. Mole
   b. Ectopic pregnancy
   c. Ovarian cyst
   d. Hydatidiform mole
5. **Prolonged infection with HPV-18 is linked with** _____
   a. Ovarian cancer
   b. Carcinoma of the cervix
   c. Endometrial cancer
   d. Uterine polyp

Answer Key

1. a   2. c   3. a   4. d   5. b

FURTHER READING

1. Anderson TJ, Page DL. Risk assessment in breast cancer. In recent advances in histopathology, number 17, Anthony PP, et al (Eds). London Churchill Livingstone, 1997. pp. 69.
2. Arver B, et al. Hereditary breast cancer: A review. Semin Cancer Biol. 2000;10: 271.
3. Ross JS. Predictive and prognostic molecular markers in breast cancer. In recent advance in histopathology, number 21, Pignatelli M, Underwood JCE (Eds). Philadelphia, Churchill Livingstone, 2005. pp. 31–50.
4. Tavassoli FA. Pathology of the breast. Edinburgh, Churchill Livingstone, 1992.

CHAPTER 13

Central Nervous System

Neena Sood, Nancy Kurien, Suresh Sharma

MENINGITIS

In meningitis, the brain and the spinal cord meninges become inflamed, usually as a result of bacterial infection. Such inflammations may involve all three meningeal membranes—the dura mater, arachnoid mater, and the pia mater.

Etiopathogenesis

- Meningitis is almost always a complication of bacteremia, especially from the following:
  - Pneumonia
  - Empyema
  - Osteomyelitis
  - Endocarditis
- Other infections associated with the development of meningitis include:
  - Sinusitis
  - Otitis media
  - Encephalitis
  - Myelitis
  - Brain abscess, usually caused by *Neisseria meningitis, Haemophilus influenzae, Streptococcus pneumoniae,* and *Escherichia coli.*
- Meningitis may follow trauma or invasive procedures, including:
  - Skull fracture
  - Penetrating head wound
  - Lumbar puncture
  - Ventricular shunting

Aseptic meningitis may result from a virus or other organism. Sometimes, no causative organism can be found.

Clinical Manifestations

- Signs of meningitis typically include:
  - Fever, chills, malaise resulting from infection and inflammation
  - Headache, vomiting, and rarely, papilledema (inflammation and edema of the optic nerve) from increased ICP.
- Signs of meningeal irritation include:
  - Nuchal rigidity
  - Positive Brudzinski's and Kernig's signs
  - Exaggerated and symmetrical deep tendon reflexes
  - Opisthotonos (a spasm in which the back and extremities arch backward so that the body rests on the head and heals)

- Other features of meningitis may include:
  - Sinus arrhythmias from irritation of the nerves of the autonomic nervous system
  - Irritability from increasing ICP
  - Photophobia, diplopia, and other vision problems from cranial nerve irritation
  - Delirium, deep stupor, and coma from increased ICP and cerebral edema
  - An infant may show signs of infection, but most are simply fretful and refuse to eat. In an infant, vomiting can lead to dehydration, which prevents the formation of a bulging fontanel, an important sign of increased ICP
  - As the illness progresses, twitching, seizures (in 30% of infants), or coma may develop. Most of the older children have the same symptoms as adults. In subacute meningitis, the onset may be insidious.

Pathological Changes

- CSF becomes turbid purulent material that interferes with CSF flow
- Swelling of brain
- Presence of thick exudates
- Presence of tubercles
- Bacterial meningitis may be associated with abscesses in the brain
- Numerous neutrophils fill the entire subarachnoid space in severely affected areas
- Gram staining reveals a number of causative bacteria
- Acid-fast bacilli may be demonstrated
- Cryptococcus meningitis due to fungus is characterized by infiltration of lymphocytes, plasma cells, and granulomas.

Diagnostic Methods

- Lumbar puncture shows elevated CSF pressure (from obstructed CSF outflow at the arachnoid villi), cloudy or milky white CSF, high protein level, positive Gram stain, and culture (unless a virus is responsible), and decreased glucose concentration
- Positive Brudzinski's and Kernig's signs indicate meningeal irritation
- Culture of blood, urine, and nose and throat secretions reveal the offending organism
- Chest X-ray may reveal pneumonitis of lung abscess, tubercular lesions, or granulomas secondary to a fungal infection
- Sinus and skull X-rays may identify cranial osteomyelitis or paranasal sinusitis as the underlying infectious process or skull fracture as the mechanism for the entrance of microorganisms
- White blood cell count reveals leukocytosis
- CT scan may reveal hydrocephalus or rule out cerebral hematoma, hemorrhage, or tumor as the underlying cause.

ENCEPHALITIS

Infection and severe inflammation of the brain, caused by different viruses are known as encephalitis.

Clinical Manifestations
- Fever
- Headache

- Vomiting
- Seizures
- **Focal neurological deficit:** Drowsiness, coma, paralysis, ataxia, and organic psychoses
- Meningeal irritation (stiff neck and back).

Pathological Changes in CNS
- Mononuclear cell infiltration by lymphocytes, plasma cells, and macrophages
- Cell lysis (cytolytic viral infection) and phagocytosis of cell debris by macrophages
- Viral inclusions, which can often be detected in infected neurons or glial cells; occasionally, these can be of diagnostic value, for example, 'owl-eye', inclusion in cytomegalovirus infection, or Negri bodies in rabies
- Reactive hypertrophy and hyperplasia of astrocytes and microglial cells, often forming cell clusters
- Edema, which is of vasogenic type.

Types of Encephalitis
Bacterial Encephalitis
Pathological changes: As follows:
- Localized area of inflammatory necrosis and edema surrounded by a fibrous capsule
- Acute and chronic inflammatory cell and septic thrombosis of vessels present
- Abscess containing pus cells.

Viral Encephalitis
Pathological changes: As follows:
- Presence of parenchymal infiltrate
- Consisting of lymphocytes, plasma cells, and macrophages
- Microscope cluster of microglial cells presentation
- Infranuclear bodies present (Negri bodies).

HIV Encephalitis
Pathological changes: As follows:
Focal irregular gelatinous areas of gray and white matter infect cerebrum, brainstem, cerebellum, and spinal cord.

STROKE
- A stroke, also known as cerebrovascular accident or brain attack, is a sudden impairment of cerebral circulation in one or more blood vessels
- A stroke interrupts or diminishes oxygen supply, and commonly causes damage or necrosis in the brain tissue. The sooner the circulation returns to normal after a stroke, the better the chances are for recovery
- However, about one-half of the patients who survive a stroke remain permanently disabled and experience a reoccurrence within weeks, months, or years. It is the leading cause of admission to long-term care.

CHAPTER 13: Central Nervous System

Etiopathogenesis
- Stroke typically results from one of the three causes:
  - Thrombosis of the cerebral arteries supplying the brain or the intracranial vessels occluding blood flow
  - Embolism from thrombi outside the brain, such as in the heart, aorta, or common carotid artery
  - Hemorrhage from an intracranial artery or vein, such as from hypertension, ruptured aneurysm, arteriovenous malformations, trauma, hemorrhagic disorders, or septic embolism
- Risk factors that have been identified as predisposing a patient to stroke include:
  - Hypertension
  - Family history of stroke
  - History of transient ischemic attacks (TIAs)
  - Cardiac disease including arrhythmia, coronary artery disease, acute myocardial infarction, dilated cardiomyopathy, and valvular disease
  - Diabetes
  - Familial hyperlipidemia
  - Cigarette smoking
  - Increased alcohol intake
  - Obesity, sedentary lifestyle
  - Use of oral contraceptives
- Cardiac causes can be distinguished between high and low-risk:
  - *High-risk:*
    - Atrial fibrillation and paroxysmal atrial fibrillation
    - Rheumatic disease of the mitral or aortic valve disease
    - Artificial heart valves, known cardiac thrombus of the atrium or ventricle
    - Sick sinus syndrome
    - Sustained atrial flutter
    - Recent myocardial infarction
    - Congestive heart failure
    - Coronary artery bypass graft (CABG) surgery
  - *Low-risk/potential:*
    - Calcification of the annulus (ring) of the mitral valve
    - Patent foramen ovale (PFO)
    - Atrial septal aneurysm
    - Atrial septal aneurysm with patent foramen ovale
    - Left ventricular aneurysm without thrombus
    - Systemic hypoperfusion
    - Hypoxemia (low blood oxygen content)
    - Venous thrombosis due to locally increased venous pressure.

Classification
Strokes can be classified into two major categories:
1. Ischemic is due to interruption of blood supply
2. Hemorrhagic is due to the rupture of a blood vessel or an abnormal vascular structure. More than 80% of the strokes are due to ischemia; the remainder is due to hemorrhage.

Ischemic Stroke

In an ischemic stroke, the blood supply to the brain is decreased, leading to dysfunction and necrosis of the brain tissue in that area. There are four reasons why this might happen:
- Thrombosis (obstruction of the blood vessel by a blood clot-forming locally)
- Embolism (due to an embolus from elsewhere in the body)
- Systemic hypoperfusion (general disease blood supply, e.g., in shock)
- A venous thrombosis.

A stroke without an obvious explanation is termed 'cryptogenic' (of unknown origin).

Thrombotic Stroke

In thrombotic stroke, a thrombus (blood clot) usually forms around atherosclerotic plaques. Since blockage of the artery is gradual, the onset of symptomatic thrombotic strokes is slower. A thrombus itself (even if non-occluding) can lead to an embolic stroke if the thrombus breaks off at which point it is called an 'embolus'.

Thrombotic stroke can be divided into two types depending on the type of vessel, the thrombus is formed by the following factors:
- Large vessel disease involves:
  - The common and internal carotids
  - Vertebral and the circle of the villus.

  A disease that may form thrombi in the large vessels include (in the descending incidence):
  - Atherosclerosis
  - Vasoconstriction
  - Aortic, carotid, and vertebral artery dissection
  - Various inflammatory diseases of the blood vessel wall (Takayasu arteritis, giant cell arteritis, vasculitis)
  - Non-inflammatory vasculopathy
  - Fibromuscular dysplasia
- Small vessel disease involves
- The smaller arteries inside the brain
- Branches of the circle of villus, middle cerebral artery, stem, and arteries arising from the distal vertebral and basilar artery.

  Diseases that may form thrombi in the small vessels include (in descending incidence):
- Lipohyalinosis (deposition of eosinophilic matter in the blood vessel as a result of high-blood pressure and aging)
- Fibrinoid degeneration (stroke involving these vessels are known as lacunar infarcts)
- Microatheroma (small atherosclerotic plaques)
- Sickle cell anemia, which can cause blood cells to clump up and block vessels, can lead to stroke. A stroke is the second leading killer of people under 20 who suffer from sickle cell anemia.

Embolic Stroke

- An embolic stroke refers to the blockage of an artery by an embolus, traveling particle, or debris in the arterial bloodstream originating from elsewhere. An embolus is most frequently a thrombus, but can also be a number of other substances including fat (e.g., from bone marrow in broken bone), air, cancer cells, or clumps of bacteria (usually from infectious endocarditis).

- Emboli most commonly arise from the heart (especially in atrial fibrillation) but may originate from elsewhere in the arterial tree

Hemorrhagic Stroke

- Intracerebral hemorrhage (ICH) is bleeding directly into the brain tissue, forming a gradually enlarging hematoma (pooling of blood); it generally occurs in small arteries or arterioles.
- Common causes are due to:
  - Hypertension
  - Trauma
  - Bleeding disorders
  - Amyloid angiopathy
  - Illicit drug use (e.g., amphetamines or cocaine)
  - Vascular malformations
- The hematoma enlarges until pressure from surrounding tissue limits its growth, or until it decompresses by emptying into the ventricular system, CSF, or the pia surface. A one-third of intracerebral bleed is into the brain's ventricles.
- A widely used classification of ischemic stroke is the **Bamford classification**, introduced in 1991. This relies on the presenting symptoms and physical examination to identify the area of the brain affected, and can be used to predict prognosis as well as underlying etiology:
  - **Total anterior circulation infarct (TACI)**
  - **Partial anterior circulation infarct (PACI)**
  - **Lacunar infarct (LACI)**
  - **Posterior circulation infarct (POCI)**
- Each of these gives a stereotypical clinical picture. Before the location of the infarction has been confirmed by diagnostic imaging (e.g., CT scan), they may be referred to as total anterior circulatory syndrome and so on (TACS, PACS, LACS, POCS).

Clinical Manifestations

The clinical features of stroke vary according to the affected artery and the region of the brain it supplies, the severity of the damage, and the extent of collateral circulation developed. A stroke in one hemisphere causes signs and symptoms on the opposite side of the body; a stroke that damages cranial nerves affects structures on the same side as the infarction.

- General symptoms of a stroke include:
  - Unilateral limb weakness
  - Speech difficulties
  - Numbness on one side
  - Headache
  - Vision disturbances (diplopia, hemianopia, ptosis)
  - Dizziness
  - Anxiety
  - Altered level of consciousness (LOC)
- **Additional, symptoms**: Are usually classified by the artery affected. Signs and symptoms associated with middle cerebral artery involvement include:
  - Aphasia
  - Dysphasia

- Visual field deficit
- Hemiparesis of the affected side (more severe in the face and arm than in the legs)
- Symptoms associated with carotid artery involvement include:
  - Weakness
  - Paralysis
  - Numbness
  - Sensory changes
  - Vision disturbances on the affected side
  - Altered LOC
  - Bruits
  - Headache
  - Aphasia
  - Ptosis
- Symptoms associated with vertebrobasilar artery involvement include:
  - Weakness on the affected side
  - Numbness around lips and mouth
  - Visual field deficit
  - Diplopia
  - Poor coordination
  - Dysphagia
  - Slurred speech
  - Dizziness
  - Nystagmus
  - Amnesia
  - Ataxia
- Signs and symptoms associated with anterior cerebral artery involvement include:
  - Confusion
  - Weakness
  - Numbness, especially in the legs on the affected side
  - Incontinence
  - Loss of coordination
  - Impaired motor and sensory functions
  - Personality changes
- Signs and symptoms associated with posterior cerebral artery involvement include:
  - Visual field deficit
  - Sensory impairment
  - Dyslexia
  - Perseveration (abnormally persistent replies to questions)
  - Coma
  - Cortical blindness
  - Absence of paralysis (usually).

Pathological Changes

- At a very early stage after cerebral infarction, no naked eye abnormalities are apparent.
- However, 24 hours after infarction the:
  - Affected tissue becomes softened and swollen
  - A loss of definition between white and gray matter

- Edema around the infarct, resulting in local mass effect
- Histology shows infiltration by macrophages, which are filled with the local product of myelin breakdown
- Reactive astrocytes and proliferating capillaries are often present at the edge of the infarct
- Eventually, all the dead tissue is phagocytosed to leave a fluid-filled cystic cavity with a gliotic wall.

Complications

Complications vary with the severity and type of stroke, but may include:
- Unstable blood pressure (from loss of vasomotor control)
- Cerebral edema
- Fluid imbalances
- Sensory impairment
- Infections such as pneumonia
- Altered LOC
- Aspiration
- Contractures
- Pulmonary embolism
- Death.

Diagnostic Methods

- Computed tomography scan identifies an ischemic stroke within the **first 72 hours** of symptom onset and evidence of a hemorrhagic stroke (lesions larger than 1 cm) immediately
- Magnetic resonance imaging assists in identifying areas of ischemia or infarction and cerebral swelling
- Cerebral angiography reveals disruption of displacement of the cerebral circulation by occlusions such as stenosis or acute thrombus, or hemorrhage
- Digital subtraction angiography shows evidence of occlusion of cerebral vessels, lesions, or vascular abnormalities
- Carotid duplex scan identifies the degree of stenosis
- Brain scan shows ischemic areas, but may not be conclusive for up to 2 weeks after a stroke
- Single-photon on emission computed tomography and positron emission tomography scans identify areas of altered metabolism surrounding lesions not yet able to be detected by other diagnostic tests
- Transesophageal echocardiogram reveals cardiac disorders, such as atrial thrombi, atrial septal defect, or patent foramen ovale, as causes of thrombotic stroke
- Lumbar puncture (performed if there are no signs of increased ICP) reveals bloody CSF when the stroke is hemorrhagic
- Ophthalmoscope may identify signs of hypertension and atherosclerotic changes in retinal arteries
- EEG helps identify damaged areas of the brain

On the basis of the history and neurological examination, as well as the presence of risk factors, a doctor can rapidly diagnose the anatomical nature of the stroke (i.e., which part of the brain is affected), even if the exact cause is not yet known.

Prehospital care professionals will typically use the face arm speech test (**FAST**) to assess stroke:
- **Face:** Look to see if there is any drooping or loss of muscle tone on the face
- **Arm:** Ask the patient to close their eyes and hold both arms out straight for 30 seconds. In a patient with a stroke, you might see one arm tending to slowly move down
- **Speech:** Listen to see if you can hear any slurring of speech not otherwise explained (e.g., alcohol) and see if they can answer simple questions (where are you? what is your name? what day of the week it is? etc.).

CNS TUMORS

- Second most common tumors in children and the sixth most common in adults
- Present clinically with localizing signs due to tissue destruction or with the non-specific effects of raised intracranial pressure
- Classified according to the cell of origin and degree of differentiation
- Survival depends on the age of the patient and the site, size, and histology of the neoplasm.

Primary Tumors

The most common group of primary CNS neoplasms are the intrinsic tumors of the brain, which account for all primary CNS neoplasms in children. In adults, intrinsic tumors account for around 65% of the primary CNS neoplasms, the majority of which are of glial origin. Intrinsic tumors occur more frequently in male patients.

Meningiomas

- Meningiomas account for around 18% of intracranial neoplasms in adults
- Female patients outnumber males by 2:1
- Meningiomas arise from cells of the arachnoid cap (a component of arachnoid villi).

Most Frequent Sites

- Parasagittal region
- Sphenoidal wing
- Olfactory groove
- Foramen magnum.

Characteristics of Meningiomas

- Smooth lobulated masses
- Broadly adherent to the dura
- Infiltration of the adjacent dura and overlying bone is common
- Invasion of the brain is exceptionally rare
- The brain may be markedly compressed by a meningioma, resulting in considerable anatomical distortion
- Histologically, meningiomas display a variety of patterns, the most characteristic of which includes sheets of fusiform cells in a composite solid and whorled pattern
- Small foci of calcification are common
- Occasionally, meningiomas are frankly malignant and may metastasize outside the CNS, for example to lungs.

Gliomas

Gliomas are tumors of the brain parenchyma that histologically resemble different types of glial cells.

The major types of tumors in this category are:
- Astrocytomas
- Oligodendrogliomas
- Ependymomas.

Astrocytoma
- Poorly defined, a gray, infiltrative tumor that expands and distorts the invaded brain.
- Infiltration beyond the grossly evident margins is always present
- The cut surface of the tumor is either firm or soft and gelatinous
- Cystic degeneration may be seen
- Some areas are firm and white, others are soft and yellow (the result of tissue necrosis)
- Show regions of cystic degeneration and hemorrhage.

Oligodendrogliomas
- Infiltrative tumors
- Contain gelatinous, gray masses
- May show cysts
- Presence of focal hemorrhage
- The tumor is composed of sheets of regular cells with spherical nuclei containing finely granular chromatin
- The tumor typically contains a delicate network of anastomosing capillaries
- Calcification, present in as many as 90% of these tumors, ranges from microscopic foci to massive depositions
- Mitotic activity is usually very difficult to detect
- With increasing cell density, nuclear anaplasia, increased mitotic activity and necrosis, the tumor becomes higher grade (anaplastic oligodendroglioma).

Ependymomas
- Typically solid or papillary masses extending from the floor of the ventricle
- Composed of cells with regular, round-to-oval nuclei with abundant granular chromatin
- Between the nuclei there is a variably dense fibrillary background
- Tumor cells may form round or elongated structures (rosettes, canals) that resemble the embryologic ependymal canal, with long, delicate processes extending into the lumen
- Anaplastic ependymomas show increased cell density, high mitotic rates, necrosis, and less evident ependymal differentiation.

Secondary Tumors

Metastatic spread of the brain tumor to other regions of the body is rare, but the brain is not comparably protected against the spread of tumors from elsewhere. Carcinomas are more commonly metastatic to the nervous system than lymphoid malignancies; sarcomas infrequently metastasize to the brain. The CNS may be involved by other neoplasms in two main ways, i.e., compression and invasion of tumors and metastatic tumors.

Compression and Invasion Tumors

Tumors arising in adjacent organs may compress and invade the CNS, producing localizing clinical signs or presenting as space-occupying lesions. The most common examples involving the brain are pituitary adenomas, which frequently cause visual impairment due to the presence of optic chiasm.

METASTATIC CNS TUMORS

- Metastatic tumors are those in which the cancer cells have traveled from the original or the primary site to the second or more distant site. Most commonly, metastasis occurs through the blood vessels and lymphatic system. Tumor cells also can be transported from one body location to another by external means, such as carriage on instruments or gloves during surgery.
- **Hematogenous spread:** Invasive tumor cells break down the basement membrane and walls of the blood vessels, and the tumor sheds malignant cells into the circulation. Most of the cells die, but a few escape the host defenses and the turbulent environment of the bloodstream. From here, the surviving mass of tumor cells, called tumor cell embolus, travels downstream and commonly lodges in the first capillary bed it encounters. For example, blood from most organs next enters the capillaries of the lungs, which are the most common site of metastasis.
- Once lodged, the tumor cells develop a protective coat of fibrin, platelets, and clotting factors to evade detection by the immune system. Then they become attached to epithelium, ultimately invading the vessel wall, interstitium, and the parenchyma of the target organ. To survive, the new tumor develops its own vascular network and ultimately spreads again.
- **Lymphatic spread:** The lymphatic system is the most common route for distant metastasis. Tumor cells enter the lymphatic vessels through damaged basement membranes and are transported to regional lymph nodes. In this case, the tumor becomes trapped in the first lymph node it encounters. The consequent enlargement, possibly the first evidence of metastasis, may be due to increased tumor growth within the node or a localized immune reaction to the tumor. The lymph node may filter out or contain some of the tumor cells, limiting further spread. The cells that escape can enter the blood from the lymphatic circulation through plentiful connections between the venous and lymphatic systems.
- **Metastatic sites:** Typically, the first capillary bed, whether lymphatic or vascular, encountered by the circulating tumor mass determines the location of the metastasis. For example, because the lungs receive all of the systemic venous return, they are a frequent site for metastasis. In breast cancer, the axillary lymph nodes, which are close to the breast, are a common site of metastasis. Other types of cancer seem most likely to spread to specific organs. This organ tropism may be a result of growth factors or hormones secreted by the target organ or chemotactic factors that attract the tumor.
- The CNS is a common site for metastases, which may occur by the hematogenous or direct spread. The most common neoplasms to metastasize to the CNS are the carcinomas of:
    - Breast
    - Bronchus
    - Kidney and colon
    - Malignant melanomas
    - Metastases often occur at the boundary between gray and white matter and may present as space-occupying lesions with or without focal signs

- Metastatic carcinoma sometimes infiltrates the subarachnoid space producing carcinomatous meningitis.

Clinical Manifestations
- Headache, dizziness, vertigo, nausea and vomiting, and papilledema secondary to increased intracranial pressure from tumor invasion and compression of surrounding tissue
- Cranial nerve dysfunction secondary to tumor invasion or compression of cranial nerves
- Focal deficits including motor deficits (weakness, paralysis, or gait disorders), sensory disturbances (anesthesia, paresthesia, or disturbance of vision or hearing) secondary to tumor invasion or compression of motor or sensory control areas of the brain
- Disturbances of higher function include defects in cognition, learning, and memory.

Local
- Dementia, personality or behavioral changes, gait disturbances, seizures, and language disorders
- Sensory loss, hemianopia, cranial nerve dysfunction, ataxia, papillary abnormalities, nystagmus, hemiparesis, and autonomic dysfunction depending on the location of the tumor.

Diagnostic Test Results
- Stereotactic tissue biopsy confirms cell type
- Neurologic assessment reveals manifestations of lesion affecting specific lobe
- Skull X-ray, CT scan, MRI, and cerebral angiography identify the location of the mass
- Brain scan reveals an area of increased uptake in the location of the tumor
- Lumbar puncture shows increased pressure and protein levels, decreased glucose levels, and occasionally, tumor cells in CSF.

MULTIPLE CHOICE QUESTIONS

1. **Tumors arising from brain parenchyma are called _____**
   a. Meningioma
   b. Adenoma
   c. Glioma
   d. Sarcoma
2. **Paralysis of all four limbs is called _____**
   a. Paraplegia
   b. Hemiplegia
   c. Paresthesia
   d. Quadriplegia
3. **An impairment in motor and sensory function of the lower extremities is called _____**
   a. Paraplegia
   b. Tetraplegia
   c. Quadriplegia
   d. Hemiplegia
4. **Increased accumulation of CSF in brain is called _____**
   a. Meningitis
   b. Hydrocephalus
   c. Brain abscess
   d. Meningioma
5. **The mass of material in the vascular system which is able to become dislodged and block the lumen of blood vessel is called _____**
   a. Thrombus
   b. Clot
   c. Embolus
   d. Hemorrhage

Answer Key
1. c   2. d   3. a   4. b   5. c

FURTHER READING

1. Brat, et al. Surgical neuropathology update: A review of changes introduced by the WHO classification of tumors of the central nervous system, 4th edition. Arch Pathol Lab Med. 2008;132:993.
2. Forastiere A, et al. Head and neck cancer. N Engl J Med. 2001;345:1890.
3. Graham DI, Lantos PL (Eds). Greenfield's neuropathology, 6th edition. London, Arnold, 1997.
4. Kapadia SB. Salivary gland tumours. In: Gupta RK (Ed). Proceedings of III International CME and Update in Surgical Pathology, Lucknow, SGPGI, 1998.
5. Kleihues P, et al. WHO classification of tumours: Pathology and genetics of tumours of the nervous system. Lyon, IARC Press, 2000.
6. Mac Donald DG, Browne RM. Tumours of odontogenic epithelium. In: Anthony PP, et al. (Eds). Recent Advances in Histopathology, number 17. London, Churchill Livingstone. 1997, pp.139.
7. Mastrianni JA, Roos RP. The prion diseases. Semin Neurol. 2000;20:337.
8. Minnerman LE, Sobin LH. WHO-histological typing of tumours of the eye and its adnexa, number 24 Geneva, WHO, 1980.
9. Seifert G. WHO histological typing of salivary gland tumours, 2nd edn. Berlin, Springer-Verlag, 1991.
10. Simpson RHW. Salivary gland tumours. In: Anthony PP, et al. (Eds). Recent Advances in Histopathology, number 17. London, Churchill Livingstone, pp. 167, 1997.
11. Vokes EE, et al. Head and neck cancer. N Engl J Med. 1993;328:184.
12. Yanoff M. Fine BS. Ocular Pathology, 4th edn. London, Mosby-Wolfe, 1996.

SECTION 3

CLINICAL PATHOLOGY

CHAPTER

- Examination of Body Cavity Fluids

CHAPTER 14

Examination of Body Cavity Fluids

Neena Sood, Nancy Kurien, Suresh Sharma

CEREBROSPINAL FLUID ANALYSIS

- Cerebrospinal fluid (CSF) is a clear, colorless fluid formed primarily in the ventricular choroid plexus by a combination of both, active process and ultracentrifugation
- Reabsorption of CSF occurs at the arachnoid villi, which are projected into the venous sinuses in dura mater
- A total volume of CSF is 90–150 mL in adults and 10–60 mL in a neonate
- Normally up to 2 mL of CSF is withdrawn by lumbar puncture under strict aseptic technique
- CSF specimen should be transported to the laboratory immediately and processed in 1 hour, otherwise cellular degradation occurs
- CSF analysis helps to detect infections of the spinal cord and brain, brain tumor, autoimmune diseases like multiple sclerosis, or, any bleeding in the brain or spinal cord.

Gross Examination

Color

Normally CSF is clear colorless like distilled water and does not have clots. The color of CSF is examined by holding the CSF tube beside a distilled water tube against a clean white paper. If a pale yellow or pink color is noted, centrifuge the sample at high speed for 5 minutes and examine the supernatant visually.

Following alternation in CSF color may be observed due to the following reasons:
- **Yellow color (xanthochromia):** Maybe due to:
  - Following subarachnoid bedding.
  - Severely jaundiced
  - High protein level >150 mg/dL.
  - *Examination errors:* Such as delay in examination and sample contamination with detergent.
- **Orange color:** Dietary hypercarotenemia.
- **Brown color:** Meningeal metastatic melanoma.
- **Red to orange:** Patient on rifampicin therapy.
- **Pink to red:** Presence of blood in CSF sample.

pH

The normal pH of the CSF is 7.28–7.32, which may be checked using pH paper.

Appearance

Generally, the appearance of CSF is crystal clear without the presence of any clots.

The following alteration in appearance may be observed:
- **Turbid/cloudiness:** Increased cell and/or bacterial counts in CSF
- **Smoky/opalescence:** Less red blood cell (RBC) and white blood cell (WBC) cells in CSF.

Presence of clot: Due to any disturbance in the blood-brain barrier, fibrinogen appears, this fibrinogen is converted to fibrin, and a clot is seen.

Microbial Examination

- Normally during microscopic examination of CSF; no RBC is seen and only lymphocytes between 0 and 8 cells/μL
- The smear of CSF also may be stained for bacterial and Ziehl-Neelsen stain for acid-fast bacilli examination
- The CSF can also be cultured for bacteria, tuberculosis, and fungus infections
- *Conditions involving neutrophils in CSF:*
  - Bacterial meningitis
  - Brain abscess
  - Brain infarct
  - Repeated lumbar puncture.
- *Conditions causing lymphocyte in CSF:*
  - Viral meningitis
  - Tuberculous meningitis
  - Parasitic meningitis.
- *Conditions causing plasma cell in CSF:*
  - Multiple myeloma
  - Tuberculous meningitis
  - Meningoencephalitis.
- *Conditions causing lymphocyte/monocyte in CSF:*
  - Viral meningitis
  - Tuberculous meningitis
  - Fungal meningitis.
- *Conditions causing malignant cell in CSF:*
  - Leukemia
  - Lymphoma
  - Metastatic tumor.

Biochemical Examination

Routine biochemical examination of CSF consists of the estimation of proteins and glucose.

Estimation of Protein in CSF

- Normal CSF protein level in an adult is **15–45 mg/dL**. An increase in CSF protein is a sensitive but non-specific indicator of CSF disease. CSF proteins may be normal during the early stage of meningitis. Significant elevation (> 150 mg/dL) occur in bacterial meningitis.
- There are various methods for estimation for CSF protein. The turbidimetric method using trichloroacetic acid for precipitation of protein is commonly used. In principle, trichloroacetic acid, when added to CSF, causes precipitation of protein and a turbid solution is obtained in a photoelectric colorimeter.

- The increased CSF proteins may be seen in:
  - **Meningitis:** Due to increased capillary permeability of the blood-brain barrier.
  - **Spinal cord tumors:** Due to mechanical obstruction to the circulation of CSF causing increased fluid reabsorption.
  - **Multiple sclerosis, neurosyphilis, subacute sclerosing panencephalitis:** Due to increased local immunoglobulin production.
  - **Guillain-Barre syndrome:** Due to both capillary permeability and increased local immunoglobulin production.
- Traumatic and subarachnoid hemorrhage.

Estimation of Glucose in CSF

> CSF Glucose is called glycorrhachia. Normal CSF glucose range is 45-80 mg/dL.

- Normal CSF glucose is two-thirds of blood glucose (CSF blood glucose ratio is 0.6)
- A sample for blood glucose should be drawn 1 hour before lumbar puncture (LP) for comparison; CSF sample should be immediately processed for glucose estimation because falsely low results due to glycolysis may occur
- The CSF glucose is measured by glucose oxidation methods
- Normal range is 45–80 mg/dL. CSF glucose less than 40 mg/dL is abnormal.
- CSF glucose is decreased due to the utilization of bacteria (pyogenic or tuberculosis), leukocytes, or cancer cells in CSF.
- Decreased CSF glucose occurs in the following conditions:
  - Acute bacterial meningitis
  - Tuberculous meningitis
  - Fungal meningitis
  - Meningeal involvement by malignant tumor (meningeal carcinomatosis)
  - Hypoglycemia.
- CSF glucose is generally normal in viral meningitis.

EXAMINATION OF SPUTUM

Transfer the specimen in a sterile Petri dish placed against a dark background. Wooden applicator sticks can be used to spread it and can be seen with the naked eye or by using the hand lens.

Macroscopic examination

Volume

A 24-hour volume of sputum is measured in patients with various lung conditions like pneumonia, tuberculosis, bronchiectasis, chronic bronchitis; lung abscesses, or bronchial asthma. An increased amount of sputum production is seen in conditions like bronchiectasis or bronchopleural fistula.

Consistency and Appearance

- A normal sputum is clear and watery and any opalescence is because of cellular material suspended in it.

- Sputum may be described as serous, mucoid, purulent, bloody, or combinations of these, e.g., seropurulent, mucopurulent.
- In pulmonary edema, the sputum is serous, frothy, and blood-tinged. Most opaque particles are masses of pus and epithelium. Other material seen in the sputum can be Curschmann's spirals (seen in sputum of patients with bronchial asthma), Dittrich's plug(seen in sputum of a patient with pulmonary gangrene, fetid bronchitis) caseous material, bronchial casts, or food substances.

Color

- Normal sputum is clear and colorless
- A yellow color indicates pus and epithelial cells as seen in the pneumonic process
- Greenish tint implies Pseudomonas as the etiologic agent
- Rust colored sputum is due to decomposed and seen in pneumococcal pneumonia or pulmonary gangrene, whereas bright red sputum is found in recent hemorrhage which can follow acute cardiac infarction, pulmonary infarction, neoplasm invasion, and rupture of vessels.

Odor

Normal sputum is odorless.

Suppurative pulmonary disorder such as lung abscess, cavitary tuberculosis, or gangrene produces the most putrid odors. A ruptured subphrenic or liver abscess may impart a fecal odor.

Other Findings

Cheesy masses: Fragments of necrotic pulmonary tissue seen in pulmonary gangrene or tuberculosis.

Bronchial casts: These are branching tree-like casts of bronchi and their size depend upon the size of bronchi from which they have been expectorated. These can be seen in untreated lobar pneumonia, fibrinous bronchitis. To recognize these casts they have to be floated on water against a black background.

Broncholiths: These are formed due to the calcification of necrotic/infected tissue within a larger bronchus or cavity. The central core of these may be a foreign body or fungus growth. Though rare, when seen, chronic tuberculosis should be kept in mind.

Dittrich's plug: It is seen in putrid bronchitis and bronchiectasis. When expectorated, are usually solitary of variable size. When crushed they are found to be made of cellular debris, fatty acid crystals, fat globules, and bacteria. These plugs are seen most commonly in chronic bronchitis, bronchiectasis, and bronchial asthma.

Foreign bodies: They are usually objects inhaled by a child. Usually, substances inhaled are peanuts and buttons. Radiologically they are difficult to see.

Parasites: Various parasites that can be seen in sputum are: *Ascaris lumbricoides, Echinococcus granulosus, Toxocara canis,* and *Paragonimus westermani.*

ANALYSIS OF GASTRIC CONSTITUENTS
- Digestive enzymes/factors
- Pepsin and hydrochloric acid (HCL) (for protein digestion)
- Renin for curdling milk and gastric lipase—a weak lipolytic ferment
- Normal gastric constituents in infants and children
- The stomach of neonates secretes a small amount of pepsin, rennin, and free acids
- Almost 4% of otherwise normal children have achlorhydria, this percentage gradually rises with age
- During the first year of life, the volume of residuum is 2–5 mL; both these rise to adult levels at 15–20 years of age.

Abnormal Gastric Constituents
Abnormal gastric constituents may include the following:
- *Blood:* An important abnormal finding
- Food remnants many hours after eating
- A large amount of mucus or bile
- Sarcinae, pyogenic bacteria, lactobacilli, and, yeast cells
- Tissue fragments, a large amount of epithelium
- Parasites and ova
- Organic acids, e.g., lactic acid, seen in absence of hydrochloric acid
- Tubercle bacilli, in pulmonary tuberculosis, by swallowing sputum containing *Mycobacterium tuberculosis.*

Routine Gastric Juice Examination
Gross Examinations
- **Amount:** Normal findings content is 50–100 mL
- **Color:**
  - Blood is red or color of coffee ground if acid hematin is formed
  - Fresh bile is yellow, old bile is green
  - In stasis, food colors may persist.
- **Odor:**
  - Normal is sour or slightly rancid
  - Fecal in intestinal obstruction
  - Ammoniacal in uremia.
- **Character:** Let stand, note the three layers:
  - Top mucus
  - Middle opalescent fluid
  - Bottom, bread-like residue.
- **Reaction:** Acidic normal
- **Rate of secretion:** Mean values for the basal rate of secretion of acid:
  - Age 20–49 years—2.5
  - Age 50–59 years—2.0
  - Age ≥ 60 years—1.5.

- Mean values for 12-hour nocturnal secretions in a normal person:
  - Volume 580 mL.
  - Free acid 29 mEq/L or 16.85 mEq/12 hours.

Chemical Examination

- **Blood:** Maybe due to one of the causes of hematemesis or may be due to trauma of passing a tube; do guaiac or benzidine tests
- **Qualitative test for free HCL (Topfer's test):** To 5 drops of gastric juice in an evaporating dish add 1 or dimethylaminoazobenzene. Cherry-red color with HCL
- Titration of acid.

ANALYSIS OF DUODENAL CONTENTS

Indications for Duodenal Drainage

- For diagnosis of biliary tract and liver disease
- For diagnostic purpose relating to parasites, pancreatic enzymes, etc.
- For therapeutic drainage in cholangitis or biliary obstruction
- Composition of bile.

Gross Chemical Characteristics

- **Volume/24 hours:** 700–1000 mL
- **Specific gravity:** 1.010 (hepatic duct) and 1.026 (gallbladder)
- **Total solid:**

Total solid	Hepatic duct	Gallbladder
Bile salts	1.8 g%	8.7 g%
Fatty acid and lipid	0.24 g%	1.8 g%
Cholesterol	0.16 g%	0.87 g%
pH	7.5	6
Sodium (Na)	134–156 mEq/L	
Potassium (K)	3.9–6.3 mEq/L	
Chlorine (Cl)	38 mEq/L	

- **Composition of pancreatic juice:**
  - *Volume/24 hours:* 500–800 mL
  - *Specific gravity:* 1.007
  - *pH:* 7–8.
- **Digestive enzymes:**
  - *Proteolytic enzymes:* Trypsin, chymotrypsin, elastase, and collagenase
  - *Peptidases:* Carboxypeptidases
  - Aminopeptidase
  - *Nucleus:* Ribonuclease and deoxyribonuclease
  - Amylolytic amylase
  - Lipolytic lipase
  - Phospholipase.

ANALYSIS OF PERITONEAL FLUID

Normally, the peritoneal cavity contains less than 100 mL of clear, straw-colored fluid.

Indications of Abdominal Paracentesis

To be done under ultrasound guidance:
- Ascites of unknown etiology
- Symptomatic ascites, e.g. dyspnea
- Possible ruptured viscus or intra-abdominal hemorrhage due to trauma
- Acute abdominal pain of unknown etiology
- Postoperative hypotension and pain of unknown etiology
- Instillation of cytotoxic drugs in ascites due to malignancy.

The chief complication of abdominal paracentesis is intestinal perforation, perforation of other viscera is rare. If aspiration reveals gross blood or intestinal contents—laparotomy must be done.

Gross Examination of Peritoneal Fluid

Color of Peritoneal Fluid

- **Pale yellow to amber in:**
  - Congestive heart failure
  - Hepatic vein obstruction
  - Cirrhosis
  - Nephrotic syndrome.
- **Similar appearance in:**
  - Ruptured urinary bladder.
- **Turbid fluid suggests peritonitis due to:**
  - Appendicitis
  - Pancreatitis
  - Strangulated/infracted intestine
  - Torn/ruptured bowel due to primary bacterial infection.
- **Blood tinged or grossly bloody fluid may be seen:**
  - Ruptured spleen
  - Ruptured liver
  - Torn mesenteric vessels
  - Aortic aneurysm rupture
  - Splenic artery, leaking aneurysm
  - Hemorrhagic pancreatitis
  - Peritoneal laceration following effort
  - Traumatic tap clears as more fluid aspirated.
- **Greenish in:**
  - Perforated duodenal ulcer
  - Perforated intestine
  - Cholecystitis
  - Perforated gallbladder
  - Acute appendicitis
  - Biliary peritonitis is usually rapidly fatal.

- **Milky fluid is due to chylous ascites, various causes are:**
  - Lymphoma
  - Carcinoma
  - Tuberculosis
  - Parasitic infestations
  - Adhesions
  - Hepatic cirrhosis
  - Nephrotic syndrome.

If surgical treatment is not indicated, elimination of long-chain fatty acids decreases the accumulation of chylous fluid abdomen, pericardium, or pleural cavity.

ANALYSIS OF PERICARDIAL FLUID

The pericardial sac under normal circumstances contains 20–50 mL of clear, straw-colored fluid. A rapid abnormal accumulation of 200 mL may produce cardiac tamponade, while gradual accumulation of 1000 mL or more may be relatively asymptomatic.

Indications for Pericardial Fluid Aspiration

- Acute or chronic cardiac tamponade
- To confirm the diagnosis and establish the cause of pericardial effusion of unknown etiology.

Complications of Pericardial Fluid Aspiration

- Cardiac arrhythmias, especially ventricular fibrillation
- Infection of pleural spaces by purulent pericardial fluid
- Laceration of an-atrium or coronary artery
- Pneumothorax
- Inadvertent injection of air into the cardiac chamber.

Gross Examination of Pericardial Fluid

- Gross appearance of pericardial fluid (PF) may be clear, cloudy, blood-tinged, grossly bloody, milky, or similar to gold paint
- **Increased amounts of normal-appearing pericardial fluid may be found in:**
  - Congestive heart failure
  - Stages of inflammation
  - Some patients with idiopathic pericarditis.
- **Cloudy appearance may be associated with:**
  - Septic/non-septic inflammation
  - Chronic effusions of any etiology
  - Myxedema
  - Idiopathic
  - Post-myocardial infarction syndrome.
- **Blood-tinged pericardial fluid seen in:**
  - Traumatic tap, but it clears on aspirating more fluid.

- **Grossly fluid may be caused by:**
  - Idiopathic hemorrhagic pericarditis
  - Post-myocardial infarction syndrome
  - Tuberculosis
  - Post-pericardiotomy syndrome
  - Systemic lupus erythematosus
  - Metastatic carcinoma
  - Bacterial pericarditis
  - Leaking aortic syndrome.
- **Milky pericardial fluid may be due to:**
  - Pericardium pericarditis from any cause, e.g., bacterial, fungal, tuberculosis, rheumatoid pericarditis, rheumatic, and myxedema.

Microscopic Examination

- Total or differential counts done as for CSF
- Increased leukocytes with a preponderance of neutrophils are characteristic of bacterial pericarditis but may also be seen in viral pericarditis or chronic post-myocardial infarction syndrome
- A high percentage of lymphocytes suggest tuberculous pericarditis
- Microbiological examination
- Cultures for bacteria, fungi, and tuberculosis should be performed in all effusions of unknown etiology.

Chemical Examination

- Pericardial fluids should be classified as transudates or exudates
- **Transudates are typically seen in:**
  - Congestive heart failure
  - Hypoproteinemic states
  - Myxedema
  - Viral pericarditis
  - Early septic/non-septic inflammation.

> For patients undergoing pericardial fluid aspiration, continue to monitor vital signs, observe for any sign of cardiac or respiratory distress.

ANALYSIS OF SEMEN

- Semen examination is an integral part of the investigation for infertility. As a result of its relative simplicity, semen examination is often requested before the more complicated and expensive examination of the female. Repeat examination should be done if once it is found to be normal.
- Semen consists of spermatozoa suspended in seminal plasma. Spermatozoa comprise about 5% of semen volume. Approximately of the semen is derived from the seminal vesicles. The viscid, neutral or slightly alkaline fluid is often yellow or even deeply pigmented using high flavin content.
- Prostate contributes 20% of the volume of semen. This milky fluid is acidic with a pH of about 6.5 largely because of the high content of citric acid. The prostatic secretion is also

rich in proteolytic enzymes and acid phosphates. These proteolytic enzymes are believed to be responsible for the coagulation and liquefaction of semen. Less than 10%–15% of semen volume is contributed by epididymis, vasa defferentia, bulbourethral and urethral gland.

Purposes of Semen Analysis

Semen examination is done for the investigation of:
- **Infertility:** The sperm count test is performed if a man's fertility is in question. It is helpful in determining if there is a problem in sperm production or quality of the sperm as a cause of infertility
- **Success of vasectomy:** The test may also be used after a vasectomy to make sure there are no sperm in the semen
- **Medicolegal cases,** e.g., rape.

Collection of Semen Sample

The sperm collection test for men who can produce semen involves the following steps:
- A man should abstain from ejaculation for several days before the test because each ejaculation can reduce the number of sperm by as much as a third.
- A man collects a sample of his semen in a collection jar during masturbation either at home or at the doctor's office. The proper collection procedure is important since the highest concentration of sperm is contained in the initial portion of the ejaculate. Specially designed condoms may be available that will enable the collection of the sample during sexual intercourse.
- The sample should be kept at body temperature and delivered promptly, because if the sperm are not analyzed within 3 hours or kept reasonably warm, a large proportion may die or lose motility.
- A semen analysis should be repeated at least three times over several months.

Gross Examination

Semen is examined grossly for the following features:
- **Color:** Normally it is whitish, grey-white, or slightly yellowish.
- **Volume**
  - Normally, the volume of semen is between 2.5 and 5 mL
  - The volume is slightly more in patients with infertility
  - The volume does not vary with the period of abstinence
  - *Viscosity:* When ejaculated, semen is fairly viscid and it falls drop by drop
  - *Reaction:* Normally, it is slightly alkaline with a pH between 7 and 8
  - *Liquefication:* It occurs because of the presence of fibrinolysin; normally liquefication occurs within 10–30 minutes.

Microscopic Examination

Semen is examined microscopically for the following:
- **Motility:** Place a drop of liquefied semen on a clean glass slide. Put a coverslip over it and examine it under the microscope, first under low power and then under high power. Normally within 2 hours of ejaculation, more than 60% of spermatozoa are vigorously

motile and in 6–8 hours 25%–40% are still motile. Following are the grades for motility of sperm:
- Motility is graded on 1–4 ranking system
- For fertility motility should be greater than 2
- Grade 1 sperm wriggle sluggishly and make little progress
- Grade 2 sperm move forward, but they are either very slow or do not move in straight line
- Grade 3 sperm move in a straight line at a reasonable speed and can home in on an egg accurately
- Grade 4 sperm are as accurate as grade 3 sperm but move at terrific speed.

- **Sperm count:** A low sperm count should not be viewed as a definitive diagnosis of infertility, but rather as one indicator of a fertility problem. A sperm count below 13.5 million was considered a strong indication of infertility, pregnancy was possible so long as any motile sperm were present. If there are no sperm cells at all in the semen, the doctor checks for obstruction in the tubes or for Sertoli cell-only syndrome in which there are no sperm-producing cells in the testes.
- **Sperm morphology:** Morphology is the shape and structure of the sperm, and of the three main sperm values may be the best predictor of fertility. Older reports indicated that about 60% of the sperm should be normal in size and shape for adequate fertility. Determining the morphology of the sperm is particularly important for the success of fertility treatments in vitro fertilization and intracytoplasmic sperm injection.

Chemical Examination

Chemical analysis of semen consists of the following test:
- **Fructose test:** This test determines androgen deficiency or ejaculatory obstruction to semen. The level of seminal fructose is low in both these conditions. Normal seminal fructose level is 150–600 mg/dL.
- **Acid phosphatase test:** This test is used for seminal stain and on vaginal aspirate in medicolegal cases. Normally semen has 2500 KA units/mL of acid phosphatase.
- Other factors may be measured such as:
  - White blood cell counts are taken to detect infection
  - Low levels of a substance called inhibin B, which appears to be produced only in the testes, may indicate blockage or other defects in the seminiferous tubules
  - Low levels of another compound, alpha-glucosidase may also indicate blockage in the epididymis.

> Azoospermia: In semen, lack of sperm cells.
> Asthenospermia: Reduced sperm motility.
> Oligospermia: Low sperm count.

Specimen Collection

- Before collecting or expectorating sputum, the mouth should be pre-rinsed and this removes contaminants from the oral cavity especially.
- For most examinations, a first-morning specimen is best as it represents the pulmonary secretions accumulated overnight.
- To obtain a good specimen, the patient's cooperation and understanding are essential. Usually, no problem arises with adults.

- Children are problematic sometimes. The undermentioned methods can be used for them:
  - A nasopharyngeal swab may be taken, which is quite representative of the bronchial pathogens
  - A cough plate is held before the child's mouth and the child is urged to cough
  - Cough swab method gives the most representative, non-contaminated sputum sample. The child's mouth is held open by using a tongue depressor. Epiglottis, is visualized and is touched with a swab to induce cough. Material expelled trachea is deposited on the swab, which can then be plated on appropriate culture media.
  - In patients who are uncooperative, cannot produce adequate sputum, induction should be tried.
- Commonly used inductants are:
  - 10% sodium chloride.
  - Acetylcysteine.
  - Sterile or distilled water aerosols.
- In persons with a history of bronchospasmodic disorders, bronchodilators should be given after indunctants are used. Acetylcysteine breaks disulfide bonds, which maintain structure mucus. Acetylcysteine, given in an aerosol form bronchodilator.
- The specimen should be collected in a disposable, impermeable container with crew cap.

URINE EXAMINATION

Urine testing, also known as urinalysis can provide the healthcare professional with valuable data about the patient's health status, including diseases of the upper urinary tract including the kidneys and the ureters, the lower urinary tract includes the bladder, and urethra, and diseases of the liver. The urinalysis can also provide information regarding systemic diseases like diabetes mellitus, metabolic disorders, and general hydration. Urine examination includes analysis of:
- Physical characteristic
- Chemical characteristics
- Microscopic analysis

Sample Collection of Urine

In Children

Collection of a urine sample can be a difficult task in infants and young children. There are four ways of urine collection in children:
- **Bagged sample:** Attach a perineal bag to collect the sample.
- **Clean catch:** By placing the baby on a sterile receptacle.
- **Mid-stream void:** Practically very difficult.
- **Suprapubic aspiration:** Invasive procedure, gives the best quality sterile sample.

In Adults

- **Midstream void:** Initial part of urine is not collected. Most useful, but the procedure must be explained in detail to the patient to avoid contamination.
- **Catheter sample:** In critically ill, non-ambulatory patients this technique is used. Sample should never be taken from a urine drainage bag, instead, it should be withdrawn from the sample collection port using an aseptic technique.

- **Supra-pubic aspiration:** Invasive procedure, that gives the best quality sterile sample in critically ill patients who cannot be catheterized.

Once the urine is collected it should be immediately transported to the laboratory, after proper labeling, with a maximum delay of 2 hours beyond which it should either be refrigerated or discarded.

A battery of tests can be done on the bedside by either using Uri sticks (commercially available) or in the laboratory by routine testing.

Physical Characteristics

Color

The color of urine is affected by many conditions including fluid balance, diet, medicines, and diseases. Dark urine is usually seen in conditions of excessive sweating, dehydration, and decreased fluid intake. Urine becomes light-colored in cases of excessive fluid intake and certain renal conditions. The dark brown color of urine may indicate the presence of bilirubin in urine. Vitamin B supplements can turn urine bright yellow. Some medicines, blackberries, beets, rhubarb, or blood in the urine can turn urine red-brown color. **Table 14.1** mentions the normal color and other characteristics of urine.

Clarity

Urine is normally clear. Bacteria, casts, mucus, blood, sperms, etc. can make urine look cloudy or turbid.

Table 14.1: Normal characteristics of urine.

S. No.	Parameter	Normal values
1.	Color	Pale yellow
2.	Odor	Slightly 'nutty'
3.	Specific gravity	1.003–1.030
4.	pH	5–7.2
5.	Proteins	Nil to traces
6.	Sugar	Nil to traces
7.	Ketone bodies	Nil to traces
8.	Bilirubin	Nil to traces
9.	White blood cells (WBCs)	0–2/High power field
10.	Red blood cells (RBCs)	0–3/High power field
11.	Nitrites	Nil to traces
12.	Sodium	150–300 mmol/24 h
13.	Potassium	50–90 mmol/24 h
14.	Calcium	15–20 mmol/24 h
15.	Phosphate	0–38 mmol/24 h

Odor

Infection with *Escherichia coli (E. coli)* bacteria can cause a bad odor, while diabetes or starvation can cause a sweet, fruity odor. Urine that smells-like maple syrup can mean maple syrup urine disease when the body cannot break down certain amino acids.

Specific Gravity

Specific gravity indicates the concentration ability of kidneys. A very high specific gravity means very concentrated urine, which may be caused by not drinking enough fluid, loss of too much fluid (excessive vomiting, sweating, or diarrhea), or substances (such as sugar or protein) in the urine. Very low specific gravity means dilute urine, which may be caused by drinking too much fluid, severe kidney disease, or the use of diuretics.

> Isosthenuria: The specific gravity of urine is the same as that of protein-free plasma. Seen in chronic renal disease.

pH

Some foods (such as citrus fruit and dairy products) and medicines (such as antacids) can affect urine pH. A high (alkaline) pH can be caused by severe vomiting, kidney disease, and a few cases of urinary tract infections. Low (acidic) pH may be due to diabetes, aspirin overdose, severe diarrhea, drinking too much alcohol, etc.

Chemical Characteristics (Table 14.2)

Protein

Protein is normally not found in the urine. Fever, hard exercise, pregnancy, and some diseases, especially kidney disease, may cause the protein to be in the urine.

Glucose

High glucose levels are observed in urine in cases of uncontrolled diabetes. Glucose can also be found in urine when the kidneys are damaged or diseased. Intravenous (IV) fluids can cause glucose to be in the urine. Too much glucose in the urine may also indicate an adrenal gland problem, liver damage, brain injury, and certain types of poisoning. Healthy pregnant women can have glucose in their urine, which is normal during pregnancy.

Table 14.2: Common tests for detecting chemical components in urine.

Components	Tests
Protein	Urine electrophoresis (detect monoclonal antibodies) Test using sulfosalicylic acid
Glucose	Benedict's test (semiquantitative) Fehling's test
Ketone bodies	Rothera's test Lestradet's test
Bilirubin	Fouchet's test Rosin's test
Urobilinogen	Ehrlich's test

Nitrites

Bacteria that cause a urinary tract infection (UTI) make an enzyme that changes urinary nitrates to nitrites. Nitrites in urine show UTI is present.

Leukocyte Esterase (WBC Esterase)

Leukocyte esterase shows leukocytes [white blood cells (WBCs)] in the urine. WBCs in the urine may indicate UTI.

Ketones

Ketones in the urine can mean an alteration in metabolic function. The presence of ketone bodies in urine is called ketonuria.

Causes of ketonuria are uncontrolled diabetes, a very low carbohydrate diet, starvation, or alcoholism. Ketones are often found in the urine when a person does not eat (fasts) for 18 hours or longer. This may occur when a person is sick and cannot eat or vomits for several days. Low levels of ketones are sometimes found in the urine of healthy pregnant women.

Microscopic Analysis

Red or White Blood Cells

Blood cells are not normally found in urine. Inflammation, disease, or injury to the kidneys, ureters, bladder, or urethra can cause blood in the urine. Strenuous exercise can also cause blood in the urine. White blood cells may be a sign of infection or kidney disease. The presence of WBC in urine is termed pyuria.

Casts

Some types of kidney disease can cause plugs of material (called casts) to form in tiny tubes in the kidneys. The casts then get flushed out in the urine. Casts can be made of RBCs (RBC casts) or waxy (waxy casts) or fatty substances (Fatty casts) or protein (hyaline casts) or trapped granular debris (granular casts), epithelial casts, or leucocyte casts. The type of cast in the urine can help show what type of kidney disease may be present.

Crystals

Healthy people often have only a few crystals in their urine. A large number of crystals or certain types of crystals may mean kidney stones are present or there is a problem with how the body is using food (metabolism).

Bacteria, Yeast Cells or Parasites

There are no bacteria, yeast cells, or parasites in urine normally. If these are present, it can mean presence of an infection.

Squamous Cells

The presence of squamous cells may mean that the sample is not of good quality. These cells indicate that during sample collection the urine stream touched the skin surface of the perineum.

Urine Dipstick Test

This is a rapid method to detect various chemical alterations in urine. In this, a dipstick with various squared columns is immersed in urine. The grades of color changes are measured against the color codes given in the packaging. The numerous chemical changes which can be detected include protein, glucose, ketone, bilirubin, nitrites, etc. The color-coded area of strip, with the indication agent should not be touched with a wet or bare hand. Once dipped in urine, it should be kept horizontally to avoid mixing up of any reagent present in colorcoded reagent zones **(Fig. 14.1)**.

Urine Culture

Normal urine is sterile, however, in cases of UTI, there may be the presence of organisms in culture. This is usually accompanied by the presence of WBCs. A patient with UTI presents with urgency, increased frequency of micturition (urination), burning sensation, while passing urine, pain during passing urine (dysuria), foul-smelling urine. The patient might complain of passing cloudy urine.

As the lower end of the urinary tract can have commensal organisms, the patient is said to have infection only when the number of bacteria per milliliter of urine is more than 1,00,000 on culture. This is known as 'significant bacteriuria'. Urine is cultured on media such as CLED (Cysteine, Lactose, Electrolyte Deficient) or a combination of blood agar and MacConkey agar.

Common Organisms

The most common organisms causing UTIs are:
- *Escherichia coli*
- *Staphylococcus saprophyticus* (sexually active females)
- *Pseudomonas aeruginosa*
- *Proteus vulgaris.*

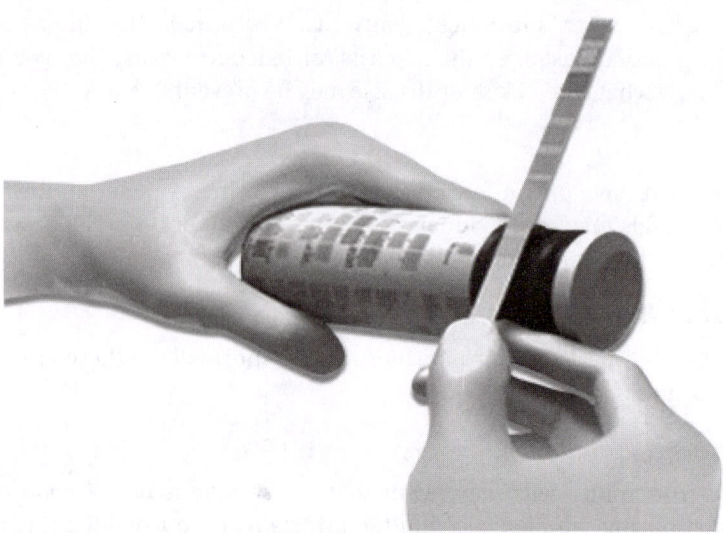

Fig. 14.1: Urine dipstick.

Culture Media

Commonly used media for urine culture are
- MacConkey agar
- MacConkey topped with glucose agar
- Blood agar

FECAL EXAMINATION

Average healthy adults defecate from three times a day to three times a week. The common pattern is once a day. The stool tends to be soft and bulky on a diet high in vegetables and small and dry on a diet high in meat.

The aim of stool analysis is to determine the presence of blood, ova and parasites, bile, fat, pathogens, or substances such as ingested drugs. Additional studies include fecal urobilinogen, nitrogen, *Clostridium difficile,* fecal leukocytes, calculation of stool osmolar gap, food residues, and other substances requiring laboratory evaluation.

Collection of Stool Specimen

Adults

One way is to catch the stool on plastic wrap that is loosely placed over the toilet bowl and held in place by the toilet seat or bedpan. Then, put the sample in a clean container with the help of a wooden spatula or spoon. Samples can also be collected by using toilet paper.

Infants and Young Children

We can line the diaper with plastic wrap. Try to place the plastic wrap in a way that separates the stool from urine, so you can get a better sample.

Swabs can also be used to collect stool specimens both in adults and children. One must be extra cautious not to mix fecal specimens with urine as there are inhibitory substances present in urine, which might alter the results.

Routine Examination

Gross examination of stool characteristics such as color, consistency, odor, helminths or parts of worms can reveal pathologies/infections affecting the gastrointestinal tract.

Normal characteristics of the stool are:
- **Color:** Brown
- **Consistency:** Well-formed and soft.

Various chemical parameters can also be checked such as fats, occult blood, etc. A few important tests have been described below.

Fecal Occult Blood

Fecal occult blood is also known as stool guaiac, the hemoccult test is a qualitative method for detection of blood in the stool. It is intended as a diagnostic aid during routine physical examination, a monitor for bleeding patients with iron deficiency anemia or recuperating from surgery, peptic ulcer, ulcerative colitis, and as a screen for colorectal cancer.

Clostridium difficile Toxin Screen

Inhibition of normal intestinal flora due to antibiotic treatment can lead to overgrowth of the bacteria, *Clostridium difficile*. The organism produces toxins that can cause tissue damage and the result is antibiotic-associated pseudomembranous colitis.

Microscopic Examination

Microscopic examination is performed to observe any presence of RBCs, WBCs, ova, cyst, larvae, etc.

Red Blood Cells

The presence of RBC indicates bleeding within the gastrointestinal (GI) tract. There are various reasons for bleeding, e.g., invasive infections, carcinoma, and inflammatory bowel diseases such as ulcerative colitis.

White Blood Cells

The presence of WBCs in stool specimens indicates some inflammatory condition affecting the GI tract, which can be due to infections, etc.

Ova and Cyst

Ova and cyst in the stool indicate intestinal parasitic infection. A simple saline mount can help to identify the causative parasite and also to start appropriate treatment. To increase the sensitivity of the test, single specimens for 3 consecutive days are recommended.

Stool Culture

Enteric bacterial infections, causing diarrhea and dysentery are important health problems throughout the world. Stool cultures are performed to detect enteric pathogens or potential pathogens. The stool has a large number of normal flora, which makes detection of pathogenic organisms difficult. Therefore, to prevent the commensal flora from growing the stool is first passed in enrichment media, which suppresses the growth of unwanted bacteria and only allows pathogenic ones to grow. The most suitable media for the recovery of pathogenic organisms from the stool specimen are MacConkey media, DCA (deoxycholate citrate agar) media, XLD (xylose lysine deoxycholate) media, etc.

Important bacteria causing gastrointestinal infections are:
- *E. coli*
- *Salmonella* species
- *Shigella* species
- *Yersinia enterocolitica*
- *Campylobacter* species.

MULTIPLE CHOICE QUESTIONS

1. In sputum analysis, the presence of Dittrich's plug indicates _____.
   a. Normal sputum
   b. Bronchiectasis
   c. Tonsillar crypts
   d. Allergic rhinitis

2. Lack of sperm cells in semen is called _____.
    a. Polyspermia
    b. Azoospermia
    c. Oligospermia
    d. Asthenospermia
3. Normal glucose range in CSF of adult is _____.
    a. 20-30 mg/dL
    b. 30-40 mg/dl
    c. 90-100mg/dL
    d. 45–80 mg/dL
4. The presence of neutrophils in CSF indicates _____.
    a. Bacterial meningitis
    b. Tuberculosis meningitis
    c. Fungal meningitis
    d. Viral meningitis
5. Blood-tinged peritoneal fluid is suggestive of _____.
    a. Ruptured spleen
    b. Pancreatitis
    c. Congestive heart failure
    d. Infracted intestine
6. Commonly used media for urine culture is _____.
    a. Chocolate agar
    b. EMB agar
    c. MacConkey agar
    d. Broth media
7. Most common causative organism of UTI is _____.
    a. *Serratia*
    b. *Pseudomonas*
    c. *Proteus mirabilis*
    d. *Escherichia coli*
8. Test to detect ketone bodies in urine is _____.
    a. Rothera's test
    b. Benedict's test
    c. Fehling's test
    d. Rosin test
9. Presence of ova and cyst on microscopic examination of stool indicates _____.
    a. Inflammation
    b. Parasitic infection
    c. Carcinoma
    d. Crohn's disease
10. The presence of WBC in urine is called _____.
    a. Pyuria
    b. Dysuria
    c. Azotemia
    d. Uremia

Answer key

1. b   2. b   3. d   4. a   5. a
6. b   7. b   8. d   9. a   10. a

FURTHER READING

1. American Thoracic Society. Diagnostic standards and classification of tuberculosis in adults and children. Am J Respir Crit Care Med. 2000;161:1376-95.
2. Burtis CA, Ashwood ER (Eds). Tietz Fundamentals of Clinical Chemistry, 4th edn. Philadelphia: WB Saunders Co. 1996.
3. Drossman DA, Shaheen NJ, Grimm IS (Eds). Handbook of Gastroenterologic Procedures 4th edn. Philadephia: Lippincott Williams and Wilkins, 2005.
4. Ellenby MS. et al. Lumbar puncture. N Engl J Med. 2006;355:e12. Downloaded from www.nejm.org on January. 14,2007.
5. Hirsh A. Male subfertility. BMJ. 2003;327:669-72.
6. Indian Council of Medical Research. What is new in the diagnosis of tuberculosis? Part I: Techniques for diagnosis of tuberculosis. ICMR Bulletin. 2002;32;No 8.
7. Laszlo A. Tuberculosis: Laboratory aspects of diagnosis. CMAJ. 1999;160:1275-9.
8. Light RW. Pleural effusion. N Engl J Med. 2002;346:1971-77.
9. Phadke AM. Clinical Atlas of Sperm Morphology. New Delhi: Jaypee Brothers Medical Publishers (P) Ltd. 2007.
10. Riordan FAI, Cant AJ. When to do a lumbar puncture. Arch Dis Child. 2003;87:235-7.
11. Rosenfeld L. Gastric tubes, meals, acid and analysis-rise and decline. Clin Chem. 1997;43:837-42.

12. Runyon BA. Care of patients with ascites. N Engl J Med. 1994;330:337-42.
13. Seehusen DA, Reeves MM, Fomin DA. Cerebrospinal fluid analysis. Am Fam Physician 2003;68:1103-8.
14. Soini H, Musser JM. Molecular diagnosis of mycobacteria. Clin Chem. 2001;47:809-14.
15. Tarn AV. Lapworth R. Biochemical analysis of pleural fluid; What should we measure? Ann Clin Biochem. 2001;38:311-22.
16. Thomsen TW, DeLaPena J, Setnik GS. Thoracentesis. N Engl J Med. 2006;355:e16. Downloaded from www.nejm.org on January 14, 2007.
17. Thomsen TW, Shaffer RW, White B, Setnik GS. Paracentesis. N Engl J Med. 2006;355:e21. Downloaded from www.nejm.org on January. 14, 2007.
18. Thunissen FBJM. Sputum examination for early detection of lung cancer. J Clin Path 2003:56:805-10.
19. Wallach J. Interpretation of Diagnostic Tests 7th edn. Philadelphia. Lippincott: Williams and Wilkins, 2000.
20. Watterson SA, Drobniewski FA. Modern laboratory diagnosis of mycobacterial infections. J Clin Path. 2000;53:727-32.
21. Wolfe MM, Soll AH. The physiology of gastric acid secretion. N Engl J Med. 1988;319:1707-14.
22. World Health Organization. (2010). WHO Laboratory Manual for the Examination and Processing of Human Semen, 5th ed. World Health Organization. https://apps.who.int/iris/handle/10665/44261.

SECTION 4

GENETICS

CHAPTERS

- Introduction to Genetics
- Emerging Paradigm of Genetics in Nursing
- Maternal and Prenatal Genetics
- Neonatal and Children Testing or Screening
- Genetic Conditions of Adolescents and Adults
- Services Related to Genetics

CHAPTER 15

Introduction to Genetics

Suresh Sharma, Sohinder Kaur

INTRODUCTION

In 1865, Gregor Mendel was the first to describe the elements of hereditary genes. His observation and analysis of the observable features of pea led him to conclude that specific traits particulate factors were passed on unchanged from a parent plant to the next generation. Scientific discoveries during the last several decades have provided more information about how genes function and how they contribute to human health and disease. Currently more than 10,371 identified genetic disorders are known to be inherited in a predictable pattern in families. Nurses are at present in all health care setting and care for individuals who may have genetic conditions or predisposition. They also ensure that these individuals have access to the most current genetic information, genetic diagnosis, treatment and management therapeutics. With this knowledge, nurses can collect appropriate family information; provide current and appropriate information and support patients, families and communities as they integrate this new information and technology into their daily lives.

CONCEPT OF GENETICS

- The term 'genetics' was introduced by Bateson in 1906. It has been derived from the Greek word 'gene', which means 'to become' or 'to grow into'. Therefore, genetics is the science of coming into being.
- "Genetics is that branch of biological sciences, which deals with the transmission of characteristics from parents to offspring".
- In other words "genetics is the study of inheritance of disease in families, mapping of disease genes to specific location on chromosomes, analysis of molecular mechanism through which genes cause disease and the diagnosis and treatment of genetic diseases".
- Traditionally genetics has been associated with childbearing decision-making and caring for children with genetic disorders. Medical genetics has focused on the inheritance of hereditary disorders affecting only a small portion of the population. Genetic services have been primarily associated with prenatal genetic counseling, identification of pediatric disorders associated with birth defects and dysmorphology and in some cases rare adult onset single gene disorders. Recent genetic and technological advances are helping us to better understand how genetic changes impact human variation as well as the development of cancer, Alzheimer's, diabetes and other multifactorial diseases that are prevalent in adults.
- The Human Genome Project, one of the most significant research endeavors of the 20th century, deserves much of the credit for the discovery of these new applications of genetic information. Specifically, research from the Human Genome Project is providing a new and better understanding of the genetic contribution to disease, the development of targeted

drug therapy (pharmacogenetics) and the development of genetic tests that identify those who may have or are at risk for genetic diseases. The results of this explosion of knowledge are the rapid paradigm shift from the 'old genetics' to the 'new genetics'. Under the 'new genetics' paradigm nearly all diseases have a genetic component (see chapter 19).
- The influence of recent genetic advances on nursing practice is especially evident in oncology. Oncology nurses practicing in cancer prevention and control apply genetic principles to their daily clinical practice. For example, they assess hereditary and non-hereditary cancer risk factors, take detailed family histories and construct pedigrees, identify individuals and families at risk for hereditary cancer syndromes, make recommendations for cancer risk reduction, surveillance and management and when appropriate, counsel and educate about the risks and benefits of genetic testing.
- This genetic revolution and shift to the 'new genetics' has created a demand for health professionals in a number of clinical specialties who understand the genetic contribution to disease risk, the impact on disease management and the genetic educational needs of patients and families. Nurses have risen to the challenge capitulating genetic nursing practice into a new era.

BASIC GENETIC TERMS

- **Genes:** Genes are genetic material on a chromosome that code for a trait. For example, one person has a gene for eye color.
- **Alleles:** They are variations of genes. Means the two genes, which occur on the same locus in the two homologous chromosomes of an individual and control the expression of a character, are called 'alleles'. For example, one person has the allele for brown eye color. Note that some alleles are dominant over others, i.e., if a person inherits both the dominant and the recessive alleles, the dominant allele will be the one expressed.
- **Gene locus:** A particular portion or region of the chromosome representing a single gene is called as locus. The alleles of gene occupy the same gene locus on the two homologous chromosomes.
- **Homologous chromosomes:** Members of the chromosome pairs with same gene number and arrangement.
- **Dominant allele:** It is one of a pair of alleles, which can express itself whether present in homozygous or heterozygous state, e.g., the gene for tallness Tt and TT, where T is dominant alleles and person will be tall in both conditions.
- **Recessive allele:** The allele of an allelic or allelomophic pair, which is unable to express its effect in the presence of its contrasting alleles in a heterozygote is called recessive alleles. For example, one has alleles of eye 'Bb' (B for brown, b for blue) here b is recessive allele therefore person will have brown eye not blue. The effect of recessive allele become known only when it is present in the homozygous state (bb), in this state person will have blue eye.
- **Codominant alleles:** The alleles, which do not show dominance-recessive relationship and are able to express themselves independently when present together are called codominant alleles. Here, in heterozygous state both alleles express themselves. As a result, the heterozygous condition has a phenotype different from either homozygous genotypes. The joint character may appear to be intermediate between the ones produced by the two homozygous genotypes.
- **Heterozygous alleles:** One alleles of the same gene pair differs from the other. For example, for eye color Bb.

- **Homozygous alleles:** Alleles that are identical or same in gene pair. For example, for eye color BB.
- **Hemizygous:** Having one copy of a particular gene. For example, for eye color only B is present.
- **Genotype:** It is the gene complement or genetic constitution of an individual with regard to one character irrespective of whether the genes are expressed or not. For example, one has the genotype Bb, since one have the allele for brown eye color (B) and the allele for blue eye color (b). An organism is said to be homozygous for a certain trait if both it carries two of the same alleles. It is homozygous dominant if it carries two dominant alleles and homozygous recessive if it carries two recessive alleles. The organism in above said example is heterozygous—it carries two different alleles.
- **Phenotype:** It is observable or measurable distinctive structure or functional characteristics of an individual with regard to one or more characters, which is a result of gene products brought to expression in a given environment. The characteristics are visible to a person (e.g. height, color of eyes, etc.), or require special test for its identification (e.g., serological test for blood group). In other words it is the expression of a gene. For example, since one has the genotype Bb with one dominant and one recessive allele, the dominant allele (B) will mask the recessive allele (b) and one will have the phenotype for brown eyes. Phenotype can be modified by environment through genotype establishes the boundaries within which the environment can modify the phenotype. For example, a fair colored person can have tanned colored skin due to excessive exposure to skin.
- **A karyotype** is a picture showing the arrangement of a full set of human chromosomes. For example, the most common karyotype for females is to have two X chromosomes and is represented as 46, XX, while males have both X and Y chromosomes represented as 46,XY.
- **Trait:** A characteristic that can be genetically determined and represents a specific characteristic of an individual. For example, hair color or blood type.
- **Recessive traits:** A trait that is masked to express as characteristic. For example, having a straight hair line, freckles on face, narrow eyes, colored eye, etc.
- **Dominant traits:** A trait that can be expressed more strongly than any other version of characteristic. For example, curly hair, wide eyes, dimples on face, black eye, etc.
- **Genome:** A complete set of person's genes or complete list of nucleotides (A,C,G and T for DNA genomes).
- **Genomics:** The study of whole genomes and the scientific study of complex diseases that are caused more by genetic and environmental factors than by individual genes, such as heart disease, asthma, diabetes and cancer.

PRACTICAL APPLICATIONS OF GENETICS IN NURSING

Nurses have a major role in the delivery of genetic services and management of genetic information and they offer care that protects patients and families from the risk associated with genetic information, including addressing family issues. Genetics nursing is practiced in different environment such as maternity, pediatrics, medical-surgical, psychiatric and community health nursing as well. It is a holistic practice that includes assessing, planning, implementing and evaluating the physical, spiritual, ethical and psychosocial aspects of patients and families who have genetic concerns. Client and family assessment helps nurses to identify genetic risk factors, detailed family history helps them to construct a pedigree, analyze the data and interpret the information correctly. Planning and implementation of care during diagnosis and management of genetic disorders. In care, provide genetic education and develop and carry out a plan of care to address genetic concerns. Nurses provide information, counseling and support services to person affected by or at risk for genetic conditions.

Advanced practice nurses may play direct roles in genetic counseling and in advanced assessment. They also may work within a particular specialty in which genetics plays a role, such as an oncology or cardiology clinic, as well as in long-term management of specific genetic disorders depending on the specialty area in which they are trained.

The past several years have transformed genetic nursing practice from a hidden practice to a recognized nursing specialty with a visible contribution to the genetic and overall health of individuals and families. Nurses have been involved in managing genetic information since the 1960's, when nurses provided services to children with genetic disorders and their families. Although in some respects, the nurse's role today in managing genetic information and caring for individuals and families at risk for or diagnosed with genetic diseases, or conditions is similar to this traditional role, the scope of practice is much broader and more encompassing. What has also changed, according to Forsman, is the amount of genetic information available and the population to which this information may be applied. We now know that genetic changes contribute to most, if not all diseases. Consequently, the scope of genetic knowledge application in nursing is limitless. "Nursing can ignore genetics no longer. The time for meaningful action is now". Major practical applications of genetics in nursing are as follows:

- **Understands genetic basis of disease:** With knowledge of genetics, nurses well understand that large proportion of total disease has genetic basis. In addition will learn about:
  - Role of different genes in causation of genetic disorders and defects.
  - Good or bad genes for health-illness continuum.
  - Role of gene and chromosomal mutation in health and illness.
  - Normal and abnormal cell division and its genetic regulation.
  - Mechanism of disease inheritance from one generation to next generation.
  - Basic mechanisms of inheritance and transmission of chromosomes and genes, including the concepts of variation and mutation.
  - Genetic factors are playing role in an individual's health.
  - Genetic contribution toward different diseases, disorders and defects.
  - Genetic contributions to common and complex conditions such as breast cancer, colorectal cancer, heart disease and hypercholesterolemia, mental illness, certain behavioral traits and Alzheimer disease.
- **Early and effective diagnosis of genetic disorders:** Genetic knowledge of nurses will equip them with:
  - Information about genetic risk, genetic testing and screening and the implications both positive and negative results.
  - Interpretations of the results of genetic tests.
  - Interpretation of genetic risks (i.e., how to explain the meaning of a one in four risk for having another child with Tay-Sachs disease).
  - Awareness of the possibility of an inherited or genetic component for a client's condition and knowledge of cardinal features of familial predisposition such as early age of disease onset, multiple family members with the same diagnosis, predisposing risk factors.

- What constitutes a proper family history specifically? What key information should be obtained and how to construct and read pedigrees.
- **Contributes toward health promotion with genetic aspect:** By learning about genetics, nurses will enhance their understands about:
  - Relationship of health and disease in respect to genetics, including how genetics and the environment interact and how genes interact with genes; this should lead to new ways of thinking about health promotion and disease prevention.
  - Healthy prenatal environment will ensure minimal risk of genetic defects among newborns.
  - Environmental interaction of an individual is an important factor in reference to gene or chromosomal mutation, which may have positive or negative impact on health of an individual.
  - Learn about pharmacogenomics that every individual have unique genetic makeup therefore responds differently with same drug; for example, a drug 'A' may be very effective to cure an illness in an individual, but same drug may bring severe hypersensitive reaction for another person.
  - An understanding of genetic contributions to human diversity including concepts such as discrimination and eugenics.
- **Prevention of genetic conditions:** Prevention is major principle of any medical discipline, similarly knowledge of genetics well enhance nurse's understanding that:
  - Several genetic disorders can be prevented with prompt and early diagnosis and treatment; for example, phenylketonuria (PKU) related mental retardation could be prevented with early newborn screening and diagnosis and diet management.
  - The genetic disorders can be prevented by selected intervention. For example, risk of neural tube defect can be minimized with administration of folic acid in first trimester of pregnancy.
- **Management and care in genetic disorders:** Knowledge of genetics will empower the nurses to manage and care patients with genetic disorders in their routine healthcare practice by building up their understanding about:
  - Genetic approaches to the therapy of genetic and complex diseases.
  - Care management of adults with childhood genetic disorders.
  - Care management of persons with adult genetic disorders such as Huntington disease.
  - Ways in which genetic knowledge is used in diagnosis and treatment applications.
- **Genetic information and counseling:** Nurses are largely involved in providing genetic information and counseling to patients and families, who are at risk or experiencing genetic disorders. Therefore, knowledge of genetics well helps them to:
  - Development of non-judgmental attitudes about genetics and related disorders.
  - What information needs to be collected before providing genetic counseling.
  - What information needs to be provided to patient and family before offering genetic counseling.
  - Role of nurses in delivering genetic information and counseling.
  - Application of traditional nursing skills such as patient education, confidentiality and counseling about genetic information. The concept of non-directive counseling can be included.

- A study says that there is huge contribution from nurse navigators trained further as Genetic Counseling Extenders (GCEs) in screening, counseling and follow up and care of the patients of various genetic disorders.
- **Referral services:** In developing countries, there is less awareness about genetic disorders and healthcare facilities offering services for testing and management of genetic disorders. Nurses are the primary healthcare providers, who can direct them to right place for their diagnosis and management. So that, genetic information will equip nurses to provide effective referral services to their genetic clients:
  - Services available to manage the genetic disorders in local or national level.
  - Knowledge about referral possibilities knowing not only who should be referred but also, how and to whom it should be done.
  - Ways to access resources relating to genetics for patient and self-education and the need to keep current.
- **Social and ethical issues in genetics:** There are several social and ethical issues, which play important role in care of patients with genetic disorders. Therefore, study of genetic will make nurses to build:
  - An awareness of social, legal and ethical issues related to genetics including effects on individuals, groups and societies, some of which are unique to genetic conditions
  - An understanding of the social and ethical ramifications of possessing a particular genotype or genetic disorder in terms of societal issues, confidentiality, freedom of choice and risks in terms of insurance and disclosure.

Impact of Genetic Conditions on Families

Genetic disorders or defects are chronic and long lasting, permanent, even after repair. A person in family with genetic problem can be a terribly very sad experience for every family member. When cause of problem in hereditary, the news can be seriously difficult to accept for parents. In many families, when they learn that family member is suffering with a genetic problem, it may cause a grief reaction, A mourning for the loss of hope and expectations, which are part of every family. The grieving, with all its feeling of anger, depression and intense sadness is not an uncommon phenomenon.

It is normal and natural reaction whenever a person experiences a loss, whether it is the any morbidity or mortality of a person in a family. Grieving and emotional impact is one dimension of the impact of genetic conditions on family; there are several other aspects of impact on family, such as cognitive, social, cultural and economic impact of genetic conditions on families **(Fig. 15.1)**.

Social Impact

Genetic conditions in a family may lead mild to serious level of social impact on the family. Some of them are:
- Social stigma
- Social discrimination
- Decreased planned family size
- Loss of geographical mobility
- Decreased opportunities for siblings
- Loss of family integrity
- Social isolation

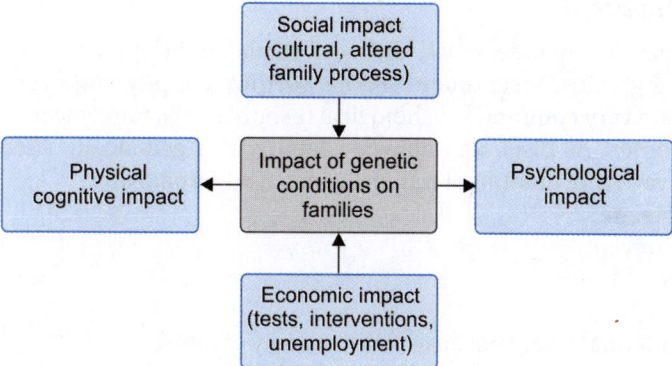

Fig. 15.1: Dimensions of impact of genetic conditions on families.

- Lifestyle alterations
- Reduction in contribution to their community by families
- Disruption of husband-wife or partner relationship
- Threatened family selfconcept
- Genetically affected persons are considered less than human being in society
- Altered family process
- Altered marriage and reproductive implications (infertility, abortions, defective child birth)
- Prenatal conflicts (whether to get pregnant or not, whether to continue pregnancy or not)
- Disruption in parent-child relationship
- Marriage partner selection problems
- Guilt regarding putting child in long term-care facilities
- Difficult child rearing
- Housing and living arrangement changes
- Cultural impact includes that genetic screening are not allowed in certain cultures, people perceive genetic conditions are the punishment of God for bad deeds

Economic Impact

The impact of burden of genetic conditions is more than just financial costs. Financial costs to the family may occur in subtle ways. These include costs of special diet, day care, household help and housing adaptations, buying special equipments and clothing and travel. If the family is not in large city, travel to major medical facilities means more than just expenses of transportation. Major economic impacts are:
- Cost of consultation charges
- Cost of genetic testing and screening
- Cost of long-term genetic therapies and repeated surgeries and transfusions
- Cost of institutionalization or long-term home of community care
- Cost of bearing additional burden and needs of other family members
- Other additional costs of care including travel and stay in city of healthcare facility; Moreover, job leave of family member accompanying for diagnosis and treatment.
- Loss of carrier opportunities and job flexibility
- In addition non-productive life, job discrimination, insurance discrimination and financial dependence on family.

Psychological Impact

Psychological reactions include shock, disbelief, denial, guilt, grieving, mourning, hostility, anger, anxiety, bargaining, resentment, shame, sorrow, self-pity and eventually adaptation and adjustment are very common psychological responses of a family who is having a person with genetic disorder. As discussed above, a family with genetically affected person may experience wide variety of emotional trauma, some of additional are:
- Loss of self-esteem
- Altered self- concept
- Hopelessness
- Helplessness
- Stress and emotional threat because of uncertainty of future
- Loss of dream and aspirations
- Coping with intolerant public attitudes

Physical and Cognitive Impact

Genetic disorders are responsible to cause variety of physical and cognitive manifestations; some of important are:
- Physical health problems
- Individual's inability to get equal opportunity to learn
- Mental retardation
- Misunderstanding regarding implications of carrier state

Factors Influence the Impact of Genetic Conditions on Families

There are various factors, which influence the impact of genetic conditions on the family and the way in which they cope. There are factors for individual families. Some of them are as follows:
- **The size, structure and stage of the development cycle of the family:** Families in which there is only one child born with congenital defects after six or seven normal ones, may be less disrupted because there are more hands to help with all that needs to be done. In general, the most successful in coping are homes in which two parents are present and they have matured in their marriage or relationship. Parents who have an affected first child early in their marriage have not yet developed their own interrelationships before having to cope with additional burden. The age of other children also determines family function. The sex of the affected children is also relevant. There is some evidence to show that father may have more difficulty in coping with severely affected sons.
- **Religious, ethnic and cultural beliefs and practices:** Some couples believe that a child who is mentally retarded or physically affected has been sent to them a special gift from God. Others, on such a discovery curse God and lose faith. If strong faith is present that comfort to family. It is also useful to know the cultural aspect of disease, disability, healing the body and death and how the individual is believed to influence or be influenced by life event.
- **Availability of and relationship with extended family members or close friends:** Having many relatives available may mean more helping hands and loving support, if the relationships are positive ones. Sometimes friends may fill the gap of relatives.

- **The prior status of the relationship between parents:** It appears that those who had a satisfactory relationship prior to the genetic problem have the best chance of remaining intact.
- **Coping resources both tangible and intangibles:** Some communities are able to form a network that provides loving support for families. Some individuals learn to draw on deep resources that they did not realize they possessed. The nurse should make every effort to identify and mobilize support from parent's group, private, public, government agencies and foundations.
- **The visibility and severity of the disorder and its meaning to the family:** In certain groups, superstitions associated with particular defect may cause the avoidance and rejection of the individual and family. Certain disorders have become more accepted than others, through the media and through the appearance of the affected person. Family may have more tolerance for a cute little girl with braces on her legs than for an 18 years adolescent who is mentally retarded and cannot control motion or drooling. Hidden disorders, such as congenital heart defects may cause burdens in the way of finances, care and concern, but not in appearance. Craniofacial anomalies until they can be corrected may cause suffering that is related to the reaction of others.
- **Variable** relating to individual family members including personalities, past experience, view of roles, attitude toward child rearing, education, etc.
- **How the family function together and has dealt with previous crisis:** This ability may be assessed by observation, interview or the use of tools such as the family APGAR or parenting stress index.
- **Lifestyle and plans of the family:** A family who travel and couple extensively may have to modify such plans. If they have a child who cannot walk or who requires special food that cannot last for a long time on trip. They can be helped to plan and modify activities in a way that may include everyone.
- **Other attributes of the disorders:** This includes the severity of the disease, its natural history, age of onset, type and frequency of treatment, the necessary for surgery or repeated hospitalization and the long-term outlook, so that future planning can occur.

Role of Nurses in Managing the Impact of Genetic Conditions on Families

Nurse need to remember that the discovery of genetic disorder or anomaly is a shattering experience for a family. It can permanently and abruptly alter the life plans of a family. Nurses can promote an effective coping among family with following interventions:
- Recognize that different people cope with such a shock in different ways; resist labeling parents as non-caring, rejecting, etc.
- Do not inject personal biases
- Build a trusting and permissive atmosphere and ascertain the support system available to the family
- Emphasize the legitimacy of parents feeling
- Work with the family in identifying and building family strength, support, limitations and other concerns, such as time, financial obligations and other children
- Raise the issues of prebirth expectations and how these may be related to present feelings, the mother may need to verbally relive the pregnancy before she can go on.

- Identify willingness and ability of parents to cope and special care procedure, such as moving the child with osteogenesis imperfecta or feeding the infant with cleft palate should be taught, help in such situation brings success in such endeavors helps to boost parents self-confidence, shows them that they can cope and gives them same sense of self-worth
- Recognize that the emotions they are experiencing are exhausting and disorganizing; decision-making may be difficult and may need to be postponed
- Observe and record the interaction of parents with each other and with child, family communication pattern, their concern, their needs, so that nursing plans and interventions are not repeated, but are built on what have occurred previously
- Help the father and mother to maintain open communication and plan for their role at home; before discharge help parents, plan for what supplies and equipments will be needed and where they can be obtained.
- Contact patient groups of person with similar affected children. These provide various type of assistance, from financial to equipments, to telephone crisis lines, to friendly listening and sharing, to coping measures, to hospital visiting and more
- Work with parents to plan a timetable that includes needs of normal sibling and for parents, tension-reducing activities
- Often provide opportunities to ask questions and voice concern
- Follow-up care and regularly scheduled session with the care coordinator is essential before parents leave the hospital
- Obtain information and refer parents to respective advanced care facilities and programs
- Plan for follow-up should include counseling for grief resolution, marital and family relationships, reproductive options discussion and genetic counseling
- Help parents and family to rebuild self-esteem and feel that they are human beings worthy of being linked
- Make it clear to family that you are willing to listen and talk and be sure that you are willing when called on
- If the parents have not raised the issue, the nurse should ask the parents, if they have considered discussing the newly diagnosed disorder with others in family and outside
- Be aware of some of the signs of successful adjustment, an intact family, the resumption of sexual relationship between partners, appropriate plans for future reproduction in light of genetic counseling and family goal, ability to help other parents, realistic plans for management of the affected child, retention of the family health practitioner and ability to relate to others are some measures that can be used.
- Remember to ask the parents, how are they doing. This will give them feeling of concerned.

REVIEW OF CELLULAR DIVISION

Cell division is a process by which a cell, called the parent cell, divides into two or more cells, called daughter cells. Cell division is usually a small segment of a larger cell cycle. This type of cell division in eukaryotes is known as mitosis and leaves the daughter cell capable of dividing again. The primary concern of cell division is the maintenance of the original cell's genome. Before division can occur, the genomic information, which is stored in chromosomes must be replicated and the duplicated genome separated cleanly between cells. A great deal of cellular infrastructure is involved in keeping genomic information consistent between 'generations'.

Another type of cell division present only in eukaryotes, called meiosis, a cell is permanently transformed into a gamete and cannot divide again until fertilization. As the cell division is the part of the cell cycle; where cell grow and divide. Therefore, it is wise to first understand about the cell cycle.

Cell Cycle

The cell cycle consists of four distinct phases—growth 1/gap 1 (G1) phase, synthesis (S) phase, gap 2/growth 2 (G2) phase (collectively known as interphase) and mitosis (M) phase. M phase is itself composed of two tightly coupled processes, mitosis, in which the cell's chromosomes are divided between the two daughter cells and cytokinesis, in which the cell's cytoplasm divides forming distinct cells. Activation of each phase is dependent on the proper progression and completion of the previous one. Cells that have temporarily or reversibly stopped dividing are said to have entered a state of quiescence called gap zero/resting (G0) phase **(Fig. 15.2)**.

M Phase

The relatively brief M phase consists of nuclear division (mitosis) and cytoplasmic division (cytokinesis). Mitosis divides genetic information during cell division.

Interphase

After M phase, the daughter cells begin interphase of a new cycle. Although the various stages of interphase are not usually morphologically distinguishable, each phase of the cell cycle has a distinct set of specialized biochemical processes that prepare the cell for initiation of cell division. Interphase is a phase of the cell cycle, which includes.

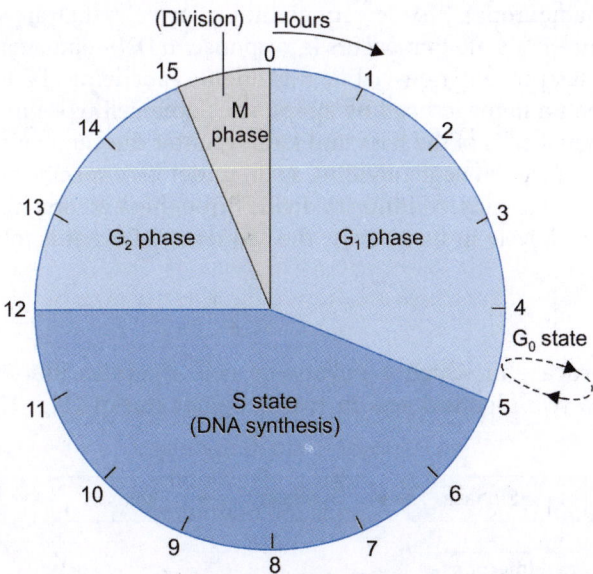

Fig. 15.2: Schematic presentation of the cell cycle (G1, gap 1; S1, synthesis 1; G2 gap 2; M, mitosis phase).

- **G1 phase:** The first phase within interphase, from the end of the previous M phase till the beginning of deoxyribonucleic acid (DNA) synthesis is called G1 (G indicating gap or growth). During this phase, the biosynthetic activities of the cell, which had been considerably slowed down during M phase, resume at a high rate. This phase is marked by synthesis of various enzymes that are required in S phase, mainly those needed for DNA replication. Duration of G1 is highly variable, even among different cells of the same species. The G1 phase is a period in the cell cycle during interphase, after cytokinesis and before the S phase.
- **S phase:** The ensuing S phase starts when DNA synthesis commences; when it is complete, all of the chromosomes have been replicated, i.e., each chromosome has two (sister) chromatids. Thus, during this phase, the amount of DNA in the cell has effectively doubled, though the ploidy of the cell remains the same. Rates of ribonucleic acid (RNA) transcription and protein synthesis are very low during this phase. An exception to this is histone production, most of which occurs during the S phase. The duration of S phase is relatively constant among cells of the same species.
- **G2 phase:** The cell then enters the G2 phase, which lasts until the cell enters mitosis. Again, significant protein synthesis occurs during this phase, mainly involving the production of microtubules, which are required during the process of mitosis. Inhibition of protein synthesis during G2 phase prevents the cell from undergoing mitosis. G2 phase is the third and final subphase in interphase of the cell cycle.

G0 Phase

- The term 'postmitotic' is sometimes used to refer to both quiescent and senescent cells. Non-proliferative cells in multicellular eukaryotes generally enter the quiescent G0 state from G1 and may remain quiescent for long periods of time, possibly indefinitely (as is often the case for neurons). This is very common for cells that are fully differentiated. Cellular senescence is a state that occurs in response to DNA damage or degradation that would make a cell's progeny non-viable; it is often a biochemical alternative to the self-destruction of such a damaged cell by apoptosis. Some cell types in mature organisms, such as parenchymal cells of the liver and kidney, enter the G0 phase semi-permanently and can only be induced to begin dividing again under very specific circumstances; other types, such as epithelial cells, continue to divide throughout an organism's life.
- Considering the cell cycle in its entirely, the sequence of event is follow the order as in **Figure 15.3**.

Mitosis

- Mitosis is the process in which a eukaryotic cell separates the chromosomes in its cell nucleus, into two identical sets in two daughter nuclei **(Fig. 15.4)**. It is generally

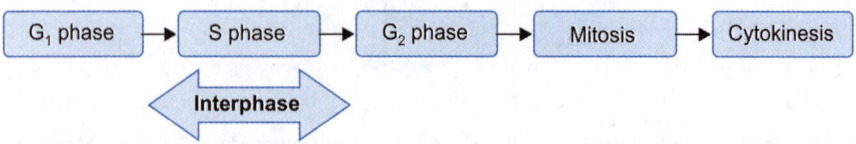

Fig. 15.3: Events of cycle in somatic cell.

followed immediately by cytokinesis, which divides the nuclei, cytoplasm, organelles and cell membrane into two daughter cells containing roughly equal shares of these cellular components. Mitosis and cytokinesis together define the mitotic (M) phase of the cell cycle—the division of the mother cell into two daughter cells, genetically identical to each other and to their parent cell.
- Mitosis occurs exclusively in eukaryotic cells, but occurs in different ways in different species. The process of mitosis is complex and highly regulated. The sequence of events is divided into phases, corresponding to the completion of one set of activities and the start of the next. These stages are prophase, prometaphase, metaphase, anaphase and telophase. During the process of mitosis, the pairs of chromosomes condense and attach to fibers that pull the sister chromatids to opposite sides of the cell. The cell then divides in cytokinesis, to produce two identical daughter cells.

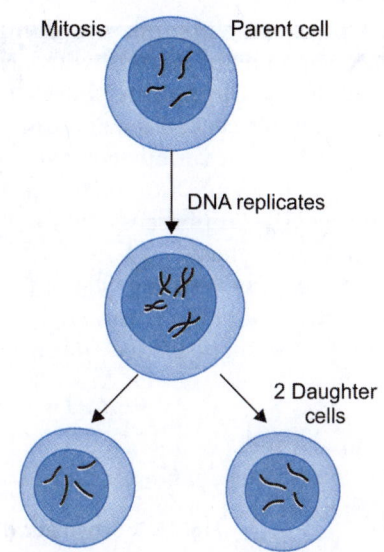

Fig. 15.4: Mitosis (DNa, deoxyribonucleic acid).

- Because cytokinesis usually occurs in conjunction with mitosis, 'mitosis' is often used interchangeably with 'mitotic phase'. Errors in mitosis can either kill a cell through apoptosis or cause mutations that may lead to cancer.

Phases of Mitosis

The mitotic phase is a relatively short period of the cell cycle. It alternates with the much longer interphase, where the cell prepares itself for cell division. Interphase is therefore not part of mitosis. Interphase is divided into three phases; G1, S and G2. During all three phases, the cell grows by producing proteins and cytoplasmic organelles. However, chromosomes are replicated only during the S phase. Thus, a cell grows (G1), continues to grow as it duplicates its chromosomes (S), grows more and prepares for mitosis (G2) and divides (M).

Prophase

It is the first stage of mitosis. During early prophase, the chromatin fibers condense and shortened into chromosome that are visible under the light microscope. The condensation process may prevent entangling of the long DNA strands as they move during mitosis. Because DNA replication took place during the S phase of interphase, each prophase chromosome consists of a pair of identical, double-stranded chromatids. A constricted region called a centromere holds the chromatid pair together. At the outside of each centromere is a protein complex known as the kinetochore. Later in prophase, tubulins in the pericentriolar material of the centrosomes start to form the mitotic spindle, a football-shaped assembly of microtubules lengthens and they push the centrosomes to the poles (end) of the cell, so that the spindle extends from pole to pole. The spindle is responsible for the separation of chromatids to opposite poles of the cell. Then, the nucleus disappears and the nuclear envelop breaks down **(Fig. 15.5)**.

SECTION 4: Genetics

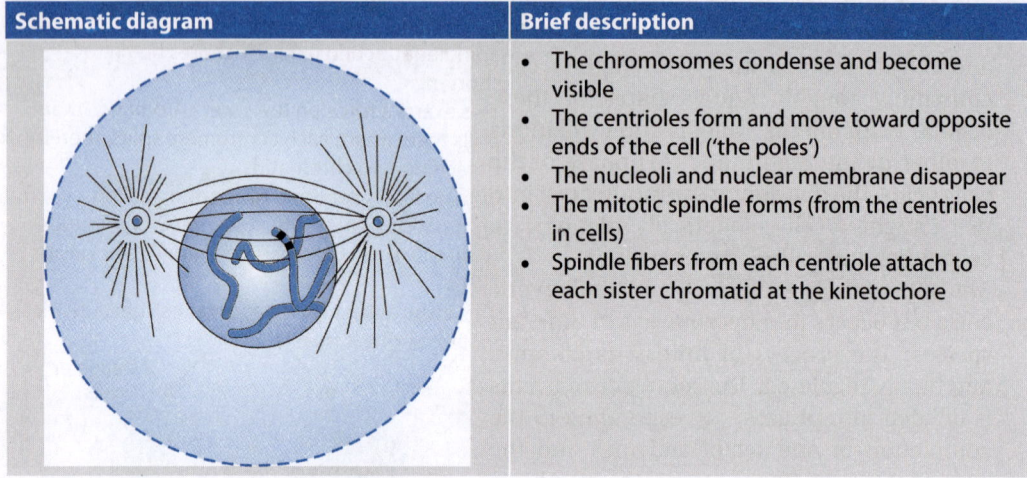

Fig. 15.5: Schematic diagram and brief description of prophase.

Metaphase

During metaphase, the kinetochore microtubules align the centromeres of the chromatid pair at the exact center of the mitotic spindle. This midpoint region in called the metaphase plate (**Fig. 15.6**).

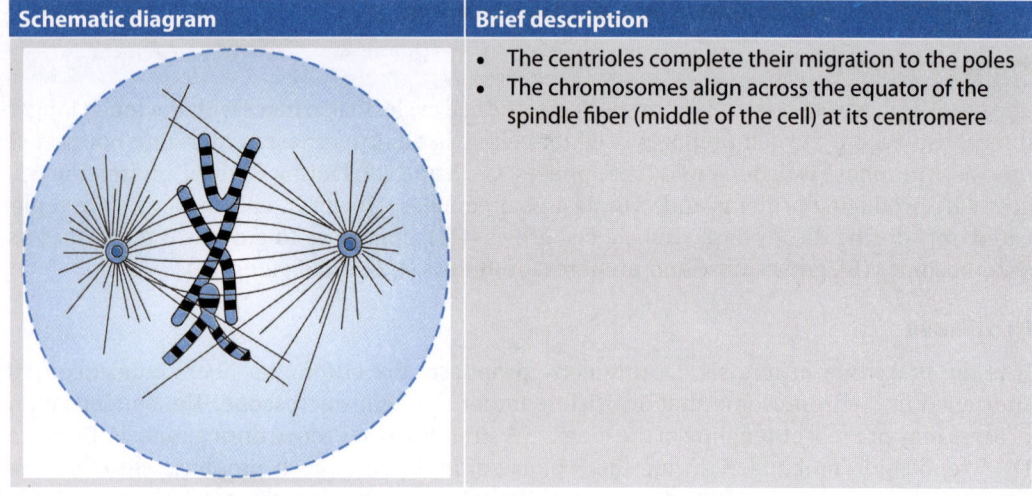

Fig. 15.6: Schematic diagram and brief description of metaphase.

Anaphase

During anaphase, the centromeres split, separating the two members of each chromatid pair, which move toward opposite poles of the cell (**Fig. 15.7**). Once separated, the chromatids are termed as chromosomes. As the chromosomes are pulled by the kinetochore microtubules lead the way, dragging the trailing arms of the chromosomes toward the pole.

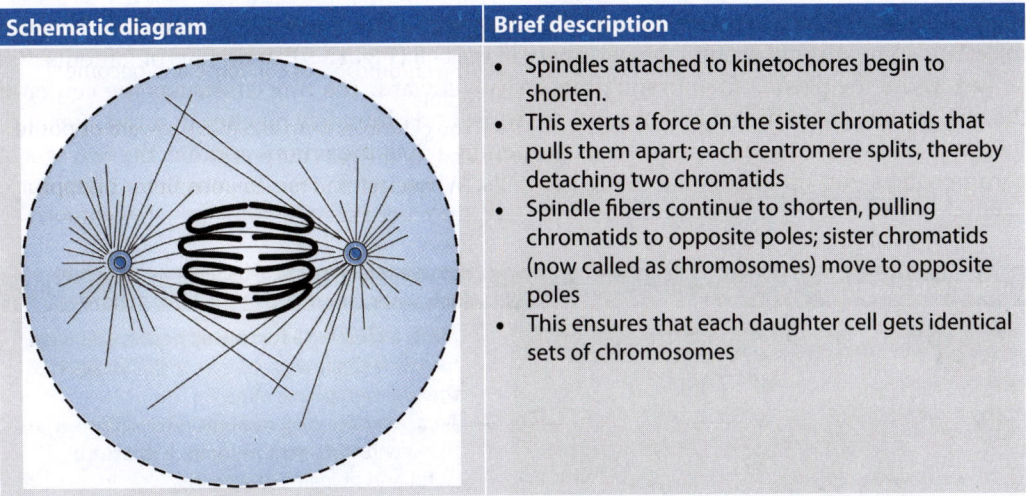

Fig. 15.7: Schematic diagram and brief description of anaphase.

Brief description (for Fig. 15.7):
- Spindles attached to kinetochores begin to shorten.
- This exerts a force on the sister chromatids that pulls them apart; each centromere splits, thereby detaching two chromatids
- Spindle fibers continue to shorten, pulling chromatids to opposite poles; sister chromatids (now called as chromosomes) move to opposite poles
- This ensures that each daughter cell gets identical sets of chromosomes

Telophase

The final stage of mitosis, telophase, begins after chromosomal movement stops **(Fig. 15.8)**. The identical sets of chromosomes now at opposite poles of the cell, uncoil and forms around each chromatin mass, nucleoli reappear in the daughter nuclei and the mitotic spindle disappears.

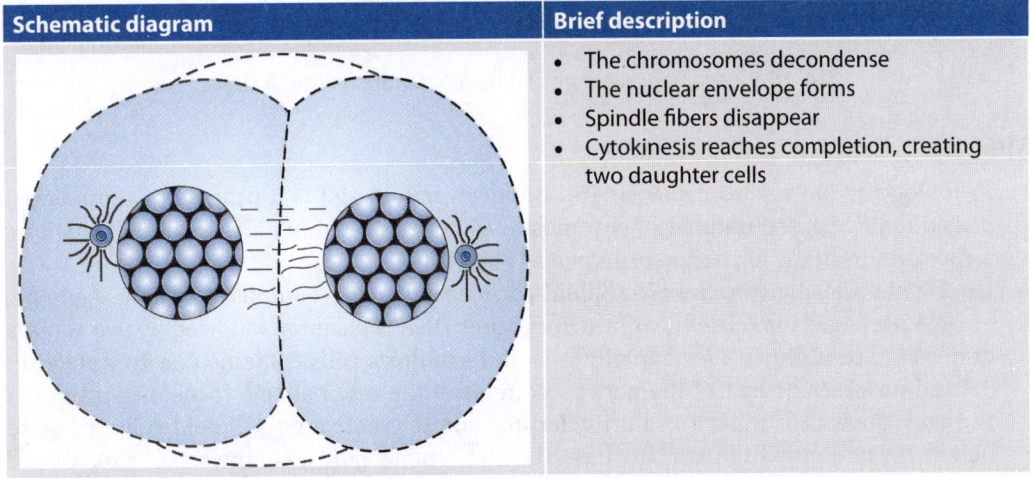

Fig. 15.8: Schematic diagram and brief description of telophase.

Brief description (for Fig. 15.8):
- The chromosomes decondense
- The nuclear envelope forms
- Spindle fibers disappear
- Cytokinesis reaches completion, creating two daughter cells

Cytoplasmic Division/Cytokinesis

Division of a parent cell's cytoplasm and organelles into two daughter cells is called cytokinesis. This process begins in late anaphase or early telophase with formation of a cleavage furrow, a slight indention of the plasma membrane. The cleavage furrow usually appears midway because the centrosomes extend around the periphery of the cell **(Fig. 15.9)**. Actin microfilaments that lie just inside the plasma membrane progressively inward. The ring constructs the center of the cell, such as tightening a belt around the waist and ultimately pinches it in two. Because the plane of the cleavage furrow is always perpendicular to the mitotic spindle, the two sets of chromosomes end up in separate daughter cells. When cytokinesis is complete, interphase begins.

Schematic diagram	Brief description
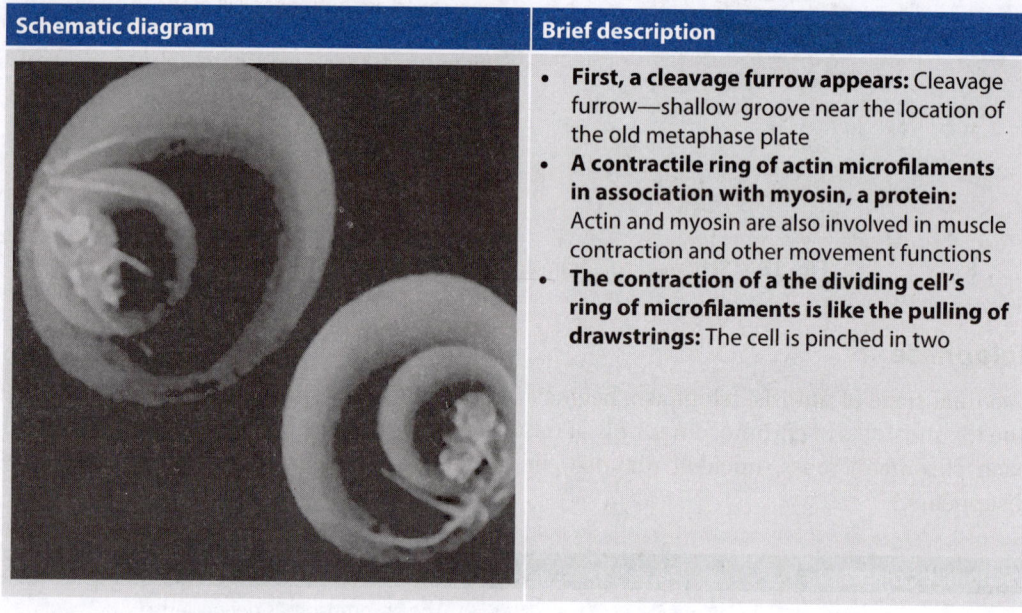	- **First, a cleavage furrow appears:** Cleavage furrow—shallow groove near the location of the old metaphase plate - **A contractile ring of actin microfilaments in association with myosin, a protein:** Actin and myosin are also involved in muscle contraction and other movement functions - **The contraction of a the dividing cell's ring of microfilaments is like the pulling of drawstrings:** The cell is pinched in two

Fig. 15.9: Schematic diagram and brief description of cytokinesis.

Meiosis

- In biology or life science, meiosis (pronounced my-oh-sis) is a process of reductional division in which the number of chromosomes per cell is cut in half. In animals, meiosis always results in the formation of gametes **(Fig. 15.10)**
- During meiosis, the genome of a diploid germ cell, which is composed of long segments of DNA packaged into chromosomes, undergoes DNA replication followed by two rounds of division, resulting in four haploid cells. Each of these cells contains one complete set of chromosomes or half of the genetic content of the original cell. If meiosis produces gametes, these cells must fuse during fertilization to create a new diploid cell, or zygote before any new growth can occur. Thus, the division mechanism of meiosis is a reciprocal process to the joining of two genomes that occurs at fertilization. Because the chromosomes of each parent undergo genetic recombination during meiosis, each gamete and thus each zygote, will have a unique genetic blueprint encoded in its DNA. Together, meiosis and fertilization constitute sexuality in the eukaryotes and generate genetically distinct individuals in populations

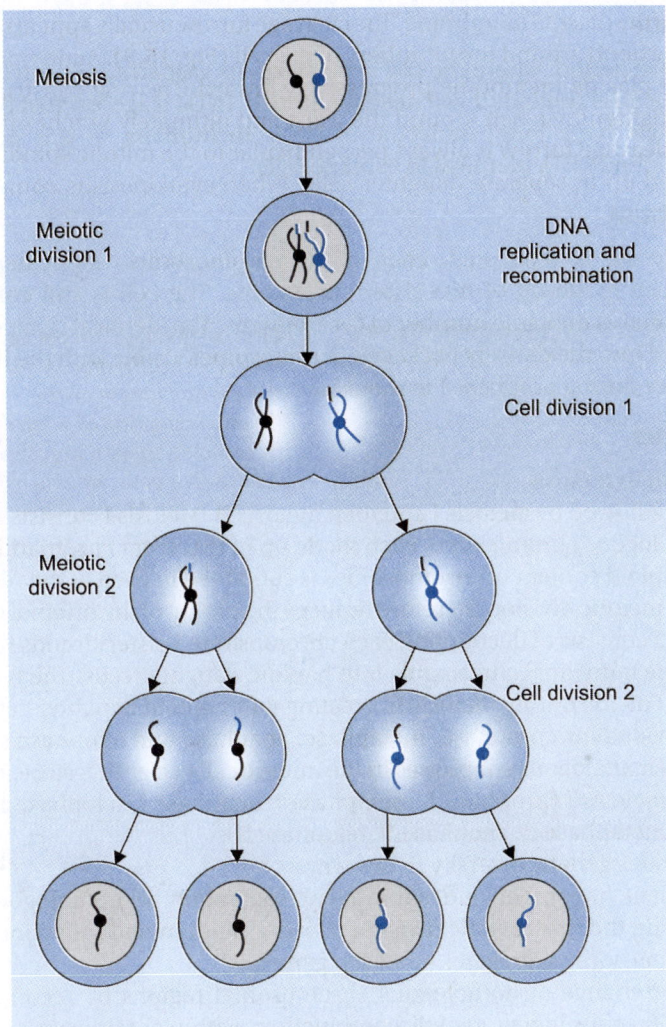

Fig. 15.10: Meiosis.

- Meiosis uses many of the same biochemical mechanisms employed during mitosis to accomplish the redistribution of chromosomes. There are several features unique to meiosis, most importantly the pairing and genetic recombination between homologous chromosomes.

Process

Because meiosis is a 'one-way' process, it cannot be said to engage in a cell cycle as mitosis does. However, the preparatory steps that lead up to meiosis are identical in pattern and name to the interphase of the mitotic cell cycle.

Interphase is divided into three phases.

1. Gap 1 (G1) Phase

This is a very active period, where the cell synthesizes its vast array of proteins, including the enzymes and structural proteins it will need for growth. In G1 stage, each of the chromosomes consists of a single (very long) molecule of DNA. In humans, at this point cells are 46 chromosomes, diploid (2N), identical to somatic cells.

2. Synthesis (S) Phase

The genetic material is replicated, each of its chromosomes duplicates, producing 46 chromosomes each made up of two sister chromatids. The cell is still considered diploid because it still contains the same number of centromeres. The identical sister chromatids have not yet condensed into the densely packaged chromosomes visible with the light microscope. This will take place during prophase I in meiosis.

3. Gap 2 (G2) Phase

G2 phase is absent in meiosis:
- Interphase is followed by meiosis I and then meiosis II. Meiosis I consists of separating the pairs of homologous chromosome, each made up of two sister chromatids, into two cells. One entire haploid content of chromosomes is contained in each of the resulting daughter cells; the first meiotic division therefore reduces the ploidy of the original cell by a factor of two. Meiosis II consists of decoupling each chromosome's sister strands (chromatids) and segregating the individual chromatids into haploid daughter cells. The two cells resulting from meiosis I divide during meiosis II, creating four haploid daughter cells. Meiosis I and II are each divided into prophase, metaphase, anaphase and telophase stages, similar in purpose to their analogous subphases in the mitotic cell cycle. Therefore, meiosis includes the stages of meiosis I (prophase I, metaphase I, anaphase I, telophase I) and meiosis II (prophase II, metaphase II, anaphase II, telophase II).
- Meiosis generates genetic diversity in two ways:
    1. Independent alignment and subsequent separation of homologous chromosome pairs during the first meiotic division allows a random and independent selection of each chromosome segregates into each gamete.
    2. Physical exchange of homologous chromosomal regions by recombination during prophase I results in new genetic combinations within chromosomes.

Meiosis-phases

Meiosis I

In meiosis I, the homologous pairs in a diploid cell separate, producing two haploid cells (23 chromosomes, n in humans), so meiosis I is referred to as a reductional division. A regular diploid human cell contains 46 chromosomes and is considered 2n because it contains 23 pairs of homologous chromosomes. However, after meiosis I, although the cell contains 46 chromosomes it is only considered n because later in anaphase I the sister chromatids will remain together as the spindle pull the pair toward the pole of the new cell. In meiosis II, an equational division similar to mitosis will occur whereby the sister chromatids are finally split, creating a total of four haploid cells (23 chromosomes, n) per daughter cell from the first division.

Prophase I

Homologous chromosomes pair (or synapse) and crossing-over (or recombination) occurs a step unique in meiosis. The paired and replicated chromosomes are called bivalents or tetrads, which have two chromosomes and four chromatids, with one chromosome coming from each parent. At this stage, non-sister chromatids may crossover at points called chiasmata (plural; singular chiasma) **(Fig. 15.11)**.

Leptotene

The first stage of prophase I is the leptotene stage, also known as leptonema, from Greek words meaning 'thin threads'. During this stage, individual chromosomes begin to condense into long strands within the nucleus. However, the two sister chromatids are still so tightly bound that they are indistinguishable from one another. The chromosomes in the leptotene stage show a specific arrangement where the telomeres are oriented toward the nuclear membrane. Hence, this stage is called 'bouquet stage' **(Fig. 15.11)**.

Zygotene

The zygotene stage, also known as zygonema, from Greek words meaning 'paired threads'. We have seen that the 46 chromosomes in each cell consist of 23 pairs (the X and Y chromosomes of the male being taken pair). The two chromosomes of each come to lie parallel to each other and are closely apposed. This pairing chromosomes also referred to as synopsis or conjugation. Two chromosomes together constitute a bivalent **(Fig. 15.11)**.

Pachytene

The pachytene stage, also known as pachynema, from Greek words meaning 'thick threads', contains the following chromosomal crossover. The two chromatids of each chromosome together become distinct. The bivalent now has four chromatids in it and is called a tetrad. There are two central and two peripheral chromatids, one from each chromosome. An important event now takes place. The two central chromatids (one belonging to each chromosome of the bivalent) become coiled over each other, so that they cross at a number of points. This is called 'crossing-over'. At the site where the chromatids cross they become adherent; the point of adhesion are called as chiasmata **(Fig. 15.11)**:

Non-sister chromatids of homologous chromosomes randomly exchange segments of genetic information over regions of homology (sex chromosomes, however, are not wholly

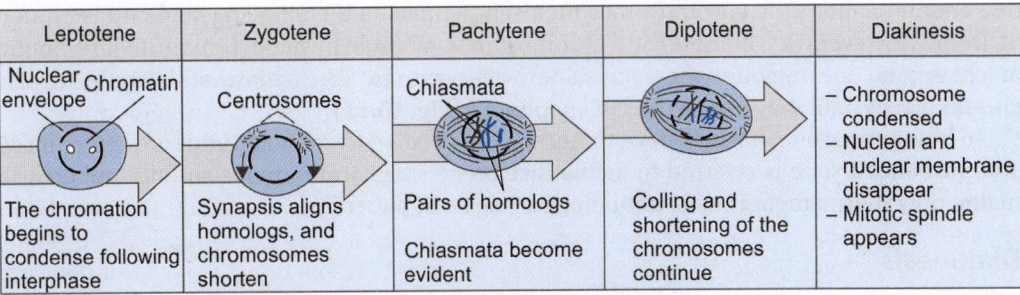

Fig. 15.11: Substages of prophase-I.

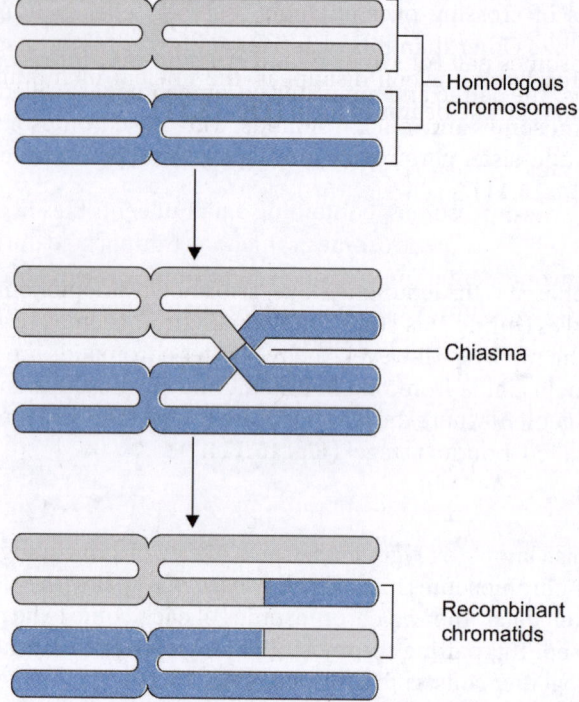

Fig. 15.12: Crossing-over (recombination).

identical and only exchange information over a small region of homology). Exchange takes place at sites where recombination nodules (the aforementioned chiasmata) have formed **(Fig. 15.12)**. The exchange of information between the non-sister chromatids results in a recombination of information; each chromosome has the complete set of information it had before and there are no gaps formed as a result of the process. Because the chromosomes cannot be distinguished in the synaptonemal complex, the actual act of crossing over is not perceivable through the microscope.

Diplotene

During the diplotene stage, also known as diplonema, from Greek words meaning 'two threads', the synaptonemal complex degrades and homologous chromosomes separate from one another a little. The chromosomes themselves uncoil a bit, allowing some transcription of DNA. However, the homologous chromosomes of each bivalent remain tightly bound at chiasmata, the regions where crossing-over occurred. The chiasmata remain on the chromosomes until they are severed in anaphase I **(Fig. 15.11)**.

In human fetal oogenesis all developing oocytes develop to this stage and stop before birth. This suspended state is referred to as the dictyotene stage and remains so until puberty. In males, only spermatogonia exist until meiosis begins at puberty.

Diakinesis

Chromosomes condense further during the diakinesis stage, from Greek words meaning 'moving through'. This is the first point in meiosis where the four parts of the tetrads are actually visible. Sites of crossing over entangle together, effectively overlapping, making chiasmata clearly visible. Other than this observation, the rest of the stage closely resembles prometaphase of mitosis; the nucleoli disappear, the nuclear membrane disintegrates into vesicles and the meiotic spindle begins to form **(Fig. 15.11)**.

Synchronous Processes

During these stages, two centrosomes, containing a pair of centrioles in animal cells, migrate to the two poles of the cell. These centrosomes, which were duplicated during S phase, function as microtubule organizing centers nucleating microtubules, which are essentially cellular ropes and poles. The microtubules invade the nuclear region after the nuclear envelope disintegrates, attaching to the chromosomes at the kinetochore. The kinetochore functions as a motor, pulling the chromosome along the attached microtubule toward the originating centriole, such as a train on a track. There are four kinetochores on each tetrad, but the pair of kinetochores on each sister chromatid fuses and functions as a unit during meiosis I.

Microtubules that attach to the kinetochores are known as 'kinetochore microtubules'. Other microtubules will interact with microtubules from the opposite centriole are called 'non-kinetochore microtubules' or 'polar microtubules'. A third type of microtubules, the aster microtubules, radiates from the centrosome into the cytoplasm or contacts components of the membrane skeleton.

Metaphase I

Homologous pairs move together along the metaphase plate, as kinetochore microtubules from both centrioles attach to their respective kinetochores, the homologous chromosomes align along an equatorial plane that bisects the spindle, due to continuous counterbalancing forces exerted on the bivalents by the microtubules emanating from the two kinetochores of homologous chromosomes. The physical basis of the independent assortment of chromosomes is the random orientation of each bivalent along the metaphase plate, with respect to the orientation of the other bivalents along the same equatorial line.

Anaphase I

Kinetochore microtubules shorten, severing the recombination nodules and pulling homologous chromosomes apart. Since each chromosome has only one functional unit of a pair of kinetochores, whole chromosomes are pulled toward opposing poles, forming two haploid sets. Each chromosome still contains a pair of sister chromatids. Non-kinetochore microtubules lengthen, pushing the centrioles farther apart. The cell elongates in preparation for division down the center.

Telophase I

- The last meiotic division effectively ends when the chromosomes arrive at the poles. Each daughter cell now has half the number of chromosomes, but each chromosome consists of a pair of chromatids. The microtubules that make up the spindle network disappear and a new nuclear membrane surrounds each haploid set. The chromosomes uncoil back into chromatin. Cytokinesis, the pinching of the cell membrane in animal cells or the formation of the cell wall in plant cells occurs by completing the creation of two daughter cells. Sister chromatids remain attached during telophase I.

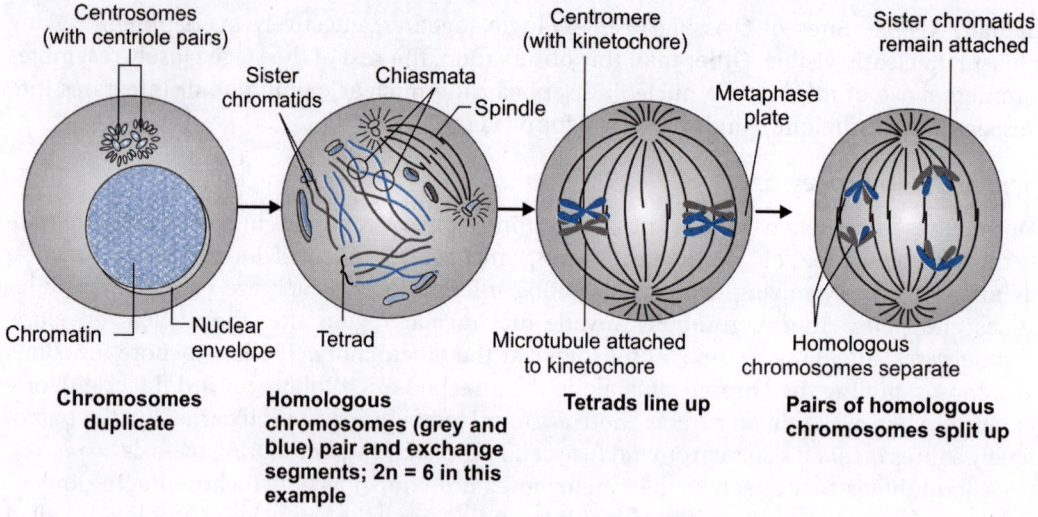

Fig. 15.13: Meiosis I (2n, diploid number).

- Cells may enter a period of rest known as interkinesis or interphase II. No DNA replication occurs during this stage **(Fig. 15.13)**.

Meiosis II

- Meiosis II is the second part of the meiotic process. Much of the process is similar to mitosis. The end result is production of four haploid cells (23 chromosomes, 1n in humans) from the two haploid cells (23 chromosomes, 1n, each of the chromosomes consisting of two sister chromatids) produced in meiosis I.
- Prophase II takes an inversely proportional time compared to telophase I. In this prophase, we see the disappearance of the nucleoli and the nuclear envelope again as well as the shortening and thickening of the chromatids. Centrioles move to the polar regions and arrange spindle fibers for the IInd meiotic division.
- In metaphase II, the centromeres contain two kinetochores that attach to spindle fibers from the centrosomes (centrioles) at each pole. The new equatorial metaphase plate is rotated by 90° when compared to meiosis I, perpendicular to the previous plate.
- This is followed by anaphase II, where the centromeres are cleaved, allowing microtubules attached to the kinetochores to pull the sister chromatids apart. The sister chromatids by convention are now called sister chromosomes as they move toward opposing poles.
- The process ends with telophase II, which is similar to telophase I and is marked by uncoiling and lengthening of the chromosomes and the disappearance of the spindle. Nuclear envelopes reform and cleavage or cell wall formation eventually produces a total of four daughter cells, each with a haploid set of chromosomes. Meiosis is now complete **(Fig. 15.14)**.

The difference between the two processes, mitosis and meiosis is given in **Table 15.1**.

Regulation of Cell Division and Growth

- A variety of genes are involved in the control of cell growth and division. The cell cycle is the cell's way of replicating itself in an organized, step-by-step fashion. Tight regulation of

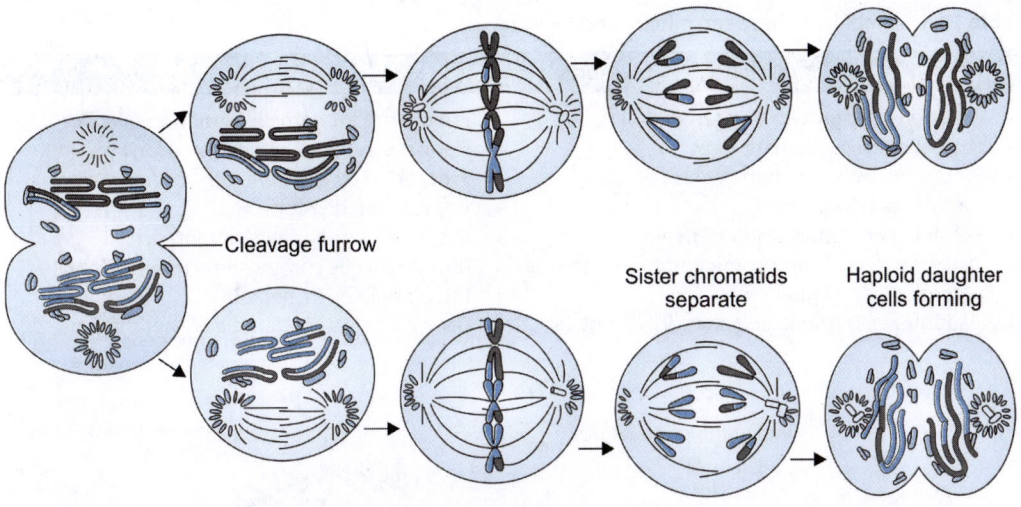

Fig. 15.14: Meiosis II.

this process ensures that a dividing cell's DNA is copied properly, any errors in the DNA are repaired and each daughter cell receives a full set of chromosomes. The cycle has checkpoints (also called restriction points), which allow certain genes to check for mistakes and halt the cycle for repairs if something goes wrong. If a cell has an error in its DNA that cannot be repaired, it may undergo programmed cell death (apoptosis) **(Fig. 15.15)**. Apoptosis is a common process throughout life that helps the body get rid of cells it does not need. Cells that undergo apoptosis break apart and are recycled by a type of white blood cell called a macrophage **(Fig. 15.16)**. Apoptosis protects the body by removing genetically damaged cells that could lead to cancer and it plays an important role in the development of the embryo and the maintenance of adult tissues.

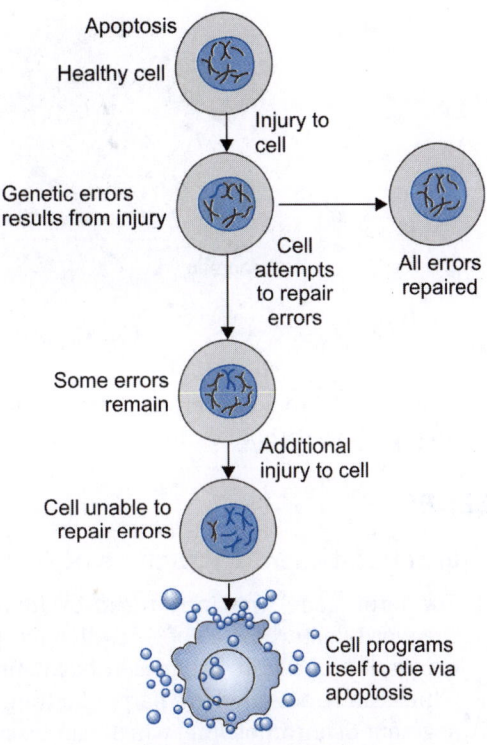

Fig. 15.15: Apoptosis.

- Cancer results from a disruption of the normal regulation of the cell cycle. When the cycle proceeds without control, cells can divide without order and accumulate genetic defects

Table 15.1: Comparison between mitosis and meiosis.

Mitosis	Meiosis
• Function is for growth and repair • Happens in most somatic cells • Proceeded by replication of chromosomes • Has one cell division • Result in two diploid daughter cells • Daughter cells chromosome number is same as parent cell (2n, diploid) • Daughter cells normally, genetically identical	• Function is for gamete formation • Happens in testes and ovary to form gametes • Proceeded by replication of chromosomes • Has two cell divisions • Results in four haploid daughter cells • Daughter cells chromosome number is half of the parent cell (n, haploid) • Daughter cells are genetically not the same

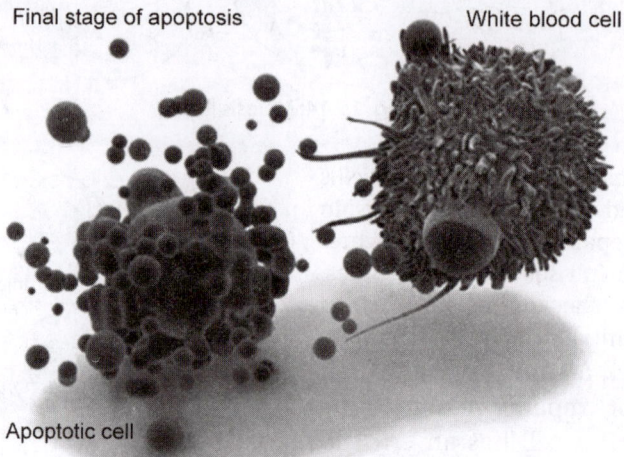

Fig. 15.16: Macrophage activity.

that can lead to a cancerous tumor. Cancer results when cells accumulate genetic errors and multiply without control.

GENES

Characteristics and Structure of Genes

- The term 'gene' was introduced by Johanssen in 1909. Prior to him Mendel had used the word 'factor' for a specific, distinct, particular unit of inheritance that takes part in expression of a trait. Johanssen has defined gene, as an elementary unit of inheritance, which can be assigned to a particular trait. Morgan's work suggested gene to be the shortest segment of chromosome, which can be separated through crossing over, can be undergo mutation and influence expression of one or more traits.
- Presently, a gene is defined as a unit of inheritance composed of a segment of DNA or chromosome situated at a specific locus (gene locus), which carries coded information associated with a specific function and can undergo crossing over as well as mutation. Some of the specific features of genes are:

- A specific portion of the DNA code is called a gene, which has genetic information.
- The term gene is often used to refer genetic material on a chromosome that code for a trait. For example, person has a gene for hair color.
- A unit of genetic material, which is able to replicate.
- It is a unit of recombination or capable of undergoing crossover.
- A unit of genetic material, which can undergo mutation.
- A unit of heredity connected with somatic structure or function that leads to a phenotype expression.
- A gene is the basic physical and functional unit of heredity.
- Genes, which are made up of DNA, act as ribonucleic acid (RNA) instructor to make molecules called proteins.
- In humans, genes vary in size from a few hundred DNA bases to more than 2 million bases. The Human Genome Project has estimated that humans have between 20,000–25,000 genes.
- Every person has two copies of each gene, one inherited from each parent. Most genes are the same in all people, but a small number of genes (less than 1% of the total) are slightly different between people. Alleles are forms of the same gene with small differences in their sequence of DNA bases. These small differences contribute to each person's unique physical features.
- Genes consists of a long strand of DNA that contain promoter, which control the activity of a gene and coding and non-coding sequence **(Fig. 15.17)**.
- Gene coding sequence determines what will be the product, while non-coding sequence can regulate the conditions of gene expression.
- When gene is active, the coding and non-coding sequence is copied in a process called transcription, producing an RNA copy of the gene's information. This RNA can then

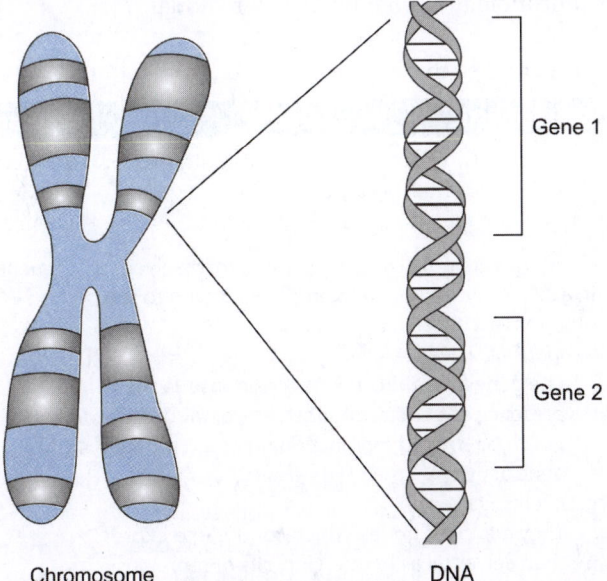

Fig. 15.17: Structure of gene—genes are made up of deoxyribonucleic acid (DNA); each chromosome contains many genes.

direct the synthesis of protein via genetic code. These RNA or proteins are known as gene products.
- Gene is a locatable region of genomic sequence, corresponding to a unit of inheritance, which is associated with regulatory region, transcribed region and/or other functional sequence regions.
- A gene is a union of genomic sequences encoding a coherent set of potentially overlapping functional products.
- The physical development and phenotype of a person can be thought of as a product of genes interacting with each other and with environment.
- Total set of genes in a person are known as genome.
- Genes is basically an instruction for human body. Each gene has a specific purpose and every single function of the human body is coded in one or more genes.
- A person's unique genetic constitutes called the genotype are made up of about 30,000–40,000 genes.
- A person's phenotype, the observable characteristics of his/her genotype, includes the physical appearance and other biological, physiological and molecular traits.

Type of Genes

Genes are of various types, classification of which depends on their characteristics and functions. Genes may carry a single copy or can have multiple copies. The genes may not always express themselves in a cell and they can function according to the requirement of the cellular activity **(Table 15.2)**.

Functions of Genes

- Genes are components of genetic material and are thus unit of inheritance.
- They control the morphology or phenotype of individual.

Table 15.2: Types of genes and their characteristics.

Type of gene	Characteristic	Example
Constitutive genes	They are those genes, which are constantly expressing themselves in a cell because their products are required for the normal cellular activities	Gene for glycolysis, adenylate pyrophos-phatase (ATPase)
Non-constitutive genes (luxury genes)	The genes are not always expressing themselves in a cell. They are switched on/off according to the requirement of cellular activities a. *Inducible genes:* The genes are switched on in response to the presence of a chemical substance or inducer, which is required for functioning of the product of gene activity b. *Repressive genes:* They are those genes, which continue to express themselves till a chemical inhibits or represses their activity	Genes for lactose system in *Escherichia coli*.

Contd...

Contd...

Type of gene	Characteristic	Example
Multigenes	It is a group of similar or nearly similar genes for meeting requirements of time and tissue-specific products	Encode the actins, hemoglobins, immunoglobulins, tubulins, interferons, histones, etc.
Repeated genes	The genes are present in multiple copies	Histone genes, *transfer RNA (tRNA)* genes, ribosomal RNA (rRNA) genes, actin genes
Single copy genes	The genes are present in single copy	
Pseudogenes	They are genes, which have homology to functional genes, but are unable to produce functional products due to intervening nonsense codons, inactivation of promoter genes	Several snRNA genes
Split genes	Split genes are those genes, which possess extra or non-essential region interspersed with essential or coding part	Present in eukaryotes
Jumping genes (transposons)	They are segments of DNA that can jump or move from one place in the genome to another	Human endogenous retroviruses (HERV), and various Ty elements of S.cerevisiae
Overlapping genes	Genes those overlap other genes	Common in DNA and RNA viruses
Structural genes:	Structural genes are those genes, which have encoded information for the synthesis of chemical substance (polypeptides for synthesis of structural and transport proteins, enzymes, hormones, several other proteins and no translated and non-coding RNAs) required for cellular machinery	*lac* Z, *lac* Y and *lac* A genes of lac operon, actin gene, etc.
Regulatory genes	Regulatory genes do not transcribe RNAs and, therefore, produce no chemicals. They are meant to controlling the function of structural genes	*Lac I* gene, *CAP* gene. etc.
Mitochondrial genes	Mitochondrial genome consists of 37 genes that encode proteins. They instruct cells to produce protein subunits of enzyme complexes of oxidative phosphorylation	MtDNA encodes for proteins in electron transport chain, e.g., NADH dehydrogenase, cytochrome b, cytochrome c oxidase and ATP synthase
Tissue specific genes	Found in only few specific genes but not in all the similar genes	*HTR1A*, specifically expressed only in brain, and *PCSK9*, specifically enriched in a number of tissues

- Replication of genes is essential for cell division
- Genes carry the hereditary information from one generation to next
- They control the structure and metabolism of the body
- Reshuffling of genes at the time of sexual reproduction produce variation
- Different linkages are produced due to crossing over
- Genes undergo mutation and change their expression
- New genes and consequently new traits develop due to reshuffling of different parts of genes
- Genes change their expression due to position effect
- Differentiation or formation of different type of cells, tissues and organs in various parts of the body is controlled by expression of certain genes and nonexpression of others
- Development or production of different stages in the life history is controlled by genes. Genes also helps in producing the enzymes which thus interacts in certain chemical reactions.

Nucleic Acid

Any of a group of complex compounds found in all living cells and viruses, composed of purines, pyrimidines, carbohydrates and phosphoric acid. Nucleic acids in the form of DNA and RNA control cellular function and heredity.

Deoxyribonucleic Acid

- DNA is a nucleic acid that contains the genetic instructions for the development and function of living things. All known cellular life and some viruses contain DNA. The main role of DNA in the cell is the long-term storage of information. It is often compared to a blueprint, since it contains the instructions to construct other components of the cell such as proteins and RNA molecules. The DNA segments that carry genetic information are called genes, but other DNA sequences have structural purposes or are involved in regulating the expression of genetic information.
- In eukaryotes such as animals and plants, DNA is stored inside the cell nucleus, while in prokaryotes such as bacteria, the DNA is in the cell's cytoplasm. Unlike enzymes, DNA does not act directly on other molecules; rather, various enzymes act on DNA and copy its information into either more DNA, in DNA replication, or transcribe it into protein. In chromosomes, chromatin proteins such as histones compact and organize DNA, as well as help in control of its interactions with other proteins in the nucleus.
- DNA is a long polymer of simple units called nucleotides, which are held together by a backbone made of sugars and phosphate groups. This backbone carries four types of molecules called bases and it is the sequence of these four bases that encodes information. The major function of DNA is to encode the sequence of amino acid residues in proteins, using the genetic code. To read the genetic code, cells make a copy of a stretch of DNA in the nucleic acid RNA. These RNA copies can then be used to direct protein synthesis, but they can also be used directly as parts of ribosomes or spliceosomes.

Ribonucleic Acid

- Ribonucleic acid is a nucleic acid polymer consisting of nucleotide monomers. RNA nucleotides contain ribose rings and uracil unlike DNA, which contains deoxyribose and thymine. It is transcribed (synthesized) from DNA by enzymes called RNA polymerases

and further processed by other enzymes. RNA serves as the template for translation of genes into proteins, transferring amino acids to the ribosome to form proteins and also translating the transcript into proteins.
- RNA is primarily made up of four different bases—adenine, guanine, cytosine and uracil. The first three are the same as those found in DNA, but in RNA, thymine is replaced by uracil as the base complementary to adenine. This base is also a pyrimidine and is very similar to thymine. Uracil is energetically less expensive to produce than thymine, which may account for its use in RNA. In DNA, however, uracil is readily produced by chemical degradation of cytosine, so having thymine as the normal base makes detection and repair of such incipient mutations more efficient. Thus, uracil is appropriate for RNA, where quantity is important, but life span is not, whereas thymine is appropriate for DNA where maintaining sequence with high fidelity is more critical.
- There are also numerous modified bases and sugars found in RNA that serve many different roles. Pseudouridine (ψ) and the DNA nucleoside thymidine are found in various places (most notably in the TψC loop of every tRNA). Another notable modified base is inosine (a deaminated guanine base), which allows a 'wobble codon' sequence in tRNA. There are nearly 100 other naturally occurring modified bases, of which pseudouridine and 2'-O-methy lribose are by far the most common. The specific roles of many of these modifications in RNA are not fully understood. However, it is notable that in ribosomal RNA, many of the post-translational modifications occur in highly functional regions, such as the peptidyl transferase center and the subunit interface, inferring that they are important for normal function. Single stranded RNA exhibits a right handed stacking pattern that is stabilized by base stacking.
- The most important structural feature of RNA that distinguishes it from DNA is the presence of a hydroxyl group at the 2'-position of the ribose sugar. The presence of this functional group enforces the C3'-endo sugar conformation (as opposed to the C2'-endo conformation of the deoxyribose sugar in DNA) that causes the helix to adopt the A-form geometry rather than the B-form most commonly observed in DNA. This results in a very deep and narrow major groove and a shallow and wide minor groove. A second consequence of the presence of the 2'-hydroxyl group is that in conformationally flexible regions of an RNA molecule (i.e., not involved in formation of a double helix), it can chemically attack the adjacent phosphodiester bond to cleave the backbone.

Biological Role of RNA

- **Messenger RNA (mRNA):** Messenger RNA is RNA that carries information from DNA to the ribosome sites of protein synthesis in the cell. Once mRNA has been transcribed from DNA, it is exported from the nucleus into the cytoplasm (in eukaryotes mRNA is 'processed' before being exported), where it is bound to ribosomes and translated into protein. After a certain amount of time, the message degrades into its component nucleotides, usually with the assistance of RNA polymerases.
- **Transfer RNA:** Transfer RNA is a small RNA chain of about 74–93 nucleotides that transfers a specific amino acid to a growing polypeptide chain at the ribosomal site of protein synthesis during translation. It has sites for amino acid attachment and an anticodon region for codon recognition that binds to a specific sequence on the messenger RNA chain through hydrogen bonding. It is a type of non-coding RNA.

- **Ribosomal RNA:** Ribosomal RNA is a component of the ribosomes, the protein synthetic factories in the cell. Eukaryotic ribosomes contain four different rRNA molecules—18S, 5.8S, 28S and 5S rRNA. Three of the rRNA molecules are synthesized in the nucleolus and one is synthesized elsewhere. rRNA molecules are extremely abundant and make up at least 80% of the RNA molecules found in a typical eukaryotic cell. In the cytoplasm, ribosomal RNA and protein combine to form a nucleoprotein called a ribosome. The ribosome binds mRNA and carries out protein synthesis. Several ribosomes may be attached to a single mRNA at any time.
- **Non-coding RNA or RNA genes:** RNA genes (sometimes referred to as non-coding RNA or small RNA) are genes that encode RNA that is not translated into a protein. The most prominent examples of RNA genes are tRNA and rRNA, both of which are involved in the process of translation. However, since the late 1990s, many new RNA genes have been found and thus, RNA genes may play a much more significant role than previously thought. In the late 1990s and early 2000, there has been persistent evidence of more complex transcription occurring in mammalian cells (and possibly others). This could point toward a more widespread use of RNA in biology, particularly in gene regulation. A particular class of non-coding RNA, micro-RNA, has been found in many metazoans (from *Caenorhabditis elegans* to *Homo sapiens*) and clearly plays an important role in regulating other genes. First proposed in 2004 by Rassoulzadegan and published in Nature 2006, RNA is implicated as being part of the germline. If confirmed, this result would significantly alter the present understanding of genetics and lead to many question on DNA-RNA roles and interactions.
- **Catalytic RNA:** Although RNA contains only four bases, in comparison to the twenty amino acids commonly found in proteins, some RNAs are still able to catalyse chemical reactions. These include cutting and ligating other RNA molecules and also the catalysis of peptide bond formation in the ribosome.
- **Double-stranded RNA:** Double-stranded RNA (dsRNA) is RNA with two complementary strands, similar to the DNA found in all 'higher' cells. The dsRNA forms the genetic material of some viruses. In eukaryotes, it acts as a trigger to initiate the process of RNA interference and is present as an intermediate step in the formation of siRNAs (small interfering RNAs). siRNAs are often confused with miRNAs; siRNAs are double-stranded, whereas miRNAs are single- stranded. Although, initially single stranded there are regions of intramolecular association causing hairpin structures in pre-miRNAs; immature miRNAs.

Comparison Between RNA and DNA

- Unlike DNA, RNA is almost always a single-stranded molecule and has a much shorter chain of nucleotides. RNA contains ribose, rather than the deoxyribose found in DNA (there is a hydroxyl group attached to the pentose ring in the 2' position whereas RNA has two hydroxyl groups). These hydroxyl groups make RNA less stable than DNA because it is more prone to hydrolysis. Several types of RNA (tRNA, rRNA) contain a great deal of secondary structure, which help promote stability.
- Such as DNA, most biologically active RNAs including tRNA, rRNA, snRNAs and other non-coding RNAs [such as the single recognition particle (SRP) RNAs] are extensively base paired to form double stranded helices. Structural analysis of these RNAs have revealed that they are not, 'single-stranded', but rather highly structured. Unlike DNA, this structure is not just limited to long double-stranded helices, but rather collections of short helices packed together into structures akin to proteins. In this fashion, RNAs can achieve chemical

CHAPTER 15: Introduction to Genetics

catalysis, such as enzymes. For instance, determination of the structure of the ribosome in 2,000 revealed that the active site of this enzyme that catalyzes peptide bond formation is composed entirely of RNA.

Figure 15.18 depicts the structure of rNa and DNa and nitrogenous bases.

Synthesis of RNA

- Synthesis of RNA is usually catalyzed by an enzyme—RNA polymerase, using DNA as a template. Initiation of synthesis begins with the binding of the enzyme to a promoter

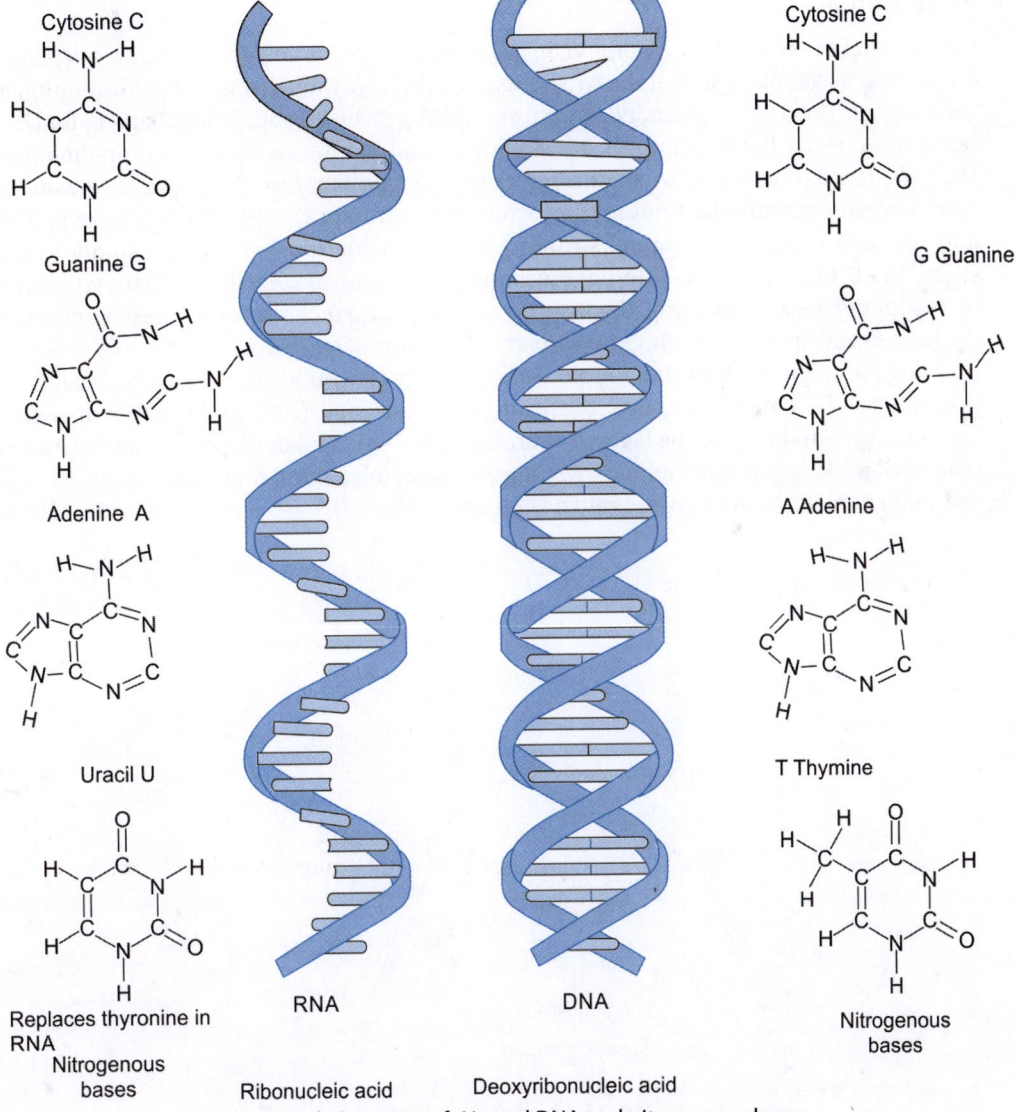

Fig. 15.18: Structure of rNa and DNA and nitrogenous bases.

sequence in the DNA (usually found 'upstream' of a gene). The DNA double helix is unwound by the helicase activity of the enzyme. The enzyme then progresses along the template strand in the 3' to > 5' direction, synthesizing a complementary RNA molecule with elongation occurring in the 5' to > 3' direction. The DNA sequence also dictates where termination of RNA synthesis will occur.
- There are also a number of RNA-dependent RNA polymerases as well that use RNA as their template for synthesis of a new strand of RNA. For example, a number of RNA viruses (such as poliovirus) use this type of enzyme to replicate their genetic material. Also, it known that RNA-dependent RNA polymerases are required for the RNA interference pathway in many organisms.

DNA Replication

- Cell division is essential for an organism to grow, but when a cell divides it must replicate the DNA in its genome, so that the two daughter cells have the same genetic information as their parent. The double-stranded structure of DNA provides a simple mechanism for DNA replication. Here, the two strands are separated and then each strand's complementary DNA sequence is recreated by an enzyme called DNA polymerase. This enzyme makes the complementary strand by finding the correct base through complementary base pairing and bonding it onto the original strand. As DNA polymerases can only extend a DNA strand in a 5' to 3' direction, different mechanisms are used to copy the antiparallel strands of the double helix. In this way, the base on the old strand dictates, which base appears on the new strand and the cell end3 up with a perfect copy of its DNA.
- In following **Figure 15.19** the double helix (blue) is unwound by a helicase. Next, DNA polymerase III (green) produces the leading strand copy (red). A DNA polymerase I molecule (green) binds to the lagging strand. This enzyme makes discontinuous segments (called Okazaki fragments) before DNA ligase (violet) joins them together.

Figure 15.20 depicts the semiconservative DNA replication.

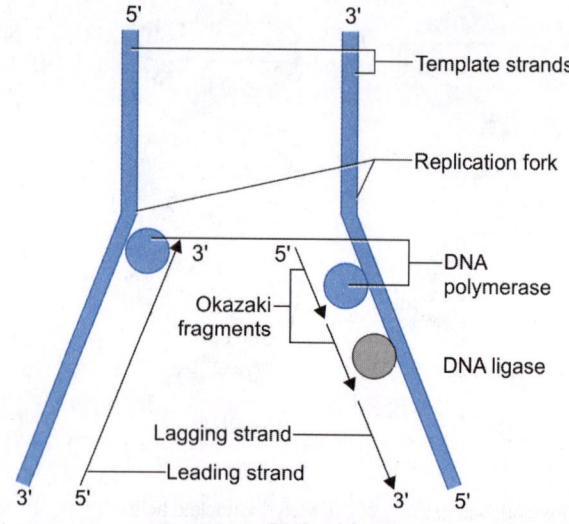

Fig. 15.19: DNA replication.

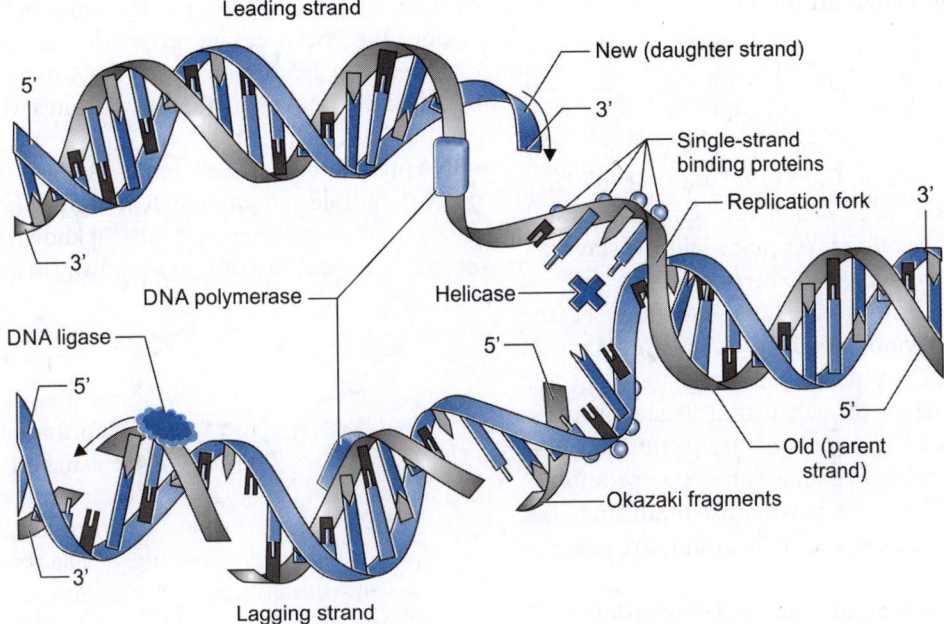

Fig. 15.20: Semiconservative DNA replication.

PROTEIN BIOSYNTHESIS

Protein biosynthesis (synthesis) is the process in which cells build proteins. The term is sometimes used to refer only to protein translation, but more often it refers to a multi-step process, beginning with amino acid synthesis and transcription, which are then used for translation. Protein biosynthesis, although very similar, differs between prokaryotes and eukaryotes **(Fig. 15.21)**.

An Overview of Protein Synthesis

Within the nucleus of the cell (light blue), genes (DNA, dark blue) are transcribed into RNA. This RNA is then subject to post-transcriptional modification and control, resulting in a mature mRNA (red) that is then transported out of the nucleus and into the cytoplasm (peach), where it undergoes translation into a protein. mRNA is translated by ribosomes (purple) that match the three-base codons of the mRNA to the three-base anticodons of the appropriate tRNA. Newly synthesized proteins (black) are often further modified, such as by binding to an effector molecule (orange), to become fully active.

Steps of the Protein Synthesis

Amino acid Synthesis

Amino acids are the monomers, which are polymerized to produce proteins. Amino acid synthesis is the set of biochemical processes (metabolic pathways), which build the amino acids from carbon sources, such as glucose. Not all amino acids may be synthesized by every organism, for example, adult humans have to obtain 8 of the 20 amino acids from their diet. The amino acids are then loaded onto tRNA molecules for use in the process of translation.

Transcription

Transcription is the process by which an mRNA template, carrying the sequence of the protein, is produced for the translation step from the genome. Transcription makes the template from one strand of the DNA double helix, called the template strand. Transcription takes place in three stages:

1. **Transcription starts with the process of initiation:** RNA polymerase, the enzyme which produces RNA from a DNA template, binds to a specific region on DNA that designates the starting point of transcription. This binding region is called the 'promoter'. As the RNA polymerase binds on to the promoter, the DNA strands are begin to unwind.
2. **The second process is elongation:** RNA polymerase travels along the template (noncoding) strand, synthesizing a ribonucleotide polymer. RNA polymerase does not use the coding strand as a template because a copy of any strand produces a base sequence complementary to the strand, which is being copied. Therefore, DNA from the noncoding strand is used as a template to copy the coding strand.
3. **The third stage is termination:** As the polymerase reaches the termination stage, modifications are required for the newly transcribed mRNA to be able to travel to the other parts of the cell, including cytoplasm and endoplasmic reticulum for translation. A 5' cap is added to the mRNA to protect it from degradation. In eukaryotes, a poly-A tail is added on the 3' end for protection and as a template for further process. Also in eukaryotes (higher organisms) the vital process of splicing occurs at this stage.

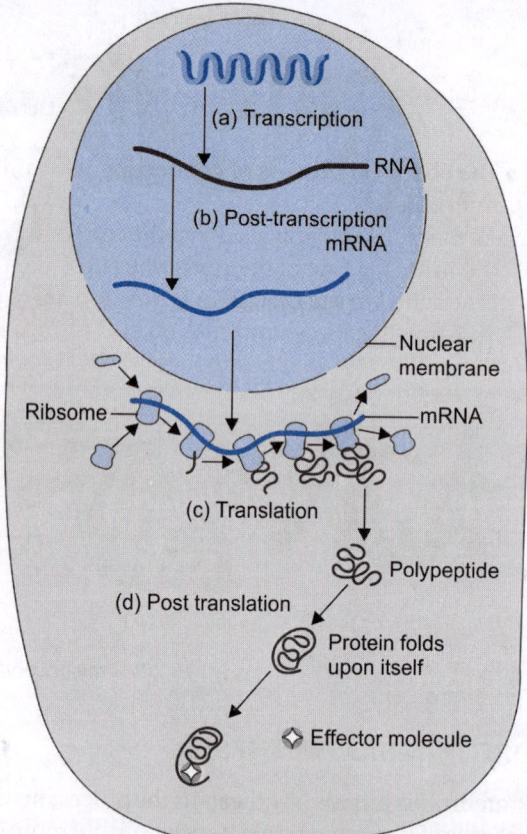

Fig. 15.21: Protein synthesis process.

Translation

During translation, mRNA previously transcribed from DNA is decoded by specialized cellular structures called ribosomes to make proteins:

- The ribosome has sites, which allow another specialized RNA molecule, known as tRNA, to bind to the mRNA. Binding of the correct tRNA to the mRNA on the ribosome is accomplished by an 'anticodon' that is part of the tRNA. Thus, the correct tRNA, chemically linked to a specific amino acid, is directed to the ribosome to be added to a growing (nascent) polypeptide. The chemical process of connecting two amino acids is shown in the picture below.

CHAPTER 15: Introduction to Genetics

$$\text{H}_2\text{N-CHR-COOH} + \text{H}_2\text{N-CHR-COOH} \rightarrow \text{H}_2\text{N-CHR-CO-NH-CHR-COOH} + \text{HOH}$$

The chemical process of connecting two amino acids resulting in a dipeptide and a water molecule.

- As the ribosome travels down the mRNA one codon at a time, another tRNA is attached to the mRNA at one of the ribosome sites. The first tRNA is released, but the amino acid that is attached to the first tRNA is now moved to the second tRNA and binds to its amino acid. This translocation continues on and a long chain of amino acid (protein) is formed. When the entire unit reaches the stop codon on the mRNA, it falls apart and a newly formed protein is released. This is 'termination'. It is important to know that during this process, many enzymes are used to either assist or facilitate the whole procedure.

Events following Biosynthesis (Protein Synthesis)

It includes post-translational modification and protein folding. During and after synthesis, polypeptide chains often fold to assume, so called, native secondary and tertiary structures. This is known as 'protein folding". Many proteins undergo post-translational modification. This may include the formation of disulfide bridges or attachment of any number of biochemical functional groups, such as acetate, phosphate, various lipids and carbohydrates. Enzymes may also remove one or more amino acids from the leading (amino) end of the polypeptide chain, leaving a protein consisting of two polypeptide chains connected by disulfide bonds.

GENETIC CODE

The genetic code is the set of rules by which information encoded in genetic material (DNA or RNA sequences) is translated into proteins (amino acid sequences) in living cells **(Fig. 15.22)**. Specifically, the code defines a mapping between trinucleotide sequences called codons and amino acids; every triplet of nucleotides in a nucleic acid sequence specifies a single amino acid. Most organisms use a nearly universal code that is referred to as the 'standard genetic code'. Even viruses, which are not cellular and do not synthesize proteins themselves, have proteins made using this standard code. For a time, therefore, the code was thought to be universal. However, there are notable exceptions. It is also possible for a single organism to translate different parts of the genome in different

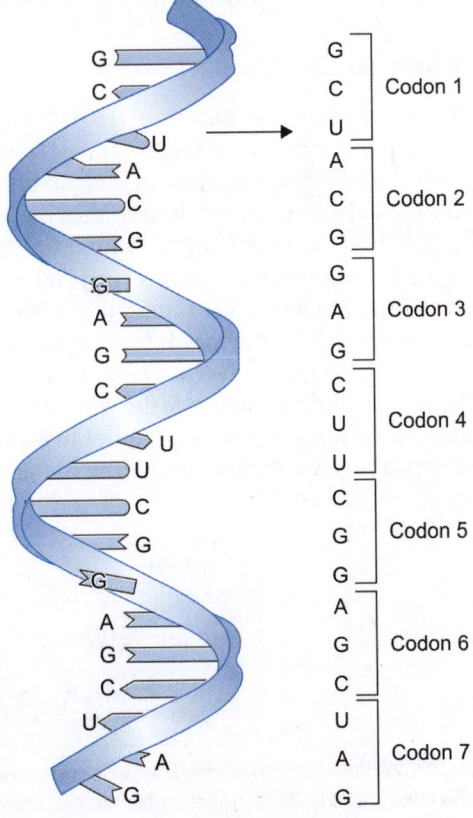

Fig. 15.22: Genetic code.

ways. For example, in humans, protein synthesis in mitochondria relies on a modified genetic code that varies from the standard one.

The position or sequence of the bases in DNA ultimately determine the position of the amino acids in the polypeptide chain whose synthesis is directed by the DNA. Therefore, the structure and properties of body proteins are determined by the DNA base sequence of a person's gene. It does this by means of a code. Each amino acid is specified by a sequence of three bases called a codon. There are 20 major amino acid and 64 codons or code words. 61 of the codon specify amino acids and 3 are 'stop' single that terminate the genetic message. One codon that specifies an amino acids usually begins the message. More than one code word may specify a given amino acid, but only one amino acid is specified by any one codon; thus the code is said to be degenerated. For example, the codons that code for the amino acid leucine are UAG, UUG, CUU, CUC, CUA and CUG, but none of these codes for any other amino acid. The relationship between the base sequence in DNA, mRNA, the anticodon in tRNA and the translation into any amino acid is shown in **Figure 15.23**.

The code is non-overlapping. Therefore, CACUUUAGA is read as CAC, UUU, AGA and specifies histidine, phenylalanine and arginine, respectively. A shorthand way of returning to specific amino acid is to use either specific group of three letters or a single letter to denote specific amino acid. To this system, for example, arginine may be referred to as 'arg' or as simply 'R', while the symbols for phenylalanine are either 'Phe' or 'F'. General genetics referred to in the reference provide more information about the code.

NAMING GENES

The Human Gene Organization (HUGO) Gene Nomenclature Committee designates an official name and symbol (an abbreviation of the name) for each known human gene. Some official gene names include additional information in parentheses such as related genetic conditions, subtypes of a condition or inheritance pattern. The Human Genomic Nomeclature Committee (HGNC) is a non-profit organization funded by the United Kingdom (UK) Medical Research Council and the United States (US) National Institutes of Health. The committee has named more than 13,000 of the estimated 20,000–25,000 genes in the human genome. The committee has accepted 30,000 symbols for naming a huge variety of genes. During the research process, genes often acquire several alternate names and symbols. Different researchers investigating the same gene may each give the gene a different name, which can cause confusion. The HGNC assigns a unique name and symbol to each human gene, which allows effective organization of genes in large databanks, aiding the advancement of research. Genetics Home Reference

DNA template	3...	AAA	TGA	CTG	...5
mRNA	5...	UUU	ACU	GAC	...5
tRNA	3...	AAA	UGA	CUG	...5
Polypeptide chain... NH_2		phe	thr	asp	COOH

Key: A=Adenine, C=cytocine, T=Thymine, U=Uracil, phe=Phenylalanine, thr=theonine, asp=aspartic acid

Fig. 15.23: Relationship among the nucleotide base sequence of deoxyribonucleic acid (DNA) mitochon-drial ribonucleic acid (mRNA), transfer ribonucleic acid (tRNA) and amino acids in the polypeptide chain production (A: adenine; C: cytocine; phe: phenylalanine; thr: threonine; T: thytmine; U: uracil).

describes genes using the HGNC's official gene names and gene symbols. Genetics Home Reference frequently presents the symbol and name separated with a colon (for example, FGFR4—fibroblast growth factor receptor 4).

CHROMOSOME

In the nucleus of each cell, the DNA molecule is packed into thread-like structures called chromosomes. Each chromosome is made up of DNA, tightly coiled many times around proteins called histones that support its structure. Chromosomes are organized structures of DNA and proteins that are found in cells. A chromosome is a singular piece of DNA, which contains many genes, regulatory elements and other nucleotide sequences. Chromosomes also contain DNA- bound proteins, which serve to package the DNA and control its functions. The word chromosome comes from the Greek (chroma, color) and (soma, body) due to their property of being stained very strongly by some dyes. Chromosomes vary extensively between different organisms. Chromosomes are packaged by proteins into a condensed structure called chromatin.

Chromosomes are not visible in the cell's nucleus not even under a microscope when the cell is not dividing. However, the DNA that makes up chromosomes becomes more tightly packed during cell division and is then visible under a microscope. Most of what researchers know today about chromosomes was learned by observing chromosomes during cell division. Each chromosome has a constriction point called the centromere, which divides the chromosome into two sections, or 'arms'. The short arm of the chromosome is labeled the 'p arm'. The long arm of the chromosome is labeled the 'q arm'. The location of the centromere on each chromosome gives the chromosome its characteristic shape and can be used to describe the location of specific genes **(Fig. 15.24)**.

In humans, each cell normally contains 23 pairs of chromosomes, for a total of 46. And 22 of these pairs, called autosomes, look the same in both males and females. The 23rd pair, the sex chromosomes, differs between males and females. Females have two copies of the X chromosome, while males have one X and one Y chromosome **(Fig. 15.25)**.

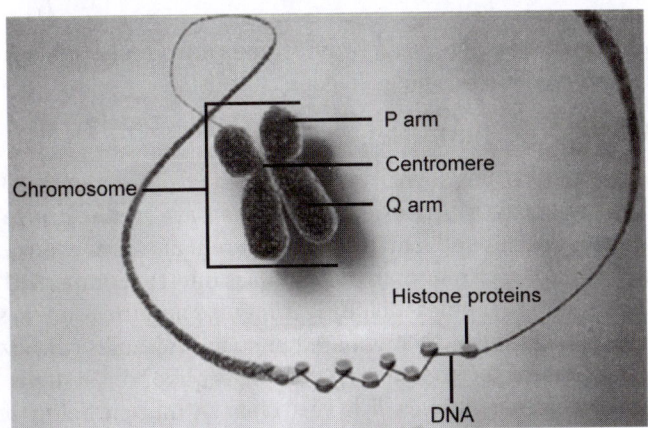

Fig. 15.24: Structure of chromosome.
(DNA: deoxyribonucleic acid)

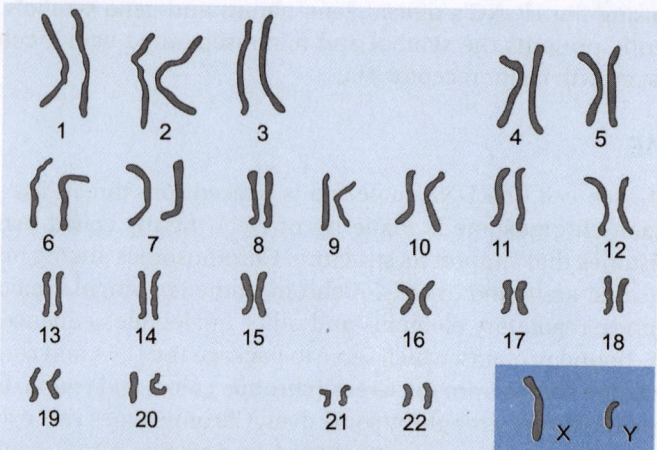

Fig. 15.25: Structure of 23 pairs of human chromosomes.

Functions of Chromosome

- Chromosomes contain genes, all the hereditary information is located in the genes
- Chromosomes control the synthesis of structural proteins and thus help in cell division and cell growth
- They control cellular differentiation
- By directing the synthesis of particular enzymes, chromosome control cell metabolism
- Chromosomes can replicate themselves or produce their carbon copies for passage to daughter cells and next generation
- Chromosomes produce nucleoli for synthesis of ribosomes
- Their haploid or diploid number respectively brings about gametophytic and sporophytic characteristics to the individual
- Chromosomes form a link between the offspring and the parents
- Some chromosomes called sex chromosomes (e.g. X and Y) determine the sex of the individual
- Through the process of crossing-over, chromosomes introduce variations
- Mutations are produced due to change in gene chemistry.

Chromosomes: Sex Determination

A sex-determination system is a biological system that determines the development of sexual characteristics in an organism. Most sexual organisms have two sexes. In many cases, sex determination is genetic—males and females have different alleles or even different genes that specify their sexual morphology. In human being, this is often accompanied by chromosomal differences. In some species of reptiles including *Alligators* and the tuatara, sex is determined by the temperature at which the egg is incubated or social variables (the size of an organism relative to other members of its population). Sex-determination systems are not yet fully understood in all the species. However, it is very clear in human being, which is very well explained by XX/XY chromosomal sex determination theory.

Chromosomal Determination of Sex

Henking (1891) discovered an X-body in the reproductive cell of firefly. Y-body was discovered by Stevens (1902). Wilson and Stevens (1905) put forward chromosome theory of sex and named the X- and Y-bodies on heterogamesis or occurrence of two types of gametes in one of the two sexes. It is of the following type:

- XX/XY type
- XX/XO type
- ZX/ZZ type
- ZO/ZZ type
- Haplodiploidy.

However, in human being XX/XY type of heterogamesis theory is applicable. In human beings, the female possess two homomorphic (isomorphic) sex chromosomes, named XX. The males contain two heteromorphic sex chromosome, i.e. XY. The Y chromosome is often shorter and heterochromatic (made of heterochromatin). Despite of difference in morphology, the XY chromosomes are homologous and synapse during zygotene phase of meiosis. It is because they have two parts, homologous and differential. Homologous region of the two help in pairing. They carry same genes, which may have different alleles. Such genes present on both X and Y chromosomes are XY-linked genes. They are inherited like autosomal genes, e.g. xeroderma pigmentation, epidermolysis bullosa. The differential region of Y chromosome carries only Y-linked or holandric genes, e.g. testis-determining factor (TDF). It is perhaps the smallest gene occupying only 14 base pairs. Other holandric genes are hypertrichosis (excessive hairness) on pinna, porcupine skin, keratoderma dissipatum (thickening of skin of hands and feet) and webbed toes. Holandric genes are directly inherited to son from his father. Genes present on the differential region of X-chromosome also find expression in male whether they are dominant or recessive, e.g. color blindness, hemophilia. It is because the male are hemizygous for these genes.

Human being have 22 pairs of autosomes and one pair of sex chromosomes. All the ova formed by female are similar in their chromosome type (22 + X). Therefore, female are homogametic. The male gametes or sperms produced by human male are of two type, (22 + X) and (22 + Y). Human males are therefore heterogametic (male digamety).

Sex of Offspring

Sex of the offspring is determined at the time of fertilization. It cannot be changed later on. It does not depend on any characteristic of the female parent because they are homogametic and produce only one type of eggs (22 + X). The male gametes are of two types androsperms (22 + Y) and gynosperms (22 + X). They are produced in equal proportion. Fertilization of the egg (22 + X) with gynosperm (22 + X) will produce female child (44 + XX), while fertilization of egg (22 + X) with androsperm (22 +Y) gives rise to male child (44 + XY). As the two types of sperms are produced in equal proportion, there are chances of getting a male or female child in a particular mating. As Y chromosome determines the male sex of the individual, it is also called as androsome **(Fig. 15.26)**.

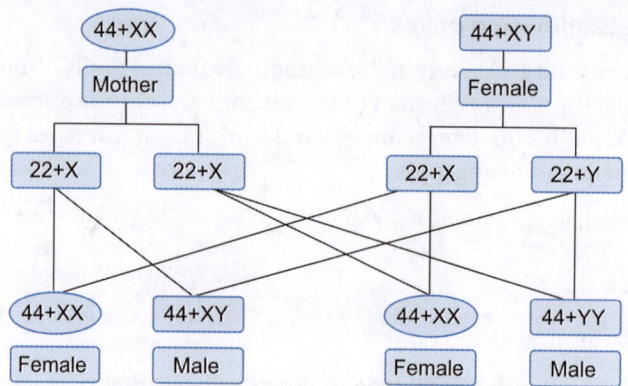

Fig. 15.26: Sex determination schematic presentation.

CHROMOSOMAL ABERRATIONS/CHROMOSOMAL MUTATION

- Chromosomal aberrations are disruptions in the normal chromosomal content of a cell and are a major cause of genetic conditions in humans, such as Down syndrome.
- In other words, they are changes in the number and/or arrangement of genes in the chromosomes.
- Change in number of chromosomes is known as aneuploidy or numerical aberration.
- Change in arrangement of genes in the chromosomes is known as structural aberration.
- Chromosomal aberrations may involve changes in single chromosome, known as intra-chromosomal aberrations.
- Chromosomal aberrations may involve changes in two chromosomes, known as inter-chromosomal aberrations.
- They are also termed as chromosomal abnormalities. Some chromosome abnormalities do not cause disease in carriers, such as translocations, or chromosomal inversions, although they may lead to a higher chance of having a child with a chromosome disorder. Abnormal numbers of chromosomes or chromosome sets, aneuploidy, may be lethal or give rise to genetic disorders.
- Chromosomal abnormalities result in a proportion of congenital anomalies, developmental and intellectual disabilities and behavioral difficulties. The majority of spontaneous abortions (about 50%–60%) are the result of chromosomal abnormalities, particularly, if they occur early, numerical changes in chromosomes are also summarized in **Table 15.3**, structural changes are summarized in **Table 15.4** and illustration in **Figure 15.27**.

Chromosomal aberrations can lead to a variety of genetic disorders. Human examples include: some of genetic disorder or genetic disease are as follows.
- **Cri-du-chat,** which is caused by the deletion of part of the short arm of chromosome 5. 'Cri -du-chat' means 'cry of the cat' in French and the condition was so-named because affected babies make high-pitched cries that sound like a cat. Affected individuals have wide-set eyes, a small head and jaw and are moderately to severely mentally retarded and very short.
- **Wolf-Hirschhorn syndrome,** which is caused by partial deletion of the short arm of chromosome 4. It is characterized by severe growth retardation and severe to profound mental retardation.

Table 15.3: Change in chromosomal number (aneuploidy) (numerical aberration).

Change	Description	Example
Monosomy	One chromosome is missing	Turner's syndrome (cells in female contain 45 chromosomes with one X chromosome rather than two)
Trisomy	One extra chromosome is present	Trisomy 21 chromosome (Down syndrome) Cells contains 47 chromosome
Tetrasomy	Two extra chromosome are present	Cells contain 48 chromosome (not compatible with life)
Triploidy	One extra chromosome set of haploid genome is present	Cells contain 69 chromosome (not compatible with life)
Tetraploidy	Two extra chromosome sets of haploid genome are present	Cells contain 92 chromosome (not compatible with life)

Table 15.4: Major changes in chromosome structure (structural aberration).

Change	Description
Deletion (del)	Part of a chromosome is missing with the accompanying DNA, can be at the end (terminal) or in the middle (interstitial); for example, del 5 p, cri-du-chat syndrome
Duplication (dup)	Part of a chromosome is duplicated along with the accompanying DNA, so that an extra piece of chromosomal material is present; for example, in cat eye syndrome, there is duplication of a certain segment of chromosome 22 resulting in iris coloboma, anal atresia and various congenital malformations
Inversion (inv)	Alteration in which a portion of the chromosome is rearranged by two breaks occurring 180° rotation of the chromosome piece between them and its reinsertion; for example, about 40% are chromosome 9; may or may not result in visible effects
Ring chromosome (r)	Formed when a segment at the end(s) of one of a pair of chromosome is lost and fuse to form a circular structure, for example, ring chromosome 14 is associated with psychomotor delay, mental retardation and dysmorphic craniofacial features; it is very rare
Translocation (t)	Transfer of a chromosome segment to another chromosome after breakage has occurred; in reciprocal translocation two chromosomes exchange piece. A Robertsonian translocation usually involve two acrocentric chromosomes whose long arms fuse. Often small fragments are lost.

Contd...

SECTION 4: Genetics

Contd...

Change	Description
	In a balanced translocation, no genetic material added or lost. Balanced reciprocal translocations usually do not cause problems. For example, translocation trisomy 21 or Down syndrome may result from the presence of 46 chromosomes that includes a translocation chromosome such as t (14t21) or t (14q21q), so that the genetic material of 47 chromosomes with genetic material of three chromosome 21s is present. There is a normal chromosome 14, two normal 21 and translocation chromosome consisting of the second chromosome 14 and extra chromosome 21q
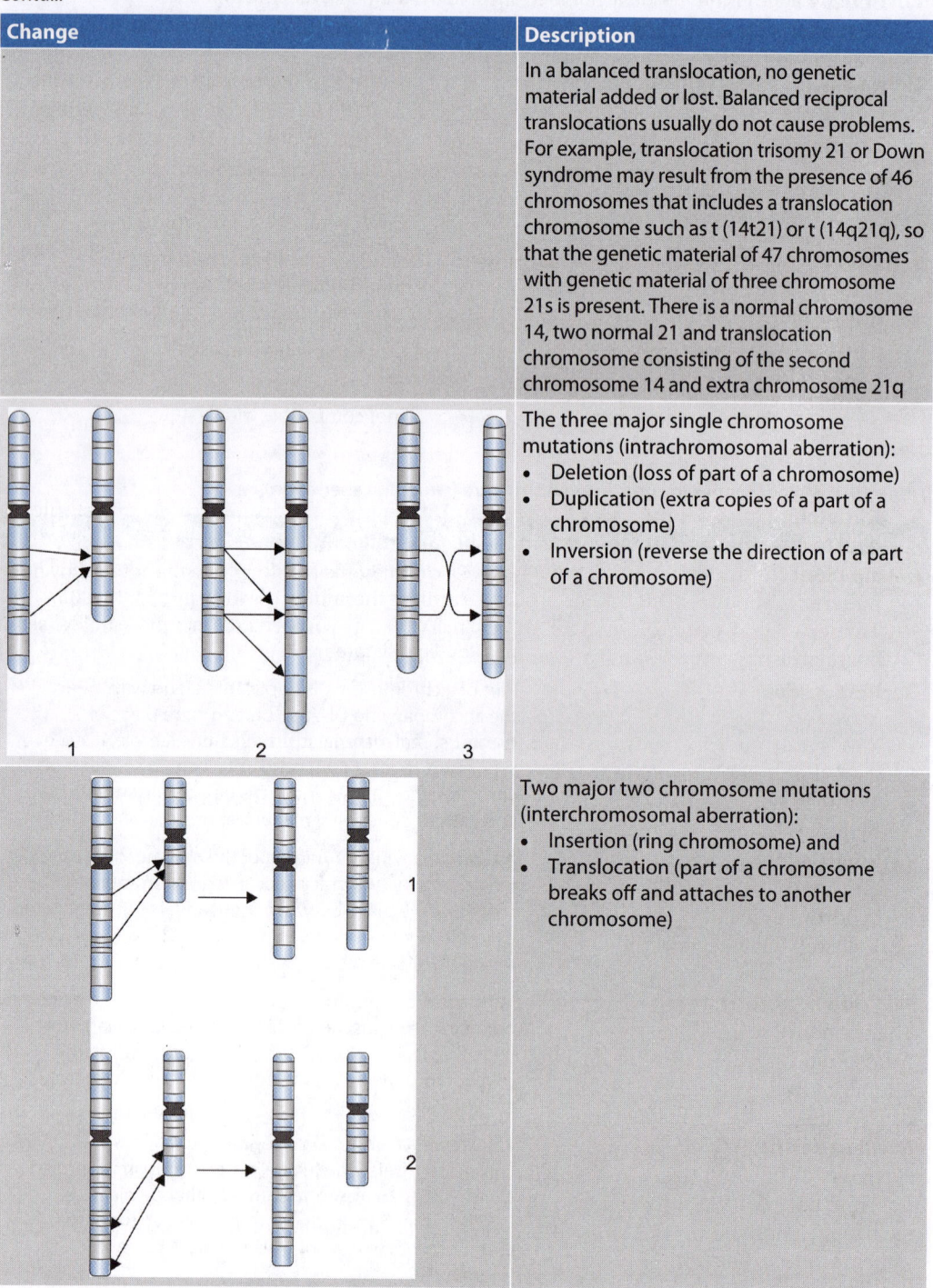	The three major single chromosome mutations (intrachromosomal aberration): • Deletion (loss of part of a chromosome) • Duplication (extra copies of a part of a chromosome) • Inversion (reverse the direction of a part of a chromosome)
	Two major two chromosome mutations (interchromosomal aberration): • Insertion (ring chromosome) and • Translocation (part of a chromosome breaks off and attaches to another chromosome)

Fig. 15.27: Chromosomal aberrations.

- **Down's syndrome,** usually is caused by an extra copy of chromosome 21 (trisomy 21). Characteristics include decreased muscle tone, stockier build, asymmetrical skull, slanting eyes and mild to moderate mental retardation.
- **Edwards syndrome,** which is the second most common trisomy after Down syndrome. It is a trisomy of chromosome 18. Symptoms include mental and motor retardation and numerous congenital anomalies causing serious health problems. About 90% die in infancy; however, those who live past their first birthday usually are quite healthy thereafter. They have a characteristic hand appearance with clenched hands and overlapping fingers.
- **Patau syndrome,** also called D syndrome or trisomy 13. Symptoms are somewhat similar to those of trisomy 18, but they do not have the characteristic hand shape.
- **Idic15, abbreviation** for isodicentric 15 on chromosome 15; also called the following names due to various researches, but they all mean the same; idic15, inverted duplication 15, extra marker, inv dup 15, partial tetrasomy 15.
- **Jacobsen syndrome,** also called the terminal 11q deletion disorder. This is a very rare disorder. Those affected have normal intelligence or mild mental retardation with poor expressive language skills. Most have a bleeding disorder called Paris-Trousseau syndrome.
- **Klinefelter's syndrome (XXY):** Men with Klinefelter's syndrome are usually sterile and tend to have longer arms and legs and to be taller than their peers. Boys with the syndrome are often shy and quiet and have a higher incidence of speech delay and dyslexia. During puberty, without testosterone treatment, some of them may develop gynecomastia.
- **Turner's syndrome (X instead of XX or XY):** In Turner's syndrome, female sexual characteristics are present, but underdeveloped. People with Turner's syndrome often have a short stature, low hairline, abnormal eye features and bone development and a 'caved-in' appearance to the chest.
- **XYY syndrome:** XYY boys are usually taller than their siblings. Like XXY boys and XXX girls, they are somewhat more likely to have learning difficulties.
- **Triple-X syndrome (XXX):** XXX girls tend to be tall and thin. They have a higher incidence of dyslexia.
- **Small supernumerary marker chromosome:** This means there is an extra, abnormal chromosome. Features depend on the origin of the extra genetic material. Cat-eye syndrome and Idic 15 are both caused by a supernumerary marker chromosome, as is Pallister-Killian syndrome.

Incidence

The incidence of the specific chromosomal abnormalities found is summarized in **Table 15.5**. Autosomal trisomies account for about 25%, sex chromosome abnormalities for about 35% and structural rearrangement for about 40%. These figures represent only a small fraction of chromosomally abnormal conception. Nature exercises considerable selections, as only small percentage of these abnormal conceptions survive to term. Between 10% and 20% of all recognized conception end in spontaneous abortions. Studies of the products of spontaneous abortion have detectable chromosomal abnormalities. Approximately, 95%–99% of all turner's syndrome embryos are spontaneously aborted, as are about 95% of those with available data, it appears that chromosome abnormalities are present in 10%–20% of all recognized conception. This may eventually be higher as techniques for determining cytogenic causes improve, more than 1,000 chromosome abnormalities have been described in live births.

Table 15.5: Incidence of selected chromosomal abnormalities in live born child.

Abnormality	Incidence
Autosomal trisomies • Trisomy 21 (Down syndrome) • Trisomy 13 (Patau syndrome) • Trisomy 18 (Edward syndrome)	 1: 650–1:1,000* 1: 4,000–1:10,000* 1: 3,500–1:7,500*
Sex-chromosome disorders • 45, X (Turner's syndrome) • 47, XXX (triple X) • 47, XXY (Klinefelter's syndrome)	 1: 2,500 – 1: 8000† 1: 850 – 1: 1,250† 1: 500 – 1: 1,000‡
Other sex-chromosome abnormalities • Male • Female	 ~1: 1,300‡ ~1: 1,300†
Structural abnormalities rearrangement (e.g. translocation, duplications)	~1: 440*

*Live births, †live female birth, ‡live male birth.

PATTERNS OF INHERITANCE

Some genetic conditions are caused by mutations in a single gene. These conditions are usually inherited in one of several straightforward patterns, depending on the gene involved. Following are the main patterns of inheritance:
- Mendelian patterns of inheritance: This includes:
  - Autosomal dominant
  - Autosomal recessive
  - *Sex linked inheritance:*
    - X-linked dominant
    - X-linked recessive
    - Y- linked (holandric) inheritance.
- Non-Mendelian patterns of inheritance:
  - Codominant pattern of inheritance
  - Mitochondrial pattern of inheritance
  - Multifactorial pattern of inheritance.

Autosomal Dominant

One mutated copy of the gene in each cell is sufficient for a person to be affected by an autosomal dominant disorder. Each affected person usually has one affected parent. Autosomal dominant disorders tend to occur in every generation of an affected family. Selective genetic disorders showing autosomal dominant inheritance are given in **Table 15.6**.

Main characteristics of autosomal dominant inheritance and disorders:
- Gene is an autosome
- One copy of the mutant gene is needed for effects
- Males and females are affected is equal number on average
- No sex difference in clinical manifestations
- Vertical family history through several generations may be seen
- There is wide variation in expression
- Penetrance may be incomplete (gene can appear in skip a generation)

Table 15.6: Selective genetic disorders showing autosomal dominant inheritance.

Disorder	Occurrence	Brief description
Aniridia	1:100,000–1:200,000	Absence of the iris of the eye to varying degree, glaucoma may develop, may be associated with other abnormalities in different syndrome
Achondroplasia	1:10,000–1:12,000	Short limbed type of dwarfism with large hands
Adult polycystic kidney disease	1:250–1:1,250	Enlarged kidney, hematuria, proteinuria, renal cysts, abdominal mass, eventually renal failure, may be associated with hypertension hepatic cyst, diverticular, cerebral hemorrhage may occur, cystic kidney seen on X-ray films
Facioscapulohumeral muscular dystrophy-la	1:100,000–3:100,000	Facial weakness, atrophy in face, upper limb and shoulder girdle and pelvic girdle muscles, speech may become indistinct—much variability in progression and age of onset
Familial hypercholes-terolemia (type-IIa)	1:200–1:500	Low-density lipoprotein (LDL) receptor mutation resulting in deviated LDL, xanthomas, archs lipoidy, corneal and coronary disease
Hereditary spherocytosis	1:4,500–1:5,000	Red cell membrane defect leading to abnormal shape, impaired survival and hemolytic anemia
Huntington disease	1:1,800–1:25,000	Progressive neurological disease due to trinucleotide repeat expansion of CAG, involuntary muscle movements with jerkiness, gait changes, lack of coordination, mental retardation with memory loss, speech problems, personality changes, confusion and deceased mental capacity usually begin in mid-adulthood
Nail-patella syndrome	1:50,00	Nail abnormalities, hypoplasia or absent patella and iliac horns, elbow dysplasia, renal lesions and disease, iris and other eye abnormalities, glaucoma, gastrointestinal problems
Neurofibromatosis 1	1:3,000–1:3,300	Café-an-lait spots, neurofibromas and malignant progression are common, complications include hypertension, variable expression
Osteogenesis imperfecta type-1	1:30,000	Fragile bones with multiple fractures, mitral valve prolapse, short stature in same cases, progressive hearing loss and Wormian bones
Polydactyly	1:100–1:300	Extra (supernumerary) digit on hand and feet
Tuberous sclerosis-I	About 1:10,000	White leaf shaped macules, seizures, intellectual delay, facial angiofibromas, erythemic nodular rash in butterfly pattern on face, learning and behavioral disorder, shagreen patches may develop retinal pathology and rhabdomyoma of the heart
Van der Woude syndrome	1:80,000–1:100,000	Cleft lip pits, missing premolars.
Von Willebrand disease	1:1,000–30:1,000	Deficiency or defect in plasma protein called von willebrand factor, leading to prolonged bleeding time, bleeding from mucous membranes. .

(CAG: cytosine-adenine-guanine)

- Increase paternal age effect may be seen
- Fresh gene mutation is frequent
- Later age of onset is frequent
- Male-to-male transmission is possible
- Normal offspring of an affected person will have normal children and grandchildren
- Least negative effect on reproductive fitness
- Structural protein defect is often involved
- In general disorders tends to be less severe than the recessive disorders
- Men and woman equally affected, variable expression, reduced penetrance (in some disorders) and advanced paternal age associated with sporadic cases.

Common examples of the autosomal dominant disorders:
- Huntington disease
- Marfan syndrome
- Hereditary breast/ovarian cancer
- Neurofibromatosis type 1
- Colon cancer.

In this example, a man with an autosomal dominant disorder has two affected children and two unaffected children (**Fig. 15.28**).

Autosomal Recessive

Two mutated copies of the gene are present in each cell when a person has an autosomal recessive disorder. An affected person usually has unaffected parents who each carry a single

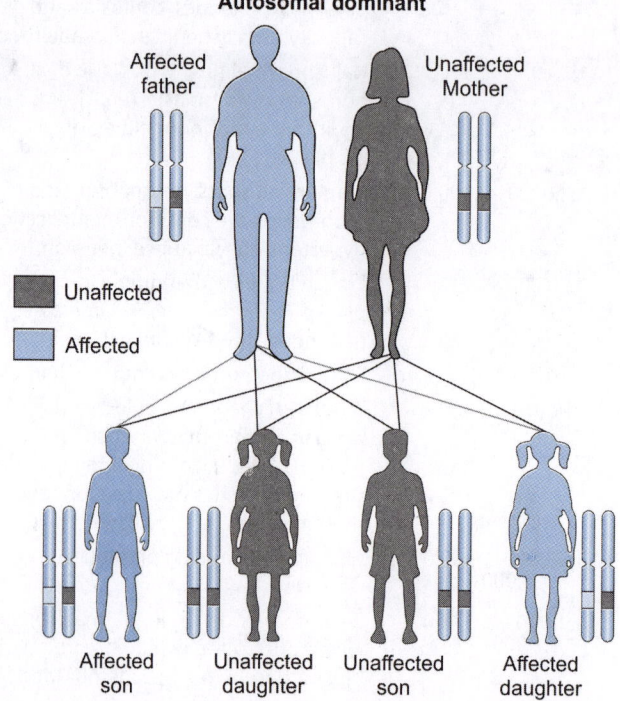

Fig. 15.28: Autosomal dominant pattern of inheritance.

copy of the mutated gene (and are referred to as carriers) **(Fig. 15.29)**. Autosomal recessive disorders are typically not seen in every generation of an affected family. Selective genetic disorders showing autosomal recessive inheritance is given in **Table 15.7**.

Main characteristics of autosomal recessive inheritance and disorders:
- Gene is located on autosome
- Horizontal occurrence seen in families
- Two copies of the mutated gene are needed for phenotypic manifestations
- Male and females are affected in equal number on average
- No sex difference in clinical manifestations
- Family history is usually negative especially for vertical transmission (in more than one generation)
- Other affected individual in family in same generation (horizontal transmission) may be seen
- Consanguinity or relatedness is more often present than in other type of inherited conditions
- Fresh gene mutation is rare
- Age of disease onset is usually early newborn, infancy, early childhood
- Greater negative effect on reproductive fitness
- Associated with particular ethnic groups.

Common examples of the autosomal recessive disorders:
- Cystic fibrosis
- Tay-Sachs disease
- Thalassemia

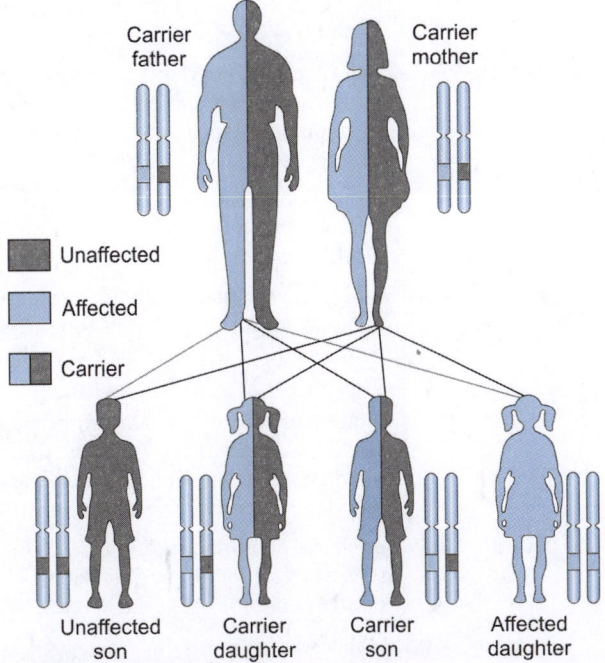

Fig. 15.29: Autosomal recessive pattern of inheritance.

Table 15.7: Selective genetic disorders showing autosomal recessive inheritance.

Disorder	Occurrence	Brief description
Albinism (tyrosinase negative)	1:15,000–1:40,000 1:85-1:630 (in Americans)	Melanin lacking in skin hair and eyes, nystagmus, photophobia, susceptible to neoplasm, strabismus, impaired vision
Argininosuccinic aciduria (ASA)	1: 60,000 - 1: 70,000	Urea cycle disorder, hyperammonemia, mild mental retardation, vomiting, seizures, coma, abnormal hair shaft
Cystic fibrosis	1:2,000- 1:2,500	Pancreatic insufficiency and malabsorption, abnormal exocrine gland, chronic pulmonary disease
Ellis-van Creveld syndrome	Rare	Short-limbed dwarfisms, polydactyly, congenital heart disease, nail anomalies
Glycogen storage disease-Ia (Von Gierke disease)	1:20,000	Glucose-6 phosphatase deficiency, bruising, hypoglycemia, enlarged liver, hyperlipidemia, hypertension, short stature
Glycogen storage disease type II (Pompe disease)	3:100,000– 4.5:100,000	Infant, juvenile and adult form acid maltase deficiency; in infant form cardiac enlargement, cardiomyopathy, hypotonia respiratory insufficiency, developmental delay, macroglossia, death from cardiorespiratory failure by about 2 years of age
Hemochromatosis	1:3,000	Iron storage and tissue damage can result in cirrhosis, diabetes, pancreatitis and other disease, skin pigmentation
Homocystinuria	1:40,000–1:1,40,000	Mental retardation, skeletal defects, lens displacement, tall risk for myocardial infraction, caused by cystathionine beta-synthase deficiency
Metachromatic leukodystrophy	1: 40,000	Arylsulfatase A deficiency leading to disintegration of myelin and accumulation of lipids in white matter of brain, psychomotor degeneration, hypotonia, adult, juvenile and infantile form
Sickle cell disease	1: 400- 1: 600	Hemoglobinopathy with chronic hemolytic anemia, growth retardation, susceptibility to infection, painful crisis, leg ulcers, dactylitis
Tay-Sachs disease	1: 3,600	Progressive mental and motor retardation with onset at about 6 months, poor muscle tone, deafness, blindness, convulsions, decelerate rigidity, death usually by 3–5 years of age
Usher syndrome	Rare	A group of syndrome characterized by congenital sensorineural deafness, visual loss due to retain-iris pigmentations, vestibular ataxia, occasionally mental retardation, speech problems; several sub types
Xeroderma pigmentosa (complementation group XP-A to XP-G)	1:60,000–1:100,000	Defective deoxyribonucleic acid (DNA) repair, sun sensitivity, freckling, atrophic skin lesions, skin cancer develops, photophobia and keratosis, death usually by adulthood

- Sickle cell anemia
- Phyenylketonuria.

In this example, two unaffected parents each carry one copy of a gene mutation for an autosomal recessive disorder. They have one affected child and three unaffected children, two of which carry one copy of the gene mutation **(Fig. 15.29)**.

SEX-LINKED INHERITANCE

X-Linked Dominant

X-linked dominant disorders are caused by mutations in genes on the X chromosome. Females are more frequently affected than males and the chance of passing on an X-linked dominant disorder differs between men and women **(Fig. 15.30)**. Families with an X-linked dominant disorder often have both affected males and affected females in each generation. A striking characteristic of X-linked inheritance is that fathers cannot pass X-linked traits to their sons (no male-to-male transmission). Selective genetic disorders showing X-linked dominant inheritance are given in **Table 15.8**.

Major characteristics of X-linked dominant inheritance and disorders:
- Mutant gene is located on X-chromosome
- One copy of the mutant gene is needed for phenotypic manifestations
- X-inactivation modifies the gene effect in females
- Often lethal in males and so many see transmission only in the female line

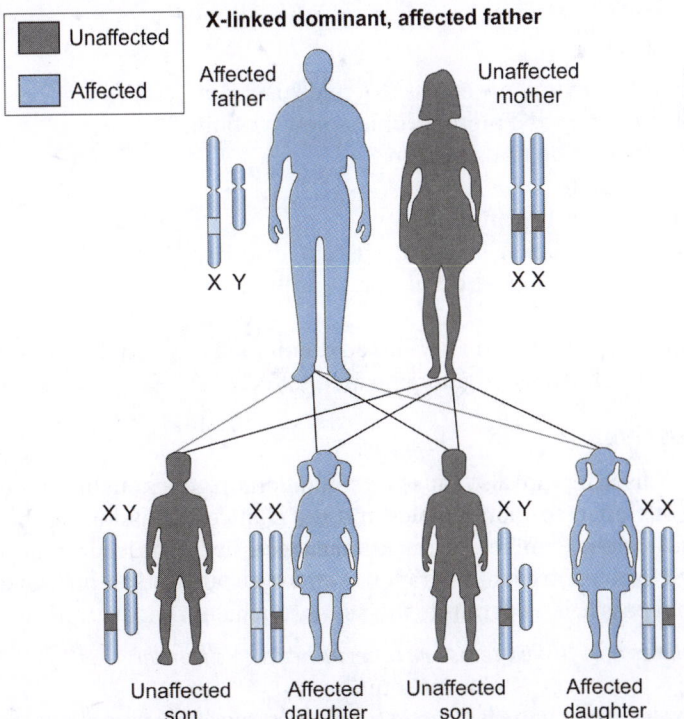

Fig. 15.30: X-linked dominant pattern of inheritance with affected father.

Table 15.8: Selective genetic disorders showing X-linked dominant inheritance.

Disorder	Occurrence	Brief description
Albright osteodystrophy	Rare	Short stature, delayed dentition, brachydactyly, hereditary hypocalcemia pseudohypoparathyroidism, many endocrine problem, muscular atrophy, mineralization of skeleton; round faces, possible intellectual disability, hypertension
Focal dermal hypoplasia	Very rare, exactly unknown	Atrophy, liner pigmentation, papillomas of skin on lips, axilla and umbilicus, digital anomalies, hypoplastic teeth, ocular anomalies (coloboma, microphthalmia)
Lucontincotia pigmenti	Very rare	Irregular swirling pigmentation of skin lesion, dental anomalies, alopecia, intellectual disability common, seizures, uveitis, retinal abnormalities
Ornithine transcarbamylase (OTC) deficiency	1: 80,000 in Japan, rare among others	Inborn error in urea cycle metabolism, failure to thrive hyperammonemia, vomiting, headache, confusion, rigidity, lethargy, seizure, coma, many males die in neonatal period
Orofaciodigital syndrome type-I	1:50,000	Cleft palate, tongue, jaw and/or lip, facial hypoplasia, intellectual disability, syndactyly, short digits polycystic kidney with renal failure
X-linked hypophosphatemia or vitamin D resistant	1: 25,000	Disorder of tubular phosphate transport, bowed legs, growth deficiency, rickets with ultimate short stature, possible hearing loss

- Affected families usually show excess of female offspring (2:1)
- Affected male have affected mother (unless new mutation)
- There is no male-to-male transmission
- There is no carrier state
- Disorders are relatively uncommon.

Common example of the X-linked dominant disorders is Fragile X syndrome. In this example, a man with an X-linked dominant condition has two affected daughters and two unaffected sons **(Fig. 15.30)**.

In this example, a woman with an X-linked dominant condition has an affected daughter, an affected son, an unaffected daughter and an unaffected son **(Fig. 15.31)**.

X-linked Recessive

X-linked recessive disorders are also caused by mutations in genes on the X chromosome. Males are more frequently affected than females and the chance of passing on the disorder differs between men and women. Families with an X-linked recessive disorder often have affected males, but rarely affected females, in each generation. A striking characteristic of X-linked inheritance is that fathers cannot pass X-linked traits to their sons (no male-to-male transmission).

Major characteristics of X-linked recessive inheritance and disorders
- Mutant gene is located on X-chromosome
- One copy of the mutant gene is needed for phenotypic effect in male (hemizygous)
- All daughters of affected males will be carriers, if the mother is normal

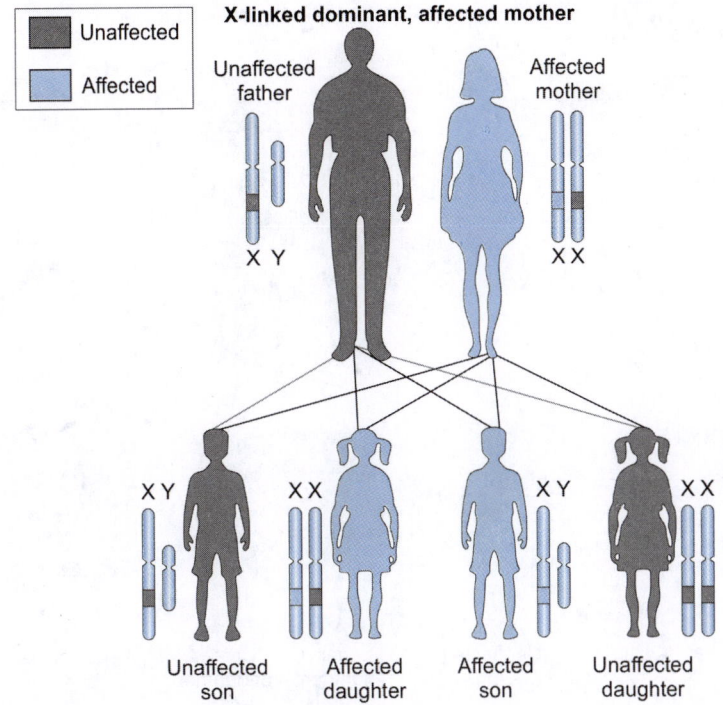

Fig. 15.31: X- linked dominant pattern of inheritance with affected mother.

- All sons of affected males will be normal, if the mother is normal
- Males are more frequently affected than females
- There are some fresh gene mutations
- There is no male-to-male transmission
- Transmission is often through heterozygous (carrier) females
- Two copies of the mutant gene are usually needed for phenotypic effect in females
- Unequal X-inactivation can lead to manifesting heterozygotic in female carriers.

Common examples of the X-linked recessive disorders
- Hemophilia
- Duchenne muscular dystrophy
- Protan and deutan form of color blindness
- Hunter syndrome
- Fabry disease.

In this example, a man with an X-linked recessive condition has two unaffected daughters who each carry one copy of the gene mutation and two unaffected sons who do not have the mutation **(Fig. 15.32)**.

In this example, an unaffected woman carries one copy of a gene mutation for an X-linked recessive disorder. She has an affected son, an unaffected daughter who carries one copy of the mutation and two unaffected children who do not have the mutation **(Fig. 15.33)**.

Few genes are known to be located on the Y chromosome and so this type of inheritance has little clinical significance. Most Y-linked genes manifest their effect with one copy and

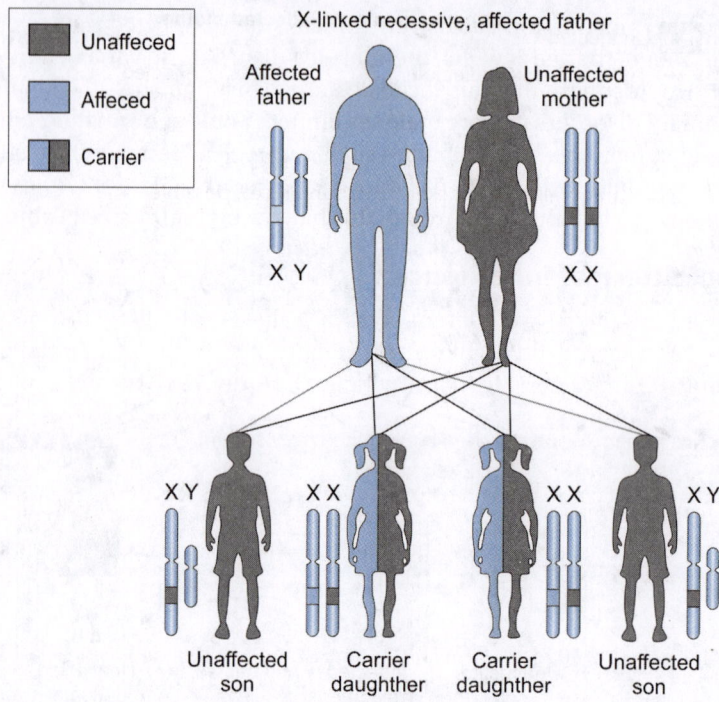

Fig. 15.32: X-linked recessive pattern of inheritance with affected father.

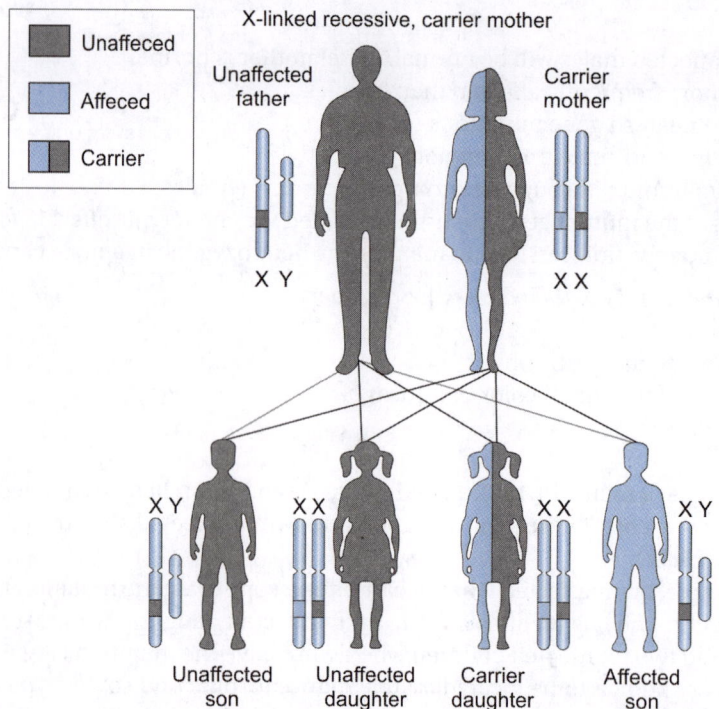

Fig. 15.33: X-linked recessive pattern of inheritance with carrier mother Y-linked (Holandric) Inheritance.

show male-to-male transmission exclusively. All sons of an affected male would eventually develop trait. Although, the age at which they develop disorders do varies. None of the affected male's daughter would inherit the trait. It can be hard to distinguish Y-linked inheritance form autosomal dominant disorders that are male sex limited. Some gene on the Y chromosome are to determine height, male sex determination such as the *'SRY'* gene for the testis determining factor, tooth enamel and size, hairy, ear and finger protein. Male infertility disorder with genetic component can be inherited through this pattern of inheritance **(Table 15.9)**.

Codominant Pattern of Inheritance

In codominant inheritance, two different versions (alleles) of a gene can be expressed and each version makes a slightly different protein **(Fig. 15.34)**. Both alleles influence the genetic trait or determine the characteristics of the genetic condition. For example:

Table 15.9: Selective genetic disorders showing X-linked recessive inheritance.

Disorder	Occurrence	Brief description
Color blindness deutan	8:100	Normal vision actually, defective color vision with green series defect
Duchenne muscular dystrophy	1:3,000–1:5,000	Eventual respiratory insufficiency and death
Fabry disease (diffuse angiokeratoma)	1:40,000	Lipid storage disorder ceramide trihexosidase deficiency, α-galactosidase deficiency, on set in adolescence to adulthood, angina, pain attacks, autonomic dysfunction, angiokeratoma
Glucosc 6-phosphate dehydrogenase (G6 PD) deficiency	1:10–1:50	Enzyme deficiency with subtype shows effect in red blood cells (RBC), usually asymptomatic unless under stress or exposed to certain drugs or infection
Hemophilia-A	1:250- 1:4,000	Coagulation disorder due to coagulation factor X deficiency
Hemophilia-B Christmas disease	14,000–1:7,000	Coagulation disorder due to coagulation factor X deficiency
Hunter syndrome	1:100,000	Mucopolysaccharide storage disorder with iduronate-2-sulfate deficiency, intellectual disability usual hepatomegaly, splenomegaly, dwarfing, stiff joints, hearing loss, mild and severe form
Lesch Nyhan syndrome	Rare	Deficiency of purine metabolism enzyme HPRT; hyperuremia, spasticity, athetosis, self-mutilation, developmental delay
X-linked ichthyosis	1:5,000–1:6,000	Symptoms usual by 3 months may be born with sheets of scales (collodion babies), dry scaling skin often appears as it unwashed, developmental delay, bone changes, vascular complications, corneal opacities, steroid sulfatase deficiency
Menkes disease	1: 200,000	Copper deficiency caused by defective transportation, short stature, seizure, spasticity, hypothermia, kinky, sparse hair (pili torti); intellectual disability

(HPRT: hypoxanthine-guanine phosphoribo syltransferase)

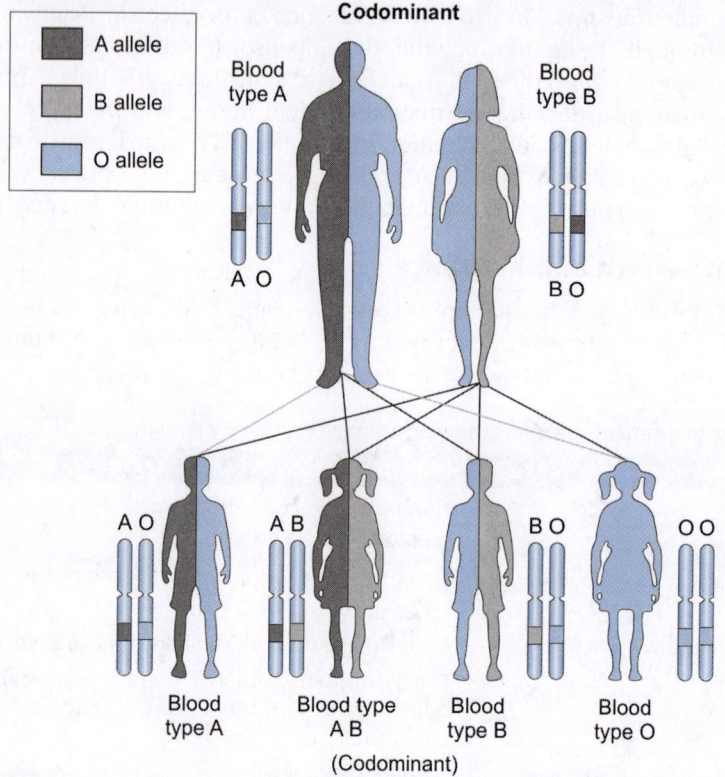

Fig. 15.34: Codominant pattern of inheritance.

- ABO blood group
- α-1 antitrypsin deficiency.

The ABO blood group is a major system for classifying blood types in humans. Blood type AB is inherited in a codominant pattern. In this example, a father with blood type A and a mother with blood type B have four children, each with a different blood type: A, AB, B and O.

Mitochondrial Pattern of Inheritance

Mitochondrial type of inheritance, also known as maternal inheritance, applies to genes in mitochondrial DNA. Mitochondria, which are structures in each cell that convert molecules into energy, each contain a small amount of DNA. Because only egg cells contribute mitochondria to the developing embryo, only females can pass on mitochondrial conditions to their children (Fig. 15.35). Mitochondrial disorders can appear in every generation of a family and can affect both males and females, but fathers do not pass mitochondrial traits to their children. For example, leber's hereditary optic neuropathy (LHON) in one family, a woman with a mitochondrial disorder and her unaffected husband have only affected children. In another family, a man with a mitochondrial condition and his unaffected wife have no affected children.

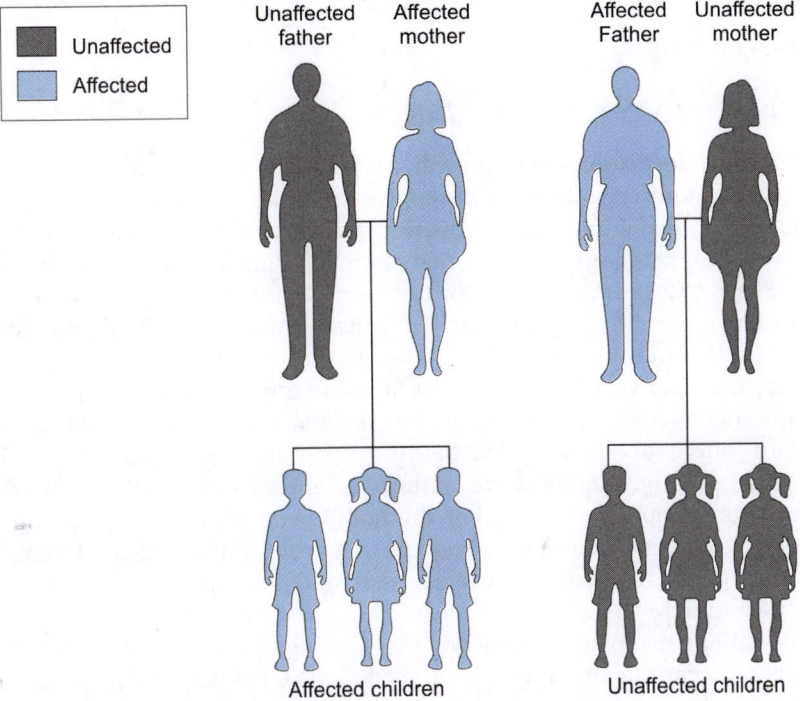

Fig. 15.35: Mitochondrial pattern of inheritance.

Multifactororial Pattern of Inheritance

Multifactororial pattern of inheritance a common cause of many birth defects as well as common adult onset conditions such as diabetes, heart disease and cancer. Multifactorial inheritance conditions are believed to be the result of multiple mutations and environmental influence that combine to cause birth defects or disease. Genetic conditions with a multifactorial cause tend to cluster in families, but do not follow the characteristic pattern of inheritance seen with single gene disorder **(Fig. 15.36)**. Example includes:
- Congenital heart disease
- Cleft lip/palate
- Neural tube defect
- Congenital hip dislocation

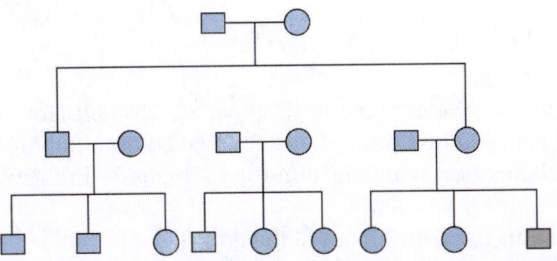

Fig. 15.36: Genetic conditions inherited in a multifactorial manner tend to cluster in families, but do not follow the characteristic pattern of inheritance seen with single gene disorders.

- Diabetes
- High blood pressure.

MENDELIAN THEORY OF INHERITANCE

Genes provide the information for the growth, development and function of our bodies. When a gene is changed, there is a different message sent to the cells. A gene change that makes the genes faulty is called a mutation. A mutated (faulty) gene may cause a problem with the development and functioning of different body systems or organs. However, some faulty genes may be beneficial. Our genes are inherited from our parents, who have inherited theirs from their parents and so on. The great majority of genes come in pairs, the exceptions being the genes on the sex chromosomes (X and Y) of a male. The term Mendelian inheritance applies when a characteristic or set of characteristics is due to the information contained in a single gene pair. The characteristic may be 'usual' or it may not, it could be a genetic condition.

Mendelian inheritance is so called because our understanding of it started with the observations of an Augustinian monk named Gregor Mendel in the 19th century. The inheritance pattern depends on whether the faulty gene is part of one of the numbered chromosomes called an autosome or on the X chromosome, which is one of the sex chromosomes. It also depends on whether the mutation that makes the gene faulty is 'recessive' or 'dominant'.

When the inheritance pattern is known it is possible to provide families and individuals with information regarding the chance (or risk) that the condition will affect themselves and other family members of future generations. Autosomal recessive inheritance, autosomal dominant inheritance, X-linked recessive inheritance and X-linked dominant inheritance are the some Mendelian patterns of inheritance.

MULTIPLE ALLOTS AND BLOOD GROUPS

Multiple Allots

More than two alternative forms of a gene present on the same locus are called 'multiple alleles'. They are produced due to repeated mutation of the same gene, but in different directions. Thus the wild type of allele for red eye color (w+ or W) in *Drosophila melanogaster* mutated to form allele for white eye (w), further mutation in both have incomplete intermediate dominance over one another. Some of these alleles are wine (ww), coral (wco), blood (wbl), cherry (wc), apricot (wa), eosine (we), buff (wb), tinged (wt), honey (wh), ecru (wec), pearl (wp) and ivory (wi). Despite the presence of several alleles of the same gene in a population, an individual can have only two alleles.

Characteristics

- There are more than two alleles of the same gene, e.g. 15 alleles for eye color in *Drosophila*, 3 alleles for blood group in human, 4 alleles for coat color in Rabbit
- All the multiple alleles occur on the same gene locus of the same chromosome or its homologue
- Chromosome contains only one alleles of the group
- An individual possesses only two alleles, while the gametes carry single allele
- Multiple alleles express different alternatives of the same character

- Different alleles show codominance-recessive or intermediate-dominance amongst themselves. However, they follow Mendelian pattern of inheritance.

Blood Group System

Immunogenetics began in 1900 when Karl Landsteiner discovered the ABO blood group system. At this time 26 such systems, plus 5 collections and 2 series are known in humans, but all are not necessarily clinical significance. A six-digit number is given to every blood group antigen in which the first three digits represent the system, collection or series and the second three digit represent the antigen. The system that are best characterized and most important are ABO, Rhesus, Kell Lewis, Duffy, MNSs, Lutheran, P, Kidd, Diego, Yt, Xg, Domfrock, Childol Rodgers and Scianna.

ABO Blood Group System

ABO blood group system in human beings is an example of multiple alleles. Human have four blood groups or blood group phenotypes; A, B, AB and O. The ABO system is the most clinically important, the major alleles present at the ABO locus chromosomes are A, B and O. Both A and B alleles are dominant to the O, but codominant to each other. The A and B alleles code for certain enzymes and glycosyltransferases and add sugar to the H substrate precursor to form the A and B glycoprotein antigen. The O allele does not produce an enzyme. These A and B antigens are not confined to the red cell, but are widely distributed through the body. There are various subtype of the A, B and O alleles with more polymorphisms being revealed by newer DNA technique, but only A1 and A2 appear to have any antigenic importance. The relationship between genotype and blood group is also shown in **Table 15.10** and example of the inheritance of the ABO blood group are illustrated in **Tables 15.11 and 15.12**.

Persons with blood group O are sometimes said to have a 'null' phenotype. Independent of the ABO system are the H and secretor systems. Person with the genotype HH or Hh produce the H substrate, which is the precursor for the A and B antigen and is modified by the enzymes produced by the A and B allele does not produce a transferase, it exerts no effect on this pathway, the H substrate is unmodifiable and more H antigen remains present. The allele h is a rare silent allele recessive to H. Person with hh who have the A and B allele do not express them due to the absence of the H substrate. The secretor (Se, se) locus determines whether the ABH antigen will be secreted in body fluids such as saliva, individuals who are nonsecretors (se, se) do not secrete ABH antigens. Approximately 80% of the white population is secretors. The secretor gene appears to have a regulatory function on the 'H' gene.

The clinical significance of this relationship is illustrated by the case of women who contacted the genetic counseling center at Postgraduate Institute of Medical Education and Research (PGIMER), Chandigarh. She was believed to have blood group O, her husband was A and her child was AB, she had been told by the local health professionals that this was not

Table 15.10: Relationship in ABO blood group system.

Blood group (phenotype)	Genotype(s)	Red cell antigen(s)	Antibodies in serum
A	AO, AA	A (+H)	Anti-B
B	BO, BB	B (+H)	Anti-A
AB	AB	A,B (+H)	None
O	OO	H	Anti-A

Table 15.11: Chart showing inheritance of blood groups by children of various parentages.

Blood group of mother	Blood group of father	O		A		B		AB	
	Blood group allele in sperm								
	Blood group allele in ova	O	O	A	O	B	O	A	B
O	O	OO (O)	OO (O)	AO (A)	OO (O)	BO (B)	OO (O)	AO (A)	BO (B)
	O	OO (O)	OO (O)	AO (A)	OO (O)	BO (B)	OO (O)	AO (A)	BO (B)
A	A	AO (A)	AO (A)	AA (A)	AO (A)	AB (AB)	AO (A)	AA (A)	AB (AB)
	O	OO (O)	OO (O)	AO (A)	OO (O)	BO (B)	OO (B)	AB (AB)	BO (B)
B	B	BO (B)	BO (B)	AB (AB)	BO (B)	BB (B)	BO (B)	AB (AB)	BB (B)
	O	OO (B)	OO (O)	AO (A)	OO (O)	BO (B)	OO (O)	AO (A)	BO (B)
Ab	A	AO (A)	AO (A)	AA (A)	AO (A)	AB (AB)	AO (A)	AA (A)	AB (AB)
	B	BO (B)	BO (B)	AB (AB)	BO (B)	BB (B)	BO (B)	AB (B)	BB (B)

*Every column presents offspring genotype of blood group and letters in parentheses are possible blood group phenotype of offspring.

Table 15.12: Example of transmission of blood group genes (ABO system*).

Parents	AO × BO	AB × OO	AA × BB	AA × BO	AB × BB	BB × OO
Offspring genotype	AB, AO, BO, OO	AO, BO	AB	AB, AO	AB, BB	BO
Theoretical proposition of each pregnancy	¼, ¼, ¼, ¼	½, ½	All	½, ½	½, ½	All
Blood group phenotype	AB, A, B, O	A, B	AB	AB, A	AB, B	B

*Not all possible combinations are shown.

possible unless her husband was not the child's father. The situation was causing considerable stress in their married relationship. Investigation demonstrated that she in fact had the B allele, but was homozygous for the rare Bombay phenotype known as hh. B antigen production was blocked by the two h alleles, even though she had one B gene. This client had contacted the genetic counseling center on her own. The health professionals involved in this case had simply accepted what they considered to be the most likely explanation, without further investigation or consultation. Rare cases of other variance are known. This is an example of why it is necessary to recognize the limits of one's own knowledge. Another approach would have been to do DNA testing to establish parentage.

A human being carries two of the three alleles, one from each parent. The maximum number of possible genotype is six for the four phenotypes. The phenotypes are tested by two antisera, anti-A and anti-B.

Table 15.13: Example of transmission of blood group genes (Rh system).

Parents	DD × dd	Dd × dd	Dd × Dd
Offspring genotype	DD	Dd, dd	DD, Dd, dd
Theoretical proposition of each pregnancy	All	½, ½	¼, ½, ¼
Blood group phenotype	Rh (+)	Rh (+), Rh (-)	Rh (+), Rh (+), Rh (-)

Rhesus (Rh) System

It was not until 1940 that Landsteiner and Wiener discovered the rhesus (Rh) system. This system has become increasingly more complex. Many variants and about 45 antigens are known and various symbols have been used to describe the major components. The most common the one proposed by Fisher, Race and Sanger, reflected the existence of three very closely linked lock C, D or d (ho d) antiserum for the 'd' antigen has been found and those who are RhD negative actually lack the gene; however 'd' is used here for convenience and E or C and E alleles are much less antigenic than D. the D alleles are considered responsible for determining Rh positivity (+) in a dominant relationship to 'd'. This inheritance pattern is illustrated in **Table 15.13**; the percentage of Rh negative individuals in the white population is approximately 15%, few native Americans or Asians are Rh negative. In the black population approximately 7% are Rh negative.

FACTS ABOUT TRANSMISSION OF GENETIC DISORDERS

When a genetic disorder is diagnosed in a family, family members often want to know the likelihood that they or their children will develop the condition. This can be difficult to predict in some cases because many factors influence a person's chances of developing a genetic condition. One important factor is how the condition is inherited. For example:

- **Autosomal dominant inheritance:** A person affected by an autosomal dominant disorder has a 50% chance of passing the mutated gene to each child. The chance that a child will not inherit the mutated gene is also 50%.
- **Autosomal recessive inheritance:** Two unaffected people who each carry one copy of the mutated gene for an autosomal recessive disorder (carriers) have a 25% chance with each pregnancy of having a child affected by the disorder. The chance with each pregnancy of having an unaffected child who is a carrier of the disorder is 50% and the chance that a child will not have the disorder and will not be a carrier is 25%.
- **X-linked dominant inheritance:** The chance of passing on an X-linked dominant condition differs between men and women because men have one X chromosome and one Y chromosome, while women have two X chromosomes. A man passes on his Y chromosome to all of his sons and his X chromosome to all of his daughters. Therefore, the sons of a man with an X-linked dominant disorder will not be affected, but all of his daughters will inherit the condition. A woman passes on one or the other of her X chromosomes to each child. Therefore, a woman with an X-linked dominant disorder has a 50% chance of having an affected daughter or son with each pregnancy.
- **X-linked recessive inheritance:** Because of the difference in sex chromosomes, the probability of passing on an X-linked recessive disorder also differs between men and women. The sons of a man with an X-linked recessive disorder will not be affected and his

daughters will carry one copy of the mutated gene. With each pregnancy, a woman who carries an X-linked recessive disorder has a 50% chance of having sons who are affected and a 50% chance of having daughters who carry one copy of the mutated gene.
- **Codominant inheritance:** In codominant inheritance, each parent contributes a different version of a particular gene and both versions influence the resulting genetic trait. The chance of developing a genetic condition with codominant inheritance and the characteristic features of that condition, depend on which versions of the gene are passed from parents to their child.
- **Mitochondrial inheritance:** Mitochondria, which are the energy-producing centers inside cells, each contain a small amount of DNA. Disorders with mitochondrial inheritance result from mutations in mitochondrial DNA. Although, mitochondrial disorders can affect both males and females, only females can pass mutations in mitochondrial DNA to their children. A woman with a disorder caused by changes in mitochondrial DNA will pass the mutation to all of her daughters and sons, but the children of a man with such a disorder will not inherit the mutation.

It is important to note that the chance of passing on a genetic condition applies equally to each pregnancy. For example, if a couple has a child with an autosomal recessive disorder, the chance of having another child with the disorder is still 25% (or 1 in 4). Having one child with a disorder does not 'protect' future children from inheriting the condition. Conversely, having a child without the condition does not mean that future children will definitely be affected.

Although the chances of inheriting a genetic condition appear straightforward, factors such as a person's family history and the results of genetic testing can sometimes modify those chances. In addition, some people with a disease causing mutation never develop any health problems or may experience only mild symptoms of the disorder. If a disease that runs in a family does not have a clear-cut inheritance pattern, predicting the likelihood that a person will develop the condition can be particularly difficult.

Estimating the chance of developing or passing on a genetic disorder can be complex. Genetics professionals can help people understand these chances and help them make informed decisions about their health.

MECHANISM OF INHERITANCE

Heredity is the transmission of genetic character from parents to the offspring. Gregor Johann Mendel (1866) proposed that inheritance is controlled by paired germinal units or factors, now called genes. They are present in all cells of the body and are transferred to the next generation through gametes. Factors or genes are thus physical basis of heredity. They represent small segment of chromosomes. Genes are passed from one generation to the next generation or from one cell to its daughter cell as components of chromosome (chromosomal basis of heredity). The genetic material present in chromosomes is DNA. Genes are the segment of DNA called citrons. Therefore, DNA is the chemical basis of heredity.

Inheritance refers to, how genetic information is passed down from one generation to next generation. The basic features of mechanism of inheritance are as follows:
- Genes or chromosomes are physical basis of inheritance
- Person inherits half of the genetic information from each parent
- Every gene has two copies of genes and each parent contributes for one copy of gene to their offspring

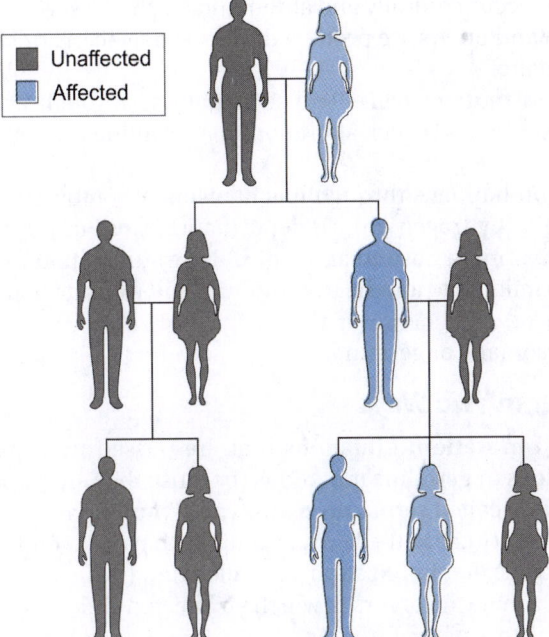

Fig. 15.37: Mechanism of inheritance.

- Genes for different traits are inherited separately from one another. For example, the gene for hair color is not linked with the gene for height. A child may have his mothers' hair color, but may not her height. For the most part, each trait is inherited separately.

A particular disorder might be described as 'running in a family' if more than one person in the family has the condition. Some disorders that affect multiple family members are caused by gene mutations, which can be inherited (passed down from parent to child). Other conditions that appear to run in families are not inherited. Instead, environmental factors such as dietary habits or a combination of genetic and environmental factors are responsible for these disorders **(Fig. 15.37)**.

GENE MUTATION (ERRORS OF TRANSMISSION)

Gene mutation are new sudden inheritable discontinuous variations, which are caused by a change in the nucleotide type and sequence of a DNA segment representing a gene. In other words, a gene mutation is a permanent change in the DNA base sequence that makes up a gene. Mutations range in size from a single DNA building block (DNA base) to a large segment of a chromosome. The first recorded gene mutations are ancon sheep (1791) and hornless (polled) cattle (1889). Following are the main features of the gene mutation:
- All genes can mutate, however, mutability differs from gene to gene
- The direction of gene mutation cannot be predictable; it can occur in any possible direction to any possible degree
- A mutated gene can mutate back to its permutation state
- Gene mutation can be lethal, harmful, neutral or advantageous
- Most of the mutations are recessive and involve loss of function; a few are dominant ones

- The gene mutation may occur naturally and automatically due to several reason, termed as spontaneous mutation and others are produced by external factors or chemicals, they are termed as induced mutations
- Individuals also possess mutator genes (cause mutations through altering polymerase activity) and antimutator genes (check alteration in nucleotide through sequence during replication)
- A spontaneous mutation happens through mechanisms of tautomerism (a base change by the repositioning of a hydrogen atom), depurination (loss of purine base—A or G), deamination (change a normal base to an atypical base), transition (a purine change to another purine or a pyrimidine to another pyrimidine) and transversion (a purine become a pyrimidine or vice versa)
- Mutation can occur in somatic or germinal cells.

Gene Mutations Occur in Two Ways

- **Germline or inherited mutation:** Mutations that are passed from parent to child are called inherited mutations or germline mutations (because they are present in the egg and sperm cells, which are also called germ cells). This type of mutation is present throughout a person's life in virtually every cell in the body. Mutations that occur only in an egg or sperm cell, or those that occur just after fertilization, are called new (de novo) mutations. De novo mutations may explain genetic disorders in which an affected child has a mutation in every cell, but has no family history of the disorder.
- **Somatic or acquired mutation:** Acquired during a person's lifetime. Acquired (or somatic) mutations occur in the DNA of individual cells at some time during a person's life. These changes can be caused by environmental factors such as ultraviolet radiation from the sun or can occur if a mistake is made as DNA copies itself during cell division. Acquired mutations in somatic cells (cells other than germ cells) cannot be passed on to the next generation. Mutations may also occur in a single cell within an early embryo. As all the cells divide during growth and development, the individual will have some cells with the mutation and some cells without the genetic change. This situation is called mosaicism.

    Some genetic changes are very rare: Others are common in the population. Genetic changes that occur in more than 1% of the population are called polymorphisms. They are common enough to be considered a normal variation in the DNA. Polymorphisms are responsible for many of the normal differences between people such as eye color, hair color and blood type. Although, polymorphisms generally have no negative effects on a person's health, some of these variations may influence the risk of developing certain disorders.

Causes of Gene Mutation

Any extracellular physical or chemical factor, which can cause mutation or increase the frequency of mutation in an individual is called as mutagen.

Physical Factors

Physical factor that cause gene mutation are two types, temperatures and high-energy radiations:
1. **Temperature:** Increase in temperature increase the rate of mutations. Rise in temperature breaks the hydrogen bonding between the two strands of DNA and hence denatures the letters.
2. **High-energy radiations:** They include neutrons, α-particles, cosmic rays, γ-particles, β-rays, X-rays, ultraviolet rays, etc. Ultraviolet rays are non-ionizing radiations, which

affect DNA by forming thymine dimers. It causes bends in DNA duplex that bring about mis replication. Other high-energy radiations are ionizing radiations. They ionize DNA constituents that can react with several biochemicals, X-rays are known to deaminate and dehydroxylate nitrogen bases, from peroxides and oxidize deoxyribose.

Chemical Factors

They are of several types. The common ones are nitrogen acid, alkylating agents, base analogues and acridines. Even some of drugs are known to cause gene mutation, like chemotherapeutic drugs for cancer.

Types or Mechanism of Gene Mutation

The smallest part of a gene that undergoes mutation is known as muton. It can be as small as a single nucleotide. Most of the gene mutations involve change in only a single nucleotide or nitrogen base. These gene mutations are called 'point mutations'. A mutation involving more than one base pair is termed as 'gross mutation'. Gene mutation usually occurs during replication of DNA. It is therefore, also called as 'copy error mutation'. During gene mutation a gene may undergo several point mutations. This produces multiple alleles. Gene mutations have varying effects on health, depending on where they occur and whether they alter the function of essential proteins. The DNA sequence of a gene can be altered in a number of ways. The main types or methods of gene mutations are as follows:

Inversion mutation

A distortion of DNA by mutagen can change the base sequence of a gene in the reverse order. The process is called inversion. The new sequence will naturally have different codones. For example, there is reverse order of DNA base after mutation **(Fig. 15.38)**.

Substitution Mutation (Replacement)

In substitution a nitrogen base is changed with another. It is of two type, transition and transversion.
1. **Transition mutation:** A nitrogen base is replaced by another of its type, i.e. one purine is replaced by another purine (adenine ↔ guanine), while one pyrimidine by another

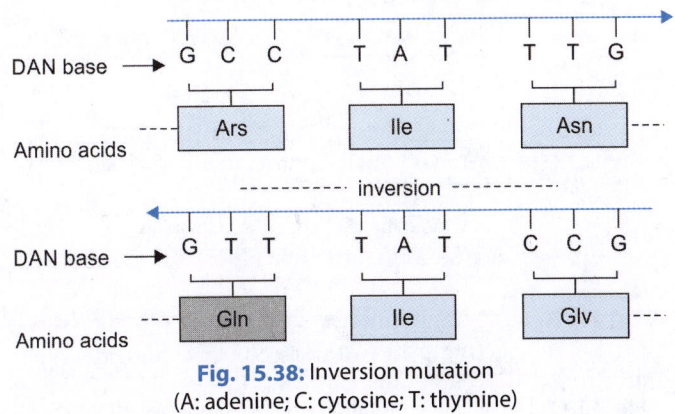

Fig. 15.38: Inversion mutation
(A: adenine; C: cytosine; T: thymine)

pyrimidine (cytosine ↔ thymine or uracil). In example, a purine (guanine) is replaced by another purine (adenine) **(Fig. 15.39)**.

2. **Transversion mutation:** Hence, a purine base is replaced or substituted by a pyrimidine base and vice versa, e.g. uracil or thymine with adenine and cytosine with guanine. For example, cytosine replaced guanine as shown in **Figures 15.40 and 15.41** thymine replaced adenine.

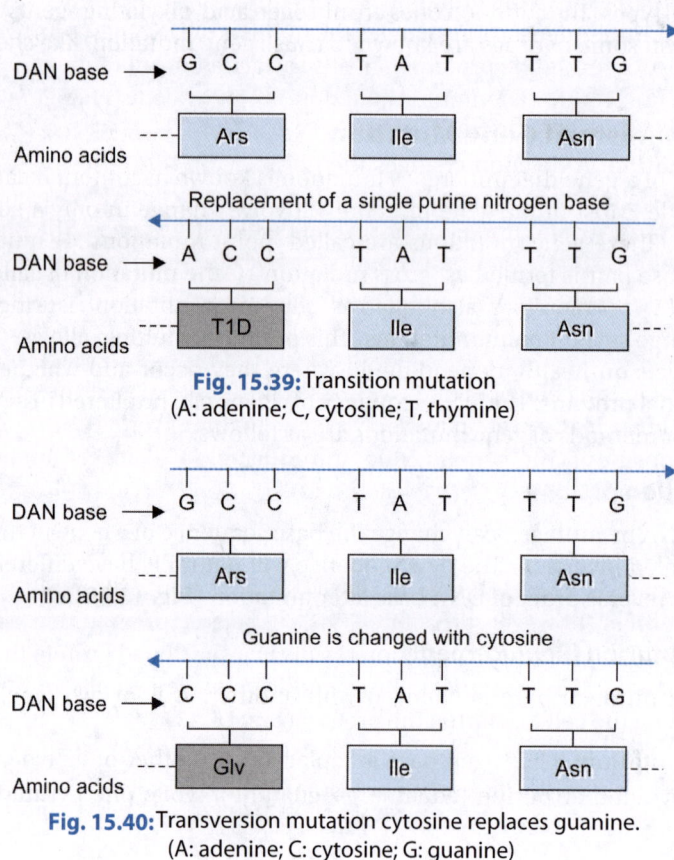

Fig. 15.39: Transition mutation
(A: adenine; C, cytosine; T, thymine)

Fig. 15.40: Transversion mutation cytosine replaces guanine.
(A: adenine; C: cytosine; G: guanine)

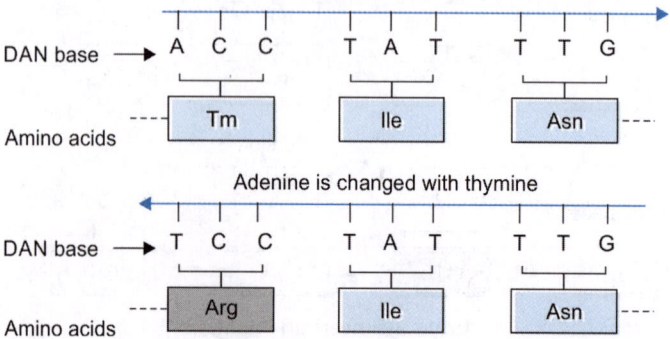

Fig. 15.41: Transversion mutation (thymine replaces adenine).

Frame-shift Mutation

They are those mutations in which the reading of the frame of base sequence shift laterally either in the forward direction due to insertion (addition) of one or more nucleotide or in the backward direction due to deletion of one or more nucleotides. Therefore, frame-shift mutations are of two kinds—insertion and deletion. A frame-shift mutation changes the amino acid sequence from the site of the mutation.

- **Insertion mutation:** An insertion changes the number of DNA bases in a gene by adding a piece of DNA. As a result, the protein made by the gene may not function properly. In this example, one nucleotide (adenine) is added in the DNA code, changing the amino acid sequence that follows **(Fig. 15.42)**.
- **Deletion mutation:** A deletion changes the number of DNA bases by removing a piece of DNA. Small deletions may remove one or a few base pairs within a gene, while larger deletions can remove an entire gene or several neighboring genes. The deleted DNA may alter the function of the resulting protein(s). For example, one nucleotide (adenine) is deleted from the DNA code, changing the amino acid sequence that follows **(Fig. 15.43)**.

Missense Mutation

This type of mutation is a change in one DNA base pair that results in the substitution of one amino acid for another in the protein made by a gene. In this example, the nucleotide adenine is replaced by cytosine in the genetic code, introducing an incorrect amino acid into the protein sequence **(Fig. 15.44)**.

Nonsense Mutation

A nonsense mutation is also a change in one DNA base pair. Instead of substituting one amino acid for another, however, the altered DNA sequence prematurely signals the cell to stop building a protein. This type of mutation results in a shortened protein that may function improperly or not at all. For example, the nucleotide cytosine is replaced by thymine in the DNA code, signaling the cell to shorten the protein **(Fig. 15.45)**.

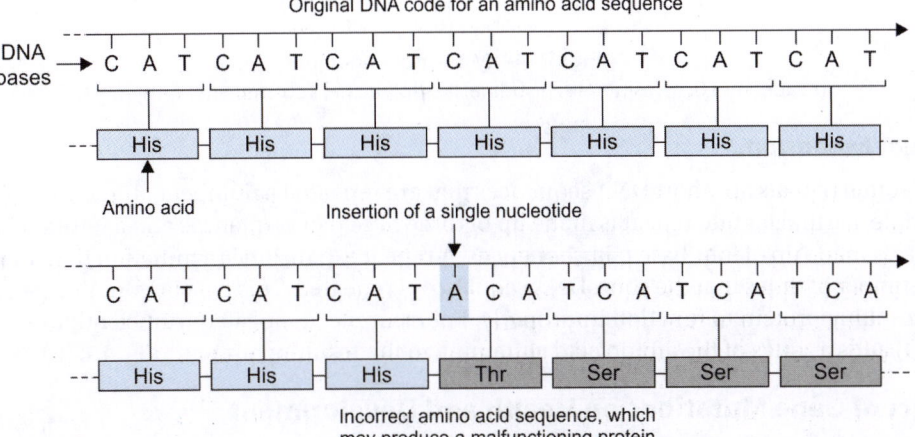

Fig. 15.42: Insertion mutation.

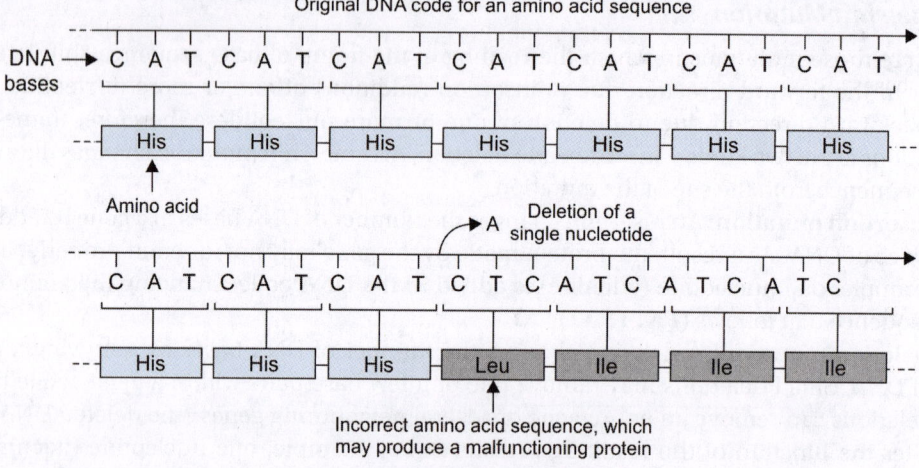

Fig. 15.43: Deletion mutation.
(A: adenine; C: cytosine; His: histidine; ile: isoleucine; Leu: peucine; T: thymine)

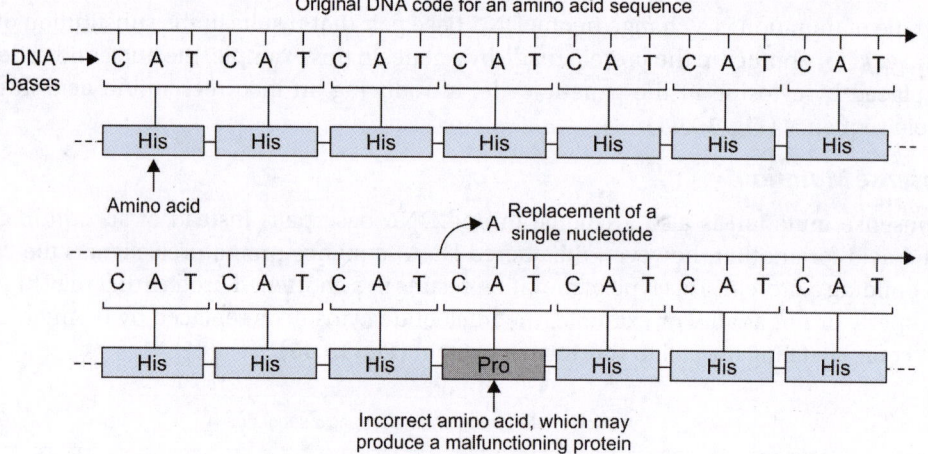

Fig. 15.44: Missense mutation.
(A: adenine; C: cytosine; His: histidine; ile: isoleucine; Leu: peucine; T: thymine)

Repeat Expansion

Nucleotide repeats are short DNA sequences that are repeated a number of times in a row. For example, a trinucleotide repeat is made up of three base pair sequences and a tetranucleotide repeat is made up of four base pair sequences. A repeat expansion is a mutation that increases the number of times that the short DNA sequence is repeated. This type of mutation can cause the resulting protein to function improperly. For example, a repeated trinucleotide sequence (CAG) adds a series of the amino acid glutamine to the resulting protein **(Fig. 15.46)**.

Effect of Gene Mutations on Health and Development

- To function correctly, each cell depends on thousands of proteins to do their jobs in the right places at the right times. Sometimes, gene mutations prevent one or more of these

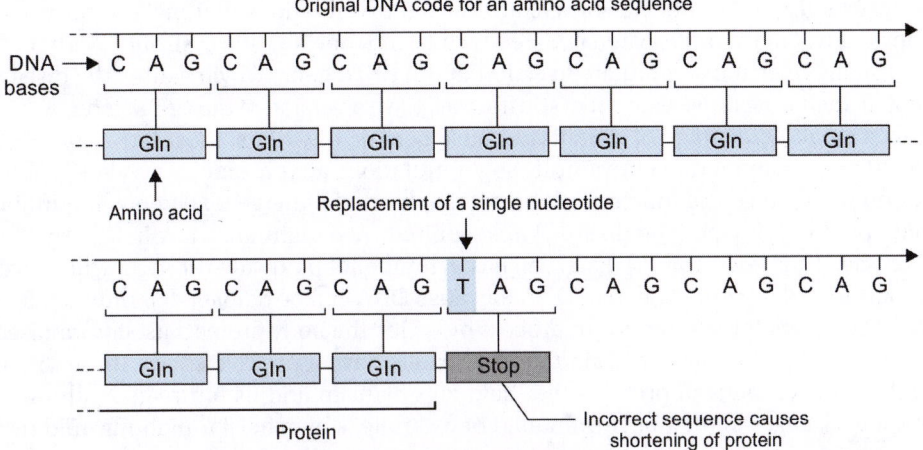

Fig. 15.45: Nonsense mutation.
(A: adenine; C: cytosine; G: guanine; Gln: glutamine; T: thymine).

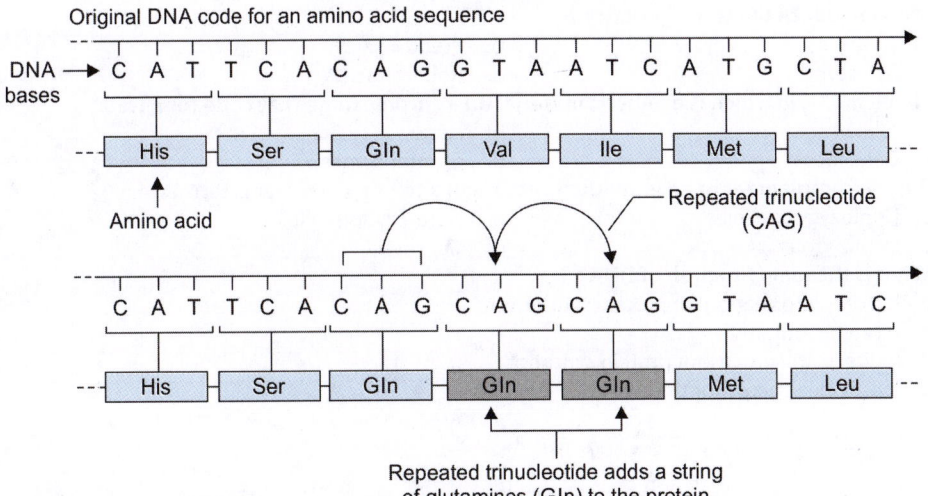

Fig. 15.46: repeat expnsion.

(A: adenine; C: cytosine; G: guanine; His: histidine; Ile: isoleucine; Leu: leucine; Ser: serine; T: thymine; Val: valine)

proteins from working properly. By changing a gene's instructions for making a protein, a mutation can cause the protein to malfunction or to be missing entirely. When a mutation alters a protein that plays a critical role in the body, it can disrupt normal development or cause a medical condition. A condition caused by mutations in one or more genes is called a genetic disorder.

- In some cases, gene mutations are so severe that they prevent an embryo from surviving until birth. These changes occur in genes that are essential for development and often disrupt the development of an embryo in its earliest stages. Because these mutations have very serious effects, they are incompatible with life. It is important to note that genes themselves do not cause disease. Genetic disorders are caused by mutations that make a gene function improperly. For example, when people say that someone has 'the cystic fibrosis gene', they are usually referring to a mutated version of the *CFTR* gene, which causes the disease. All people, including those without cystic fibrosis, have a version of the *CFTR* gene.

- Only a small percentage of mutations cause genetic disorders; most have no impact on health or development. For example, some mutations alter a gene's DNA base sequence, but do not change the function of the protein made by the gene. Often, gene mutations that could cause a genetic disorder are repaired by certain enzymes before the gene is expressed (makes a protein). Each cell has a number of pathways through which enzymes recognize and repair mistakes in DNA. Because DNA can be damaged or mutated in many ways, DNA repair is an important process by which the body protects itself from disease.

A very small percentage of all mutations actually have a positive effect. These mutations lead to new versions of proteins that help an organism and its future generations better adapt to changes in their environment. For example, a beneficial mutation could result in a protein that protects the organism from a new strain of bacteria.

MULTIPLE CHOICE QUESTIONS

1. **Who introduce the term 'genetics'?**
   a. Aristotle
   b. Freud
   c. Bateson
   d. Robert Koch
2. **Name the term which is a genetic material on a chromosome that code for a trait.**
   a. Allele
   b. Gene
   c. Gene locus
   d. Chromosomes
3. **A gene complement of an individual with regard to one character is termed as:**
   a. Homozygous alleles
   b. Heterozygous alleles
   c. Hemizygous
   d. Genotype
4. **What is the main function of DNA?**
   a. It stores information for protein synthesis
   b. It can be mutated
   c. It directs the process of protein synthesis
   d. It provides energy for the cell

Answer Key

1. c   2. b   3. d   4. d

FURTHER READING

1. American Society of Human Genetics/American College of Medical Genetics. Points to consider: Ethical, legal and psychosocial implications of genetic testing in children and adolescents. Am J Hum Genet. 1995;57:1223-41.
2. Beauchamp TL, Childress JF. Principles of Biomedical Ethics. New York: Oxford University Press; 1994.
3. Billings PR, Kohn MA, de Cuevas M, et al. Discrimination as a consequence of genetic testing. Am J Hum Genet. 1992;50:476-82.
4. Bove C, Fry ST, MacDonald DJ. Presymptomatic and predisposition genetic testing: ethical and social considerations. Semin Oncol Nurs. 1997;13:135-40.
5. Clayton (Ed). 50 Years of DNA. Palgrave MacMillan Press, 2003. ISBN 978-1-40-391479-8.
6. Enkins J. Educational issues related to cancer genetics. Semin Oncol Nurs. 1997;13(2):141-4.
7. Fiers W, Contreras R, Duerinck F, et al. Complete nucleotide-sequence of bacteriophage MS2-RNA: primary and secondary structure of replicase gene. Nature. 1976;260(5551):500-7.

8. Havens DMH, Kovner R. Genetic testing: how it is transforming the role of health professionals and the implications for pediatric nurse practitioners. J Pediatric Health Care. 1997;11(4):193-7.
9. Holtzman NA, Watson MS. Promoting safe and effective genetic testing in the United States: Final report of the task force on genetic testing. J Child Fam Nurs. 1999;2(5):388-90.
10. Judson, Horace Freeland. The Eighth Day of Creation: Makers of the Revolution in Biology, Cold Spring Harbor Laboratory Press, 1996. ISBN 978-0-87-969478.
11. Lippman-Hand A, Fraser FC. Genetic counseling: provision and reception of information. Am J Hum Genet. 1979;(2):113-27.
12. Love RR, Evans AM, Josten DM. The accuracy of patient reports of a family history of cancer. J Chronic Dis. 1985;38(4):289-93.
13. MacDonald DJ. The oncology nurse's role in cancer risk assessment and counseling. Semin Oncol Nurs. 1997;13(2):123-8
14. Matloff ET, Peshkin BN. Complexities in cancer genetic counseling: Breast and ovarian cancer. Principles and Practice of Oncology Updates. 1998;12:1-11.
15. Michie 5, Bron F, Bobrow M, et al. Nondirectiveness in genetic counseling: an empirical study. Am J Hum Genet. 1997;60(1):40-7.
16. National Human Genome Research Institute. Avaibale from: https://www.genome.gov/genetics-glossary/Dominant/ revised 19.01.2022.
17. National Society of Genetic Counselors. Code of Ethics. 1992.
18. National Society of Genetic Counselors. Position Statements. 1991.
19. Offit K. Clinical Cancer Genetics: Risk Counseling and Management. New York: Wiley-Liss publication;1998, 249.
20. Olby, Robert. The Path to The Double Helix: Discovery of DNA, first published in October 1974 by MacMillan, with Foreword by Francis Crick; ISBN 978-0-48-668117-7; the definitive DNA textbook, revised in 1994, with a 9 page postscript.
21. Peters J, Stopfer J. Role of the genetic counselor in familial cancer. Oncology. 1996;10:159-75.
22. Rassoulzadegan M., et al. Nature, doi:10.1038/nature04674, 2006.
23. Reilly PR, Boshar MF, Holzman SH. Ethical issues in genetic research: Disclosure and informed consent. Nat Genet. 1997;15:16-20.
24. Ridley, Matt. Francis Crick: Discoverer of the Genetic Code (Eminent Lives) first published in June 2006 in the USA and then to be in the UK September 2006, by HarperCollins Publishers; 192 pp, ISBN 978-0-06-082333-7.
25. Rieger PT. Overview of cancer and genetics: Implications for nurse practitioners. Nurse Practitioner Forum. 1998;9:122-33.
26. Rothenberg K, Fuller B, Rothstein M, et al. Genetic information and the workplace: Legislative approaches and policy changes. Science. 1997;275:1755-7.
27. Rothenberg KH. Genetic discrimination and health insurance: A call for legislative action. J Am Med Womens Assoc. 1997;52:43-44.
28. Rowland LP. Molecular basis of genetic heterogeneity: Role of the clinical neurologist. J Child Neurol. 1998; 13:122-32.
29. Savage R, Armstrong D. Effect of a general practitioner's consulting style on patients' satisfaction: A controlled study. BMJ. 1990;301:968-70.
30. Scanlon C, Fibison W. Managing Genetic Information: Implications for Nursing Practice. Washington DC: American Nurses Association; 1995.
31. Schneider KA. Counseling About Cancer: Strategies for Genetic Counselors. Denni sport: Graphic Illusions; 1994.
32. Shiloh S, Saxe L. Perception of risk in genetic counseling. Psychological Health. 1989;3:45-61.
33. Walker AP. Historical perspective and philosophical perspective of genetic counseling. In: Emery AEH, Rimoin DL, Connor JM, (Eds). Principles and Practice of Medical Genetics, 3rd edition. New York: Churchill-Livingstone; 1996.
34. Wertz DC, Fanos JH, Reilly PR. Genetic testing for children and adolescents. Who decides? JAMA. 1994;272:875-81.

CHAPTER 16

Emerging Paradigm of Genetics in Nursing

Suresh Sharma

INTRODUCTION

In a last few years, genetic nursing practice has been transformed from a nearly hidden specialty to a recognized specialty practice with formal recognition, publication of scope and standards of practice, and most recently the availability of credentialing for genetic nurses. All areas of nursing practice have been impacted by recent advances in genetic knowledge and technology. Nearly all diseases are now recognized to have a genetic component. Nurses now provide education to patients about hereditary risk for developing disease, counsel about the benefits and risks associated with genetic testing, and manage disease risk based on genetic information.

The recent development of commercial testing for susceptibility genes (such as the predisposition genes for hereditary breast and ovarian cancer (HBOC) syndrome, have had a great impact on nursing's role in the identification and management of individuals at risk for developing many diseases. These developments have led to tremendous changes in genetic nursing practice. Nurses have been involved in managing genetic information since 1960's, when nurses provided services to children with genetic disorders and their families. Although in some respects, the nurse's role today in managing genetic information and caring for individuals and families at risk for or diagnosed with genetic diseases or conditions is similar to this traditional role, the scope of practice is much broader and more encompassing. What has also changed, according to Forsman, is the amount of genetic information available and the population to which this information may be applied. We now know that genetic changes contribute to most, if not all diseases. Consequently, the scope of genetic knowledge application in nursing is limitless. "Nursing can ignore genetics no longer. The time for meaningful action is now".

There is an opportunity for nursing to practice health promotion tailored to highly specific and uniquely personal predispositions; in other words, for individualized health care, nurses can offer care that protects patients and families from the risks associated with genetic information, including addressing family issues. Nurses are also needed to refer patients to genetic specialists and assist patients in making choices as a genetic health care. Every nurse is needed; do not miss the revolution. All nurses have a role in the delivery of genetic services and the management of genetic information. Nurses require genetic knowledge to identify, refer, support and care for persons affected by or at risk for genetic conditions.

"Genetic nursing is a holistic practice that includes assessing, planning, implementing, and evaluating the physical, spiritual, ethical and psychosocial aspects of patients and families who have genetic concerns." Genetic nurses practice in many different environments. Genetic nursing practice includes client and family assessment to identify genetic risk factors and intervention, information, service and referral needs; take a detailed family history and construct a pedigree, analyze the assessment data, provide genetic education, and develop and carry out a plan of care to address genetic concerns. In addition, nurses in genetics provide genetic counseling, order and interpret genetic tests if within their scope of practice, and provide surveillance and management of persons affected by or at risk for genetic conditions.

In oncology, for example, areas of responsibility begin with risk assessments for cancer in patients and family members. This assessment includes a detailed family history, construction of a pedigree and assessment of hereditary, environmental and lifestyle cancer risk factors. Once these risk factors are determined, the information is interpreted to the patient. Recommendations for cancer prevention and early detection can be tailored to the specific risks identified. If genetic testing for a cancer susceptibility gene is appropriate, the individual/family should be informed about the risks and benefits associated with the test, and the potential risks and benefits associated with the screening and prevention measures. The nurse also needs to explore possible psychosocial responses to the potential outcomes of a genetic test. This education may be done individually or with several family members. If testing is pursued, results are disclosed in person. At that point, a tailored plan for prevention and early detection is written and given to the family or individual. Long-term follow-up includes assessment of adjustment to the test results, and compliance and follow-through with the plan for cancer prevention and early detection.

GENETIC NURSING PRACTICE MILESTONES

Genetic nursing practice has seen several memorable milestones in less than 5 years. In the past, there has been minimal recognition of the important role that nurses can play in genetics. The International Society of Nurses in Genetics (ISONG) has clearly been the leader in working with nursing leaders to promote genetic nursing practice and develop a credentialing process for genetic nurses. Through these efforts, only 5 years ago, the American Nurses Association established genetic nursing as an official specialty of nursing practice.

- **1960:** Nurses published about the nurse's role in genetics and conducting genetics research
- **1984:** Genetic Nursing Network was formed which later became ISONG
- **1988:** International Society of Nurses in Genetics (ISONG) was incorporated
- **1997:** Genetic nursing designated an official nursing specialty by American Nurses Association
- **1998:** Statement on the scope and standards of genetics clinical nursing practice published by ISONG and ANA
- **2001:** ISONG approved the formation of Genetic Nursing Credentialing Commission (GNCC)
- **2001:** Credentialing of the first Genetics Advanced Practice Nurses APNG(c)
- **2002:** GNCC goes online at www.geneticnurse.com, develops a logo and becomes incorporated
- **2002:** GCN credential is first offered by GNCC
- **2009:** Development of the graduate-level genomic nursing competencies. Thirty-eight competencies are organized, some of the examples are risk assessment and interpretation; genetic education, counseling, testing, and results; interpretation; clinical management; ethical, legal and social issues (ELSI); professional role, leadership; and research, etc.
- **2014:** GNCC transition credentialing by portfolio to ANCC
- **2015:** ANCC awards new AGN-BC (Advanced Genetics Nursing Certification) credentials
- **2017:** ANCC close their portfolio credentialing process-renewals only

- **October 2017-June 2019:** ISONG recognized the need to provide another entity for credentialing of Genetic Nurses. Henceforth, 21 volunteer nurses were called to develop the Nurse Portfolio Credentialing Commission (NPCC)
- **2018:** The Nurse Portfolio Credentialing Commission (NPCC) was established
- **July 2019:** Portfolio assessment program for the NPCC by volunteer group was developed
- **December 2019:** Complete operation of www.nurseportfolio.org and portfolio submission for credentialing occurred April, 2020: First group of genetics/genomics, specialty nurses, credentialed as ACGN (Advanced Clinical Genetic Nurse).

ROLES OF NURSES IN GENETICS

Following are the main role of nurses in field of the genetics:
- Planning, implementing, administering (managing), and evaluating screening and testing programs
- Monitoring and evaluating clients with genetic disorders in a similar manner to other disorders by working with families under stress caused by problems related to a genetic condition
- Coordinating care and services for individuals or families affected by genetic conditions, managing home care and therapy for persons with genetic disease
- Follow-up on positive newborn screening tests
- Interviewing clients with possible genetically related conditions
- Assessing needs and interactions in clients and families affected by genetic disease
- Taking comprehensive and relevant family histories and create appropriate pedigrees to interpret the risk areas affecting current generations
- Assessing the client and family's sociocultural or ethnic health beliefs and practices, as they relate to the genetic problem
- Assessing the client and family's strengths and weaknesses, and family functioning
- Providing health teaching and education related to genetic serving as an advocate for a client and family affected by a genetic disorder
- Participating in public education about genetics through IEC (information, education and communication)
- Developing an individualized plan of care, including anticipatory guidance for a person with a genetic condition
- Interpret genetic testing results and values and communicate it to the clients and families.
- Explaining the purpose, meaning, and implications of genetic tests and results
- Reinforcing and interpreting genetic counseling and testing information
- Supporting families when they undergo counseling and make decisions
- Recognizing the possibility of a genetic component in a disorder and taking appropriate referral action, appreciating and ameliorating the social impact of genetic problems on the patient, family and members of the community
- Participate and conduct research in nursing genetics and genomics, publish the results to lay greater evidence-based results about genetic nursing practice.

IMPORTANCE OF GENETICS IN NURSING CURRICULUM

Nursing programs traditionally include certain non-nursing courses like general biology, microbiology, sociology/anthropology, ethics, pharmacology and genetics depending on the design of the curriculum.

Genetic concepts must be in all courses in the nursing program. They must be included in both didactic teaching and clinical applications. They must include practical and relevant examples with applications. Before making decisions about how and where to include genetic content in the nursing curriculum, it is important first to appraise the content to which students are actively exposed. In a nursing program, sometimes there is more genetic content than is realized. For example, when listing genetic content in a survey, if one school did not include discussing cystic fibrosis as genetic under chronic illness for children, the first step is to meet with the instructors of courses both within nursing and outside nursing and find out what content is already present. If a particular topic is not covered, which the nursing program believes is important, they can request that it should be added. If the nursing program believes that a course in molecular biology or human genetics or an interdisciplinary course that focuses on genetics is needed, then they can work directly and collaboratively with the relevant department(s) to design a course that can be added to the basic nursing curriculum. It is also important that the nursing program examine what knowledge the students should have retained from prior learning. It may not be necessary to reteach the content completely such as meiosis, mitosis and typical patterns of inheritance, etc.

The **Figure 16.1** depicts that bidirectional interaction of nursing with genetics and genomics mainly through new specialty, new technology ad new lens. Similarly, nursing genetics can advance through advocating for clients and human responses available for the clients in this genomic era. In the midst of this bidirectional interaction of nursing with genetics and genomics, evolution may lead to paradigm shift which gives rise to challenging and innovative opportunities and ideas. Thus, acquisition of constant knowledge to action should be gained from innovations, adopters and environment.

Some other ideas for including genetic content within nursing curricula for both nursing and non-nursing courses are listed later with examples. Graduate programs can use similar ideas by providing more complexity and depth for topics and by incorporating genetic content at a higher level into the specialty courses. The exact nature depends on the area of specialization.

Important knowledge for the basic nursing graduate in regard to genetics includes the following:
- Basic mechanisms of inheritance and transmission of chromosomes and genes, including the concepts of variation and mutation. Non-mendelian mechanisms should be included.

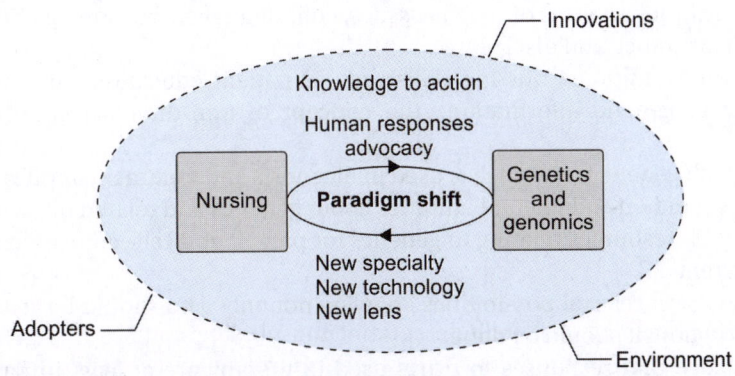

Fig. 16.1: Interaction of nursing with genetics and genomics.

A major issue is how much of this should be retaught, as it typically is in maternal child health or obstetrics and pediatrics? Should a separate course on molecular biology required for nursing be taught within the university or should all undergraduate students, regardless of major, have an interdisciplinary course that relates knowledge from biology, anthropology, philosophy, sociology and other disciplines to genetically related issues?

- Information about the common inherited genetic disorders, for example, cystic fibrosis, Down syndrome, phenylketonuria, sickle cell anemia and hemochromatosis. Disorders that are particularly frequent in persons who reside in the geographic location of school should be included
- An understanding of genetic contributions to human diversity, including concepts such as discrimination and eugenics
- Ways of thinking about health and disease in relation to genetics, including how genetics and the environment interact and how genes interact with genes. This should lead to new ways of thinking about health promotion and disease prevention
- Information about genetic contributions to common and complex conditions such as breast cancer, colorectal cancer, heart disease and hypercholesterolemia, mental illness, certain behavioral traits and Alzheimer disease
- Care management of adults with childhood genetic disorders
- Care management of persons with adult genetic disorders such as Huntington disease
- An understanding of genetic approaches to the therapy of genetic and complex diseases
- Interpretation of genetic risks (i.e., how to explain the 1 in 4 risk of having another child with Tay-Sachs disease)
- What constitutes a proper family history specifically, what key information should be obtained and how to construct and read pedigrees
- Information about genetic risk, genetic testing and screening, and the implications—both positive and negative
- How to interpret the results of genetic tests
- Awareness of the possibility of an inherited or genetic component for a client's condition and knowledge of cardinal features of familial predisposition such as early age of disease onset, multiple family members with the same diagnosis and predisposing risk factors
- An awareness of social, legal and ethical issues related to genetics, including effects on individuals, groups and societies, some of which are unique to genetic conditions
- An understanding of the social and ethical ramifications of possessing a particular genotype or genetic disorder in terms of societal issues, confidentiality, freedom of choice, and risks in terms of insurance and disclosure
- Application of traditional nursing skills such as patient education, confidentiality, and counseling to genetic information. The concept of non-directive counseling can be included
- Ways in which genetic knowledge is used in diagnosis and treatment applications
- Development of non-judgmental attitudes about genetics and related disorders
- Ways to access resources relating to genetics for patient and self- education and the need to keep current
- Knowledge about referral possibilities knowing not only who should be referred but also how and to whom it should be done
- The knowledge that responses to drugs used in therapy are at least in part genetically determined

- Advanced practice nurses may play direct roles in genetic counseling and in advanced assessment. They also may work within a particular specialty in which genetics plays a role, such as an oncology or cardiology clinic, as well as in long-term management of specific genetic disorders depending on the specialty area in which they are trained. An example of the latter is the nurse who works in a sickle cell clinic. The graduate curriculum should include a higher level of the concepts discussed previously as well as advanced material related specifically to the specialization.

BARRIERS AND APPROACHES FOR IMPLEMENTATION OF GENETICS IN NURSING

Numerous barriers including genetic content in basic nursing education have been identified. The most commonly encountered barrier is lack of time. Knowledge continues to expand, but until recently, nursing programs have continued with essentially the same program length. The intensity of the curriculum has increased and has become denser at a time when many students have less time to spend on learning or are less qualified than previously. Faculty barriers include perceived lack of knowledge, insecurity in their knowledge, not perceiving genetic content as important and not recognizing the broad scope of genetics, as it influences health care, but treating the genetic approach as a collection of rare disorders to be memorized. Lack of supporting reviews and translational research related to genetic nursing practice is another significant barrier.

Potential approaches to addressing these barriers can include the following:
- **Educating faculty:** As the nursing faculty is aging, education in genetics may have taken place some time ago and must be refreshed
- **Instilling confidence in faculty:** The faculty must be confident that they can understand material and are interpreting it correctly. This can be addressed through continuing education and workshops. Faculty must feel secure with content to teach it
- Providing rewards and incentives for faculty
- Expanding on what is already in the curriculum after determining what already exists
- Using genetic examples that may be central or incidental. For example, a person who has a particular genetic condition could be the focus of a surgical case study in which the genetic condition is not central, but the genetic information is included
- Emphasizing a life span approach for genetic disorders
- Emphasizing the relevance of genetic examples and using contemporary examples, for example, cloning or DNA testing as used in the OJ
- Offering continuing education/workshops for faculty that may include hands on demonstrations
- Seeking consultation/advice to get started with concrete examples
- Recognizing need for frequent updating
- Identifying an advocate or point person in school. This person may be educated to become a resident expert
- Working with course instructors and the curriculum committee to achieve goals
- Identifying resources for information about instruction and online information, courses available for faculty updating, core knowledge and curriculum developed for other disciplines and for teaching tools such as genetic games and deconstructions that are not only informative but also fun. Many scientific supply houses have these products.

ASSUMPTIONS REGARDING GENETICS AND HEALTH CARE IN FUTURE

Some of the guiding principles or basic assumptions in relation to genetics inform that health care must be weighed before considering what core genetic knowledge is needed for practicing nurses. These assumptions include the following:

- Nurses in all areas of practice will encounter clients with traditional genetic disorders and common disorders with a genetic component
- Most disorders, if not all, have a genetic basis to a greater or lesser extent, even conditions such as fractures. To a degree, a mutant gene can be thought of as an etiologic agent
- Traditional genetic disorders are seen across the lifespan. Many inherited biochemical disorders have infant, childhood and adult forms. Other disorders typically appear or are noticed in adulthood, such as Huntington's disease and hemochromatosis
- The previously existing genetic condition of a particular client influences the choice of care and treatment for any new health problem for which he/she is seeking consultation
- The so-called common or complex diseases such as cancer and heart disease have a genetic component evident in origin, diagnosis, treatment, management and preventive approaches
- Humans are diverse not only because of cultural and social factors but also because of genetic variation. This is not inherently bad or good, but a fact that influences how we all respond to foods, drugs, medications and chemicals in the environment, and profoundly affects how people respond to healthcare interventions, because all people have different degrees of possible health
- Assessment for genetic risk for specific conditions preceding options of testing followed by counseling will become more prevalent and include persons at risk for common diseases such as heart disease, various types of cancers and Alzheimer disease, in addition to those already in common use, such as prenatal diagnosis
- Technologic advances are such that persons with genetic disorders that appear in infancy or childhood and formerly caused early death are living not only to early adulthood but later also. For example, some adults with sickle cell anemia have lived into their 80s. Healthcare providers must deal with how the genetic disorder impacts the appearance and management of common health problems and aging and vice versa. For example, how will co-illness with type 2 diabetes mellitus influence the course of disease and response in an adult with cystic fibrosis? How will common conditions such as hypertension be managed against the background of a previously existing genetic disease?
- Ways of thinking about health promotion and disease prevention will change
- Many diseases will be diagnosed and treated using knowledge from genetics
- Genetic information that influences health care through the lifespan will be available prenatally.

Genetic knowledge makes it possible to individualize aspects of health care such as prevention and treatment in new ways. In the not too distant future, it will be possible to predict the diseases for which a fetus or newborn will have a genetic predisposition, and a fetus or newborn will have a predicted genetic future that may be subject to modulation.

Genetics often has been associated with tertiary health care and rare genetic disorders in the minds of many nurses. Genetics plays and will continue to play a greater role in the common and complex disorders such as various cancers, infectious diseases, Alzheimer's disease, heart disease and chronic obstructive pulmonary disease, and in relatively common genetic conditions that have significant organ effects, such as hemochromatosis. Clients who see primary care providers such as advanced practice nurses will seek genetically related information and may require assessment for genetic risk at multiple points in the life span from prenatal to the older age group. On the basis of such risk assessment, they may choose genetic testing. Studies have demonstrated that a significant percentage of healthcare professionals misinterpret the results of genetic testing. Often they may not know that it is available for a condition relevant to their client or may not recognize that their client is at risk. The curriculum in nursing and other healthcare professions is deficient in genetic content.

MULTIPLE CHOICE QUESTIONS

1. **In which year nurses publish about nurse's role in genetics?**
   a. 1947
   b. 1950
   c. 1960
   d. 1964
2. **International Society of Nurses in Genetics (ISONG) was incorporated in which year?**
   a. 1960
   b. 1980
   c. 1988
   d. 1995
3. **What is the role of nurse in genetic?**
   a. Planning, implementing, administering (managing), and evaluating screening and testing programs
   b. Following-up on positive newborn screening tests
   c. Providing health teaching and education related to genetic serving as an advocate for a client and family affected by a genetic disorder
   d. All of the above

Answer Key

1. c
2. c
3. d

FURTHER READING

1. Anderson G, Monsen RB, Prows CA, et al. Preparing the nursing profession for participation in a genetic paradigm in health care. Nursing Outlook. 2000;48(1):23–7.
2. Anderson G, Yetter C, Monsen R. Genetics, nursing and public policy: Setting an international agenda. Policy, Politics and Nursing Practice. 2000;1(4):245–55.
3. Forbes NP. The nurse and genetic counseling. Nurs Clin North Am. 1966;1(4):679–88.
4. Forsman I. Evolution of the nursing role in genetics. Journal of Obstretics Gynecology and Neonatal Nursing. 1994;23(6):481–85.
5. Frank T. Hereditary risk of breast and ovarian carcinoma: The role of the oncologist. The Oncologist. 1998;3:403–12.
6. Greco K, Anderson G. Redressing Policy in Cancer Genetics: Moving Toward Transdisciplinary Teams. Policy, Politics and Nursing Practice. 2002;3(2):129–39.
7. Greco K. ISONG news. MEDSURG Nursing 2002;11(3):152.
8. Greco, K. Cancer genetics nursing practice: Impact of the double helix. Oncology Nursing Forum Supplement. 2000;27(9):29–36.
9. International Society of Nurses in Genetics and the American Nurses Association. Statement on the scope and standards of genetics clinical nursing practice. Washington DC: American Nurses Association; 1998.
10. Jenkins JF, Prows C, Dimond E, et al. Recommendations for educating nurses in genetics. Journal of Professional Nursing. 2001;17(6):283–90.
11. Lashley F. Nursing and genetics: The past and the future. In: Lashley F (Ed). The Genetics Revolution: Implications for Nursing. Washington DC: American Academy of Nursing; 1997.

12. Lashley FR. Integrating genetics content in undergraduate nursing programs. Biological Research for Nursing 1999;1(2):113–8.
13. Mahon SM. The role of the nurse in developing cancer screening programs. Oncology Nursing Forum. 2000;27: (9 Suppl): 19–27.
14. National Coalition of Health Professional Education in Genetics (NCHPEG). Retrieved 01/03/03 from http://www.nchpeg.org
15. National Institutes of Nursing Research (2003b, April). Abstract retrieved 01/03/03 from http://www.nih.gov/ninr/news-info/geneventposter.pdf
16. National Institutes of Nursing Research (2003a, June). Retrieved 01/03/03 from http://www.nih.gov/ninr/research/dir/sgi.html
17. Nussbaum RL, McInnes RR. Huntington FW. Thompson & Thompson Genetics in Medicine, 6th edition. Philadelphia: WB Saunders; 2001.
18. University of Iowa, College of Nursing (nd). Retrieved 01/03/03 from http://www.nursing.uiowa.edu/centers/gnirc/clingenet.html.
19. https://nurseportfolio.org/about-npcc-1
20. https://nurseportfolio.org/credentials-offered
21. J Hu et al./International Journal of Nursing Sciences 5 (2018) 336e342338
22. https://pubmed.ncbi.nlm.nih.gov/28824901/

CHAPTER 17

Maternal and Prenatal Genetics

Suresh Sharma, Vandana Mehta

INTRODUCTION

The complete sequencing of the human genome in 2003 has opened doors for new approaches to health promotion, maintenance and treatment. Maternal and prenatal genetic is one of the most important health promotion, maintenance and treatment field of the genetics. Genetic research is now leading to a better understanding of the genetic components of common diseases, such as cancer, diabetes and stroke, and creating new gene-based technologies for screening, prevention, diagnosis and treatment of both rare and common diseases. Nurses are on the forefront of care and therefore will participate fully in genetic-and genomic-based practice activities such as collecting family history, obtaining informed consent for genetic testing and administering gene-based therapies. This new direction in healthcare calls for all nurses to be able to effectively translate genetic and genomic information to patients with an understanding of associated ethical issues.

GENETICS AND INFECTION

Maternal infections during pregnancy are known to cause deleterious effect on health and development of growing fetus. In case of any infection host response in the form of increased level of cytokines and chemokines. It is observed in various studies that increased level of maternal serum cytokines interlukin-8 (IL-8) during second trimester can increase the risk of schizophrenia among offspring. 'TORCH' infections generally refer to a group of maternally acquired communicable diseases that include Toxoplasmosis, Other (varicella, Venezuelan equine encephalitis, mumps, coxsackie, parvovirus, HIV), Rubella, Cytomegalovirus and Herpes. These infections are well known to cause harmful effect on developing fetus **(Table 17.1)**.

The following list describes many of the features that can be seen in children who are exposed to TORCH infections during pregnancy.

Maternal Infections

Following is the brief description of selected common maternal infections and their effect on growing fetus.

Toxoplasmosis

Toxoplasmosis is caused by a parasite, which is transmitted by raw or uncooked meat or through infected cat feces. It is also associated with a mononucleosis-like illness. However, unlike CMV, prior infection does confer immunity. Transmission rate to the fetus is 15–20% in the first trimester, but rises to 60% in the third trimester. However, sequelae are more severe with first trimester infection and are similar to those seen with CMV infections:

Table 17.1: Maternal infection, observed on effects and preventive measure.

Infections	Observed effects	Preventive measures
Cytomegalovirus (CMV)	Birth defects, low birth weight, growth retardation, developmental disorders	Good hygienic practices such as handwashing
Hepatitis B virus	Low birth weight, prematurity	Vaccination
Human immunodeficiency virus (HIV)	Low birth weight, childhood cancer	Practice universal precautions
Human parvovirus B19	Miscarriage still births, transient effusions, fetal hydrops, severe anemia	Good hygienic practices such as handwashing
Rubella (German measles)	Birth defects, low birth weight, visual or hearing impairment, heart defects, calcium deposits in the brain	Vaccination before pregnancy if no prior immunity
Toxoplasmosis	Miscarriage, birth defects, developmental disorders	Good hygiene practices such as handwashing
Varicella-zoster virus (chicken pox)	Birth defects, low birth weight, prematurity and spontaneous abortion	Vaccination before pregnancy if no prior immunity

Screening for the absence or presence of IgG or IgM specific antibodies is important for diagnosing acute toxoplasma infection in pregnancy. Maternal toxoplasmosis infection will bring various effects on developing fetus such as:

- Central nervous system disorders
- High risk of schizophrenia
- Congenital hepatosplenomegaly
- Retinitis
- Brain cyst and mental retardation
- Risk of epilepsy.

Varicella

Varicella infection during pregnancy is associated with a less than 10% risk for fetal embryopathy. The effects include microcephaly, growth disturbances, ocular abnormalities and limb defects with cicatricial skin scarring in a dermatomal pattern when the mother is infected in the first half of pregnancy. Shingles (or herpes zoster) may be associated with similar findings, but in a much smaller percentage of exposed infants.

Congenitally acquired varicella is associated with overwhelming illness in approximately 25% of babies who are exposed to near the time of birth. The highest risk is for those infants to develop a rash between 5 and 10 days of age. Varicella Zoster IG antibodies (VZIG) may be given to the at-risk newborn. Varicella infection may result in the following defects in fetus:

- Microcephaly
- Eye defects
- Limb hypoplasia

- Risk of spontaneous abortion
- Neonatal infection
- Fetal death

Mumps

The data are limited, but suggests an increased rate of pregnancy loss. There is also some evidence for a small risk of endocardial fibroelastosis in the newborn.

Measles (Rubella)

Based on a small amount of data, there does not appear to be an increase in the rate of birth defects in exposed fetuses.

HIV/AIDS Infection

HIV infection in the mother is currently not felt to be associated with a fetal embryopathy. However, the perinatal transmission rate is approximately 30%. Recent evidence suggests that use of AZT (zidovudine) during pregnancy dramatically reduces the fetal transmission rate.

Syphilis

If syphilis is not treated well, it can lead to the following fetal anomalies:
- Blindness
- Mental retardation
- Hypoplastic nose and limb deformities
- Anemia
- Skin rashes.

Rubella

First described in 1941, this prototype of congenital infections is characterized by congenital heart defects, cataracts, deafness and mental retardation. Maternal infection in the first eight weeks of pregnancy is associated with an 85% risk for congenital rubella syndrome (CRS). The risk decreases to that of the general population by approximately 20 weeks gestation. Despite an active immunization program, it is estimated that 6–10% of postpubertal women are seronegative.

Data collected by the CDC suggests that inadvertent use of rubella vaccination in pregnancy or in the three months prior to pregnancy is not associated with congenital rubella syndrome or any increase in the rate of birth defects. However, theoretical risks dictate that the rubella live-virus vaccine be avoided during pregnancy. It is highly recommended that nonrubella immune new mothers be vaccinated prior to discharge from the hospital. Maternal rubella infection can cause serious central nervous system and heart anomalies in growing fetus, such as:
- Congenital heart anomalies.
- Mental retardation.
- Deafness.
- Blindness.
- Childhood psychotic disorders.

Rubella infection brings serious health effect on fetus. Therefore, preconception screening and vaccination need to be provided to all women, and they should avoid pregnancy for at least three months after rubella vaccination.

Cytomegalovirus (CMV)

Cytomegalovirus is a member of the herpes virus family and is ubiquitous in the environment. It is associated with a mononucleosis-like illness that may be indistinguishable from other viral illnesses:

- Between 1 and 4% of nonimmune pregnant women have a primary CMV infection during pregnancy. There is 40% probability that the infection is transmitted to the fetus. The risk for congenital infection appears to be highest when the maternal infection has occurred in the first half of pregnancy. Of those fetuses that are infected, 10–15% have clinically apparent disease at birth, typically including microcephaly, hepatosplenomegaly and chorioretinitis. The mortality in symptomatic newborns is 20–30%.
- Primary infection does not confer total immunity for future pregnancies. However, poor outcome of infected fetuses is substantially less when the infection occurs in a mother who has previously had a CMV infection. Testing for CMV during pregnancy can be difficult. A single high titer does not differentiate between a primary and nonprimary infection. Therefore, either two analyses of four weeks apart looking for rising titers or both IgG and IgM titers can be obtained. IgM is often available only at reference laboratories. Due to the difficulties in testing, routine screening of all pregnant women is not recommended.

Herpes Simplex Virus (HSV)

- The greatest concern for fetal embryopathy (growth, cognitive and ocular abnormalities) is from primary infection in the first half of pregnancy. Although it is very rare, infection of the fetus has also been reported with recurrent maternal infections:
  - The more common scenario accounting for 80% of neonates with HSV, is infection in the intrapartum period which can lead to skin lesions, encephalitis, and disseminated-disease involving many organ systems [central nervous system (CNS), lung, liver, adrenals, skin, eye and/or mouth]. In addition, because of infection elevated maternal IgG antibodies are known to cause various psychotic mental disorders among offspring. LSCS should be considered if the patient has active genital lesions at the time of delivery. Treatment of the newborn with antiviral medications has been effective.

Fifth Disease (Erythema Infectiosum)

Fifth disease is caused by human parvovirus B19. It produces a mild illness in children and adults consisting of a facial rash (slapped cheek appearance), 'lacy' body rash, malaise, flu-like symptoms and joint pain (especially in adults). It is spread by respiratory droplets. The incubation period is approximately two weeks. Fifty percent of the adult population is immune by virtue of the fact that they had fifth disease in childhood. However, since this is a mild illness in children, previous infection is generally not documented:

- Human parvovirus affects red blood cell precursors causing anemia. In pregnant women, this can lead to nonimmune fetal hydrops. The risk for fetal death from hydrops in an infected woman is 5% or less. In utero transfusions have been successfully used. However,

there have also been several case reports of spontaneous resolution of hydrops with a normal fetal outcome. At this time, there does not appear to be a significant risk for birth defects in the fetus.
- Pregnant women can be tested for the presence of IgG and IgM, specific for parvovirus to determine if they have been infected during the pregnancy. However, testing should be limited to those with significant exposure, an unidentified maternal rash-like illness or fetal hydrops.

Bacterial Infection

Listeria, a bacterium if causes infection in a pregnant mother may cause selected following fetal abnormalities, such as:
- Spontaneous abortion.
- Intrauterine fetal death.

Soft cheese, cold deli meats and raw seafood usually cause this infection; therefore, these foods should be avoided during pregnancy.

Role of Nurses

- Nurse need to assess the mother during antenatal for any possibility of infection.
- Refer for antenatal or prenatal screening to rule out any possibility of maternal infection.
- Obtain information during preconception counseling that women is immunized with rubella vaccine, and inform them to avoid pregnancy for at least 3 months after rubella vaccination.
- Inform the mother about the possible effects of infection on developing fetus.
- Provide emotional support to mother during periods of stress due to own illness secondary to infection and fear of possible negative effects of infection on fetus.
- Monitor maternal and fetal well-being during episode of infection.
- Provide medical therapies to treat maternal infections and save the fetus from deleterious effects of maternal infection.

CONSANGUINITY ATOPY

'Consanguinity' comes from two Latin words; con meaning shared and sanguis means blood. Consanguinity describes a relationship between two people who share a common ancestor or a 'shared blood' relationship. For example, a relationship between two cousins. The most common form of a consanguineous relationship or marriage is between first cousins and some societies can account for a large proportion of relationships. In other words, consanguinity is defined as the marriage between close relatives.

Traditionally, some cultures have practised and continued to practise marriage between relatives such as cousins as a means of strengthening family ties and retaining property within the family. The incidence of consanguinity reported in India is 5–60% and uncle-niece and first cousin are the more commonly occurring relationships in Indian population. In India, consanguineous marriages are more common among Muslims and South Indian hindu families. The consanguineous marriages are common between first cousins, where preferential patrilateral parallel cousin marriage (where a boy marries his father's brother's daughter or sister's daughter) is often favored.

Genetic Aspect of Consanguinity

- The **Table 17.2** presents proportion of genes shared between close blood relatives. Where it is illustrated that first cousins, share approximately one-eighth (1/8th) of their genes in common and are referred to as 3rd degree relatives.
- Children from a first cousin marriage will be genetically identical for one-sixteenth (1/16th) of their genetic material. If any of these identical genetic sites are comprised of recessive disease-causing genes, the child will be affected with that disease.
- In general, unrelated individuals have only a small risk for having children with a recessive genetic disorder. This is because there is only a small chance that each parent would carry the same recessive gene and that both parents would pass this same gene to their child. When individuals are consanguineous (related), they have inherited some of their genetic information from the same family member. This leads to an increased chance that they would carry the same recessive gene and have a child with a recessive genetic disorder.
- Usually two unrelated people will not carry the same faulty gene copy:
  - Children of unrelated parents are at low risk of inheriting from each of their parents a copy of the same faulty gene that could result in a genetic condition.
  - They have a risk of between 2 and 3% (2 to 3 out of every 100 births) of having a child with a birth defect or disability, many of which will be genetic.
- People who are blood relatives share a greater proportion of the same genes than unrelated people do because they have a common ancestor such as a grandparent from whom they inherited their genes through their parents.
- The closer the biological relationship between relatives, it is more likely that they will have the same faulty gene in common.
- Children of parents who are blood relatives generally have as mall increased risk over that of unrelated parents of inheriting from each of their parents a copy of the same faulty gene that could result in a genetic condition:
  - *For example, if parents are first cousins,* the risk is a little higher (about twice), i.e., 5–6% (5 to 6 out of every 100 births).
  - The chances of having a baby with a problem would be higher, and parents are more likely to share the same faulty gene copy, if their parents and/or grandparents are also close blood relatives.
- This risk applies only to immediate offspring of related individuals and not to their grandchildren or other family members.
- The increased risk for genetic health problems is related to the possibility of passing on recessive genes.

Table 17.2: Proportion of genes shared between close blood relatives.

Relationship of each other	Relationship type	Proportion of similar genes
Identical twin (monozygotic)	—	All (100%)
Nonidentical (dizygotic) twin, brothers and sisters, parents and children	First degree	1/2 (50%)
Uncles and aunts, nephew and nieces, grandparents and half brothers and half sisters	Second degree	1/4 (25%)
First cousin, half uncles, aunts and half nephews and nieces	Third degree	1/8 (12.5%)

- Genetic diseases are inherited in several different ways: Dominant, recessive and X-linked.
- Children born to a consanguineous couple are primarily at higher risk for a recessive genetic disease.
- A recessive disease is a genetic condition caused by inheriting two copies of a nonworking gene.
- When couples belong to certain ethnic groups in which there is a known increased incidence of a specific genetic disease, it may be possible to screen them for this disease to determine if one or both are carriers. It is not possible to screen for all recessive diseases, however, the increased risk for an affected child cannot ever be removed entirely.

Negative Effects of Consanguinity

The risk that those marrying a relative are more likely to have offspring with birth defects or a disabling condition is nearly always exaggerated and perceived as being higher than it actually is. All parents who are unrelated carry a risk of between 2 and 3% of having a child with a birth defect or disability. Where parents are first cousins and there is no family history of a specific condition or where there is no other history of parents being related in previous generations, the risk is approximately double that for unrelated parents. So, the total risk of having a child with a genetic condition where parents are first cousins is around 5-6%. However, in societies with a tradition of first cousin marriage and where marriages are usually contracted within the community, many couples are often more closely related than first cousins and consequently their risk may be significantly higher.

Role of Nurses

- **Being nonjudgmental:** A nonjudgmental attitude toward consanguineous couples is essential to foster good working relationships between the healthcare provider and communities where consanguineous marriage is prevalent.
- **Premarital genetic counseling:** It important to provide premarital genetic counseling to closely related couple who are planning to have marriage. Ensure that couples referred for premarital counseling are aware that it is not possible to provide blood tests looking for general 'genetic compatibility', apart from a few basic carrier tests for a limited range of specific conditions.
- **Preconceptional counseling:** Plan to provide genetic counseling for a couple who are close blood relatives and are thinking of becoming parents. Do not wait to refer for preconception screening a consanguineous couple until a pregnancy is underway, especially if they have a family history of a possible autosomal recessive condition.
- **Prenatal testing:** Refer the couple for prenatal testing and counseling for early diagnosis and intervention of genetically abnormal fetus. Do not imply that a child's condition is their parents' fault; even if a couple is consanguineous and the child has two identical copies of a mutant gene, no one chooses to pass on an illness and no one is 'to blame'.
- **Support:** Support the couple and family during prenatal diagnosis and help them to take crucial decisions if needed.
- **Education and awareness:** Implement public awareness programs about negative effects of consanguineous marriages.

PRENATAL NUTRITION AND FOOD ALLERGIES

- Role of prenatal nutrition play in causation of food allergy among children is still full of mysteries and controversies. Many researches in the field of prenatal nutrition and food allergy of children have not yielded much significant results. But one thing is clear: Childhood is a crucial turning point. This is when the immune system takes shape, it can go down one of two paths where one leads to allergies and the other leads to tolerance. Experts argue about the best ways to protect baby from allergies during pregnancy **(Fig. 17.1)**.
- Prenatal nutrition is an area that needs a lot more research, but suggested that pregnant women might want to 'pick foods wisely' because what a pregnant woman eating today may not only nourish her body, but may have an impact on her growing fetus. Recent research suggests that when moms-to-be eat apples during pregnancy, their offspring have lower rates of asthma. And, mothers who consume fish during pregnancy may lower their child's risk of developing the allergic skin condition called eczema. "There are influences that occur in utero that can have lasting impact," said Dr Jennifer Apple yard, chief of allergy and immunology at St John Hospital and Medical Center in Detroit. "More and more, we are finding influences for later health develop earlier than we anticipated."

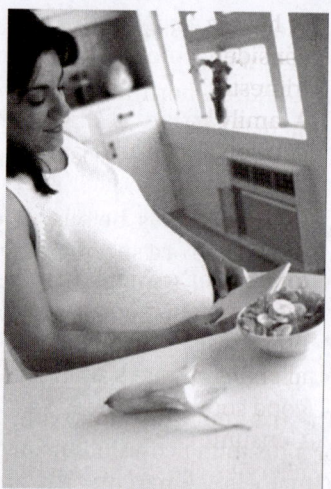

Fig. 17.1: Prenatal nutrition.

- Dutch researchers recently followed 1,253 children from before birth to age 5. Their mothers completed food questionnaires during their pregnancies, and their children's health was assessed. The children's diets were also assessed. Women who consumed the most apples during pregnancy, more than four a week had children who were 37% less likely to have ever wheezed than children of mothers who had the lowest consumption of apples during pregnancy. Additionally, youngsters born to apple-loving moms were 46% less likely to have asthma symptoms and 53% less likely to have doctor- confirmed asthma than those whose mothers shunned the fruit. The mechanism behind apples' apparent protective effect needs further study, but may have something to do with the flavonoids and other antioxidants contained in apples, said Dr Devang Doshi, Director of Pediatric Allergy and Immunology at Beaumont Hospital in Royal Oak, Michigan.
- The study published in the journal Thorax, also found that mothers who ate fish more than once a week had children who were 43% less likely to have eczema than women who never ate fish. "This was a good study, but we need a lot more evidence still," said Doshi, who pointed out that the children in the study generally had well-balanced, nutritious diets, and that may have played a role as well.

Facts of Prenatal Nutrition and Food Allergies in Children

- The verdict is still out on whether nutrition during pregnancy can affect baby's tendency toward food sensitivities or allergies. "The fairest answer is that we do not really know for sure," says Scott H Sicherer, MD, associate professor of pediatric allergy at The Elliot and Roslyn Jaffe Food Allergy Institute at Mount Sinai School of Medicine in New York. Even so, the American Academy of Pediatrics (AAP) recommends that mothers at high risk

of having an infant with food allergies, who have a family history of food allergy, should consider avoiding peanuts, one of the most highly allergenic of all foods, during the third trimester.
- A family history of allergies is the single most important factor that predisposes a person to develop allergic disease.
- If one parent has allergic disease, the estimated risk of the child to develop allergies is 48%; the child's risk grows to 70% if both parents have allergies.
- Eating peanuts during pregnancy and/or while breast feeding may increase the child's risk for developing a peanut allergy and other food allergies; especially if parents have a family history of allergies. Peanuts are the one food that one might avoid during pregnancy. While other research studies argue that until the parents does not have family history of food allergies, women during pregnancy and breast feeding can enjoy peanut safely, since it is a good source of protein and folic acid, which is essential during pregnancy.
- Consumption of tuna sandwich or milkshake during pregnancy will give baby food allergies, which can be avoided.
- This genetic tendency, called 'atopy', occurs when allergic individuals' immune systems essentially go into overdrive when they come into contact with an allergen. An allergen refers to any substance such as pollen, mold or animal dander, which can trigger an allergic response. Food allergies in children can cause a variety of problems that range from eczema to life-threatening allergic reactions.

Prevention of Food Allergy

Here are some recommendations from the American Academy of Pediatrics (AAP) for prevention of food allergy among children:
- **Don't eat peanuts during pregnancy:** It has been shown to increase the incidence of peanut allergy in children. Studies are inconclusive regarding other allergens, such as eggs, milk and fish, and given the essential role of these foods in providing balanced prenatal nutrition, no dietary restrictions are currently recommended.
- **Breastfeed exclusively for six months:** By doing so, one reduce infant's exposure to cows' milk and soy, the primary components in most infant formula. Exclusive breast feeding has been shown to lower rates of infant eczema and good immune system. If it is not possible to breastfeed exclusively, choose hypoallergenic formula brands, such as Enfamil's Nutramigen and Similac's Alimentum.
- **Avoid peanuts while breastfeeding:** Again, studies show lower levels of allergy when nursing mothers avoid peanuts. Research results for other foods a remixed, so the American Academy of Pediatrics suggests that avoidance diets while nursing be determined on a case-by-case basis.
- **Wait to start solid foods:** Allergic eczema has been found to be more common in kids fed solids before 6 months. Wait until child is 6 months old to introduce solid foods. Especially if you have a family history of food allergies, taking steps to prevent early exposure to foods that can cause allergies is a good idea. As a child grows older and the digestive system matures, the body is less likely to absorb food or food components that trigger allergies. Experts believe that waiting to introduce solid foods until your child is 6 months old may help prevent allergies to those foods.
- **Delay introducing allergenic foods:** The American Academy of Pediatrics suggests that children not be fed cow's milk until they are 1year old. Eggs should be avoided until 2, and tree nuts, peanuts and fish (e.g., cod, whitefish and shellfish) until kids are 3 years old.

- In fact, cutting out foods to protect the child from allergies can have unwanted consequences. A scientific review article published in 2000 in the Cochrane Database of Systematic Reviews concluded that avoiding cow's milk and eggs during pregnancy does not protect children from developing allergies to foods or to anything else. The only noticeable result was that some women struggled to gain enough weight while pregnant. However, it is suggested to introduce cow's milk after one year, which will prevent the chances of developing milk allergy.
- Introduce egg stage 2. This may help prevent the child from developing an egg allergy.
- Introduce nuts and seafood stage 3. This may help prevent the child from developing an allergy to these foods (do not give the child whole nuts until he/she has molars and can chew them well).
- **Avoid mixing of food items:** Introduce all new foods gradually and one at a time. Before introducing mixed foods that could cause an allergic reaction, introduce each new food on its own. Do not mix foods until you are sure each individual food is tolerated.
- **Avoid uncooked food:** Give child cooked or homogenized foods. Many foods are less likely to cause an allergic reaction after they are cooked. However, be careful. A few foods such as cod and celery still contain allergy-causing proteins after cooking.
- **Avoid infection causing agents:** Soft, unpasteurized cheeses like feta, Brie, Camembert and goat as well as ready-to-eat meats like hot dogs and deli meats may contain Listeria, a bacteria that cause mild flu-like symptoms in most adults, but can be very dangerous for unborn babies. Listeriosis, the infection caused by the bacteria in a pregnant mother can cause miscarriage, premature birth or severe illness or death of a newborn.

Last but not least a question arises that, what a pregnant woman should eat? "The general consensus is that women should consume a good, well-balanced diet with lots of fruits and vegetables, and not to overindulge in any one food," in addition peanuts can be avoided.

ROLE OF PRENATAL NUTRITION IN PREVENTION OF GENETIC DISORDERS

Prenatal nutrition plays a major role in prenatal genetics. The discovery that folic acid supplementation to pregnant mother can reduce the risk of neural tube defects is a dramatic success story. Many of genetic disorders and birth defects are preventable through balanced prenatal and intranatal diet of the mother. Following are some of the examples:
- **Folic acid:**
  - *Down syndrome:* A recent landmark study indicated that mothers of children with Down syndrome have an imbalance in folate metabolism that may be explained, in part, by a common genetic variation in an enzyme involved in the folic acid pathway. Further studies are expected to see if maternal folic acid supplementation will reduce the incidence of the disorder. If folic acid does prove to reduce incidences of Down syndrome, then this means the chromosome abnormality found in the disorder is a feature associated with the syndrome, but was not the singular cause. Interestingly, before 'bad' genes started getting the sole blame for most birth defects, medical doctors used to think that 'maternal nourishment' was a factor in Down syndrome. Unfortunately somewhere along the line this view fell out of favor. On the mineral front, a number of studies on Down syndrome have linked the syndrome to zinc deficiencies.

A 1994 study has shown zinc supplementation had a positive effect on Down syndrome patients.
- *Cleft palate:* Reduced significantly through maternal supplementation of folic acid.
- *Spinal bifida:* Reduced significantly through maternal supplementation of multi-vitamins with folic acid.

- **Magnesium:**
  - *Mitral valve prolapse (MVP):* Mitral valve prolapse (MVP) is a common feature of most inherited connective tissue disorders, yet also a common finding among the population on general. Geneticists consider mitral valve prolapse syndrome to be an inherited collagen disorder with overlapping features similar to Marfan syndrome. It is listed in the Marfan nosology as a differential diagnosis to be considered instead of Marfan syndrome. Nutrition oriented research studies, however, show the majority of people with mitral valve prolapse are magnesium deficient and that magnesium supplementation frequently reduces or alleviates MVP symptoms.
  - *Cerebral palsy:* Recent research shows that very low-birth-weight babies have a lower incidence of cerebral palsy (CP) when their mothers are treated with magnesium sulfate soon before giving birth. The findings come from a study sponsored by the National Institute of Neurological Disorders and Stroke (NINDS) and the California Birth Defects Monitoring Program (CBDMP).
- **Zinc supplementation:**
  - *Wilson's disease:* People with this inherited disorder have excess copper accumulate in their bodies. Zinc supplementation therapy is used to reduce copper levels and has been successful in treating the disorder.
- **Iron supplementation:**
  - *Blue sclera:* A feature of a wide variety of connective tissue disorders including Ehlers-Danlos syndrome, osteogenesis imperfecta and Marfan syndrome. Most cases of blue sclera have been linked to iron deficiency.

Further understanding of maternal nutrition and birth defects may follow the more typical course of studies of nutrition. Causes of maternal (and hence fetal) nutrient deficiencies include primary deficiencies that arise because of low intake of essential nutrients, a problem that is generally more common in developing as compared industrialized countries and secondary (conditioned) nutrient deficiencies that arise due to genetic factors, nutrient interactions, toxicants including medications and other chemicals, diseases and physiological stressors.

MATERNAL AGE

- Women are born with all of the eggs, which they will use in their lifetime. The eggs age with the individual and as women get older, their risk increases for having a chromosomally abnormal pregnancy. Once a woman is 35 year old at the time of delivery, she is of advanced maternal age.
- Chromosomes are the inherited structures in the cells of the body. Normally, there are 46 chromosomes in each cell, arranged into 23 pairs. Chromosomal abnormalities involving an entire missing or extra chromosome are not inherited and are not caused by an exposure during pregnancy. Instead, they are caused by random mistakes in cell division at the time of conception and can occur in anyone's pregnancy. The chance for such an event to occur does increase with a woman's age.

Genetic Aspect of Advanced Maternal Age

- Many women today are waiting until later in life to have children. However, an older mother may be at increased risk for miscarriage, birth defects and pregnancy complications such as twins, high blood pressure, gestational diabetes, and difficult labors. The risk of having a baby with chromosomal abnormalities increases with maternal age. Listed below are the risks for having a baby with Down syndrome, one of the most common chromosomal birth defects, as well as the overall risks for having a baby with any type of chromosome abnormality, including Down syndrome **(Table 17.3)**:
- It is possible that risks may be higher as many statistics report only live births and do not take into account pregnancies with chromosomal abnormalities that were terminated or ended due to natural pregnancy loss. There are approximately 400 different types of chromosome abnormalities that have been observed in humans, however, many are rare. The risk for Down syndrome makes up almost half of the maternal age risk for chromosome abnormalities.
- Common chromosomal abnormality have been seen in children born from mothers with advanced age are as follows:
    - *Down syndrome (trisomy 21):* The most common chromosomal abnormality in live borns is Down syndrome (trisomy 21). Down syndrome is caused by an extra chromosome 21; thus, an affected individual has three rather than two copies of chromosome 21. It is this extra genetic material that causes the features of Down syndrome, including mental retardation, a characteristic facial appearance and other health problems.
    - In general, for women under the age of 40, after having one child with Down syndrome, the chance of having another baby with Down syndrome is 1%. After age 40, the recurrence risk for Down syndrome is based on the age of the mother at delivery. It is important to know that about 75% of babies with Down syndrome are born to women under the age of 35. This is because women under the age of 35 have more babies than women over 35. The physician may refer parents to a genetic specialist or genetic counselor who can explain the results of chromosomal tests in detail.
    - Some studies have shown a higher chance of miscarriage (early pregnancy loss) in older mothers. When considering all women, about half of first trimester miscarriages occur because of a chromosomal abnormality in the fetus. Because these abnormalities increase with maternal age, miscarriage is also more likely.
    - Two other chromosomal abnormalities which are more likely to occur in women of advanced maternal age are trisomy 18 and trisomy 13, resulting from three copies of chromosomes 18 or 13 respectively. Babies with these chromosomal abnormalities have severe mental retardation and serious birth defects. Most infants with these

Table 17.3: Maternal age risks for chromosome abnormalities.

Maternal age	Down syndrome	Any other
15–24 years	1/1,300	1/500
25–29 years	1/1,100	1/385
35 years	1/350	1/178
40 years	1/100	1/63
45 years	1/25	1/18

birth defects do not survive their 1st year of life. Although more severe than Down syndrome, they are also far less common. Other chromosomal abnormalities seen in live borns occur with the sex chromosomes, the X and the Y. An extra or missing X or Y chromosome may cause mild physical differences, learning disabilities, behavioral and sometimes fertility issues.
- Details of various other genetic disorders seen among children born from parents with advanced age are illustrated in **Table 17.4**:

Role of Nurses
- Nurses need to ensure that any woman pregnant and over the age of 30, should talk with physician about individual health and discuss plans for helping and development of baby to maintain a healthy pregnancy.

Table 17.4: Genetic disorders associated with increased parents age.

Disorders	Description	Inheritance mechanism
Achondroplasia	Short limbed type of dwarfism with large hands	AD*
Acrodysostosis	Intellectual disability, short limbs with deformities especially in arms and hands growth deficiency, small head, nose and maxilla	AD
Apert syndrome	Craniofacial deformities such as craniostenosis, skeletal deformities especially 'sock' feet and syndactyly	AD
Basal cell nevus syndrome	Nevi that become malignant, rib and spine anomalies, variable degree of intellectual disabilities, eye abnormalities	AD
Crouzon craniofacial dysostosis	Hypoplasia and abnormalities of skull and face craniosynostosis, premature suture closer, shallow eye orbits	AD
Marfan syndrome	Elongated thin extremities, cardiovascular complications, especially of aorta, ocular anomalies, especially lens	AD
Oculodentodigital	Digital anomalies such as incurved fifth figure or syndactyly, tooth eventual hypoplasia. Other dental abnormalities, microphthalmos, glaucoma possible	AD
Treacher Collins syndrome (mandibulofacial dysostosis)	Molar and mandibular hypoplasia, hypoplasia conductive deafness ear malformations, lower eyelid defects, limb abnormalities	AD
Waardenburg syndrome	Bilateral perception deafness, pigment disturbance of hair and eyes (e.g., white lock of hair and uniform light-colored iris or heterochromic irises) lateral displacement of inner canthus of eye, many have other anomalies	AD
Progeris progeria	Thin skin, alopecia, growth deficiency, atherosclerosis appearance of premature aging	AD AR†
Duchene muscular dystrophy	Progressive muscular disease with weakness	XR‡
Hemophilia-A	Coagulation disorders with deficiency of factor VIII	XR

(*AD: autosomal dominant; †AR: autosomal recessive; ‡XR: X-linked recessive)

- Pregnant mother with age of above 35 years should be referred for prenatal testing to diagnose or rule out chromosomal abnormalities and other genetic birth defects. Testing may include blood tests, ultrasound, chorionic villus sampling (testing the tissues around the fetus) or amniocentesis (withdrawing a sample of the amniotic fluid).
- Nurses should provide details about the prenatal testing and support the women during prenatal testing.
- Nurses should help the women and family to take decision about prenatal testing and termination of pregnancy if fetus is found to be with chromosomal abnormalities.
- Nurses should plan and implement pre- and intra-conception counseling about ill effects of advanced parental age.

MATERNAL DRUG THERAPY

The use of drugs in pregnant and lactating women requires a thorough understanding of the unique interactions between the mother, fetus/infant and the pharmacologic agents that are used in therapy. Any agent that is consumed by a woman may have adverse effects on the fetus/infant. There exists a paucity of data and information for most drugs relative to pregnancy and lactation. Conclusions that can be drawn remain speculative and the use of any drug during pregnancy and lactation requires extreme caution. Factors involved in fetal drug exposure include the dynamic changes of maternal physiology related to drug absorption, distribution, metabolism and excretion. Placental transfer of drug occurs with almost all agents, each to varying degrees. The notion that the placenta provides an impervious barrier must be dismissed. The least understood of factors involving potential fetal harm is teratogenicity. The mechanisms and types of teratogenic agents are poorly understood in humans. Most drugs are present in the breast milk and, therefore, carry some degree of potential harm. Minimizing exposure is a goal that can be obtained when taking into account the maternal physiology, basic pharmacokinetic factors, physiochemical interactions between drug and membranes, and the chemical composition of breast milk.

The topic of 'drug safety in pregnancy' embraces the effect of drugs on the pregnancy, fetus or neonate and the effects of the pregnancy on drug disposition. Almost all drugs cross the placenta to some extent and may pose risk to the developing fetus. A few exceptions exist (e.g., insulin, heparin) which are very large molecules that do not cross biological membranes readily.

Effects of Pregnancy on Drug Disposition (Pharmacokinetics)

The physiological changes that occur with pregnancy may affect pharmacokinetics. These effects vary with the drug and with the individual, are generally difficult to predict and frequently poorly studied.

Oral availability: Gastrointestinal motility maybe reduced during pregnancy and this may result in delayed absorption of orally administered drugs. However, in the vast majority of cases this is unlikely to be of clinical significance as the total amount of drug that is systemically available will not change appreciably.

Distribution: Maternal water and fat content increases in pregnancy and may increase the volume of distribution of drugs. This should impact only on those drugs that are initiated with a loading dose, when higher doses may be required.

Plasma albumin concentrations decrease in pregnancy and may result in reduced protein binding of some drugs. For most drugs these changes should not impact on drug dosing because the unbound (active) concentration should not change. However, problems may arise when drug concentrations are used to tailor drug therapy (e.g., anticonvulsants). Routine measured drug concentrations are usually the total concentrations, i.e., bound plus unbound (free). Total drug concentrations may decline in pregnancy so for drugs such as phenytoin it is important to measure unbound concentrations just prior to and during pregnancy. Total phenytoin concentrations must not be used to make dosage adjustments in pregnant women. Interpretation of phenytoin concentrations during pregnancy is very complicated and specialist consultation is usually required.

Metabolism/elimination: Maternal drug clearance often increases because of changes that include increased renal and hepatic blood flow and enzyme induction. This generally means that increased maintenance doses of both metabolized and renally eliminated drugs may be required in pregnancy. For example, drugs that are extensively renally eliminated (e.g., penicillins) will have enhanced clearance in pregnancy because of increased glomerular filtration rates. Increased hepatic metabolism of drugs is variable, but can be expected to result in increased dosage requirements in the third trimester for agents such as phenytoin and methadone.

Effects of Drug on Pregnancy, Fetus or Neonate (Teratogenicity)

First-trimester drug exposure has the largest risk of malformations and ideally all drug therapy should be stopped before attempting conception. Accidental drug exposure is a frequent occurrence because approximately half of all pregnancies are unplanned. Major malformations are thought to affect 2–4% of all live births. In the majority of cases, the cause of the abnormalities cannot be identified. Exogenous factors such as drugs are thought to cause only 1%–5% of all malformations (i.e., affecting <0.2% of all live births). The percentage of pregnancies affected by drugs is small, but largely preventable.

It is difficult to predict which pregnancies exposed to teratogens will result in malformation. This is because most known teratogens only cause problems in a small percentage of exposed pregnancies. Accurate timing of the exposure can help in the assessment of fetal risk as some drugs cause only specific abnormalities at a certain time period in the pregnancy (**Box 17.1**). For example, folic acid antagonists (e.g., carbamazepine) will not cause neural tube defects if exposure to the drug occurred after the fourth week postconception by which time neural tube closure has occurred. However, folic acid antagonists may cause other types of malformations beyond this time.

A number of drugs are suspected of being teratogenic, but only a few have been identified with certainty. Perhaps the best known of these drugs is thalidomide, which was shown to give rise to a full range of malformations including phocomelia (short flipper-like appendages) of all four extremities. Other drugs known to cause fetal abnormalities are the antimetabolites that are used in the treatment of cancer, the anticoagulant drugs (warfarin), several of the anticonvulsant drugs. Some drugs affect a single developing structure, for example, Propylthiouracil can impair thyroid development. More recently vitamin A and its derivative (the retinoids) have been targeted for concern because of their teratogenic potential.

Fetal abnormalities such as cleft palate, heart defects, retinal and optic nerve abnormalities and CNS malformations were observed in women ingesting therapeutic doses of the drugs

Box 17.1: Stages of fetal development during pregnancy.

- *Pre-embryonic (days 0–17 postconception):* Drug exposure during this time is not usually considered to pose risk of malformations. An 'all or nothing response' is said to occur. There is early abortion or no adverse effect on fetal development. However, the half-life of the drug must be considered because many drugs remain in the maternal circulation for a long period after discontinuation
- *Embryonic (days 18–56 postconception):* This is the most important time in terms of risk of fetal malformations
- *Fetal period (days 56 – term):* The risk of malformations is lower, but some abnormalities may still occur because development of organs/tissues such as the central nervous system, teeth and genitalia continues. For example, ethanol exposure may affect central nervous system development and tetracyclines may adversely discolor deciduous teeth and suppress bone growth

during the first trimester of pregnancy. There is also a concern about teratogenic effect of vitamin A, such as those contained in some dietary supplements or vitamin pills. It is currently recommended that doses greater than 10,000 IU should be avoided **(Box 17.2)**.

In 1983, the US Food and Drug Administration established a system for classifying drugs according to possible risk to the fetus. According to the system, drugs are put into five categories A, B, C, D and X. Drugs in category-A are the least dangerous and category B, C and D are increasingly more dangerous. Those in category-X are contraindicated during pregnancy, because of proven teratogenicity. Because many drugs are suspected of causing fetal abnormalities and even those that were once thought to be safe are now being viewed critically. It is recommended that women in their childbearing years avoid unnecessary use of drugs. This pertains to nonpregnant women as well as pregnant women because many developmental defects occur early in pregnancy. As happened with thalidomide, the damage to the embryo may occur before pregnancy is suspected or confirmed **(Table 17.5)**.

Role of Nurses

- Educate mother to remember following basic principles regarding drug therapy during maternity period:
    - Avoid all drugs in pregnancy where possible, especially in the first trimester.
    - Herbal and other complementary therapies are often perceived by the lay public as 'safe'. Unfortunately, data on many of these products are very limited and in sufficient

Box 17.2: Drugs considered to be human teratogens (not exhaustive).

Teratogenic drugs	
• ACE inhibitors	• Misoprostol
• Androgens	• Penicillamine
• Antineoplastics (some)	• Phenytoin
• Carbamazepine	• Tetracyclines
• Carbimazole	• Thalidomide
• Danazol	• Valproic acid
• Diethylstilbestrol	• Vitamin A and derivatives, e.g., isotretinoin
• Ethanol	• Warfarin
• Lithium	

Table 17.5: Harmful or teratogenic effect selected drugs on fetal.

Drugs	Reported effects
ACE inhibitors	Renal dysfunction, oligohydramnios, intrauterine growth retardation
Antibiotic	
Aminoglycosides	As streptomycin
Chloramphenicol	Gray baby syndrome, hypothermia, failure to feed, collapse and death
Streptomycin	Ototoxic to fetal ear, VIII cranial nerve damage, other aminoglycosides
Tetracycline	Yellow/brown discoloration of tooth enamel hypoplasia, inhibits bone growth
Anticancer drugs	
Alkylating agent	Chlorambucil has been associated with renal agenesis, busulfan has association with growth retardation, cleft palate, microphthalmia and increased incidence of multiple malformations, all apparently cause a risk of increased spontaneous abortion
Aminopterin	Cranial dystosis, hydrocephalus, hypertelorism, micrognathia, limb and hand defects, multiple congenital malformations
Antimetabolites	Cyclophosphamides have been associated with increased incidence of multiple malformations, especially skeletal defects and cleft palate
Methotrexate	Increased incidence of miscellaneous congenital malformations, especially of the central nervous system and limbs
Anticoagulants Warfarin	Fetal warfarin syndrome, facial abnormalities, nasal hypoplasia, respiratory difficulties, hypoplastic nails, microcephaly, hemorrhage, ophthalmic abnormalities, bone stippling, developmental delay
Anticonvulsants	
Phenytoin	Fetal hydantoin syndrome, growth retardation, metal deficiency, dysmorphic features, short nasal bridge, mild hypertelorism, cleft lip and palate, cardiac defects, transplacental carcinogenesis (neuroblastomas)
Trimethadione	Apparent syndrome of developmental delay, v-shaped eyebrow and paramethadione, low-set ears, high or cleft palate, irregular teeth, cardiac defects, growth retardation, speech difficulties, increased risk of spontaneous abortion
Valporic acid	Spinal bifida
Antimalarial	
Chloroquine	Slight risk of chorioretinitis, may cause ototoxicity
Quinine	Deafness, limb anomalies, visceral defects, visual problems, other multiple congenital anomalies
Antithyroid	
Iodides and thiouracils	Depression of fetal thyroid, hypothyroidism, goiter
Carbimazole	Scalp defects, dysmorphic defects, other possible anomalies
Antidepressants	Withdrawal reactions
Antihypertensives	Fetal hypoxia with excessive treatment due to decreased placental perfusion
Corticosteroids	Fetal adrenal suppression
NSAIDs	Premature closure of the ductus arteriosus, renal impairment
Opioids	Withdrawal reactions

- to determine their safety in pregnancy. In general, herbal remedies should be avoided during pregnancy.
- Consider tapering and discontinuing unnecessary pharmacotherapy prior to attempting conception. Remember that some drugs or their metabolites may have long half-life and persist for some time after stopping therapy.
- Many conditions are self-limiting and do not require drug treatment. Reassurance or lifestyle measures (e.g., avoidance of migraine triggers) may be sufficient.
- Where possible, delay treatment until after results of laboratory testing (e.g., swabs), or until after delivery (e.g., for treatment of hypercholesterolemia).
- If drug therapy is needed, select drugs with the most established safety record. For example, amitriptyline (or nortriptyline) or fluoxetine should be selected over moclobemide or nefazodone for depression.
- Use the lowest effective dose for the shortest possible time.
- Poor control of some maternal disease states may carry significant risk to the development of the fetus. In addition, the severity or frequency of some maternal diseases (e.g., migraines) may improve in pregnancy allowing a reduction in the dosage of some drugs or cessation of treatment.
- Teach women that over the counter products including vitamins, herbs or iron are considered drugs and should not be taken without discussion with her healthcare provider.
- Educate women as to the dangers of self-medication in pregnancy.
- It is also important to realize that some mothers may be very anxious about the risks that their drug therapy poses to their baby. This may lead to noncompliance with drug therapy or unnecessary pregnancy terminations.

- Before administering any drug to any women in fertile age, does not forget to ask about her pregnancy status.
- Consider every drug as unsafe during pregnancy and try to avoid as far as possible.
- Question any prescription of the doctor, if you find that drug prescribed may be teratogenic.
- Provide preconception or prenatal counseling about harmful effects of drugs on fetus if taken during pregnancy.
- Integrate the previous information into school health programs.
- Provide teaching related to nonpharmacological management to common conditions, such as common cold, can be managed by rest, steam inhalation and plenty of water, anxiety can be managed by relaxation techniques instead of medication.
- Involve the client in decision making, if drug therapy is being considered, as an informal pattern in her own care.
- Instruct the woman to keep an accurate list of all medication ingested during pregnancy with the reason for it.
- Maintain are cord of all prescription or recommended drugs with the same information. This should be in a handy form for easy reference as part of the patient profile. If drug therapy is necessary, the lowest effective therapeutic dose of the least toxic agent should be used.
- The risk and benefit should always be considered and doses should be individualized.
- Question any drug that appears contraindicated in pregnancy, because the practitioner prescribing it may not know that the patient is pregnant.

EFFECTS OF RADIATION, DRUGS AND CHEMICALS

The concept of the fetus as totally protected by placenta barrier was cracked by the association of specific birth defects with rubella infection and shattered by the thalidomide disaster of the early 1960s. Exposures to radiation, chemicals and drugs during pregnancy can be teratogenic (harmful for embryo or fetus) **(Fig. 17.2)**.

The term 'teratogen' is often used to describe those agents acting during pregnancy that cause structural or functional damage to the unborn child, in contrast to 'mutagen', which damage genetic material. Low risk teratogens are defined as agents that produce congenital defect in less than 10 infants among 1,000 maternal exposure (Shepard, 2002). Term such as embryotoxic, fetotoxic or developmental toxicity may also be used. The term 'fetus' as used in this chapter also includes the embryo. The stage of development of the embryo determines the susceptibility to teratogens. The period during which the embryo is most susceptible to teratogenic agents is when rapid differentiation of tissues are taking place, usually from 15 to 60 days postconception. In a given exposure during pregnancy, a teratogen can have any of the following consequences:
- No apparent effect
- Prenatal or perinatal death

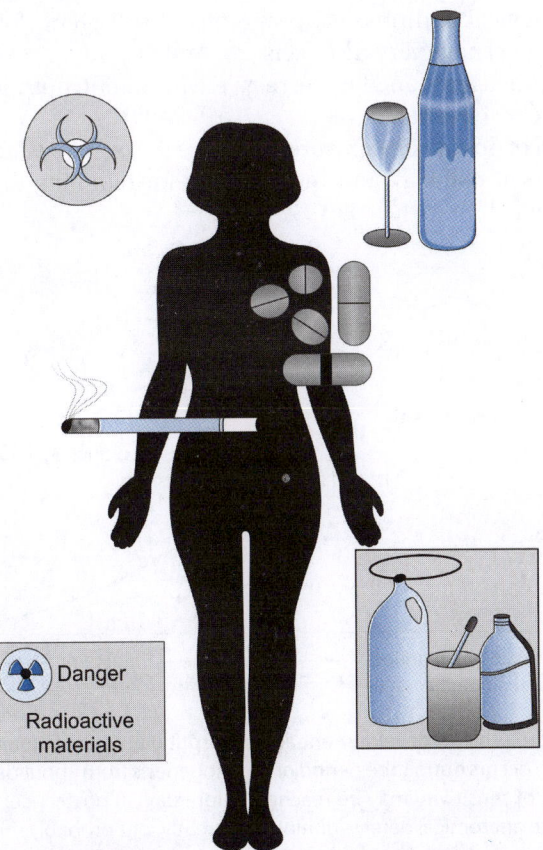

Fig. 17.2: Radiation, drugs and chemicals exposure.

- Congenital anomalies
- Altered fetal growth (e.g., growth retardation)
- Postnatal functional, behavioral deficits, aberrations and
- Carcinogenesis

Factors Influence the Effect of the Teratogens

Complex and multifaceted maternal and fetal factors influence the effect of drugs, radiations and chemicals on fetus:
- Agents often act differently in different species and on individuals with same species (e.g., differentiating genetic constitution, variability in metabolic pathway, etc.) this applies to both the mother and fetus.
- The age of the fetus at the time of exposure, generally when exposed to agents affecting the period from fertilization to implantation, the result is either death or regeneration during period of organogenesis. The result is usually gross structural alteration and after organogenesis in the fetal period are the results are usually related to alteration in cell size and number, although the CNS and external genitalia remain vulnerable through most of pregnancy (**Fig. 17.3**).
- The agent access to and disposition within the fetus.
- The chemical, biological and physical properties of the agent (for microorganism type, virulence and number) have varying effects.
- Interaction with other agents and factors (e.g., environment, nutritional, other drugs, etc.) can have negative consequences.
- Level and duration of dosage or exposure influence the agent's effect.
- Maternal biochemical pathway and mechanisms for handling drugs and chemical are altered by pregnancy.

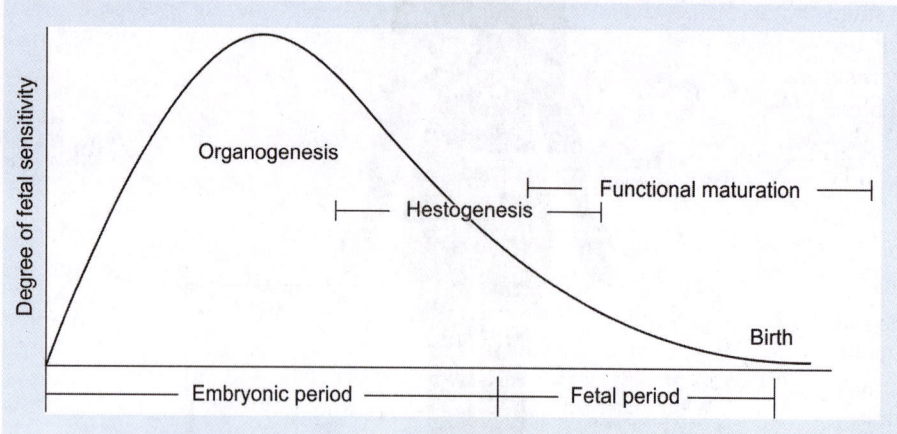

Fig. 17.3: Period of fetal growth and development and susceptibility to deviation (the highest sensitivity, at least to structure deviation occurs during the period of organogenesis from about days 18–20 until about days 55–60. The absolute peak of sensitivity may be reached before day 30 postconception. As organogenesis is completed susceptibility to anatomical defects diminished greatly, but probably minor structural deviation is possible until histogenesis is completed late in the fetal period are more likely to involve growth or functional aspects because these are the predominantly developed mental features at this time).

- The degree of interference with maternal system and the extent of modulation that occurs determine the effect on the fetus.
- The genetic constitution of both mother and fetus, dizygotic twins have been born with one having anomalies typical of a drug effect, whereas the other was normal.

Drugs and chemical, can cause fetotoxic effect not only by direct fetal interaction but also through interference with maternal system (circulatory, endocrine, excretory, appetite regulatory, etc.).

Effects of Chemicals and Drugs

Environmental chemicals and drugs can cross the placenta and cause damage to the developing embryo and fetus. Some of the best documented environmental teratogens are the organic mercurial, which cause neurologic deficits and blindness. Sources of exposure to mercury include contaminated food (fish) and water. The precise mechanism by which chemicals and drugs exert their teratogenic effects is largely unknown. They may have cytotoxic (cell killing), antimetabolic or growth-inhibiting properties, often their effects depend on the time of exposure (in terms of embryonic or fetal development) and extend of exposure (dosage).

Drugs including alcohol and illicit drugs, top the list of chemical teratogens, most drugs can cross placenta and expose the fetus to both the pharmacologic and teratogenic effects. Factors that affect placental drug transfer and drug effect on the fetus includes:
- The rate at which chemical or drug cross the placenta. Lipid soluble drugs tend to cross the placenta more rapidly and enter the fetal circulation. The molecular weight of a drug also influences the rate and amount of chemical or drug transferred across the placenta. Drugs with molecular weight less than 500 can cross placenta easily depending on lipid solubility and degree of ionization, those with a molecular weight of 500–1,000 cross the placenta with more difficulty and those with molecular weight greater than 1,000 cross very poorly.
- The stage of placental and fetal development at the time of chemical or drug exposure.

Illicit use of psycho stimulants during pregnancy is an increasing problem in modern society, resulting in increased number of adverse pregnancy outcomes such a miscarriages, vaginal bleeding and cognitive effects in newborns **(Table 17.6)**.

Table 17.6: Fetal effect of chemicals and drugs used during pregnancy.

Drugs	Effects on fetus
Alcohol	Microcephaly, heart defects, mental retardation fetal alcohol syndrome (FAS)
Tobacco	Miscarriage, premature labor, fetal intrauterine growth retardation (IUGR)
Cocaine and Methamphetamine	Miscarriage, premature labor, fetal IUGR, fetal withdrawal symptoms (tremors, sleeplessness, muscle spasm, and sucking difficulties), learning difficulties
Heroin and other narcotics	Premature birth, low-birth-weight babies, hypoglycemia, fetal respiratory distress, intracranial hemorrhage, withdrawal symptoms (irritability, vomiting, diarrhea, joint stiffness)
Marijuana	Premature birth, low-birth-weight babies
Phencyclidine	Withdrawal symptoms (lethargy, altering tremors)
Organic solvent chemicals inhalants (Paints, glues, etc.)	Varying degree birth as well as microcephaly, heart defects, growth and mental retardation

Alcohol: The features of FAS occur in 30–40% of babies born to chronic alcoholics. Another 50–70% of such babies may suffer from fetal alcohol effects (FAE), which is milder than FAS. To be diagnosed with FAS a baby must have the following features:
- Growth retardation
- Central nervous system problems
- Characteristic facial appearance (small head, flat facial profile, thin upper lip)
- Other major birth defects (heart, gastrointestinal, etc.) are possible
- Children with FAS have failure to thrive, mild-to-moderate mental retardation and behavior problems. FAS is the most preventable cause of mental retardation.

Thalidomide: Well-known teratogen leading to limb defects in exposed babies. This medication to prevent morning sickness is not used anymore. This is one of the notorious component that causes not only the malformation of limbs but also other internal and external organs. Twenty four to 36 days after fertilization is the critical period for exposure of thalidomide effect.

Cigarette smoking: Constant exposure to cigarette smoke decreases the amount of oxygen crossing the placenta and can lead to low birth weight and premature babies.

Cocaine, street drugs: Women addicted to street drugs are at increased risk for having babies born addicted to these drugs. The biggest risks to the babies are not from the drugs themselves, but due to poor maternal nutrition and lack of prenatal care. Prenatal cocaine exposure is not associated with a syndrome (a group of seemingly unrelated birth defects found to have a single cause). Studies are still on-going, looking at long-term effects of exposures in school age children. Cocaine is a vasoconstrictor, which causes blood vessels to shrink. There are many prenatal complications due to even one exposure to cocaine:
- Miscarriage
- Placental abruption
- Vascular defects (limb reduction)
- In utero strokes
- Increased risk for sudden infant death syndrome (SIDS)
- Infant drug withdrawal.

Anticonvulsants: Exposure to antiseizure medications is associated with fetal anticonvulsant syndrome. Approximately 10% of children exposed to Dilantin and other seizure medications will have some growth and mental retardation, digit hypoplasia (shortening) and a characteristic face. Use of valproic acid and carbamazepine in early pregnancy are associated with a 1% risk for spina bifida.

Lithium: Exposure to lithium is associated with an increased risk for congenital heart defects (retinoids).

Vitamin A: Women taking oral vitamin A have a high risk of having a baby with major birth defects including hydrocephaly (excess fluid in the brain), small head size, mental retardation, malformed ears, facial abnormalities and heart defects. Topical vitamin A has not proven to increase the risk for birth defects.

Role of Nurses
- Be proactive, do preconception counseling, which should include assessment of current alcohol and drug use, environmental exposure and smoking, and provide education.
- Females of reproductive age seen in various settings should be taught that medication and social drugs exposure of certain type can affect the fetus, especially in the 1st month

or trimester when she may not realize she is pregnant. This should include the danger of medication sharing.
- Encourage the client to tell physician, nurse and other health practitioners involved in her care that she is pregnant.
- Identify those most likely to be users of medications and drugs (including alcohol, caffeine and cigarettes) and inform those who are considering pregnancy or who are already pregnant of the hazards.

Effects of Radiation

Every healthy woman without personal or a family history of reproductive or developmental problems begins her pregnancy with a 3% risk for birth defects and a 15% risk for miscarriage. These are background risks for all healthy pregnant women. Radiation enhances reproductive risk among these women. Heavy doses of ionizing radiation have been shown to cause microcephaly, skeletal malformations and mental retardations. There is no evidence that diagnostic level of radiation causes congenital abnormalities. However, some of the institution still prefers to ask for pregnancy status of a woman before any radiological investigation. Other institutions may require a pregnancy test before any extensive diagnostic X-ray studies.

In routine radiation risk is caused by medical radiation procedures, effect of which is discussed in further discussion of this topic, other sources of radiation which impose the reproductive risk of nonionizing radiation, includes electromagnetic fields emitted from computers, microwave communication systems, microwave ovens, power lines, cellular phones, household appliances, heating pads and warming blankets, airport screening devices for metal objects, and diagnostic levels of ultrasound has been studied extensively. Two national committees of scientists evaluated the risk from these nonionizing radiation sources. Both of the committees published books on the subject. The first came out in 1993 from the Oak Ridge Associated University panel created by the White House while the second was the product of the committee of the National Academy of Sciences. Both of these groups concluded that the reproductive risk of nonionizing radiation is minimal even if existent.

Genetic Aspect of Radiation

This discussion presents facts about effects of radiation in reference to gene damage:
- It is generally believed that radiation is teratogenic. However, Muller's study concluded that no new or unique mutations are produced by radiations, in the range of 25–400 R, the frequency of mutation was linear. The majority of radiation-induced mutations were recessive; both parents would have carried the genes for an effect to be observed in the offspring and there was no dose rate or dose frequency effect.
- Epidemiological studies have not demonstrated radiation-induced genetic effects. A largest population study of the atomic bomb survivors and their offspring concluded that blood screening of 27,000 children of atomic survivors for 28 specific disorders that may have been caused by radiation exposure demonstrated only two mutations. However, vivo radiation studies have shown significant teratogenic effect on genes of organisms.
- Principle effects of irradiation on the fetus includes:
  - Prenatal or neonatal death
  - Congenital abnormalities
  - Intrauterine growth retardation
  - Low intelligence (low IQ)
  - Genetic abnormalities

- Spontaneous abortion
- Cancer induction.
- Throughout most of pregnancy, the embryo/fetus is assumed to beat about the same risk for carcinogenic effects as children. Radiation has been shown to increase the risk for leukemia and many types of cancer in adults and children.
- Data on the effect of irradiation in utero were obtained by offspring from the atomic bomb survivors; revealed that microcephaly, mental and growth retardation were main abnormalities seen. Abnormalities in eye, genitals and skeletal system occurred less often. Children from Hiroshima and Nagasaki who were irradiated in utero between 8 and 25 weeks postconception demonstrated lower IQ. Also these children were found with microcephaly.
- Based on the Law of Bergonie and Tribondeau (developing embryo is very radiosensitive) and embryo's response to radiation depends on **(Fig. 17.4)**:
  - *Total radiation dose:* Radiation less than 100 mGy is considered safe for fetus. Malformations have a threshold of 100–200 mGy or higher and are typically associated with CNS problems. Fetal doses in excess of 100 mGy can result in some reduction of IQ (intelligence quotient). Fetal doses in the range of 1,000 mGy can result in severe mental retardation and microcephaly, particularly during 8–15 weeks and to a lesser extent at 16–25 weeks.
  - *Rate of frequency radiation:* Fetal doses of 100 mGy are not reached even with three pelvic computed tomography (CT) scans or 20 conventional diagnostic X-ray examinations.
  - *Quality of radiation.*
  - *Stage of fetal development:* During 8–25 weeks postconception the CNS is particularly sensitive to radiation.

Effects of Medical Radiation Procedures

- Ionizing radiation is the kind of electromagnetic radiation produced by X-ray machines, radioactive isotopes (radionuclides) and radiation therapy machines. There is potential for the embryo or fetus to be exposed during the diagnostic or therapeutic procedures for women who are pregnant and have X-rays, fluoroscopy, radiation therapy or are administered liquid radioactive materials.
- Most diagnostic procedures expose the embryo to less than 5 rad or 50 mGy. This level of radiation exposure will not increase reproductive risks (either birth defects or miscarriage).

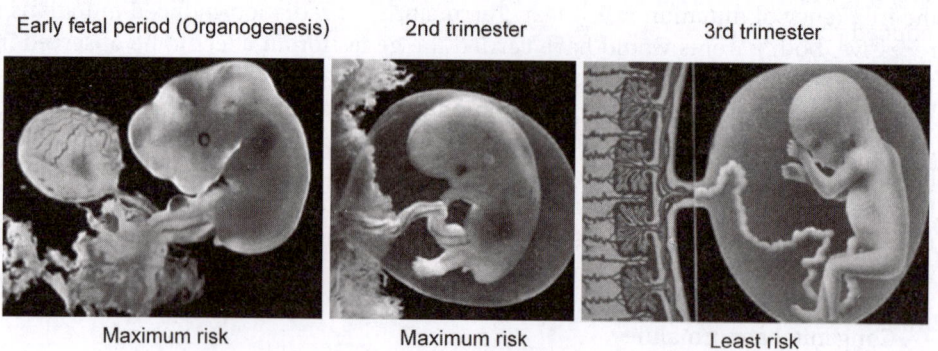

Fig. 17.4: Radiation risk during different stages of fetal developments.

According to published information, the reported dose of radiation result in an increased incidence of birth defects or miscarriage is above 20 rad or 200 mGy.
- A pregnant medical worker may work in a radiation environment as long as there is reasonable assurance that the fetal dose be kept below 1 mGy during pregnancy. 1 mGy is approximately the dose that all person receive annually from penetrating natural background.
- Another important consideration is the stage of pregnancy in which the radiation exposure occurred:
  - *In the first two weeks postconception* or the second two weeks from the last menstrual period, the embryo is very resistant to the malforming effects of X-rays. The embryo is, however, sensitive to the lethal effects of X-rays although doses much higher than 5 rad or 50 mSv is necessary to cause a miscarriage.
  - *From third to eighth week of pregnancy,* the embryo is in the period of early embryonic development, but is not affected by either birth defects, pregnancy loss or growth retardation unless the exposure is substantially above the 20 rad (200 mGy) exposure.
  - *From eighth to fifteenth week of pregnancy,* the embryo or fetus is sensitive to the effects of radiation on the CNS. But here again, the exposure has to be very high. The threshold has been estimated to be higher than 30 rad (300 mSv) before an effect can be seen on the IQ of the developing embryo. General diagnostic studies do not reach these levels and, therefore, these effects are rarely of concern for patients.
  - *Beyond 20th week of pregnancy* when the fetus is completely developed, it has become more resistant to the developmental effects of radiation. In fact, the fetus is probably no more vulnerable to many of the effects of radiation than the mother in the latter part of pregnancy. But the most important thing is that practically none of the diagnostic radiological procedures will affect an embryo at this late stage of pregnancy and certainly there is no risk for birth defects or miscarriage from the range of exposures that occur from diagnostic studies.
- *Minimizing risk of medical radiation procedures:* Healthcare providers need to follow following principles to minimize the harmful effects of radiation on growing fetus.
- All medical radiation practices (occupational and patient related) should be justified before performing (more benefit than risk).
- Medical radiation exposures should be justified for each patient before they are performed.
- After it is decided to do a medical radiation procedure, the fetal radiation dose should be reduced while still obtaining the required diagnostic information.
- Radiation therapy and interventional fluoroscopically-guided procedures may give fetal doses in the range of 10–100 mGy or more depending on the specifics of the procedure, which is considered safe during pregnancy.
- After higher dose medical procedures have been performed on pregnant patients, fetal dose and potential fetal risk should be estimated by a knowledgeable person.
- Most nuclear medicine diagnostic procedures are done with short-lived radionuclides (such as technetium-99m) that do not cause large fetal doses.
- Often, fetal dose can be reduced through maternal hydration and encouraging voiding of urine.
- Some radionuclides do cross the placenta and can pose fetal risks (such as iodine-131). Therefore, use of such radionuclides should be discouraged.

- The fetal thyroid accumulates iodine after about 10 weeks gestational age. High fetal thyroid doses from radioiodine can result in permanent hypothyroidism.
- If pregnancy is discovered within 12 h of radioiodine administration, prompt oral administration of stable potassium iodine (60–130 mg) to the mother can reduce fetal thyroid dose. This may need to be repeated several times.
- A number of radionuclides are excreted in breast milk. It is recommended that breast-feeding is suspended as follows:
  - Completely after ^{131}I therapy
  - Three weeks after ^{131}I, ^{125}I, ^{67}Ga, ^{22}Na, and ^{201}Tl therapy
  - Four weeks after ^{67}Ga
  - Twelve hours after iodine-labelled hippurates and 99mTc compounds except labelled red blood cells, DTPA, and phosphonates.

Radiation Exposure and Termination of Pregnancy

- High fetal doses (100–1,000 mGy) during *late pregnancy* are not likely to result in malformations or birth defects since all the organs have been formed.
- A fetal dose of 100 mGy has a small individual risk of radiation-induced cancer. There is over a 99% chance that the exposed fetus will *NOT* develop childhood cancer or leukemia.
- Termination of pregnancy at fetal doses of less than 100 mGy is *NOT* justified based upon radiation risk.
- At fetal doses in excess of 500 mGy, there can be significant fetal damage, the magnitude and type which is a function of dose and stage of pregnancy.
- At fetal doses between 100 and 500 mGy, decisions should be based upon individual circumstances.

Role of Nurses

- Nurses should be proactive in assessment of a women regarding pregnancy before conducting any radiodiagnostic or radiotherapeutic interventions.
- Estimate risk-benefit ratio for any radiological intervention.
- Take an informed consent from patient after discussing the potential expected risk of medical radiation on fetus before any medical radiation procedure.
- Provide radiation protective devices to pregnant women during radiodiagnostic procedures, like lad jackets during X-ray studies.
- Provide antenatal education to women about reproductive risk of exposure to radiation.
- Conduct several school health programs to enhance awareness of children about reproductive risk of exposure to radiation sources in prepregnant age (potential effect of radiation on ova and sperms).

PRENATAL TESTING AND DIAGNOSIS

- Prenatal genetic testing generally refers to tests that are done during pregnancy to either screen for or diagnose a birth defect. The main goal of prenatal genetic testing is to provide families with information to make informed choices about pregnancy and reproduction, and to assist the healthcare providers in providing the best care and management of women during pregnancy.

- Some prenatal genetic tests are screening tests. They cannot diagnose a birth defect, but only determine if the fetus has a high or low risk for a particular problem. One example is maternal serum screening. Maternal serum screening test for Alpha fetoprotein (AFP) is conducted to identify pregnancies at increased risk for open neural tube defects. Down syndrome and trisomy 18, etc. These screening tests do not always give a definitive prenatal diagnosis and may just show the probability of a problem with the fetus. In most cases, further diagnostic tests are required to confirm and diagnose the fetal abnormality.
- Other prenatal tests are diagnostic and can diagnose certain fetal problems with a high degree of accuracy. Amniocentesis is an example of a prenatal diagnostic test performed on amniotic fluid (fluid surrounding the developing baby during pregnancy). As the fetus grows and sheds cells, those cells can be found in the amniotic fluid and can be used to study the chromosomes. This test identifies fetal chromosome abnormalities. If, for example, an extra chromosome 21 is seen, a diagnosis of Down syndrome is made.

Purposes of Prenatal Diagnosis
- To enable timely medical and surgical treatment of a condition before or after birth.
- To give the parents the chance to abort a fetus with the diagnosed condition.
- To give parents the chance to 'prepare' for a baby with a health problem or disability or for the likelihood of a stillbirth.
- Having this information in advance of the birth means that healthcare staff can better prepare themselves and parents for the delivery of a child with a health problem.

Indications for Prenatal Testing and Diagnosis

In general, genetic testing is offered to couples or individuals identified as being at risk for a particular genetic problem. Some of the risk factors that healthcare providers consider in deciding who should be offered testing include family history, medical history and ethnicity. Prenatal diagnosis is therefore offered to all pregnant women if they have positive antenatal screening results. However, some women may be offered definitive prenatal diagnosis from the outset without any preceding screening tests, for example:
- Family history of an inherited condition, mental retardation or birth defects
- History of previous pregnancy with fetal abnormality
- Mother has been exposed to viral illness such as toxoplasmosis or rubella during pregnancy
- Mother has been exposed to teratogens, such as certain drugs or radiation during pregnancy
- Woman has type 1 diabetes mellitus, epilepsy or myotonic dystrophy
- Women 35 or older who are pregnant or are planning to become pregnant
- Abnormal ultrasound findings
- Couples who are close blood relatives such as first cousins
- Ethnicity, for example, Asians have higher risk of sickle cell anemia
- Unexplained or multiple miscarriages
- Positive maternal serum screening, such as AFP Tetra.

The primary aim of a prenatal diagnosis is to provide an accurate diagnosis that will allow the widest possible range of informed choice to those at increased risk of having children with genetic disorders or with congenital abnormalities.

Prenatal Screening

The following antenatal screening tests are offered:
- **Screening for potential for neonatal infection:** Testing for hepatitis B, HIV, syphilis is offered to all women at antenatal visit. This means that effective postnatal intervention can be offered to infected women to decrease the risk of mother-to-child-transmission.
- **Screening for hemolytic disease of the newborn:** Maternal blood group and RhD status are checked at antenatal visit. Assessment for atypical red cell alloantibodies is also carried out at visit and again at 28 weeks to screen for the possibility of the development of hemolytic disease of the newborn. All nonsensitized pregnant women who are RhD negative are offered routine antenatal anti-D prophylaxis.
- **Screening for sickle cell and thalassemia:** Maternal blood testing for disease and carrier status is carried out and, if necessary, paternal blood testing is undertaken so that the probability of the fetus being affected can be assessed.
- **Down syndrome screening:** All pregnant women should be offered this screening. This is done using nuchal translucency, serum screening or both combined, depending on the gestation of pregnancy.
- **Fetal anomaly screening:** An ultrasound scan is performed between 18 and 20 weeks to screen for structural anomalies including skeletal, genitourinary, gastrointestinal, CNS and other organ defects. There is no evidence that ultrasound causes harm to the fetus or the mother.
- **Abdominal palpation and measurement of symphysis-fundal distance:** This is a screening test to help detect babies that are small-or large-for-gestational-age and to help detect poly or oligohydramnios, which may suggest an underlying problem with the fetus that requires further investigation and definitive prenatal diagnosis.

Types of Prenatal Testing and Diagnosis

Prenatal testing and diagnosis is offered to women whose prenatal screening test is positive or indicate high risk. Women who have had a previous fetal abnormality or who have a family history of an inherited condition may be offered these diagnostic tests from the outset. Types of prenatal tests are of broadly of two categories, i.e., noninvasive prenatal tests (ultrasound, fetal echocardiography and fetal radiology) and invasive prenatal tests (amniocentesis, chorionic villus sampling, fetal blood sampling, maternal blood tests, fetal tissue sampling, and fetoscopy) as discussed in detail below:

NONINVASIVE TESTS

Ultrasound

Ultrasound has become the standard in fetal evaluation because it is safe and noninvasive.

It can confirm pregnancy, determine fetal age, growth and development, identify placental implantation site, determine fetal viability or death, confirm multiple gestation, identify masses associated with pregnancy, assess amniotic fluid volume and placental calcification, and facilitate the use of more invasive studies, diagnostics and treatment. When assessing for specific congenital anomalies or abnormalities in early pregnancy, the uterus and bladder must be differentiated. To facilitate this, clients are instructed to consume approximately 32–48 Oz of fluid 1–2 hours before the procedure and are encouraged not to void until the procedure is completed. Some discomfort due to the pressure exerted by the transducer over a full bladder is expected. A full bladder is typically not necessary for clients in the late stages of pregnancy **(Fig. 17.5)**.

Fetal Echocardiography

This is performed through the maternal abdomen when there is suspicion of a congenital cardiac defect. This procedure provides information regarding blood flow velocity and direction, size, position, valves and chambers of the heart. No specific patient preparation is necessary and no discomfort is involved in the procedure. Client preparation and counseling regarding expected and actual study findings and emotional support to assuage any anxiety about the procedure are necessary **(Fig. 17.6)**.

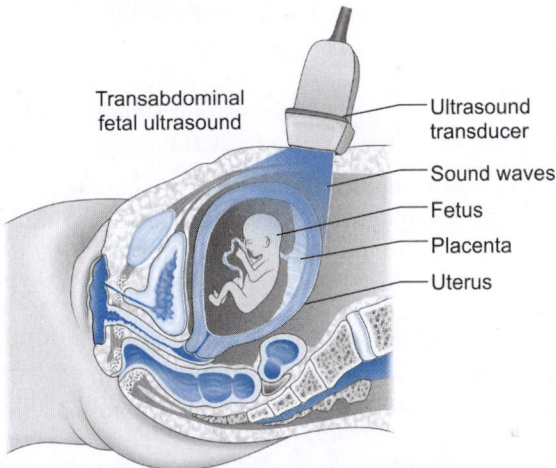

Fig. 17.5: Transabdominal fetal ultrasound.

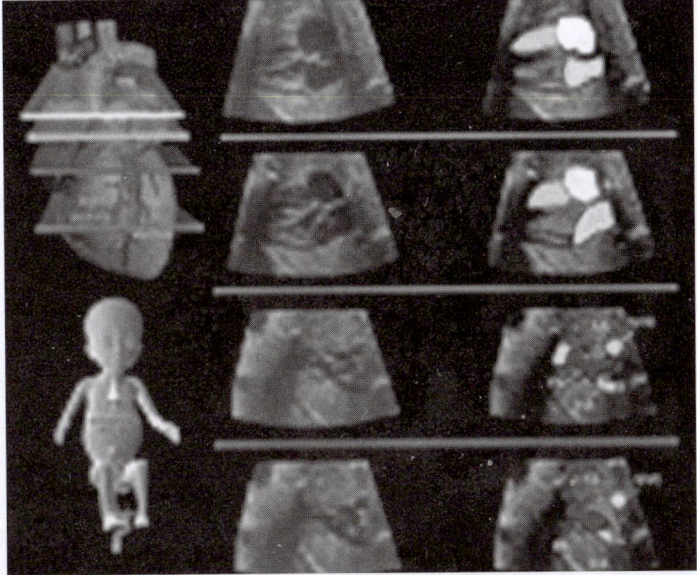

Fig. 17.6: Fetal echocardiography.

Fetal Radiology

In suspected skeletal dysplasia, X-rays can be taken around the same time as the routine anomaly ultrasound scan. Prenatal magnetic resonance imaging (MRI) is also used to assess fetuses with spina bifida, look for associated malformations, and along with ultrasound scanning help to predict neurological deficit and ambulatory potential. Fetal echocardiography can also be carried out if cardiac defects are suspected, for example if there is a family history or in maternal diseases with an increased risk of fetal heart defects such as diabetes. CT and MR imaging can be used during pregnancy. Concern has been raised as to the long-term side effects, particularly with MR imaging due to the high noise level transferred to the fetus. Risks of the technology and the lack of a long history of its use must be weighed against the benefits of determining a problem in utero.

INVASIVE TESTS

Amniocentesis

Amniocentesis is the sampling of amniotic fluid during pregnancy. Amniocentesis involves the insertion of a needle through the maternal abdominal and uterine walls and into the amniotic space. Approximately 10–20 mL of amniotic fluid is aspirated. The procedure is performed under ultrasound guidance at approximately 16–20 weeks gestation. Fetal cells are retrieved for analysis **(Fig. 17.7)**. It can be done:
- Early in pregnancy (early amniocentesis between 12 and 14 weeks gestation)
- Later in pregnancy (midtrimester amniocentesis between 16 and 18 weeks gestation)
- The fluid extracted contains cells from the amnion and fetal skin, lungs and urinary tract.

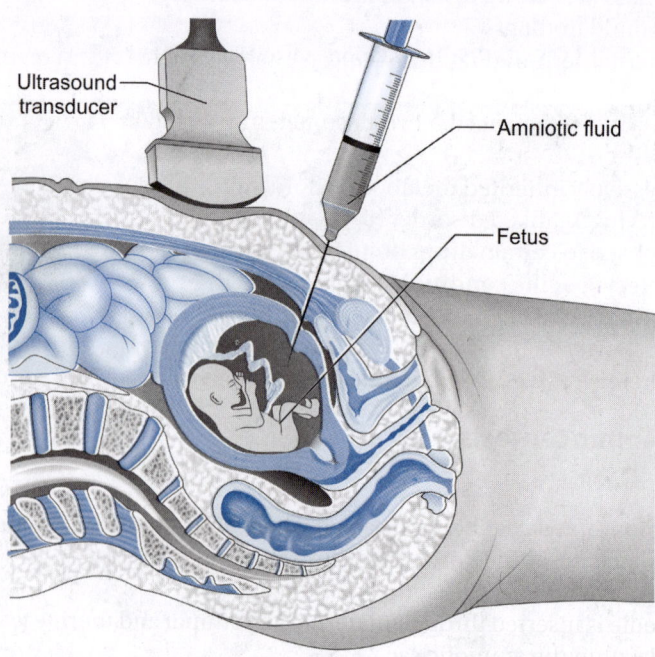

Fig. 17.7: Amniocentesis.

Analysis of Amniocentesis

These fetal cells are grown in culture media allowing analysis for the following:
- **Cytogenetic analysis:** Analysis for chromosomal abnormalities such as Down Syndrome can be carried out using cell culture and karyotyping. More recently, rapid aneuploidy techniques using PCR have been used to detect Down syndrome, which provide results much more quickly than karyotype analysis from cultured cells, which usually takes 13–14 days.
- **Molecular genetic tests:** If a disease-causing mutation has been identified in a family, molecular genetic tests can be performed to detect genetic diseases such as cystic fibrosis (CF).
- **Biochemical analysis:** Enzyme levels can be assayed to detect inborn errors of metabolism. Alpha-fetoprotein (AFP) and acetylcholinesterase levels can be measured to help identify and distinguish between neural tube defects (NTDs), anencephaly, and ventral wall defects, such as gastroschisis and omphalocele that may have been suspected during anomaly scanning. Hormone level scan be assessed to diagnose adrenogenital syndrome.

Indications for Amniocentesis

- Advanced maternal age (> 35 years) the most common indication.
- **Previous child with:**
  - Neural tube defect (1 in 20 subsequent pregnancies affected).
  - Chromosomal abnormalities.
  - A birth defect.
- **Positive antenatal screening tests, including for example:**
  - Fetal ultrasound findings.
  - Raised maternal serum AFP (ultrasound now also used in NTD screening).
- **History of:**
  - Parent carrying a balanced chromosomal translocation (1 in 4–10 chance fetus affected).
  - Risk of recessively inherited metabolic disorder.
  - Mother carrying X-linked disorder (to determine fetal sex).
  - Mother exposed to certain drugs or infections (which can cause fetal malformations).
- **Analysis to detect specific conditions from:**
  - DNA (e.g., fragile X, sickle cell disease, cystic fibrosis).
  - Enzymatic activity in amniocytes (e.g., Tay-Sachs disease).
  - Fluid biochemistry (e.g., in congenital adrenal hyperplasia-17-OH-progesterone).

Procedure of Amniocentesis

Technique

- Rhesus immunoprophylaxis should be given where appropriate (fetomaternal transfusion is a risk in amniocentesis and chorionic villus sampling)
- Preferably performed under ultrasound guidance
- 22G spinal needle is inserted through maternal abdominal and uterine walls into pocket of amniotic fluid within the amniotic sac
- About 10–20 mL of fluid is aspirated (or approximately 1 mL per week of gestation)

- A cell filtration system may be used
- Smaller volumes may be aspirated where advanced laboratory techniques require less material.

Mid Trimester Amniocentesis

- Normally performed in second trimester from 14 to 16 weeks gestation
- There is relatively more amniotic fluid (enough amniotic fluid for reliable cell culture- about 20 mL)
- There is still time to terminate the pregnancy (if results indicate this to be advisable).

Early Amniocentesis

- This has been conducted at weeks 9–14
- Less fluid is removed and ultrasound guidance is essential
- Carries higher risk of loss of pregnancy (around 7%) and talipes equinovarus
- Preferred over chorionic villus sampling (CVS) where CVS unreliable (in twin pregnancies).

Diagnostic Testing of Amniotic Fluid

The following tests can be performed on aspirated amniotic fluid:

- **On the amniotic fluid:**
  - AFP and acetylcholinesterase levels (for NTD).
  - Bilirubin levels (for gestational assessment and to detect isoimmune hemolysis).
  - Tests of lung maturity (various but lecithin to sphingomyelin ratio for example).
  - Enzyme analysis (many and varied including for inborn errors of metabolism).
- On fetal cell sextracted from amniotic fluid testing for genetic and chromosomal disorders:
  - Direct metaphase visualization of chromosomes (for example, for Prader-Willi syndrome).
  - Direct DNA analysis techniques (for example, for Tay-Sachs disease, phenylketonuria, Duchenne muscular dystrophy and cystic fibrosis).
  - Indirect DNA analysis (for example, used to detect linkage disorders when the exact gene is not known).

Risks and Complications of Amniocentesis

- Uterine cramping.
- Uterine bleeding (about 2%).
- Amniotic fluid leakage (about 3%).
- There is a risk of maternal rhesus sensitization in susceptible pregnancies.
- Amnionitis (only about 0.1%).
- Increased risk of miscarriage.
- Failure of cell culture from 1 up to 5% if performed under 12 weeks' gestation.
- Anxiety for parents caused by delay in diagnosis (may make choices for termination of pregnancy difficult).

Chorionic Villus Sampling

Chorionic villus sampling (CVS) or chorionic villus biopsy (CVB), diagnostic procedure in which a sample of chorionic villi from the developing placenta is removed from the uterus

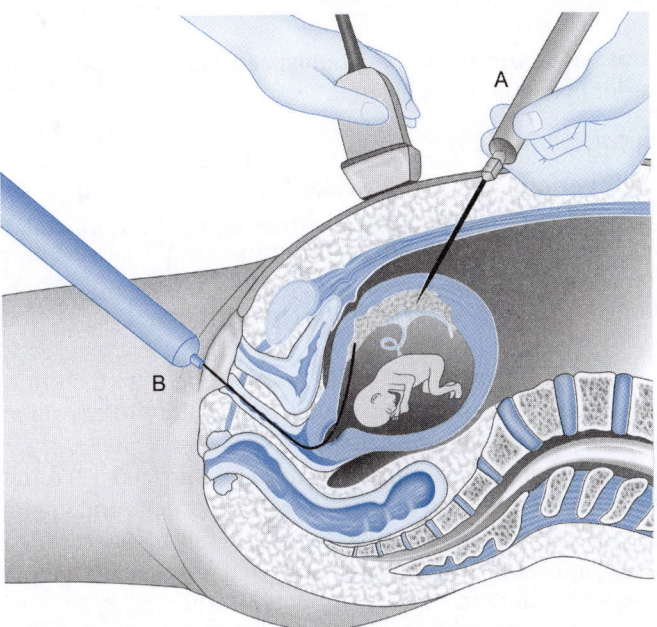

Fig. 17.8: Chorionic villus sampling (CVS) (A) transabdominal needle and (B) transcervical cannula.

of a pregnant woman, using a fine needle inserted through the abdomen (A-approach in **Fig. 17.8**) or a thin plastic catheter inserted into the vagina and through the cervix (B-approach in **Fig. 17.8**). Chorionic villi are finger like projections of a membrane (the chorion) that surrounds the fetus. The villi develop from the fertilized ovum or egg and have a genetic composition similar to that of the fetus. Cells in the sample are grown in the laboratory and studied to detect the presence in the fetus of such genetic birth defects as Tay-Sachs disease and Down syndrome since it allows the examination of the fetal karyotype and/or genotype. The sex of the child can also be as certained.

Indications of CVS

Aim of procedure: Prenatal diagnosis of chromosomal/single-gene abnormalities. Most likely to be used in the following situations:
- Advanced maternal age
- Past history of genetic/chromosomal abnormality
- Familial chromosomal rearrangement
- Biochemical/molecular diagnosis of a familial genetic disorder.

CVS cannot be used to screen for structural problems such as NTDs, which have no known metabolic or molecular basis (unlike amniocentesis). Women should have serum AFP and other diagnostic tests to detect this condition.

Contraindications of CVS

- Previous or suspected NTDs (as not the appropriate test)
- Active bleeding

- Infection
- **Transcervical route of sampling:** Cervical polyps, fibroids, fundal placenta, retroverted uterus with posterior placement of placenta.

Procedure and Practical Points of CVS

- Procedure is usually performed at 10–13 weeks.
- Written consent should be obtained.
- Sample obtained either by ultrasound-guided transabdominal needle or transcervical cannula aspiration/biopsy forceps.
- Results are obtained within 7–14 days (direct preparation 1 week, long-term culture 2 weeks).
- Thus, CVS allows earlier diagnosis than with amniocentesis (which may only be safely conducted in the second trimester) and earlier opportunity to consider termination of pregnancy in the event of a fetal abnormality.
- Use of biopsy forceps rather than cannula aspiration for transcervical route seems to make the procedure technically easier and to be preferred by patients and operators alike.
- Diagnostic accuracy 97.5–99.6%, depending on abnormality being screened for. It is slightly less accurate than amniocentesis because of placental mosaicism (the placenta can have populations of cells with different karyotype/genotype in about 0.8–1.6% of cases). If results from direct preparation are inconclusive then amniocytes need to be cultured.

Risk and Complications with CVS

- Repeat procedures are required in 1–10% of cases due to laboratory failure, mosaicism, ambiguous results, insufficient sample or maternal cell contamination. The latter occurs more frequently in transcervical CVS.
- In a low-risk population, background pregnancy loss is about 2% and second trimester amniocentesis increases this risk by a further 1%.
- Miscarriage rates following CVS are higher than after second trimester amniocentesis. However, there is some evidence to suggest this continues to improve over time probably relating to improvements in technique.
- Transcervical CVS carries a higher risk of pregnancy loss.
- Transcervical CVS is more technically demanding than transabdominal route and more likely to lead to sample failures and multiple insertions.
- On the whole, second trimester amniocentesis is safer than transcervical sampling or early amniocentesis.
- Where early diagnosis is needed, transabdominal CVS is preferred to early amniocentesis/transcervical CVS.
- Where transabdominal CVS is not technically possible then transcervical CVS or second trimester amniocentesis should be used.
- Amniotic fluid leakage.
- Vaginal bleeding (higher for transcervical vs transabdominal route).
- Sepsis (rare).
- CVS at 8–9 weeks was reported to be associated with an increased incidence in limb deficiencies (oromandibular limb hypoplasia and isolated limb disruption) in the fetus and so procedure no longer performed this early.

Fetal Blood Sampling (FBS)

Fetal blood sampling technique uses ultrasound guidance to obtain fetal blood cells from the umbilical cord. It enables karyotyping/chromosome analysis as well as being used for the assessment and treatment of rhesus isoimmunization. Intrauterine blood transfusions may be performed using this technique. Fetal viral infection can be confirmed by immunoglobulin assessment of fetal blood and some hematological and metabolic abnormalities can be detected. The fetal loss rate is 1–3%. In the past, fetal blood sampling was used only during labor through the mother's open cervix to test blood from the fetal scalp for oxygenation. Today, in many perinatal care centers, fetal blood sampling is performed by specially trained perinatologists as part of diagnosis, treatment and monitoring fetal problems at various times during pregnancy. Fetal blood sampling is known by several names depending on the sampling site used to collect the specimen including cordocentesis, also known as percutaneous umbilical blood sampling (PUBS).

Indications of FBS

Fetal blood sampling is used presently for the following indications:
- Diagnosis of genetic disorders particularly those that need fetal DNA sample that cannot be diagnosed by other prenatal diagnostic methods, these may include hemoglobinopathies (although DNA analysis of amniotic fluid cells or CVS largely replaced FBS), certain immunologic deficiencies, disorders and certain coagulation disorders.
- **Diagnosis of chromosomal abnormalities:** For the purpose of rapid chromosome analysis (in 24 hours) particularly if ambiguous results, mosaicism or culture failure results from amniocentesis or CVS.
- To diagnose and treat severe fetal anemia or other blood problems such as Rh disease.
- Diagnosis of fetal infection such as toxoplasmosis, cytomegalovirus, rubella (usually done after 22 weeks).
- Evaluation of nonimmune hydrops fetalis.
- To perform certain fetal blood biochemistry testes such as acid-base status of fetus.
- Evaluation of twin-to-twin transfusion syndrome.
- To give certain medications to the fetus.
- To check for fetal oxygen levels in later pregnancy.

Procedure of Blood Sampling

There are several ways blood can be obtained from the fetus. After cleansing the mother's abdomen with antiseptic, a long, thin needle is inserted into the mother's uterus guided by ultrasound. Blood may be taken from the following sources:
- Blood vessels of the umbilical cord (also called cordocentesis, or percutaneous umbilical blood sampling, or PUBS).
- A fetal blood vessel usually in the liver or heart.
  Fetal blood transfusions are performed using a similar technique. The fetus either receives blood or has unhealthy blood exchanged for healthy blood to treat some problems. In this case, it may be necessary to give a sedative medication to keep the baby from moving. After a fetal blood sampling procedure, mothers will need rest in the hospital and have the fetal heart rate monitoring for few hours.

Risks and Complications with Fetal Blood Sampling

Fetal blood sampling is a very complex procedure that must be performed by a specially trained physician. It is used when other tests or procedures are not possible or not effective **(Table 17.7)**.

Maternal Blood Tests

- Maternal serum AFP levels can be measured to aid the diagnosis of NTDs between 15 and 22 weeks. They are also raised in abdominal wall defects, but amniotic fluid analysis of acetylcholinesterase can help to differentiate between these conditions. AFP screening involves obtaining a venous sample of maternal blood. Screenings are usually performed between 15 and 22 weeks gestation. Elevated AFP levels may be indicative of NTD, multiple gestation, Rh incompatibility or isoimmunization, low gestational age or other congenital anomalies such as congenital nephrosis, duodenal atresia, esophageal atresia, tetrology of Fallot or hydrocephaly. Low AFP levels may be indicative of trisomy 13, 18 or 21.
- The determination of AFP levels is also done in conjunction with triple marker screening. This consists of testing for AFP, human chorionic gonadotropin and serum estriol levels. Triple marker screening is especially useful in testing for trisomies. Depending on the results of either of these studies, other studies may be recommended. Sensitive counseling, education, and support by nurses specially trained in this field can help clients make informed decisions regarding the tests, their outcomes, and any additional steps that may be needed.
- The triple screen is a blood test typically performed between 15 and 20 weeks of pregnancy to detect women whose pregnancies may be at higher risk for three types of problems: open NTDs, Down syndrome and trisomy 18 (chromosome abnormalities).
    - The triple screen measures the levels of three chemicals in the mother's blood; two are hormones produced by the placenta and the other is AFP, a protein made in the baby's liver and secreted into the amniotic fluid surrounding the baby. All three chemicals cross the placenta and enter the mother's blood stream, where they can be measured. Openings along the baby's body, such as along the spine or in the abdominal wall, allow more than normal amounts of AFP to leak from the baby and enter the amniotic fluid, increasing the level of AFP in the mother's bloodstream **(Box 17.3)**.

Fetal Tissue Sampling

Another invasive type of testing involves fetal tissue sampling. This can also be carried out for skin, muscle, liver and other fetal organ analysis. Fetal tissue sampling is indicated for

Table 17.7: Risks and benefits of fetal blood sampling.

Risks	Benefits
• Bleeding from the fetal blood sampling site • Changes in the fetal heart rate • Infection • Leaking of amniotic fluid • Fetal death	• Specialized information about the health of the fetus can often be obtained • Fetuses with severe blood damaging diseases can be treated before birth

Box 17.3: Key points of maternal blood tests.

- This test is routinely done to assess neural tube defect
- AFP screening involves obtaining a venous sample of maternal blood
- Test is usually performed between 15–22 weeks
- Elevated AFP level may be indicative of:
    - Neural tube defect
    - Multiple gestation
    - Rh incompatibility/isoimmunization
    - Low gestation age
    - Fetal abdominal wall problems (e.g., omphalocele, gastroschisis)
    - Fetal kidney disease
    - Placental problems
    - Other congenital anomalies such as (nephrosis, duodenal atresia, esophageal atresia, tetralogy of Fallot and hydrocephaly)
- Low level of AFP may be indicative of:
    - Trisomy 13, 18 or 21
- Triple marker screening includes AFP, human chorionic gonadotrophin (hCG) and serum estriol level estimation in maternal venous sample
- Triple marker screening is done to detect trisomies

disorders that are not diagnosable through amniocentesis or CVS and are at increased risk for congenital anomalies. The procedure may be performed at 16–22 weeks gestation and fetal skin, liver or muscle tissue may be sampled. Skin specimens approximately 2 mm in diameter typically are taken from the buttocks, back, thorax and occasionally the scalp. In cases in which potential liver enzyme abnormalities may exist and are not diagnosable by other means, liver biopsy is indicated; however, few have been performed. A muscle biopsy might be indicated when DNA analysis is inconclusive or carrier status cannot be ascertained and there is a risk for such conditions as the X-linked recessive Duchenne muscular dystrophy, Beck muscular dystrophy, or mitochondrial myopathies; few have been performed to date.

Fetal tissue sampling is performed under the guidance of ultrasound with the client mildly sedated in order to decrease fetal movement. Procedural risks include spontaneous abortion, amniotic fluid leakage, maternal or fetal infection or injuries, preterm labor or delivery, hemorrhage due to anterior abdominal wall, uterine or placental injuries and cosmetic or functional injuries **(Box 17.4)**.

Fetoscopy

Fetoscopy allows visualization of the fetus using endoscopic techniques. It is usually carried out between 18 and 20 weeks gestation. It allows fetal inspection for structural abnormalities, fetal blood sampling to detect and possibly allow intervention in conditions such as hemophilias, thalassemia and sickle cell disease, as well as fetal skin and liver biopsy. The development of a thin gauge embryo fetoscopic technique (TGEF) for endoscopy in the first trimester, with advances in optical system, may revitalized prenatal diagnosis by direct visualization when that in needed. The transabdominal approach is most common, as transvaginal approaches are associated with high fetal losses. This method may also be used to access the embryo for blood and tissue sampling for fetal therapy.

Box 17.4: Key points of fetal tissue sampling.

- This is an invasive type of testing, involves fetal tissue sampling
- Sample may be taken from skin, liver or muscle tissue
- This is performed for disorders that are not diagnosable through amniocentesis or CVS and are at risk for congenital anomalies
- The procedure may be performed at 16–22 weeks gestation
- Skin specimens approximately 2 mm in diameter typically taken from the buttocks, back, thorax and occasionally the scalp
- In case where potential liver enzyme abnormailites may exist and are not diagnosable by other means liver biopsy is indicated
- A muscle biopsy might be indicated when DNA analysis is inconclusive or carrier status cannot be ascertained and there is a risk for such conditions as the X-linked recessive Duchene muscular dystrophy, Beck muscular dystrophy or mitochondrial myopathies
- Fetal tissue sampling is performed under the guidance of ultrasound with client is mildly sedated in order to decrease fetal movement
- Potential risk involved are spontaneous abortions, amniotic fluid leakage, maternal or fetal infection or injury, preterm labor, hemorrhage, cosmetic or functional injury, etc.

PREIMPLANTATION PRENATAL DIAGNOSIS

Preimplantation genetic diagnosis (PGD) (or also known as embryo screening) refers to procedures that are performed on embryos prior to implantation, sometimes even on oocytes prior to fertilization. PGD is considered an alternative to prenatal diagnosis. Its main advantage is that it avoids selective pregnancy termination as the method makes it highly likely that the baby will be free of the disease under consideration. PGD thus is an adjunct to assisted reproductive technology and requires in vitro fertilization (IVF) to obtain oocytes or embryos for evaluation.

Indications of PGD

Currently, there are mainly two groups of patients for which PGD is indicated:
- The first group consists of couples with a high risk of transmitting an inherited condition. This can be a monogenic disorder, meaning the condition is due to a single gene only, (autosomal recessive, autosomal dominant or X-linked disorders) or a chromosomal structural aberration (such as a balanced translocation). PGD helps these couples identify embryos carrying a genetic disease or a chromosome abnormality, thus avoiding the difficult choice of abortion. In addition, there are infertile couples who carry an inherited condition and who opt for PGD as it can be easily combined with their IVF treatment.
- The second group consists of couples who undergo IVF treatment and whose embryos are screened for chromosome aneuploidies. The technique is not used to obtain a specific prenatal diagnosis but rather for screening, properly referred to as preimplantation genetic screening (PGS) to increase the chances of an ongoing pregnancy. The main indications for PGS are an advanced maternal age, a history of recurrent miscarriages or repeated unsuccessful implantation. It has also been proposed for patients with obstructive and nonobstructive azoospermia.

Genetic Analysis Techniques of PGD

Fluorescent in situ hybridization (FISH) and polymerase chain reaction (PCR) are the two most commonly used technologies in PGD, although other approaches have been proposed or are currently in development (such as whole genome amplification and comparative genomic hybridization). PCR is generally used to diagnose monogenic disorders and FISH is used for the detection of chromosomal abnormalities (for instance, aneuploidy screening or chromosomal translocations). Recently a method was developed allowing to fix metaphase plates from single blastomeres. This technique in conjunction with FISH, m-FISH can produce more reliable results, since analysis is done on whole metaphase plates.

Ethical Issues of Prenatal Testing

- The option to continuing or aborting pregnancy is the primary choice after most prenatal testing. Rarely, fetal intervention corrective procedures are possible.
- Are the risks of prenatal diagnosis, such as amniocentesis worth the potential benefit?
- Some fear that this may lead to being able to pick and choose what children parents would like to have. This could lead to choice in sex, physical characteristics and personality in children. Some feel this type of eugenic abortion is already underway (sex-selective, etc.).
- Knowing about certain birth defects such as spina bifida and teratoma before birth may give the option of fetal surgery during pregnancy or assure that the appropriate treatment and/or surgery be provided immediately after birth.
- Questions of the value of mentally or physically disabled people in society.
- How to ensure that information about testing options is given in a nondirective and supportive way?
- Those parents are well informed if they have to consider abortion or continuing a pregnancy.

Role of Nurses

Nurses' role in prenatal genetic testing will be different in invasive and noninvasive prenatal testing based on the nature of the test. However, some of the general responsibilities are as follows:

- Provide detailed information about the test including purposes, risk-benefit ratio, procedure of test, expected results, cost of test, expected risks, total time needed in getting results, etc.
- Help the patient to manage preprocedure anxiety.
- Take an informed written consent from the patient.
- For early pregnancy ultrasonography advise the patient to consume 900–1200 mL water 1–2 hours before procedure.
- Administer Rho (D) immunoglobulin to Rh negative mothers before every invasive test, which involve risk of fetal blood comes in contact with mother.
- Administer prophylactic antibiotic in invasive tests as per institution's policy.
- In fetal tissue sampling, sedate the patient by administering 5–10 mg diazepam as per order.
- Consult the patient and family about expected results of the test.
- Provide relaxing and comforting environment to reduce anxiety.
- Provide emotional support before, during and after the procedure.
- Offer counseling services as per need of the patient and family.
- Inform about follow-up and test result availability contacts, etc.

INFERTILITY

Infertility primarily refers to the biological inability of a man or a woman to contribute to conception. Infertility may also refer to the state of a woman who is unable to carry a pregnancy to full term. There are many biological causes of infertility, some of which may be bypassed with medical intervention. Generally, worldwide it is estimated that one in seven couples have problems conceiving, with the incidence similar in most countries independent of the level of the country's development.

There are strict definitions of infertility used by many doctors. However, there are also similar terms, e.g., subfertility for a more benign condition and fecundity for the natural improbability to conceive. Infertility in a couple can be due to either the woman or the man, not necessarily both.

Reproductive endocrinologists, the doctors specializing in infertility, consider a couple to be infertile if:
- The couple has not conceived after 12 months of contraceptive-free intercourse if the female is under the age of 34.
- The couple has not conceived after 6 months of contraceptive-free intercourse if the female is over the age of 35.
- The female is incapable of carrying a pregnancy to term.

Subfertility

A couple that has tried unsuccessfully to have a child for a year or more is said to be subfertile meaningless fertile than atypical couple. The couple's fecundability rate is approximately 3–5%. Many of its causes are the same as those of infertility. Such causes could be endometriosis or polycystic ovarian syndrome.

Primary vs Secondary Infertility

Couples with primary infertility have never been able to conceive, while on the other hand, secondary infertility is difficulty conceiving after already having conceived and carried a normal pregnancy. Technically, secondary infertility is not present if there has been a change of partners.

Causes

Common causes of infertility are:
- Ovulation problems
- Tubal blockage
- Male associated infertility
- Age-related factors
- Uterine problems
- Previous tubal ligation
- Previous vasectomy
- Unexplained infertility.

Factors

Factors that can cause male as well as female infertility are.
Genetic factors: A Robertsonian translocation in either partner may cause recurrent spontaneous abortions or complete infertility.

General factors: Diabetes mellitus, thyroid disorders, adrenal disease.

Hypothalamic-pituitary Factors
- Kallmann syndrome
- Hyperprolactinemia
- Hypopituitarism.

Environmental factors: Toxins such as glues, volatile organic solvents or silicones, physical agents, chemical dusts and pesticides.

Genetic Basis of Infertility

- Fertility, similar to other bodily functions is the concerted action of numerous processes that result in normal quality sperm. As molecular genetics has advanced, so has our knowledge about the genetics of male infertility. *Most recently, it has become obvious that more men may have a genetic basis for infertility than was previously thought.* Genetics may contribute to infertility by acting at a variety of physiologic levels including hormonal balance, sperm production and sperm motility. An understanding of the genetic basis for reproductive failure is essential to treat and counsel infertility patients. Although treatments of genetically caused infertility are limited. Because of this, it is important to be conversant in genetic issues to better inform patients:
    - About their conditions.
    - About the risks of possible transmission to their offspring.
  The *Y chromosome* is a small, but intensely studied chromosome that is known to carry the genes that determine both testis development and spermatogenesis. It has 60 million base pairs and consists of a long arm (Yq) and a short arm (Yp). On the short arm can be found the gene for *testis determining factor (TDF)* and on the long arm, one or more genes that may control spermatogenesis, is known as *Azoospermia factor (AZF genes)*.
- The long arm (Yq) of the Y chromosome has recently become the focus of renewed interest as it is now recognized that 7% of oligospermic and 15% of azoospermic men may harbor a small gene deletion on this arm. An exact relationship between the gene, its protein product and spermatogenesis is still unclear.

Genetic Diseases Resulting in Infertility

The genetic diseases resulting in infertility topic will be discussed by dividing the reproductive tract into three components, pretesticular, testicular and post-testicular, and examining specific genetic abnormalities that affect each portion of the tract.

Genetic Conditions with Pretesticular Effects

Pretesticular effects are generally hormonal in nature, because spermatogenesis is largely controlled by hypothalamic-pituitary axis. Several syndromes are known to affect the hypothalamus and pituitary gland. Most of these result from single gene deletions:

Kallman's syndrome causes male hypogonadism because of a deficiency in hypothalamic gonadotropin-releasing hormone (*GnRH*). It occurs in 1/50,000 persons and is most commonly an X-linked recessive disease. The clinical features include anosmia, facial asymmetry, color blindness, renal anomalies and cryptorchidism. The hallmark of the syndrome is a delay in pubertal development. Patient's have severely atrophic testes (<2 cm) with biopsies showing germ cell arrest and Leydig cell hypoplasia. Hormone evaluation reveals a low testosterone, low LH and low FSH. These men can be fertile when given FSH and LH. In females, the symptoms include amenorrhea and dyspareunia along with inability to experience hot flashes.

Prader-Willi syndrome is another very rare condition (1/20,000) characterized by obesity, retardation, small hands and feet and hypogonadism. Again, a deficiency of GnRH is the problem. This condition is caused by the loss of function of genes in particular region of chromosome 15. Similar to Kallman's syndrome, spermatogenesis can be induced with exogenous FSH and LH.

Bardet-Biedl syndrome is another rare form of hypogonadotropic hypogonadism that results from GnRH deficiency. It is characterized by retinitis pigmentosa, polydactyly and hypogonadism. Hypogonadism presents similar to Kallman's syndrome except the patient has genetic obesity. The hypogonadism can be treated with follicle-stimulating hormone (FSH) and luteinizing hormone (LH).

Sickle cell anemia is associated with the inheritance of BS-globin genes and is found in 1/600 African-Americans. Men with sickle cell anemia have decreased testosterone and either increased or decreased LH and FSH. Although high or low levels of gonadotropins would appear to implicate very different diseases, it may be that pituitary and testicular microinfarcts from sickle disease account for these two disparate presentations of hypogonadism.

β-Thalassemia patients have mutations in the β-globin gene that leads to an imbalance in the alpha- and beta-globin composition hemoglobin. The trait is present in 3–5% of Mediterranean and African peoples. Clinical features range from mild anemia (trait) to iron overload (major thalassemia). Infertility may result from the deposition of iron in the pituitary gland and testis.

Cerebellar ataxia can be associated with hypogonadotropic hypogonadism. This is a rare condition, which can result from consanguineous unions. Cerebellar involvement includes abnormalities of speech and gait. These patients are eunuchoid-looking with atrophic testis. Hypothalamic-pituitary dysfunction is thought to cause infertility; the basis for the dysfunction may be from pathological changes in cerebral white matter.

Genetic Conditions with Testicular Effects

Conditions that directly affect the testicle tend to result from structural or numerical chromosomal abnormalities. Unlike with pretesticular conditions that are treatable with hormone replacement, the testicular effects are at present largely untreatable. Assisted reproductive technology, however, can provide biological children for men with these conditions, but it virtually ensure that the genetic disease will be transmitted.

Klinefelter's syndrome is the most common genetic reason for azoospermia accounting for 14% of cases. It has a classic triad: small, firm testes, gynecomastia and azoospermia. In this abnormality of chromosomal number, 90% of men carry an extra X chromosome (47XXY) and 10% of men are mosaic with a combination of XXY/XY. Paternity with this syndrome is rare, but more likely in the mosaic form of the disease. Testes biopsies show sclerosis and hyalinization. Hormones usually demonstrate a decreased testosterone and frankly elevated LH and FSH. This syndrome may present with increased height, decreased intelligence, varicosities, obesity, diabetes, leukemia, increased likelihood of extragonadal germ cell tumors and breast cancer.

XYY syndrome is another abnormality of chromosomal number that can result in infertility. Typically, men with *47, XYY* are tall and 2% exhibit aggressive, often criminal behavior. Hormone evaluation reveals an elevated FSH and normal testosterone and LH. Semen analyses show either severe oligospermia or azoospermia. Testis biopsies demonstrate maturation arrest or Sertoli cell-only syndrome.

XX male syndrome presents as a male with azoospermia. Typically, there are normal male external and internal genitalia. Patients usually present with gynecomastia at puberty. Hormone evaluation shows elevated FSH, LH and low or normal testosterone. Testis biopsy reveals an absence of spermatogenesis with hyalinization, fibrosis and Leydig cell clumping. The most obvious explanation is that the SRY or testis determining region is translocated from the Y to the X chromosome so that testis differentiation is present. However, the *Azoospermia gene (AZF)* is not similarly translocated, resulting in azoospermia.

Noonan's syndrome presents phenotypically as a *male Turner's syndrome (45, X0)*. However, the karyotype is normal 46, XY and the chromosomal abnormality not yet identified. Typically, the semen have dysmorphic features like webbed neck, short stature, low set ears and wide set eyes. At birth, 75% will have cryptorchidism that limits fertility in adulthood. If testis is fully descended, then fertility is possible and likely.

Immotile cilia syndrome is a heterogeneous group of disorders in which sperm motility is reduced or absent. The sperm defects are from abnormalities in the motor apparatus or axoneme of sperm and other ciliated cells. Various defects in the dynein arms cause deficits in ciliary and sperm activity. *Kartagener's syndrome* is a subset of this disorder that presents with the triad of chronic sinusitis, bronchiectasis and situs inversus. Most immotile cilia cases are diagnosed in childhood due to respiratory and sinus difficulties. Cilia present in the retina and ear may also be defective and lead to retinitis pigmentosa and deafness in *Usher's syndrome*. Men with immotile cilia characteristically have *necrospermia* or completely nonmotile but viable sperms in normal numbers. Depending on the ciliary defect, there can be some sperm motility and forward progression. Sperm nuclear material is thought to be unaffected. Serum hormones are normal as is the test is biopsy. The hypo-osmotic sperm swelling test can determine whether nonmotile sperms are viable and may help these men to conceive.

Azoospermia gene: It has recently been discovered that approximately 10–15% of men with azoospermia will have structural changes in the Y chromosome. This idea was originally postulated in 1976 based on small structural changes in the Y chromosome seen on karyotyping. This led to the concept that an 'azoospermic factor (AZF)' existed and its absence or mutation accounted for the azoospermia. Since then, an explosion in molecular genetics technology has allowed far more sophisticated analysis of the Y chromosome. Presently, the DAZ (deleted in Azoospermia) region is the most likely candidate gene and is the subject of intense study at UCSF by Dr Renee Reijo. *The exact function of these genes in spermatogenesis is not clear, as the gene products are only beginning to be recognized. It is expected, however, that men who acquire or inherit these gene deletions will certainly pass them on to offspring if assisted reproductive technology is used to achieve biological pregnancies.*

Genetic Conditions with Post-testicular Effects

The post-testicular portion of the reproductive tract includes the epididymis, vas deferens, seminal vesicles and associated ejaculatory apparatus. Genetic conditions in these organs are mainly of polygenic or multifactorial nature. This discussion will exclude conditions that present with ambiguous genitalia or intersex.

Cystic fibrosis is the most common fatal autosomal recessive disorder in the United States. It is associated with more than 600 possible genomic mutations. The disease is associated with fluid and electrolyte abnormalities *(abnormal chloride-sweat test)* and presents with chronic lung obstruction and infections, pancreatic insufficiency and infertility. Interestingly, 98% of men with CF have wolffian duct abnormalities, i.e., the body and tail of the epididymis, vas deferens, seminal vesicles and ejaculatory ducts are atrophic, fibrotic or completely absent. Serum hormones and spermatogenesis are usually normal. Most afflicted patients die in their twenties of pneumonia or related problems. Gene therapy is being actively applied to this disease. A blood test for CF genetic mutations is available.

Congenital absence of the vas deferens (CAVD) accounts for 1–2% of all cases of infertility and up to 5% of azoospermic men. On physical examination, no palpable vas deferens is observed on one or both sides. Similar to CF, the rest of the wolffian duct system may also be abnormal and unreconstructable. Recently, this disease has been demonstrated to be a *form fruste of CF*. However, the vast majority of the semen fail to demonstrate any symptoms of CF. In cases of bilateral vasal absence, 65% of patients will harbor a detectable CF mutation. In addition, 15% of the semen will have renal malformations, most commonly unilateral renal agenesis. Inpatients with unilateral CAVD, the incidence of detectable CF mutations is generally lower and that of renal agenesis approaches 40%. Serum hormones are normal as in spermatogenesis. Epididymal sperm aspiration is very effective in procuring sperm from these men for use with IVF since virtually all of these men will have an intact caput epididymis.

Young's syndrome presents with the clinical triad of chronic sinusitis, bronchiectasis and obstructive azoospermia. The obstruction is located in the epididymis, usually near the junction the caput and corpus. Since obstruction may not occur until after puberty, fertility is possible in some patients. The pathophysiology of the condition is unclear, but may involve abnormal ciliary function or abnormal mucus quality and sludging within the epididymis. Serum testosterone, FSH and LH are normal, as are the testis biopsies. Reconstructive surgery can be attempted, but usually meets with lower success rates than observed with other obstructed conditions.

Idiopathic epididymal obstruction is a relatively uncommon, but well-recognized condition found in otherwise healthy azoospermic men. It is successfully treated with epididymovasostomy. There is a *recent evidence linking this condition with CF*: in one series, 37% of men so obstructed were seen to harbor a CF gene mutation. This implies that up to one-half of patients with idiopathic obstruction at the level of the epididymis may in fact have a genetic predisposition or reason for the problem.

Myotonic dystrophy is the most common reason for adult-onset muscular dystrophy. This usually presents with cataracts, muscle atrophy and various endocrinopathies. Most men with this condition are noted to have testis atrophy, but fertility has been reported. Infertile men may have elevated FSH and LH with low or normal testosterone, and testis biopsies show seminiferous tubule damage in 75% of cases.

Adult polycystic kidney disease is an autosomal dominant disorder associated with numerous cysts of the kidney, liver, spleen, pancreas, epididymis seminal vesicle and testis. Disease onset usually occurs in the 3rd or 4th decade with symptoms of abdominal pain, hypertension and renal failure. About 10–40% of patients will also have cerebral berry aneurysms. Infertility with this disease is usually secondary to *obstructing cysts in the epididymis or seminal vesicles*. Serum hormones are normal and spermatogenesis is undisturbed.

Diagnosis of Infertility

- **Detailed fertility history** including frequency and timing of sexual intercourse, duration of infertility and any previous fertility events, childhood illness and any problems of development, any serious illness (diabetes, respiratory infection, cancer, previous surgeries), sexual history including STDs, any exposure to toxins such as chemicals or radiation, history of any medications and allergies, any family history of reproductive problems.
- **Physical examination:** Testicular or reproductive examination.
- **Postejaculatory urine sample.**
- **Semen analysis.**
- **Blood test for;** gondola hormonal level or infection.
- **Postcoital tests (Cervical penetration test) to;** evaluate the effect of a women's cervical mucus on man's sperms.
- **Sperm antibody test.**
- **Testicular biopsy.**
- **Ultrasound.**
- **Fertilization tests, including** the hamster test, the human zona penetration test and acrosome reaction test.
- **Genetic testing including** preimplantation genetic diagnosis (PGD) that examines all the chromosomes in a human embryo and detect defective genes such as those for cystic fibrosis, at the very earliest stages. Genetic analysis to determine DNA fragmentation in the sperm may be a better way of predicting outcome of pregnancy.

Medical Management of Infertility

- Provide higher antioxidant vitamin C and vitamin A diet.
- Hormonal monitoring and ovulation period intercourse.
- Provide stress management advices and interventions.
- **Advise for life style changes:** Man who wants to achieve higher sperm counts need some of the following life style modification as given below:
  - Avoid smoking, drugs and increase intake of coffee.
  - Get sufficient rest and exercise, and avoid excessive exercises.
  - Manage stress with yoga, meditation and spiritual interventions.
  - Prevent overheating of testis.
  - Assisted reproductive technologies (ART) management.
- It refers to methods used to achieve pregnancy by artificial or partially artificial means, which includes:
  - *Artificial insemination (AI):* This is when sperm is placed into a female's uterus (intrauterine) or cervix (intracervical) using artificial means rather than by natural copulation.
  - *In vitro fertilization (IVF):* In vitro fertilization (IVF) is the technique of letting fertilization of the male and female gametes (sperm and egg) occur outside the female body **(Fig. 17.9)**.

- *Intracytoplasmic sperm injection (ICSI):* This is beneficial in the case of male factor infertility where sperm counts are very low or failed fertilization occurs with previous IVF attempt(s). The ICSI procedure involves a single sperm carefully injected into the center of an egg using a microneedle.
- *Gamete intrafallopian transfer (GIFT):* In this a mixture of sperms and eggs is placed directly into a woman's fallopian tubes using laparoscopy following a transvaginal ovum retrieval.
- *Zygote intrafallopian transfer (ZIFT):* In this egg cells are removed from the woman's ovaries and fertilized in the laboratory; the resulting zygote is then placed into the fallopian tube.

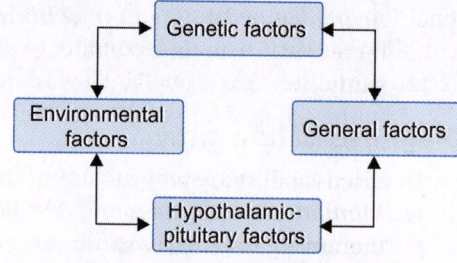

Fig. 17.9: Factors affecting fertility.

- **Other techniques:**
  - *In vitro maturation:* In this process follicles are harvested a few days before ovulation. These maturing follicles are removed and healthy embryo is produced. This allows the fertilization without the use of fertility drugs.
  - *Blastocyte transfer:* In this instead of implanting the standard 2–3 days embryo in the uterus, the procedure implants blastocyte, which are more complex 5 days old embryo.
  - *Ooplastic transfer:* This is one of the controversial and experimental procedure that use the women's own egg and a female donor's egg and the male's sperm for fertilization. Genetic materials from the donor's egg plus the sperm are added to the women's own egg. This has been successful in a few cases and long-term effects are unknown.
- **Complementary and alternative treatments:** Three complementary or alternative female infertility treatments have been scientifically tested with results published in peer-reviewed medical journals:
  - *Group psychological intervention:* A 2000 Harvard Medical School study examined the effects of group psychological intervention on infertile women. The two intervention groups; a support group and a cognitive behavior group had statistically significant higher pregnancy rates than the control group.

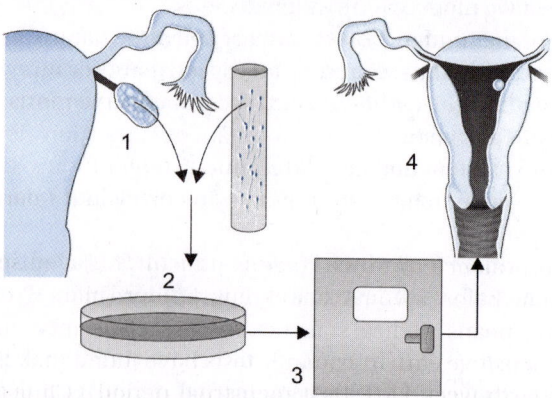

Fig. 17.10: In vitro fertilization.

CHAPTER 17: Maternal and Prenatal Genetics

- *Acupuncture:* Acupuncture performed 25 minutes before and after IVF embryo transfer increased IVF pregnancy rates in a German study published in 2002. In a 2006 similar study conducted by The University of South Australia, the acupuncture group's odds (although not statistically significant) were 1.5 higher than the control group. Although definitive results of the effects of acupuncture on embryo transfer remain a topic of discussion, study authors state that it appears to be a safe adjunct to IVF.
- *Manual physical therapy:* The Wurn technique, a manual manipulative physical therapy treatment was shown in peer reviewed publications to improve natural and IVF pregnancy rates in infertile women in a 2004 study, and to open and return function to blocked fallopian tubes in a 2008 study. The therapy was designed to address adhesions restricting function and mobility of the reproductive organs.

A scoping review of 148 studies from BMC complementary medicine and therapies in 2018, with the title "Evidence for the use of complementary and alternative medicines during fertility treatment: a scoping review" states that highest evidence is found related to role of acupuncture in improving men and women infertility though few other studies emphasized about various other CAM therapies such as Chinese herbal medicine, herbal medicine, massage and hypnosis.

Role of Nurses

- Infertility has significant psychological and social impact; therefore, nurses need to provide psychological support during throughout diagnosis and treatment of infertility.
- Provide information about causes of infertility including genetic causes, and possible treatment modalities. For example, artificial reproductive technique (ART), etc.
- Take written consent for diagnostic and therapeutic interventions.
- Assist the physical in diagnostic and therapeutic interventions.
- Provide discharge teaching and follow-up information.
- Teach about healthy life style modification and effective stress management strategies.

SPONTANEOUS ABORTIONS

- Spontaneous abortion refers to a clinical condition describing the loss of the intrauterine product prior to the viability of the fetus, conventionally accepted as 20 weeks of intrauterine life or 500 g of fetal body weight.
- In other words spontaneous abortion or miscarriage is the natural or spontaneous end of a pregnancy at a stage where the embryo or fetus is incapable of surviving, generally defined in humans at prior to 20 weeks of gestation. Miscarriage is the most common complication of early pregnancy. The medical term 'spontaneous abortion' is used in reference to miscarriages because the medical term 'abortion' refers to any terminated pregnancy, deliberately induced or spontaneous, although in common it refers specifically to active termination of pregnancy.
- Determining the prevalence of miscarriage is difficult. Many miscarriages happen very early in the pregnancy, before a woman may know she is pregnant. Treatment of women with miscarriage at home means medical statistics on miscarriage miss many cases. Prospective studies using very sensitive early pregnancy tests have found that 25% of pregnancies are miscarried by the sixth week LMP (last menstrual period). Clinical miscarriages (those occurring after the sixth week LMP) occur in 8% of pregnancies.

Types of Spontaneous Abortions

Early pregnancy loss: Very early miscarriage; those which occur before the sixth week LMP (last menstrual period) are medically termed as early pregnancy loss or chemical pregnancy

Clinical spontaneous abortion: Miscarriages that occur after the sixth week LMP are medically termed as clinical spontaneous abortion.

Alternatively the following terms are used to describe pregnancies that do not continue:
- **An empty sac** is a condition where the gestational sac develops normally, while the embryonic part of the pregnancy is either absent or stops growing very early. Other terms for this condition are blighted ovum and anembryonic pregnancy.
- **An inevitable abortion** describes where the fetal heart beat is shown to have stopped and the cervix has already dilated open, but the fetus has yet to be expelled. This usually will progress to a complete abortion.
- **A complete abortion** is when all products of conception have been expelled. Products of conception may include the trophoblast, chorionic villi, gestational sac, yolk sac and fetal pole (embryo); or later in pregnancy the fetus, umbilical cord, placenta, amniotic fluid, and amniotic membrane.
- **An incomplete abortion** occurs when tissue has been passed, but some remains in utero.
- **A missed abortion** is when the embryo or fetus has died, but a miscarriage has not yet occurred. It is also referred to as *delayed miscarriage*.

The following two terms consider wider complications or implications of a miscarriage:
1. **A septic abortion** occurs when the tissue from a missed or incomplete abortion becomes infected. The infection of the womb carries risk of spreading infection (septicemia) and is a grave risk to the life of the woman.
2. **Recurrent pregnancy loss (RPL)** or *recurrent miscarriage* (medically termed as habitual abortion) is the occurrence of three consecutive miscarriages. If the proportion of pregnancies ending in miscarriage is 15%, then the probability of two consecutive miscarriages is 2.25% and the probability of three consecutive miscarriages is 0.34%. The occurrence of recurrent pregnancy loss is 1%. A large majority (85%) of women who have had two miscarriages will conceive and carry normally afterwards.

Etiology

There are many reasons for pregnancy loss. It is important to realize that in many cases, no cause for past miscarriage(s) is identified. Most causes of miscarriage are not under our control. It is important to remember that women who have a miscarriage(s) still have a good chance for a successful future pregnancy.

Genetic Causes

Fetal chromosomal abnormalities: Approximately 50% of first trimester miscarriages are due to a chromosome abnormality in the fetus. Chromosomes are the inherited structures in the cells of our bodies. There are 46 chromosomes in each cell, arranged into 23 pairs. A baby has two copies of every chromosome—one inherited from the mother in the egg and the other inherited from the father in the sperm. Each chromosome holds hundreds to thousands of genes, which are responsible for growth and development. An extra chromosome or a missing chromosome can cause miscarriage usually in the first or second trimester of pregnancy or can lead to a child with learning difficulties or mental retardation and birth defects. Chromosome abnormalities involving a missing or extra chromosome are not inherited or caused by an exposure during pregnancy. Instead, they result from a chance mistake in cell division at the time of conception. This error is a random event that can occur in any one's pregnancy. Once a couple has had a pregnancy affected by a chromosome abnormality, there is a slightly greater chance for their future pregnancies to be affected with chromosome abnormalities. In some cases prenatal diagnosis, such as chorionic villus sampling (CVS) or amniocentesis are offered in future pregnancies.

Inherited chromosomal rearrangements: An inherited problem with the chromosomes can also cause miscarriage. A parent can have a rearrangement (a 'translocation') of his or her chromosomes in which the chromosomes are structured differently. The parent should have no health problems because, although his or her chromosomes are rearranged, they are balanced, i.e. there are no missing or extra pieces of the chromosomes. However, because of the way the chromosomes are passed from parent to child, the baby may inherit extra or missing pieces of a chromosome. Extra and missing genetic material leads to 'chromosomal imbalance' and can cause mental retardation and birth defects in a live born or cause a miscarriage. For couples who have had multiple miscarriages, the chance that one of the parents has a chromosomal rearrangement is approximately 2%-4%. While parents who carry chromosomal rearrangements are at increased risk to have further miscarriages or babies born with health problems, they can also produce healthy children. Chromosome studies can be performed on parents' blood to see if either parent is a carrier of a chromosomal rearrangement.

Gene mutation: Another genetic cause of miscarriage is a change (mutation) in a single gene (or several genes) on the chromosomes. This can cause specific genetic diseases or birth defects. Mutations can occur spontaneously in pregnancies or can be inherited from parents who themselves are healthy. Birth defects associated with these conditions can sometimes be detected during pregnancy by a sonogram. If there is a history of a specific disorder in a parent or family member, single gene disorders can be tested for prenatally in some cases.

Maternal Health Issues

Other reasons for pregnancy loss are related to maternal health. An abnormally shaped uterus can lead to pregnancy loss. Health problems such as hormonal imbalance, poorly controlled diabetes, lupus and other immune system abnormalities, kidney and heart disease, and hypertension can create difficulties in carrying a pregnancy to term. These causes of miscarriage can be evaluated by blood tests and an ultrasound examination (sonogram) of the uterus. Your doctor can evaluate you for these problems.

Environment

Another cause of pregnancy loss is an environmental exposure during pregnancy. For example, exposure to drugs, alcohol or high levels of radiation can lead to miscarriage. Infections can cause miscarriage. The risk of miscarriage may be greater in women who smoke.

Clinical Manifestations
- Vaginal bleeding.
- Pain does not strongly correlate with miscarriage.
- Blood clots with embryotic tissue passes.
- Early abrupt disappearance of early signs of pregnancy.

Diagnosis of Spontaneous Abortion

- History of per vaginal bleeding during pregnancy.
- Ultrasound examination.
- Serial human chorionic gonadotropin (HCG) testing.
- Genetic testing for aborted fetal tissue.

Management of Spontaneous Abortion

- No treatment is necessary for a diagnosed complete abortion (as long as ectopic pregnancy is ruled out). However, in cases of an incomplete abortion, empty sac or missed abortion, there are three treatment options:
  - *With no treatment (watchful waiting),* most of these cases (65–80%) will pass naturally within 2–6 weeks. This path avoids the side effects and complications possible from medications and surgery.
  - *Medical management* usually consists of using misoprostol (a prostaglandin, brand name Cytotec) to encourage completion of the miscarriage. About 95% of cases treated with misoprostol will complete within a few days.
  - *Surgical treatment* (most commonly vacuum aspiration, sometimes referred to as a D and C or D and E) is the fastest way to complete the miscarriage. It also shortens the duration and heaviness of bleeding, and is the best treatment for physical pain associated with the miscarriage. In cases of repeated miscarriage or later-term pregnancy loss, D and C is also the best way to obtain tissue samples for pathology examination.
- Genetic counseling for the couple and family, if there is genetic cause involved in causation of abortion.

Role of Nurses

- Spontaneous abortion has significant psychological and social impact; therefore, nurses need to provide psychological support during diagnosis and treatment of spontaneous abortion.
- Provide information about causes of spontaneous abortion including genetic causes, and possible treatment modalities.
- Take written consent for diagnostic and therapeutic interventions.
- Assist the physician in diagnostic and therapeutic interventions.
- Provide discharge teaching and follow-up information.
- Teach about healthy lifestyle modification and effective stress management strategies.

NEURAL TUBE DEFECTS

Complete fusion of the neural tube usually occurs between days 18 and 26 after ovulation. Neural tube defects are malformations of the neuroectoderm and are associated with abnormalities of surrounding mesodermal structures. In other words, NTD is an opening in the spinal cord or brain that occurs very early in human development. The early spinal cord of the embryo begins as a flat region, which rolls in to a tube (the neural tube) 28 days after the baby is conceived. When the neural tube does not close completely, an NTD develops. NTDs develop before most women know they are even pregnant.

Types

There are two types of NTDs:
1. **Open NTDs:** Open NTDs are more common type. Open NTDs occur when the brain and/or spinal cord are exposed at birth through a defect in the skull or vertebrae (back bones). Examples of open NTDs are spina bifida (myelomeningocele), anencephaly and encephalocele.
2. **Closed NTDs:** Closed NTDs occur when the spinal defect is covered by skin. Common examples of closed NTDs are lipomyelomeningocele, lipomeningocele and tethered cord. Lastly, spina bifida occulta (SBO) is potentially another form of an NTD in which there is a typically benign (or nonsymptom-causing) bony change in one or more vertebrae, but not involving the nerves within the spinal column. The incidence of SBO is not well defined; however, it is more common than the NTDs described above. The cause and potential similarities, or, link to NTDs, has not been established.

Table 17.8 presents the types of presentation of NTD under two board category i.e. cranial presentation and spinal presentation.

Epidemiology

- Incidence has declined significantly in the last 30 years and now occurs in approximately 0.8/1,000 total births.
- Anencephaly and spina bifida accounts for up to 95% of all neural tube defects with equal prevalence.

Risk Factors

Neural tube defects are considered a complex disorder, because they are caused by a combination of multiple genes and multiple environmental factors **(Fig. 17.11)**. The known risk factors include:
- **Family history:** One type of malformation puts other family members at risk of all types of defect. Studies of twins with NTDs have shown both identical twins have NTDs more than both fraternal twins. Studies of families show that the chance of having a second family member born with an NTD after one child is born with an NTD increases.
- May occur as part of a number of different syndromes and chromosomal disorders. NTDs are a feature (or symptom) of known genetic syndromes, such as trisomy 13, trisomy 18, certain chromosome rearrangements and Meckel-Gruber syndrome.
- Diet low in folic acid.
- Maternal drug therapy with sodium valproate and folic acid antagonists, e.g., some anti-epileptics, trimethoprim.

Table 17.8: Types of presentation of neural tube defects.

Cranial presentation	Spinal presentations
- Anencephaly - Encephalocele (meningocele or meningomyelocele) - Congenital dermal sinus	- Spina bifida - Spina bifida occulta - Myelomeningocele - Meningocele - Congenital dermal sinus - Caudal agenesis

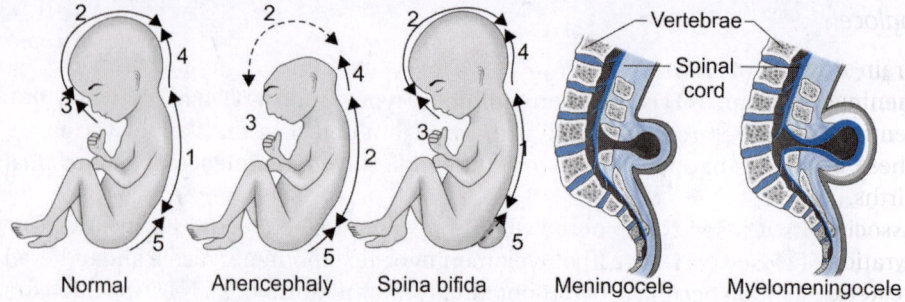

Fig. 17.11: Neural tube defects.

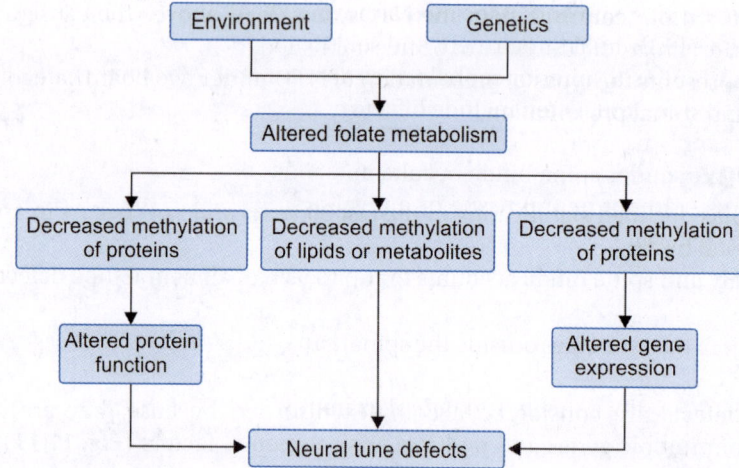

Fig. 17.12: Genetic and environmental etiology of neural tube defect.

- Dysraphism is used to describe situations where there is continuity between the posterior neuroectoderm and cutaneous ectoderm.

Presentation and Management

The different types of presentation of the NTD the illustrated in **Fig. 17.12**.

Cranial Dysraphism

Anencephaly:

- Cranial vault is absent **(Fig. 17.13)**.
- Most cases are now terminated following prenatal diagnosis.
- In live born babies, initial neurological examination may appear normal if brainstem structures are relatively intact and may have seizures.
- Infants usually die within hours or days.

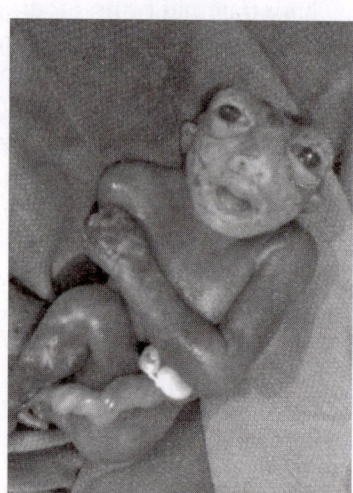

Fig. 17.13: Anencephaly.

Cephaloceles

- Brain matter herniates through a defect in skull. A cranial meningocele contains only meninges, encephalocele contains brain tissue; a ventriculocele contains part of the ventricle within the herniated part of the brain.
- These are rarer than anencephaly or spina bifida, with an incidence of 1-3/10,000 live births.
- Associated with other brain abnormalities, e.g., agenesis or corpus callosum or abnormal gyration and may be part of a recognized syndrome.
- Posterior cephaloceles are commonest in Western countries with most being occipital encephaloceles of variable size occurring above or below the tentorium. If below, then they are associated with severe cerebellar defects, e.g., Chiari III malformation.
- Depending on size, site and associated abnormalities, there may be visual, sensorimotor disturbance, intellectual impairment and seizures.
- In some parts of Asia, anterior cephaloceles are more common and may protrude into the nose, ethmoid or orbit. Often include olfactory tissue and frontal lobe tissue.
- Spinal dysraphism.
- Spina bifida includes spina bifida occulta and spina bifida cystica, which may be either a meningocele without neural tissue or a myelomeningocele where the spinal cord forms part of the cyst wall.

Meningocele

- Protrusion of the meninges outside the spinal canal accounts for 5% of cases of spina bifida cystica.
- No associated hydrocephalus and neural examination is often normal.

Myelomeningocele

- Occurs in 80-90% of spina bifida cystica cases.
- About 80% are lumbosacral consisting of a sac covered with a thin membrane that may leak CSF **(Fig. 17.14)**.
- Level of lesion is best assessed by determining upper limit of sensory loss, but at all levels there is disturbance of bladder and bowel control.
- Higher lesions are associated with bladder outlet obstruction with consequent dilatation of the upper urinary tract and chronic pyelonephritis.
- Hydrocephalus occurs in approximately 90% of cases at birth even with normal head circumference.
- Usually associated with Chiari II malformation, but may also be due to aqueduct stenosis or have no clear cause.
- Usually detected by ultrasound.
- If signs of progressive ventricular dilatation or rising intracranial pressure, usually needs insertion of a ventriculoperitoneal shunt.

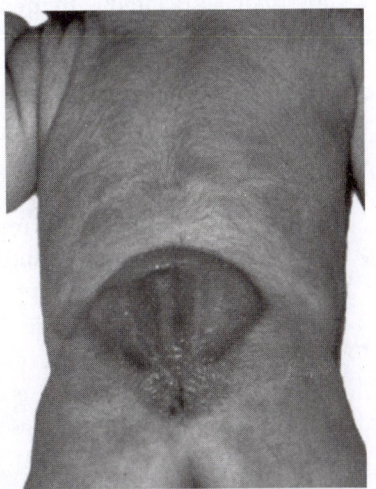

Fig. 17.14: Myelomeningocele.

Chiari II Malformation
- Occurs in approximately 70% of cases of myelomeningocele.
- Consists of downward protrusion of the medulla below the foramen magnum overlap the spinal cord.
- This causes the medulla to be kinked and the cerebellar vermis to be indented, fourth ventricle elongated and midbrain distorted.
- Problems include palsies and central apnea.
- Treatment by closure of the defect remains controversial and is not always performed.

Spina Bifida Occulta
- Defect of the posterior arch of one or more lumbar or sacral vertebra (often L5 and S1).
- Often found incidentally on X-ray in children admitted to hospital; may be considered as a normal variant.
- However, if examination reveals a nevus, hairy patch, dimple, sinus or subcutaneous mass, then MRI of the spinal cord is recommended even if no associated problems with sphincter or limb control.
- Can cause asymmetrical lower motor neurone weakness associated with wasting, deformity and diminished reflexes.
- May also be progressive gait disturbance with spasticity and impaired bladder control.

Dorsal Dermal Sinuses
- Often found in the occipital and lumbosacral areas and can connect the skin surface to the dura or to an intradural dermoid cyst.
- If open can produce recurrent meningitis so should be explored and removed if possible before infection occurs.

Lipomyelomeningocele
- Seen as a bulge in the lumbosacral region normally lateral to the mid-line.
- This is a lipoma or lipofibroma attached to the spinal cord, which is low lying.
- Are often associated with meningocele.

Diastematomyelia
- Sagittal cleft dividing the spinal cord in the two halves each surrounded by its pia mater.
- The cord may be transfixed by a bony or cartilaginous spur.
- Usually occurs in low thoracic or lumbar regions.
- Overlying skin abnormality is present in 75% of cases and X-rays show abnormalities in most cases including abnormal segmentation of vertebrae, spina bifida and scoliosis.
- Neurosurgery is normally indicated if abnormality involves cord or nerve roots with the objective of reducing pressure over spinal cord for normal growth and prevent further damage.

Prenatal Screening

Alpha-fetoprotein in maternal serum: Best detected at 16–18 weeks of pregnancy, but may not detect closed defects and is less sensitive if a woman is taking valproate.

Ultrasound: It is recommended for all at-risk women (positive serum AFP, previously affected child) can detect anencephaly from 12th week and spina bifida from 16–20 weeks (may occasionally be missed especially in L5-S2 region).

Amniocentesis: It is only used when unable to obtain adequate ultrasound images; used to measure AFP and neuronal acetylcholinesterase.

Investigations
- Magnetic resonance imaging is the study of choice for imaging neural tissue and for identifying contents of the defect in the newborn.
- CT scan allows direct visualization of the bony defect and anatomy.
- Ultrasound is used antenatally for screening.

Management
- Affected children will be getting treatment from a multidisciplinary team to address any associated physical, developmental, hearing, visual and learning difficulties that may occur in association with the NTD.
- The newborn with an open NTD should be kept warm and the defect covered with a sterile saline dressing.
- The baby should be positioned in the prone position to prevent pressure on the defect.
- Open NTDs should be closed promptly.
- *Hydrocephalus:* Ventriculoperitoneal shunt placed at the time of myelomeningocele closure.
- *Symptomatic Chiari malformations:* Suboccipital craniotomy and decompression of the posterior fossa and tonsils.
- Laminectomy and placement of a syringosubarachnoid stent to divert the CSF out of the central canal.

Complications
- Infections.
- Associated motor and sensory problems, particularly lower limb.
- Associated learning disability, developmental delay and hearing impairment.
- Bladder and bowel dysfunction.

Prevention
- Periconceptional folic acid supplementation can prevent most NTDs if widely used. Supplementation must begin before conception, for it to be effective.
- To prevent first occurrence, women who are planning to become pregnant should take 400 µg folic acid daily before conception and during first 12 weeks of pregnancy. However, women who have had a previous NTD pregnancy are recommended to take an even higher dosage of folic acid prior to planning a pregnancy. They should increase the daily dose of folic acid from 0.4 mg to 4.0 mg, one month prior to conception through the first three months of pregnancy. The 4.0–0.5 mg of folic acid should be obtained only through a prescription from the doctor.
- Food fortification with the addition of folate to grain products is considered the most effective method of ensuring adequate intake of folic acid in pregnant women.

Role of Nurses
- Provide proper position to child to prevent further neurological damage.
- Ensure infection control measures in every contact with child to prevent infection.

- Keep the defect covered with sterile wet gauze to prevent infection.
- Involve the parents in care of child, ask parents to hold the chills and look to enhance parent-child relationship.
- The parents of a child with congenital defects must be provided a high level of support and effective nurse-parents relationship is essential for effective outcome of total healthcare.
- Encourage the patients to ask as many as questions and provide answers for every question in simple and positive language by providing expected hope.
- Discussion with parents about causes of disorder and expected outcome and prognosis based on severity of NTD.
- Discuss about possible treatment modalities.
- Take or assist physical to take required sample to detect associated chromosomal abnormalities.
- Plan about discharge, provide discharge teaching and discuss about follow-up care.

DOWN SYNDROME

Down syndrome is a common genetic disorder characterized by mental retardation, dysmorphic facial features and a host of structural abnormalities. It is so called after John Langdon Haydon Down, an English physician, 1828–1896. It is also known as Mongolism or trisomy 21 chromosome **(Fig. 17.15)**.

One of the commonest genetic disorders affecting 1 in 800 live births. Down syndrome is a chromosomal condition related to chromosome 21. Most cases of Down syndrome result from trisomy 21, which means each cell in the body has three copies of chromosome 21 instead of the usual two copies. The extra genetic material disrupts the normal course of development, causing the characteristic features of Down syndrome. A small percentage of cases occur when only some of the body's cells have an extra copy of the chromosome. These cases are called mosaic Down syndrome. Although uncommon, Down syndrome can also occur when part of chromosome 21 becomes attached (translocated) to another chromosome before or at conception. Affected people have two copies of chromosome 21, plus extra material from chromosome 21 attached to another chromosome. These cases are called translocation Down syndrome. Incidence of Down syndrome cases are observed as the following:

- The underlying genetic defect is trisomy 21 in 94% of cases
- Mosaicism (2.4%) and translocations (3.3%) also occur
- About 75% of these translocations are de novo errors.

Risk Factors

- Family history.
- *Age of mother:*
  - 1:385 risk at 35 years.
  - 1:106 risk at 40 years.
  - 1:30 risk at 45 years.

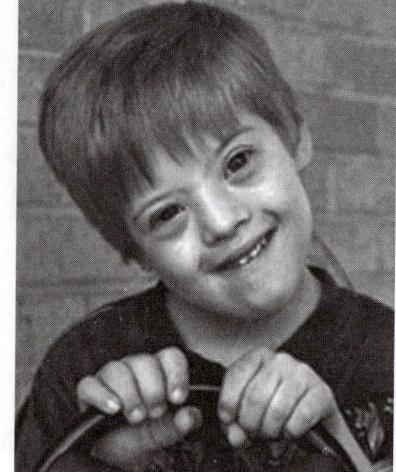

Fig. 17.15: Child with Down syndrome features.

Clinical Manifestation

At birth there are a wide range of associated physical features. Not all babies have typical facies. Frequently the first feature noticed is hypotonia **(Box 17.5)**.

Soon after birth all babies with Down syndrome should be assessed for congenital heart disease by echocardiogram. They should also have auditory evoked potential testing (before 6 months of age) to check for hearing loss, and also be checked for congenital cataracts and glaucoma **(Table 17.9)**.

Prenatal Screening and Diagnosis

- There is a large amount of published research on Down syndrome screening. It looks at combinations of markers ± ultrasound [nuchal translucency (NT) scans measure the thickness of skin at the nuchal fold at around 10–12 weeks gestation], used in the first or second trimesters. Screening aims to identify women at higher risk than that predicted on the basis of age alone. If the woman chooses to, after counseling on associated risks, she may proceed to invasive testing, e.g., chorionic villus sampling or amniocentesis to establish fetal karyotype:
  - The integrated test offers the most effective and safe method of screening for women who attend in the first trimester. This test comprises nuchal translucency scanning and pregnancy associated plasma protein-A (PAPP-A) at 11 completed weeks of pregnancy, and AFP, unconjugated estriol (uE3), free beta or total human chorionic gonadotropin (hCG) and inhibin-A in the early second trimester. With this method at an 85% detection rate, it has been estimated that there would be six amniocentesis-caused miscarriages of unaffected fetuses per 100,000 women screened, compared with 35 using the combined test or 45 with the quadruple test.
  - If PAPP-A, hCG and nuchal translucency scanning (NT) are used as a first trimester screening test, it is commonly referred to as the combined test.
  - When hCG and AFP are used between 14 and 20 weeks as a screening test, this is often called double test.
  - If uE3 is added to the double test combination, it becomes known as the triple test.
  - The addition of inhibin A to the triple test comprises the quadruple test.

Box 17.5: Neonatal features of Down syndrome.

- Brachycephaly
- Oblique palpebral fissures
- Gap between hallux and second toes
- Loose skin on nape of neck
- Hyperflexibility
- Ears set low, folded or stenotic meatus
- Protruding tongue (small narrow palate)
- Flat nasal bridge
- Muscular hypotonia
- Epicanthic folds
- Ring of iris speckles—brushfield spots
- Short little finger
- In-curved little finger
- Short broad hands
- High-arched palate
- Single palmar crease
- Congenital heart defects (CHD)
- Transient myelodysplasia of the newborn*
- Duodenal atresia*

*Highly specific for Down syndrome.

Table. 17.9: Associated conditions in a child with Down syndrome.

Cardiological disorders	Hematological disorders
Atrioventricular canal defects (AVSD)	Impaired cellular immunity (greater risk of infections, e.g., pneumonia)
Ventricular septal defects (VSD)	Increased risk of acute leukemia
Isolated secundum atrial septal defects (ASD)	Polycythemia and transient myeloproliferative disorder (TMD)
Isolated persistent patent ductus arteriosus (PDA)	
Tetralogy of Fallot	
Orthopedic disorders	**Ophthalmological disorders**
Atlantoaxial instability	Cataracts
Hyperflexibility	Refractive errors
Scoliosis	Strabismus
Hip dislocation after 2 years	Nystagmus
Patellar subluxation or dislocation	Congenital glaucoma
Foot deformities	Keratoconus
Gastrointestinal disorders	**Neurological disorders**
Esophageal atresia or tracheoesophageal fistula	Mental retardation (severe retardation to 'low normal')
Duodenal atresia	Behavioral problems
Pyloric stenosis	Seizures occur in 5–10%
Meckel's diverticulum	In older patients an Alzheimer's type picture develops in >60% of those over 60 years of age
Hirschsprung's disease	
Imperforate anus	
Gastroesophageal reflux	
Dental problems	
Celiac disease	
ENT disorders	**Endocrine disorders**
Conductive, sensorineural or mixed hearing loss	Hypothyroidism
More susceptible to otitis media, sinusitis and pharyngitis	
Obstructive sleep apnea	

- First trimester prenatal screening using a combination of maternal serum biochemistry and fetal nuchal translucency thickness has been shown to achieve detection rates over 90%.
- A disintegrin and metalloprotease 12 (ADAM 12) is a glycoprotein synthesized by placenta. It has been shown to be a potential first trimester maternal serum marker for Down syndrome (DS). ADAM 12 and PAPP-A measured at 8–9 weeks and combined with NT and

free beta-hCG measured at 12 weeks has been predicted to give a detection rate of 97% at a 5% false-positive rate.
- First trimester screening for trisomy 21 in twin pregnancies is possible and practical using a combination of nuchal translucency thickness and maternal serum biochemistry.
- Amniocentesis (at 14–16 weeks) is 99.5% accurate. Chorionic villus sampling (CVS) can be performed earlier (10–13 weeks) but accuracy is less (96–98%). Both procedures have an operator specific miscarriage risk.

Role of Nurses
- The parents of a child with Down syndrome must be provided a high level of support and nursing interventions are essentials for effective outcome of total health care.
- Conduct a counseling sessions with parents in presence of expert counselor.
- Encourage the patient to ask as many as questions and provide answers for every question in simple and positive language by providing expected hope.
- Ensure that parents hold and be with child to enhance early parent-child bond.
- Help the parents to learn about available community resources and association, which can help them to care for child.
- Teach the parents about care of child at home.
- Discuss about further diagnosis of associated health problems.
- Plan about discharge, provide discharge teaching and discuss about follow-up care.
- Offer counseling about future pregnancy and needed prenatal testing.

MULTIPLE CHOICE QUESTIONS

1. **The increased level of maternal serum cytokines interlukin-8 (IL-8) during second trimester can increase the risk of which condition?**
   a. Miscarriage   b. Stillbirth
   c. Schizophrenia   d. Neural tube defects
2. **Fifth Disease is caused by which organism?**
   a. Human papilloma virus   b. Human Parvovirus
   c. Staphylococcus   d. Streptococcus
3. **Consanguinity means relationship between two people who share common_____.**
   a. Ancestor   b. Region
   c. State   d. None of these
4. **Which of the following is the teratogenic drugs?**
   a. Oxytocin   b. Phenytoin
   c. Pantoprazole d. Paracetamol

Answer Key
1. c   2. b   3. a   4. b

FURTHER READING
1. Alfirevic Z, Gosden CM, Neilson JP. Chorion villus sampling versus amniocentesis for prenatal diagnosis. Cochrane Database Syst Rev. 2000;(2):CD000055.
2. Alfirevic Z, Sundberg K, Brigham S. Amniocentesis and chorionic villus sampling for prenatal diagnosis. Cochrane Database Syst Rev. 2003;(3):CD003252.
3. Alfirevic Z, von Dadelszen P. Instruments for chorionic villus sampling for prenatal diagnosis. Cochrane Database Syst Rev. 2003;(1):CD000114.

4. Alteneder RR, Kenner C, Greene D, et al. The lived experience of women who undergo prenatal diagnostic testing due to elevated maternal serum alpha-fetoprotein screening. MCN Am J Matern Child Nurs. 1998;23:180-6.
5. American Academy of Pediatrics Committee in Infectious Diseases. Parvovirus, erythema infectiosum, and pregnancy. Pediatrics. 1990;85:131.
6. Amniocentesis Guideline, Royal College of Obstetricians and Gynecologists. 2005.
7. Antenatal care - Routine care for the healthy pregnant woman, NICE Clinical guidance. 2003.
8. Baird PA, Sadovnick AD. Life tables for Down syndrome. Hum Genet. 1989;82(3):291-2.
9. Bender PL. Genetic family history assessment. AACN Clinical Issue. 1998;9:467-83.
10. Birnbacher R, Messerschmidt AM, Pollak AP. Diagnosis and prevention of neural tube defects. Curr Opin Urol. 2002;12(6):461-4.
11. Blackburn ST. Assessment and management of neurologic dysfunction. In Comprehensive Neonatal Nursing Care: A Physiologic Perspective, 2nd edition. Philadelphia: WB Saunders; 1998:564-607.
12. Brambati B, Tului L. Chorionic villus sampling and amniocentesis. Curr Opin Obstet Gynecol. 2005;17(2):197-201.
13. Breeze AC, Lees CC, Kumar A, et al. Palliative care for prenatally diagnosed lethal fetal abnormality. Arch Dis Child Fetal Neonatal Ed. 2007;92(1):F56-8.
14. Burke SS, Matsumoto AR: Pastoral care for perinatal and neonatal health care providers. Journal of Obstetric, Gynecologic, and Neonatal Nursing. 1999;28:137-41.
15. Busby A, Abramsky L, Dolk H, et al. Preventing neural tube defects in Europe: population based study. BMJ. 2005;330(7491):574-5.
16. Caughey AB, Hopkins LM, Norton ME. Chorionic villus sampling compared with amniocentesis and the difference in the rate of pregnancy loss. Obstet Gynecol. 2006;108(3 Pt 1):612-6.
17. Centers for Disease Control. Risks Associated with Human Parvovirus B19 Infection. Morbidity and Mortality Weekly Report. 1989;38:81-7.
18. Centini G, Rosignoli L, Kenanidis A, et al. A report of early (13 + 0 to 14 + 6 weeks) and mid-trimester amnioceenteses: 10 years' experience. J Matern Fetal Neonatal Med. 2003;14(2):113-7.
19. Chen H. Down's Syndrome. [online] e-medicine. Available from Jan 2006.
20. Chi C, Hyett JA, Finning KM, et al. Non-invasive first trimester determination of fetal gender: a new approach for prenatal diagnosis of haemophilia. BJOG. 2006;113(2):239-42.
21. Chitty LS, Kagan KO, Molina FS, et al Fetal nuchal translucency scan and early prenatal diagnosis of chromosomal abnormalities by rapid aneuploidy screening: observational study.BMJ. 2006;25;332(7539):452-5.
22. Cochrane DD, Wilson RD, Steinbok P, et al Prenatal spinal evaluation and functional outcome of patients born with myelomeningocele: information for improved prenatal counselling and outcome prediction. Fetal Diagn Ther. 1996;11(3):159-68.
23. Conover E: Hazardous exposures during pregnancy. Journal of Obstetric, Gynecologic, and Neonatal Nursing. 1994;23:524-532.
24. Coulson CC, Katz VL, Kuller JA. Triple-marker screening for aneuploidy. In: Kuller JA, Chescheir NC, Cefalo RC (Eds). Prenatal Diagnosis and Reproductive Genetics. St. Louis: Mosby; 1996.8495.
25. Delisle MF, Wilson RD. First trimester prenatal diagnosis: amniocentesis. Semin Perinatol.1999 Oct;23(5):414-23.
26. Dhallan R, Guo X, Emche S, et al. A non-invasive test for prenatal diagnosis based on fetal DNA present in maternal blood: a preliminary study. Lancet. 2007:10;369(9560):474-81.
27. Driscoll KM. The application of genetic knowledge: Ethical and policy implications. AACN Clinical Issues. 1998;9:588-99.
28. Dwyer ML. Genetic research and ethical challenges: Implications for nursing practice. AACN Clinical Issues. 1998;9:600-05.
29. Felblinger DM, Akers MC. Marfan's syndrome in pregnancy: Implications for advanced practice nurses. AACN Clinical Issues. 2000;9:563-8.
30. Fischbach FA Manual of Laboratory and Diagnostic Tests, 5th edition. Philadelphia: IB Lippincott; 1996.

31. Foley SM, Sommers MS: Molecular genetics: From bench to bedside. AACN Clinical Issues. 1998;9:491-8.
32. Fowler K, Stango S, Pass R, et al. The Outcome of Congenital Cytomegalovirus Infection in Relation to Maternal Antibody Status. N Engl J Med. 326:663-7.
33. Haddow JE. Antenatal screening for Down's syndrome: Where are we and where next? Lancet. 1998;352:336-7.
34. Hanshaw J, Dudgeon J, Marshall W. "Viral Diseases of the Fetus and Newborn, 2nd edition. W.B. Saunders; Philadelphia; 1985:92–131.
35. Hiatt PW, Grace SC, Kozinetz CA, et al. Effects of viral lower respiratory tract infection on lung function in infants with cystic fibrosis. Pediatrics. 1999;103:619-26.
36. Hoffman DE, Wulfsberg EA. Testing children for genetic predispositions: Is it in their best interest? Journal of Law and Medical Ethics. 1995;23:331-44.
37. Indian Journal of Human Genetics. May-August 2005;11(2):108-10.
38. Jones KL, Johnson K, Chambers C. Offspring of Women Infected With Varicella During Pregnancy: A Prospective Study. Teratology. 1994;49:29-32.
39. Kennedy SJ, Blough RA, Kenner CA, et al. An assessment of two training interventions designed to increase the knowledge of obstetrical nurses and nurse-midwives about the maternal serum triple screen. Prenat Diagn. 1998;18:713-20.
40. Kenner C, Dreyer L, Amlung S. Newborn genetic screening: Blessing or curse? Neonatal Network.1999;18:11-20.
41. Kenner C. National Coalition for Health Professional Education in Genetics. AACN Clinical Issues.1998;9:582-7.
42. Koren G (Ed). Maternal-fetal toxicology, a clinician's guide, 2nd edition. Marcel Dekker: New York; 1994.
43. Koren G, Pastuszak A, Ito S. Drugs in pregnancy. N Engl J Med. 1998;338:1128-37.
44. Kramer MS. The epidemiology of adverse pregnancy outcomes: an overview. J Nutr. 2003;133(5 Suppl 2):1592S-1596S.
45. Kuller JA, Chescheir NC, Cefalo RC. Prenatal Diagnosis and Reproductive Genetics. St. Louis: Mosby; 1996.
46. Kunk RM. Expanding the newborn screen: Terrific or troubling? MCN Am J Matern Child Nurs. 1998;23:266-71.
47. Laigaard J, Spencer K, Christiansen M, et al. ADAM12 as a first-trimester maternal serum marker in screening for Down syndrome. Prenat Diagn. 2006;26(10):973-9.
48. Lashley FRC. Clinical Genetics in Nursing Practice, 2nd edition. New York: Springer; 1998.
49. Laurent C. Antenatal screening and counseling: The midwife's role. Nursing Times.1998;94:52-5.
50. Lea DH, Jenkins JF, Francomano CA. Genetics in Clinical Practice: New Directions for Nursing and Health Care. Sudbury, MA: Jones and Bartlett; 1998.
51. Mangels KJ, Tulipan N, Tsao LY, et al Fetal MRI in the evaluation of intrauterine myelomeningocele. Pediatr Neurosurg. 2000;32(3):124-31.
52. Mann K, Fox SP, Abbs SJ, et al. Development and implementation of a new rapid aneuploidy diagnostic service within the UK National Health Service and implications for the future of prenatal diagnosis. Lancet. 2001;358(9287):1057-61.
53. March of Dimes Birth Defects Foundation: Stat book: Statistics for Monitoring Maternal and Infant Health. White Plains, NY: March of Dimes Foundation; 1997.
54. McCombs J, Cramer MK. Pregnancy and lactation: therapeutic considerations. In: DiPiro JT, Talbert RL, Yee GC, et al (Eds). Pharmacotherapy. A pathophysiologic approach, 4th edition. p1298-312. Appleton and Lange: Stamford; 1999.
55. NBDPN. Advances and Opportunities for Birth Defects Surveillance, Research, and Prevention. 1999:123-30.
56. Pastuszak A, Levy M, Schick B, et al. Outcome After Maternal Varicella Infection in the First 20 Weeks of Pregnancy. N Engl J Med. 1994;330:901-5.
57. Penticuff J. Ethical issues in genetic therapy. Journal of Obstetric, Gynecologic, and Neonatal Nursing. 1994;23:498-501.

58. Philip J, Silver RK, Wilson RD, et al. Late first-trimester invasive prenatal diagnosis: results of an international randomized trial. Obstet Gynecol. 2004;103(6):1164-73.
59. Pickier RH, Munro CL. Blastomere analysis: Issues for discussion. Journal of Obstetric, Gynecologic, and Neonatal Nursing. 1994;23:379-82.
60. Raff BA. Nursing and genetics for the 21st century. Journal of Obstetric, Gynecologic, and Neonatal Nursing. 1994;23:477-86.
61. Raines DA. Ethical implications of genetic testing. NursClin North Am. 1998;33:275-86.
62. Remington J, Klein J (1990). "Infectious Diseases of the Fetus and Newborn Infant." WB Saunders, Co.
63. Rice E. The human genome project and gene therapy: A genetic counselor's perspective. J Prenat Neonatal Nurs. 1998;12:16-25.
64. Richmond S, Atkins J. A population-based study of the prenatal diagnosis of congenital malformation over 16 years. BJOG. 2005;112(10):1349-57.
65. Roche ML, Kuller JA. Autosomal disorders: Cystic fibrosis, Tay-Sachs disease, and Huntington disease. In: Kuller JA, Chescheir NC, Cefalo RC (Eds). Prenatal Diagnosis and Reproductive Genetics.Mosby St. Louis; 1996:53-63.
66. Rose PG, Fraire AE. Multiple primary gynecologic neoplasms in a young HIV-positive patient. Journal of Surgical Oncology. 1993 Aug;53(4):269-72.
67. Rosenberg KD, Gelow JM, Sandoval AP. Pregnancy intendedness and the use of periconceptional folic acid. Pediatrics. 2003;111(5 Part 2):1142-5.
68. Ross U: Developmental disabilities: Genetic implications. Journal of Obstetric, Gynecologic, and Neonatal Nursing. 1994;23:502-5.
69. Rubin P (Ed). Prescribing in pregnancy, 2nd edition. BMJ Publishing Group: London; 1995.
70. Saito H, Sekizawa A, Morimoto T, et al. Prenatal DNA diagnosis of a single-gene disorder from maternal plasma. Lancet. 2000;356(9236):1170.
71. Schaap AH, van der Pol HG, Boer K, et al. Long-term follow-up of infants after transcervical chorionic villus sampling and after amniocentesis to compare congenital abnormalities and health status. Prenat Diagn. 2002;22(7):598-604.
72. Schardein JL. Chemically induced birth defects, 2nd edition. Marcel Dekker: New York; 1993.
73. Seaver L, Hoyme HE (1992). Teratology on Pediatric Practice. Pediatric Clinics of North America. 39.
74. Shaw C, Lammer EJ. Maternal periconceptional alcohol consumption and risk for orofacial clefts. J Pediatr. 1999;134:298-303.
75. Sommers MS, Beery T. Foundations of genetics: Genetic structure, function, and therapeutics. AACN Clinical Issues. 1998;9:467-48.
76. Spencer K, Nicolaides KH. Screening for trisomy 21 in twins using first trimester ultrasound and maternal serum biochemistry in a one-stop clinic: a review of three years experience. BJOG. 2003;110(3):276-80.
77. Spencer K, Nicolaides KH. Screening for trisomy 21 in twins using first trimester ultrasound and maternal serum biochemistry in a one-stop clinic: a review of three years experience. BJOG. 2003;110(3):276-80.
78. Spencer K, Spencer CE, Power M, et al. Screening for chromosomal abnormalities in the first trimester using ultrasound and maternal serum biochemistry in a one-stop clinic: are view of three years prospective experience. BJOG. 2003;110(3):281-6.
79. Spencer K, Spencer CE, Power M, et al. Screening for chromosomal abnormalities in the first trimester using ultrasound and maternal serum biochemistry in a one-stop clinic: are view of three years prospective experience. BJOG. 2003;110(3):281-6.
80. Stranc LC, Evans JA, Hamerton JL. Chorionic villus sampling and amniocentesis for prenatal diagnosis. Lancet. 1997;349(9053):711-4.
81. Theis JWG, Koren G. Maternal and fetal clinical pharmacology. In: Speight TM, Holford NHG (Eds). Avery's Drug Treatment, 4th edition. Adis International Limited: Auckland; 1997.
82. Theorell CJ, Dengenhardt M. Assessment and management of metabolic dysfunction. In Comprehensive Neonatal Nursing Care: A Physiologic Perspective. Philadelphia: WB Saunders; 1998:409-75.
83. Tritos NA. Kallmann Syndrome and idiopathic hypogonadotropic hypogonadism clinical presentation. Available from. https://emedicine.medscape.com/article/122824-clinical/Accessed Jan 19, 2021.

84. Troy ES. The genetic privacy act: An analysis of privacy and research concerns. Journal of Law and Medical Ethics. 1997;25:256-72.
85. Von Dadelszen P, Sermer M, Hillier J, et al. A randomised controlled trial of biopsy forceps and cannula aspiration for transcervical chorionic villus sampling. BJOG. 2005;112(5):559-66.
86. Wald NJ, Rodeck C, Hackshaw AK, et al. SURUSS in perspective. Semin Perinatol. 2005 Aug;29(4):225-35.
87. Waliman CM. Newborn genetic screening. Neonatal Network. 1998;17:55-60.
88. Wapner RJ, Evans MI, Davis G, et al. Procedural risks versus theology: chorionic villus sampling for Orthodox Jews at less than 8 weeks' gestation. Am J Obstet Gynecol. 2002;186(6):1133-6.
89. Wendy C. Tetragons and their effects. Available from: http://www.columbia.edu/itc/hs/medical/humandev/2004/Chpt23-Teratogens.pdf/Accessed Jan 19, 2021
90. Whitley, et al. Predictors of Morbidity and Mortality in Neonates With Herpes Simplex Virus Infections. N Engl J Med. 1991;423:450-4.
91. Williams JK. Genetic testing: Implications for professional nursing. J Prof Nurs. 1998;14:184-8.
92. Wright L. Prenatal diagnosis in the 1990s. Journal of Obstetric, Gynecologic, and Neonatal Nursing.1994;23:506-15.

CHAPTER 18

Neonatal and Children Testing or Screening

Suresh Sharma, Jyoti Arora

INTRODUCTION

Neonatal testing can be performed to diagnose disorder or screen for a potential pathologic condition among newborns. In some states of USA, four conditions are tested for, whereas other states require more than 20 different tests. The most common tests are homocystinuria, phenylketonuria, hypothyroidism and galactosemia. Hemoglobinopathies have been added in several states. The rationale behind the state mandate is that the risk to the infant is minimal, whereas the lifelong benefit is tremendous. Because many of these conditions involve errors of metabolism (formerly referred to as inborn errors of metabolism), they have a distant possibility of causing mental retardation, organic failure to thrive and even death, if undetected and untreated. The quality of life for the infant and the family can be impacted positively with early detection, and the cost to society is decreased related to less extraordinary services that are required when treatment is expeditious and successful.

Other neonatal tests focus on chromosomal changes, such as those seen with trisomy conditions. These are conditions in which the infant has three of any one chromosome instead of the normal two. The total number of chromosomes should be 46; however, in the infant with a trisomy, there is an extra chromosome when the karyotype is examined. This extragenetic material may have no clinical impact or may be severe enough, as in the case of trisomy 13 (three of chromosome 13) that death is inevitable. The diagnosis of this condition may facilitate informed family decisions about treatment. In another instance, such as with the infant diagnosed with trisomy 21 (Down syndrome), the diagnosis may allow parents to gain access to the services to foster early growth and development, to help the child reach maximum potential. In addition, a diagnosis of trisomy 21 early in life clues the healthcare professional to look for related problems, such as congenital leukemia and cardiac anomalies.

MEANING AND PURPOSE

Neonatal and children testing may be offered or conducted within the context of general or targeted neonatal and children population screening programs, or be offered to specific children at risk, but the term 'genetic testing' commonly referred to the use of specific tests for individuals who are believed to be at increased risk for a specific genetic conditions, because of their family history or symptom manifestations.

The task force on genetic testing defines a genetic test as 'the analysis of human DNA, RNA, chromosomes, protein and certain metabolites in order to detect heritable disease-related genotypes, mutations, phenotypes or karyotypes for clinical purpose.'

Genetic test or screening may be done for:
- Detecting or diagnosing a present disease state
- Determining carrier state

- Determining disease susceptibility
- Detecting abnormalities in the fetus
- The prediction of disease in usually asymptomatic person that may include late onset or adult disorders.

Although there can be difference in the use of the term 'screening'—an accepted definition is 'the presumptive identification of an unrecognized disease or defect in an apparently healthy individual'. Genetic screening was more specifically defined by the committee for the study of inborn errors of metabolism (1975) of the National Academy of Sciences and this is the accepted definition. Essentially, it is a search for:

- Child who poses genotype that is associated with the development of genetic disease. The usual purpose is such that the treatment can be instituted or the natural course of the disease can be altered. An example of this is screening newborn for phenylketonuria (PKU) in order to restrict their diet to prevent mental retardation.
- Person with certain genotype are known to predispose the individual to illness. An example of this is the identification of individuals with G6PD deficiency, who after being identified, can avoid the precipitation of hemolytic anemia by avoiding certain foods and drugs.
- Person who are heterozygous carriers of recessive inheritance genes that in autosomal recessive disorders (in double dose), can cause genetic disease in their descendants. An example of this would be screening program for the detection of Tay-Sachs carriers. This type of screening provides information to an individual so that he/she can make reproductive plan for the future genetic counseling, including reproductive options and the availability of prenatal diagnosis is an essential component of this type of screening.
- Person with polymorphism (variability) not known to be associated with a disease state. This allows for the gathering information related to the genetic makeup of the population. This may begin as research and later have therapeutic value. A common example is in the observed variation of human blood groups.

NEWBORN SCREENING

Genetic knowledge from the human genome project and the development of new technologies have led to a new era in newborn screening; which is one of the great genetic public health success stories. Newborn screening is a program identifying babies at risk of having any developmental, genetic, and metabolic disorders. Once PKU (phenylketonuria) was found to be associated with a type of mental retardation, which could be prevented if a low phenylalanine (PHE) diet was instituted soon after birth, a search began for a method to reliability test to detect PKU in newborn. Eventually Robert Guthrie developed such a test using blood taken from drops placed on filter paper and dried. Testing was based on a bacterial growth inhibition assay using the dried blood spot. This test became the base for screening virtually for the entire newborn population. If an abnormal screening test was identified, a low PHE diet could be initiated and effective treatment put in place for those whose diagnosis was confirmed. Recently, newer technology, such as tandem mass spectrometry (MS/MS) and the expansion of molecular- and DNA-based techniques have identified additional mutations that has expanded the scope of genetic screening among neonates and children.

The major reason for newborn screening is to identify apparently healthy newborn at risk through newborn screening programs, to provide early treatment for certain disorders as soon as possible and thereby prevent serious health consequences, especially severe mental retardation.

Important Elements in Newborn Screening

- Inclusion of new neonates before hospital discharge according to State Law guidelines
- Provision to include neonates not tested before discharge and those born outside the hospital as possible
- Education of parents about screening at appropriate educational level, considering cultural beliefs, religions, that involves, how the test results will be communicated
- Informed parental consent within state laws
- Collection of appropriate specimens at proper time
- Reliable, accurate, standardized testing in centralized laboratory is ideal
- Provision for re-screening, if tested early, re-screening should be done at about 3 weeks of age for PKU
- Communication of positive screening results to local physician and parents quickly (by telephone with letter of confirmation). Ideally have counseling and psychosocial support available to help parents and family with stressful situation
- Follow up all newborns with positive screening test results
- Insure means of accurate diagnosis are available for all with confirmed positive screening tests
- Provision of genetic and other counseling that is culturally competent and educationally appropriate
- Provision of for treatment and ongoing management of infant and family.

Common Disorders Screened in Newborns

- **Phenylketonuria (hyperphenylalaninemia):** It was the first disorder to be included in mass newborn screening in the early 1960s. Worldwide, more than 10 million newborns are now screened for PKU each year. The amino acid PHE is essential for protein synthesis in human. A complex reaction is involved in the hepatic conversion of phenylalanine to tyrosine and blockage causes elevations, collectively referred as hyperphenylalaninemia. Need for education of parents, informed consent for testing and provision of genetic counseling services as integral part of treatment programs.
- **Congenital hypothyroidism:** Screening for congenital hypothyroidism was carried out by measuring thyroid stimulating hormone (TSH) on dried blood spots by fluoroimmunoassay using DELFIA (Dissociation-Enhanced Lanthanide Fluorescence Immunoassay) kits.
- **Galactosemia:** Lactose (milk sugar) is a disaccharide composed of glucose and galactose. Defects in enzyme involved in the metabolism of galactose can result in galactosemia.
- **Homocystinuria:** It is a disorder of amino acid metabolism. It may result from impaired activity or deficiency of cystathionine-B-synthase (CBS) or methionine synthetase.
- **Maple syrup urine disease:** Also known as branched-chain keto aciduria, because the basic defect is in the second step (decarboxylation) of the metabolism of leucine, isoleucine and valine, which are the amino acids having branched chain and the corresponding keto acids
- Hemoglobinopathies and sickle cell disease.
- **Tyrosinemia:** A genetic disorder featured by disruptions in multistep process that breaks down the amino acid tyrosine which is a building block of most proteins.
- **Biotinidase deficiency:** Inherited disorder characterized by inability of body to recycle the vitamin biotin.
- **Congenital adrenal hyperplasia:** It encompasses a group of autosomal recessive disorders each of which involves a deficiency of an enzyme (21-hydroxylase) that is involved in the

synthesis of cortisol, aldosterone, or both. Deficiency can be due to mutations of deletions of CYP21A which is most common form of CAH.
- **Medium-chain Acyl-CoA dehydrogenase deficiency:** Enzyme that is involved in mitochondrial fatty acid ß-oxidation.
- **Cystic fibrosis:** An inherited disorder causing severe damage to the lungs, digestive system as well as other organs in the body by affecting the cells that produce mucus, sweat and digestive juices.
- Congenital hearing loss.
- Other fatty acid oxidation defects, organic acidemia, amino acidemias and other metabolic defects.
- Other disorders, such as diabetes mellitus, hyperlipidemia, familial hypercholesterolemia, neuroblastoma, fragile X-syndrome and other chromosomal diseases, Alpha 1-antitrypsin deficiency, Duchenne muscular dystrophy, hemochromatosis, *BRCA* and other gene mutations predisposing for cancer, Tay-Sachs disease, tuberous sclerosis and Huntington's disease.

GENETIC TESTING AND SCREENING IN CHILDREN

Of the 100,000 genes contained in the human genome, 15% have been localized through the efforts of the Human Genome Project (HGP). Within a short time, 100% of the human DNA sequence will be determined. This effort is comparable to reading an expansive book series that consists of 3 billion letters. Rapidly advancing technology allows new genes to be identified at an exponential rate. Newly characterized genes can cause children and adolescents to have or be more susceptible to cancer, neurodegenerative, cardiac, psychiatric and immune disorders and dyslipidemias, deafness, skeletal dysplasias and multiple system syndromes. A complete list today would be out of date tomorrow. Although identifying a disease-causing gene mutation may initiate our understanding of the disorder it confers; our understanding of the possible psychological and social ramifications for the individual or family is far less clear. The gap between discovering genetic cause and dealing with the effects of genetic testing is monumental.

It is conceivable that in the near future, armed with a web page that lists all the disease-causing genes, a family could present to their healthcare provider and request to be tested for diseases X, Y and Z. On the surface, requesting genetic testing seems harmless. It is as easy as obtaining blood for any medical test. But the testing of children imposes some inherent conflicts, some of which are subtle and others more controversial. Decisions about whether to provide genetic testing become increasingly murky for a professional, as the requests advance from testing a child for carrier status for an autosomal recessive disorder to testing a girl for a sex-linked mutation, to testing an asymptomatic child for a disease not expected to manifest itself until adulthood, to testing a child for a susceptibility to a particular disorder **(Fig. 18.1)**. The rapidly advancing ability to provide testing in the current environment makes careful consideration on the part of the providers imperative.

Approach to Genetic Testing in Children

In the past decade, the American Society of Human Genetics and the American College of Medical Genetics have developed guidelines for genetic testing in children. These guidelines have been endorsed by International Society of Nurses in Genetics. Currently, genetic testing of minors falls into several categories parallel to those as shown in **Figure 18.1**.

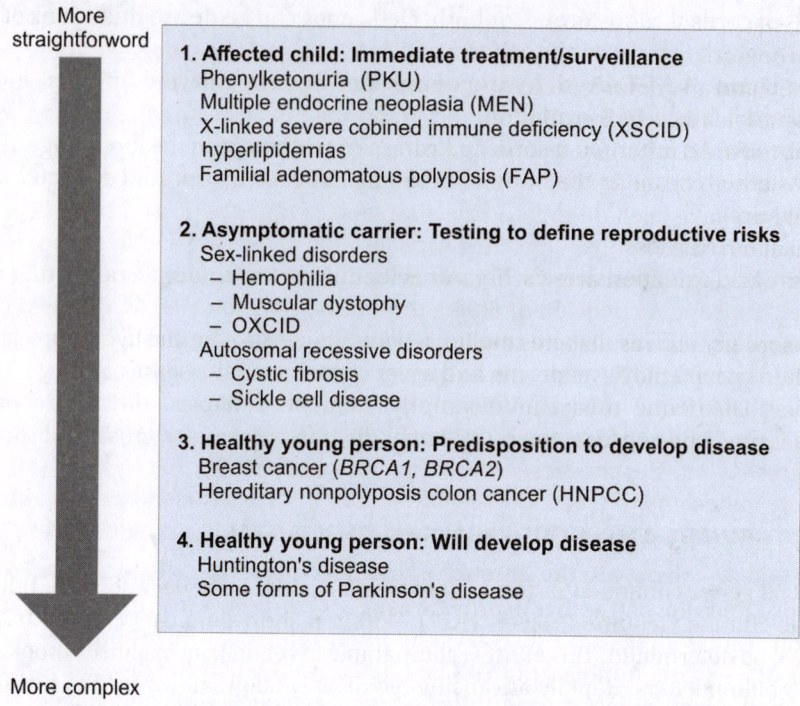

Fig. 18.1: Categorization of genetic disorders in children.

Category I—testing for a disorder for which there is immediate known benefit of treatment or preventive measures:

In this instance, greater harm occurs if testing is not done. Children at genetic risk of developing cancer may stand to gain tremendous benefits from testing that would allow preventive measures or detection early enough to achieve a cure. Those children who are known to have the gene for multiple endocrine neoplasia, develop medullary thyroid cancer that can become clinically apparent between the ages of 2 and 30. In younger individuals, the tumor is more aggressive, with metastases to liver, lung and bone. Affected children as young as 23 months have had life-preserving thyroidectomies. In this instance, genetic testing has replaced biochemical testing.

Another identifiable gene with associated inheritable childhood cancers is familial adenomatous polyposis which is manifested by multiple, premalignant adenomatous polyps in the colon and gastrointestinal tract (GIT). Untreated polyps develop into colorectal cancer. Individuals with familial adenomatous polyposis are also predisposed to adenomas that occur in the duodenum, brain and thyroid, and these children are at increased risk of developing hepatoblastoma. Colonic visualization beginning at the age of 2 has been recommended to detect and remove polyps. Youngsters who are found not to have the gene can be spared from the invasive and costly endoscopic screening.

Category II—testing for the benefit of future reproductive choice without immediate health benefit:

There are number of questions comes to our mind like, what are the benefits or the harms of learning this information at this time? The burden to advocate about whether testing best serves the child is on the professional. What if parents request testing for a daughter of 12 or 15 years? There are obvious cognitive, developmental and decision-making skills that differ between a 4-year-old child and an adolescent. A child who already has experienced the death of siblings, has heard the stories told by her mother and grandparents or has participated as a marrow donor, may weigh the confirmation of being a carrier much differently than a child without that experience. Potential consequences to individual and family dynamics as a result of DNA-based testing of children have been described. The alteration in parent-child bonding is possible, if the parent misinterprets the meaning of the carrier status and withdraws from the child or the child is rejected because she shares carrier status with a rejected spouse. A minor may undergo changes in self-concept. Anxiety about dating or marriage may be increased. Will the parents be able to convey genetic results and implied risks accurately to the child? In contrast, testing may be justified if the family's anxiety is so high that the child is suffering. Perhaps bad news may be preferential to living in a dysfunctional environment caused by uncertainty. What about the child as a future adult who has the right to explore the potential risks and benefits of carrier testing for herself when she chooses? However, adolescents do not necessarily wait until the age of majority to become parents; knowing their carrier status as teenagers might influence their sexual behavior, but they might indulge in thinking "It will never happen to me".

Category III and IV—testing in the absence of medical benefits:
In this category, decision of whether to provide genetic testing becomes increasingly complex. Predisposition testing identifies a disease gene in an individual that increases the risk for that disorder in a person, but does not confer 100% certainty that the disorder will occur. In fact, the individual who carries a predisposition gene may never become affected with that disorder. Examples of these disorders currently include familial breast cancer and hereditary nonpolyposis colon cancer. Identifying a predisposition gene in a family is not the same as knowing who will develop the disorder or how severe it will be. Other modifying genes or environmental influences determine the clinical manifestation of predisposition genes. Predisposition testing may have a role in identifying individuals who would benefit from increased surveillance and early detection. In children, however, little current evidence shows benefit for testing before the recommended age for initiating surveillance measures.

Presymptomatic testing identifies the gene alteration in an individual before the clinical manifestation of the disorder appears, with extremely high certainty that the disorder will manifest itself in adulthood. Huntington's disease, some forms of Parkinson's disease and polycystic kidney disease are examples of disorders that can be identified by genetic testing before symptoms are clinically evident. Although treatments are under development, no current intervention arrests the progression or cures these disorders. If this testing is done on at-risk family members who are minors, several harmful consequential events are conceivable. Insurability for the affected child in current environment in India could be compromised. Through stigmatization, the child may not be encouraged to meet his/her full potential or resources for educational pursuits could be diverted away from the child. Prospects for future employment might be threatened. Unrelated illnesses may be ignored, inadequately evaluated or misdiagnosed because of the underlying assumption that symptoms are related to the genetic disorder for which the child is known to have the gene.

Many unanswered questions remain about the psychological impact of genetic testing in children. Genetic testing may relieve uncertainty. Understanding how families manage uncertainty might help to identify, which families would benefit from childhood testing. Improvement in the parents' ability to cope might benefit the child.

Should Children be Tested/Screened?

Should children be tested for susceptibility to genetic diseases, presence of the genes for late-onset diseases and/or carrier state? The issue of genetic testing and screening of children has been an area of great controversy. Some centers and groups have condemned such testing and refused to provide such services to children even with parent's consent, while others are more liberal. Newborn screening already tests infants for some disorders that do have a direct therapeutic benefit. The issues to be considered are, personal issues, such as medical, psychosocial, reproductive issue and issue with a broader impact, such as those affecting insurance, carrier and future employment. A thought report by the ASHG/ACMG (1995) discusses many related issues. In a study in Great Britain, pediatricians were more likely than geneticists to allow such testing at the request of parents or adoption agencies. There was great variation according to condition. In a study by Tibben (1992), parents were more favorable toward genetic testing than were health professionals. Michie, et al. (1996) reported on a family in which testing for familial adenomatous polyposis was done for the 2- and 4-year-old sisters. Their hypothesis was that 'complying with requests for predictive DNA testing (including pre-test and post-test counseling) in parents wishing to reduce uncertainty about their children in future health is associated with good psychological outcome regardless of the test results'.

Reasons for considering testing in children commonly evolve from the diagnosis of a genetic disorder within a family, particularly one that has onset in late childhood, adolescence or adulthood, rather than the necessity for diagnosis of a genetic disorder because of an immediate health implication. Some reasons for such testing include:

- The institution of preventive measures or therapy that can treat or ameliorate the severity, or influence the natural history of the disease is a question (a direct timely medical benefit or evidence-based risk reduction program are the most compelling reasons for testing).
- Sparing the child from the unpleasantness and trauma of continued testing for disorders, such as familial cancer when a child may not possess the gene is question.
- Knowledge for the parents in terms of their own financial and reproductive planning give the future outbreak for their present children.
- The elimination of the uncertainty of knowing whether or not they possess a gene of a serious disorder such as Huntington's disease or disorder, or adult polycystic kidney disease.
- The psychological benefit of a negative test for a positive result, the chance for parents to adjust to diagnose and plan ways to control disease and cope with the news at the appropriate time for their child.
- The opportunity for life planning based on this information, including choices related to education, career, lifestyle and reproductive decisions. For example, a child at risk for retinitis pigmentosa could choose a career that did not require visual activity or child with familial hypertrophic cardiomyopathy could receive early drug therapy for prevention of arrhythmia.

Some of the reasons given for not performing such testing include:

- The child may not be able to understand the ramifications of testing, such as future insurability risks and possible effects on education and employability.
- The child may not be able to give informed consent or even assent, thus taking away the child's right to decide.
- The potential psychological consequences of learning that one has genetic disorder or is a carrier, such as lowered self-esteem, changes in family dynamics and in parent-child bounding, loss of confidentiality of the child's condition, since the parents will know the status.

Table 18.1: Qualities of an ideal screening test or procedure.

• Rapid	• Specific	• Uses easily available specimens and materials
• Inexpensive	• Safe	• Reproducible
• Simple	• Accepted	• Causes minimal discomfort
• Sensitive	• Valid	

- Stigmatization and labeling
- The potential negative psychological consequences of learning that one does not have a disorder and developing 'survivor guilt' or feeling alienated from a affected sibling or family member.

The qualities of an ideal screening test or procedure is given in **Table 18.1**.

CONGENITAL ABNORMALITIES

A congenital abnormality (congenital anomaly, congenital malformation, birth defect) is a condition, which is present at the time of birth, which varies from the standard presentation. In other words, it is a type of congenital disorder, which is primarily structural in nature.

About 3% of newborns have a 'major physical anomaly', meaning a physical anomaly that has cosmetic or functional significance. Congenital anomalies involving the brain are the largest group of 10 per 1,000 live births, compared to heart at 8 per 1,000, kidneys at 4 per 1,000, and limbs at 1 per 1,000. All other physical anomalies have a combined incidence of 6 per 1000 live births. Congenital anomalies of the heart have the highest risk of death in infancy, accounting for 28% of infant deaths due to congenital anomaly, while chromosomal anomalies and respiratory anomalies each account for 15% and brain anomalies about 12%.

Types

- A limb anomaly is called dysmelia. These include all forms of limb anomalies, such as amelia, ectrodactyly, phocomelia, polymelia, polydactyly, syndactyly, polysyndactyly, oligodactyly, brachydactyly, achondroplasia, congenital aplasia or hypoplasia, amniotic band syndrome and cleidocranial dysostosis.
- Congenital anomalies of the heart include patent ductus arteriosus, atrial septal defect, ventricular septal defect and tetralogy of Fallot. Helen Taussig has been a major force in research on congenital anomalies of the heart.
- Congenital anomalies of the nervous system include neural tube defects, such as spina bifida, meningocele, meningomyelocele, encephalocele and anencephaly. Other congenital anomalies of the nervous system include the Arnold-Chiari malformation, the Dandy-Walker malformation, hydrocephalus, macrocephaly, megalencephaly, lissencephaly, polymicrogyria, holoprosencephaly and agenesis of the corpus callosum.
- Congenital anomalies of the gastrointestinal system include numerous forms of stenosis and atresia and imperforate, etc.

Causes

- **Sporadic or unknown causes:** The cause of 40–60% of congenital anomalies in humans is unknown. These are referred to as sporadic, a term that implies an unknown cause, random occurrence regardless of maternal living conditions, and a low recurrence risk for

future children. For 20–25% of anomalies, there seems to have a 'multifactorial' cause, meaning a complex interaction of multiple minor genetic anomalies with environmental risk factors.
- **Genetic causes:** Includes the inheritance of abnormal genes from the parents as well as new mutations in one of the germ cells that gave rise to the fetus. Only 12–25% of anomalies have a purely genetic cause. Of these, the majority are chromosomal anomalies.
- **Environmental causes:** They are referred to as teratogenic. These are generally the problems with the mother's environment. Teratogens can include dietary deficiencies, toxins or infections. About 10–13% of anomalies have a purely environmental cause (e.g., infections, illness or drug abuse in the mother). For example, dietary deficiency of maternal folic acid is associated with spina bifida. Ingestion of harmful substances by the mother (e.g., alcohol, mercury or prescription drugs, such as phenytoin) can cause recognizable combinations of birth defects. Several infections (TORCH infection), which a mother can contract during pregnancy can also be teratogenic.

Genetic Testing/Screening

- Detailed physical examination
- Blood biochemistry of children
- Molecular genetic tests (direct DNA testing)
- Fluorescence in situ hybridization (FISH)
- Ultrasonography
- Echocardiography
- Electrocardiogram (ECG)
- Radiological examination [X-rays, computed tomography (CT) scan and magnetic resonance imaging (MRI), etc.]

Management

Usually surgery is required, however it depends on the extent of congenital anomaly.

DEVELOPMENTAL DELAY

Child development refers to the process in which children go through changes in skill development during predictable time periods called developmental milestones. Developmental delay occurs when children have not reached these milestones by the expected time period. For example, if the normal range for learning to walk is between 9 and 15 months, and a 20-month-old child has still not begun walking, this would be considered a developmental delay. Developmental delays can occur in all five areas of development or may just happen in one or more of those areas. Additionally, growth in each area of development is related to growth in the other areas. So if there is a difficulty in one area (e.g., speech and language), it is likely to influence development in other areas (e.g., social and emotional).

"Developmental delay is a significant lag in a child's physical, cognitive, behavioral, emotional or social development in comparison with norms". In other words, developmental delay refers to when a child's development lags behind established normal ranges for his/her age.

At least 8% of all children from birth to 6 years, have developmental problems and delays in one or more areas of development. This includes delay in speech and language development, motor development, social-emotional development and cognitive development. Some have global delays, which mean they lag in all developmental areas.

Risk Factors for Developmental Delay

Risk factors for developmental problems fall into two categories:
1. **Genetic factor:** Children are placed at genetic risk by being born with a genetic or chromosomal abnormality. A good example of a genetic risk is Down syndrome, a disorder that causes developmental delay because of an abnormal chromosome.
2. **Environmental factor:** Environmental risk results from exposure to harmful agents either before or after birth, and can include things, such as poor maternal nutrition or exposure to toxins (e.g., lead or drugs), or infections that are passed from mother to her baby during pregnancy (e.g., measles or HIV). Environmental risks also include a child's life experiences. For example, children who are born prematurely, face severe poverty, mother's depression, poor nutrition or lack of care are at increased risk for developmental delays.

Risk factors have a cumulative impact upon development. As the number of risk factors increases, a child is put at greater risk for developmental delay.

Warning Signs of a Developmental Delay

There are several general 'warning signs' of possible delay. These include:

Behavioral Warning Signs

- Does not pay attention or stay focused on an activity for as longer time as other children of the same age do
- Focuses on unusual objects for long periods of time; enjoys this more than interacting with others
- Avoids or rarely makes eye contact with others
- Gets unusually frustrated when trying to do simple tasks that most children of the same age can do
- Shows aggressive behaviors and acting out, and appears to be very stubborn compared with other children
- Displays violent behaviors on a daily basis
- Stares into space, rocks body or talks to self, more often than other children of the same age
- Does not seek love and approval from a caregiver or parent.

Gross Motor Warning Signs

- Has stiff arms and/or legs
- Has a floppy or limp body posture compared to other children of the same age
- Uses one side of body more than the other
- Has a very clumsy manner compared with other children of the same age.

Vision Warning Signs

- Seems to have difficulty following objects or people with her eyes
- Rubs eyes frequently
- Turns, tilts or holds head in a strained or unusual position when trying to look at an object
- Seems to have difficulty in finding or picking up small objects dropped on the floor (after the age of 12 months)
- Has difficulty focusing or making eye contact
- Closes one eye when trying to look at distant objects

- Eyes appear to be crossed or turned
- Brings objects too close to eyes to see
- One or both eyes appear abnormal in size or coloring.

Hearing Warning Signs

- Talks in a very loud or very soft voice
- Seems to have difficulty in responding when called from across the room, even when it is for something interesting
- Turns body so that the same ear is always turned toward sound
- Has difficulty understanding what has been said or following directions after once she has turned 3 years of age
- Does not startle to loud noises
- Ears appear small or deformed
- Fails to develop sounds or words that would be appropriate at her age.

In addition, because children usually acquire developmental milestones or skills during a specific time frame or 'window', we can predict when most children will learn different skills. If a child is not learning a skill that other children are learning at the same age that may be a 'warning sign' that the child may be at risk for developmental delay.

Screening of Developmental Delay

- A developmental screening test is a quick and general measurement of skills. Its purpose is to identify children who are in need of further evaluation. A screening test is only meant to identify children who might have a problem. The screening test may either overidentify or under identify children with delay. As a result, simply using a screening test cannot make a diagnosis. If the results of a screening test suggest that child may have a developmental delay, the child should be referred for a developmental evaluation to higher center.
- The most popular developmental screening scale or procedures are based on pioneering work of Gesell and his colleagues. Some of the currently used popular developmental screening tools are detailed below.

Battelle Developmental Inventory Screening Test

The Battelle Developmental Inventory Screening Test (BDIST) can be used to screen children aged 12–96 months, using a combination of direct assessment, observation and parental interview.

Bayley Infant Neurodevelopmental Screener

The Bayley infant neurodevelopmental screener (BINS) is a recently developed test designed for screening high-risk infants aged 3–24 months. It uses 10–13 directly elicited items per 3- to 6-month range to assess neurodevelopmental skills and developmental accomplishments (measures motor and mental maturation).

Child Development Inventories

The child development inventory (CDI), formerly known as the Minnesota child development inventory, was created to provide a systematic, standardized method for parents to report on their children's strengths, problems and present development. The original 300-item instrument has been broken down into instruments that apply to three age intervals. The CDI measures a child's development in eight areas, namely—social, self-help, gross motor, fine motor, expressive language, language comprehension, letters and numbers. It consists of a 300-item booklet and answer sheet for the parent to complete and a profile sheet for recording the results.

Denver Developmental Screening Test

- The Denver Developmental Screening Test (DDST) was introduced in 1967. Research has consistently found it lacking in sensitivity. In response to this criticism, a revised version, the Denver II was released in 1992. The Denver II is the most commonly used developmental screening tool. It combines direct observation and parental report. The tool consists of 125 items, organized into four developmental domains, namely—gross motor, fine motor/adaptive, language and personal/social.
- The summary of the most important development milestone as DDST is shown in **Table 18.2**.

Table 18.2: Key developmental milestone.

Gross motor		Fine motor	
Age	**Milestones**	**Age**	**Milestones**
3 months	Neck holding	4 months	Grasp a rattle or ring when placed in hand
5 months	Sitting with support		
8 months	Sitting without support		
9 months	Standing with support	5 months	Reaches out to an object and hold it with both hands
10 months	Walking with support		
11 months	Crawling (creeping)		
12 months	Standing without support	7 months	Holding objects with crude grasp from palm (palmer grasp)
13 months	Walking without support		
18 months	Running		
24 months	Walking upstairs	9 months	Holding small objects, such as a pellet between index finger and thumb (pincer grasp)
36 months	Riding tricycle		
Language		**Personal/social**	
Age	**Milestones**	**Age**	**Milestones**
1 month	Turn head to sound	2 months	Social smile
3 months	Cooing	3 months	Recognizing mother
6 months	Monosyllables ('ma', 'ba')		
9 months	Bisyllables ('mama', 'baba')	6 months	Smile at mirror image
12 months	Two words with meaning	9 months	Wave 'bye-bye'
18 months	Ten words with meaning		
24 months	Simple sentences	12 months	Play a simple game
36 months	Telling a story	36 months	Knows gender

Early Intervention Services for Developmental Delay

Early intervention services include a variety of different resources and programs that provide support to families to enhance a child's development. These services are specifically tailored to meet a child's individual needs. Services include:
- Assistive technology (devices a child's need)
- Audiology or hearing services
- Counseling and training for a family
- Educational programs
- Medical services
- Nursing services
- Nutrition services
- Occupational therapy
- Physical therapy
- Psychological services
- Respite services
- Speech/language.

DYSMORPHISM

"Any congenital, structural or developmental defect is known as dysmorphism; this usually occurs due to abnormal embryogenesis or morphogenesis".

Embryogenesis is a process by which the embryo is formed and develops. It starts with the fertilization of the ovum and egg, which after fertilization, is then called zygote. The zygote undergoes rapid mitotic division, the formation of two exact genetic replicates of the original cell, with no significant growth and cellular differentiation, leading to development of an embryo. Morphogenesis is one of three fundamental aspect of developmental biology along with the control of cell growth and cellular differentiation. Morphogenesis is concerned with the shapes of tissue, organs and entire organism, and the positions of the various specialized cell type. Therefore, abnormality in embryogenesis and morphogenesis may leads to dysmorphism.

Types of Dysmorphism

- **Major dysmorphism:** Are the severe type of developmental defects, which produces functional disability and early life mortality. Incidence of these defects is about 2–3% in neonates.
- **Minor dysmorphism:** Nearly 10–12% newborns have such defects, which are basically cosmetic defects and do not produce any functional disability. For example, nevus, pigmentation, preauricular skin tags, etc.

Etiology

- Chromosomal or genetic causes of these anomalies include inheritance of abnormal genes from the parents, as well as new mutations in one of the germ cells that gave rise to the fetus.
- Environmental causes of dysmorphic anomalies are referred to as teratogenic. Teratogens can include dietary deficiencies, toxins or infections. For example, dietary deficiency of maternal folic acid is associated with spina bifida. Ingestion of harmful substances by

the mother (e.g., alcohol, mercury or prescription drugs, such as phenytoin) can cause recognizable combinations of birth defects. Several infections (TORCH infection), which a mother can contract during pregnancy can also be teratogenic.
- Unknown causes, in some situation even cause can be established for a defect.

Common Dysmorphic Syndromes
- **Syndromes with craniofacial dysmorphism:**
  - Moebius sequence
  - Frontonasal dysplasia sequence
  - Goldenhar syndrome
  - Craniosynostoses syndrome
  - Carpenter syndrome
- **Syndromes with physical overgrowth:**
  - Fragile X syndrome
  - Marshall-Smith syndrome
  - Weaver-Smith syndrome
- **Syndromes with CNS and neuromuscular defects:**
  - Prader-Willi syndrome
  - Myotonic dystrophy syndrome
- **Syndromes with chromosomal abnormalities:**
  - Down syndrome (trisomy 21)
  - Edward syndrome (trisomy 18)
  - Patau syndrome (trisomy 13)
  - Turner's syndrome (monosomy of X).

Genetic Testing/Screening
- Detailed physical examination
- Blood biochemistry of children
- Molecular genetic tests (direct DNA testing)
- Fluorescence in situ hybridization (FISH)
- Ultrasonography
- Echocardiography
- Electrocardiogram
- Radiological examination (X-rays, CT scan and MRI, etc.)

Management
Depending on the extent of defect, it may not require any management or may require several surgeries.

ROLE OF NURSES IN GENETIC TESTING FOR NEONATES AND CHILDREN
- **Collect thorough family history:** Nurses must take a thorough family history. This includes information about family history, exposures and lifestyles, if clues are to be uncovered as to the relative risk a family may have for a specific condition. Asking about unaffected as well as affected family members can suggest an inheritance pattern for a specific problem

SECTION 4: Genetics

- **Newborn screening coverage:** Nurses are key players in increasing newborn screening coverage as they are the front liners and must be knowledgeable about basic genetics concepts to explain these conditions to the parents. Nurses who work in neonatal and children areas have the responsibility to assist with testing procedures, support the client and family, and provide appropriate education and clarification of information.
- **Address parents questions and respect their values:** Nurses should discuss what the results could potentially mean for the newborn and the family. Nurses' awareness of how personal values may color personal perceptions of the family's situation is imperative to avoid imposing personal values on the family.
- **Acts as advocate:** Nurses translate complex genetic information to allow the family to be competent in the use and application of that information. Many healthcare professionals feel uncomfortable with genetic interpretations; yet the family feels so even more. They have a key role in liaising and advocating the needs of patients and families.
- **Acts as case manager:** They guarantee coordinated care between medical and allied medical specialties needed in patient management and they also ensure continuity of care including the transition from pediatric to adult care.
- **Provides intensive care:** If the neonate requires intensive care or if the condition is detected early in neonatal period, the family and the nurse may benefit from pastoral care. From the family's perspective, this element of spirituality, if important to them, may help them cope. For the healthcare professional, it may facilitate working with families whose beliefs and values may differ from their own.
- **Accurate information:** Offer detailed information and support for both parents and child during testing.
- **Referral:** Provide referral and follow-up services, if required. Nurses helps families to make informed decisions, decreases their anxiety and provide information about the reasons for testing and referral to appropriate healthcare facility for testing.

MULTIPLE CHOICE QUESTIONS

1. **Name the condition in which there is a defect in the second step (decarboxylation) of the metabolism of leucine, isoleucine and valine:**
   a. Homocystinuria
   b. Maple syrup urine disease
   c. Tyrosinemia
   d. Galactosemia
2. **FISH stands for:**
   a. Fluorescent in situ hybridization
   b. First induced strand hybrid
   c. F1 insertion segment homolog
   d. Flanking insertion sequence hybrid
3. **Denver developmental screening test (DDST) was introduced in which year?**
   a. 1942
   b. 1950
   c. 1964
   d. 1967
4. **Down syndrome is a:**
   a. Trisomy 21
   b. Trisomy 18
   c. Trisomy 13
   d. Monosomy of X
5. **Edward syndrome is a:**
   a. Trisomy 21
   b. Trisomy 18
   c. Trisomy 13
   d. Monosomy of X

Answer Key

1. b
2. a
3. d
4. a
5. b

FURTHER READING

1. ASHG/ACMG. ASHG/ACMG report points to consider: Ethical, legal and psychosocial implications of genetic testing in children and adolescents. Am J Hum Genet. 1995;57:1233–41.
2. Buckley RH, Schiff S, Schiff RI, et al. Hematopoietic stem-cell transplantation for the treatment of severe combined immunodeficiency. N Engl J Med. 1999;340:508–59.
3. Clayton E. Genetic testing in children. J Med Philos. 1997;22:233–51.
4. Collins F. Shattuck lecture. Medical and societal consequences of the Human Genome Project. N Engl J Med. 1999;34:28–37.
5. Fanos J. Developmental tasks of childhood and adolescence: Implications for genetic testing. Am J Hum Genet. 1997;71:22–8.
6. Garber J, Diller L. Screening children at genetic risk of cancer. Curr Opin Pediatr. 1993;5:712–5.
7. Geiger J, Thompson NW. Thyroid tumors in children. Otolaryngol Clin North Am. 1996;29:711–9.
8. Gross RH, et al. Early Management and Decision Making for the Treatment of Myelomeningocele. Pediatrics. 1983;72(4):450–8.
9. http://www.ncbi.nlm.nih.gov/Omim/searchomim.html
10. Kennedy F. The problem of social control of the congenital defective education, sterilization, euthanasia. American Journal of Psychiatry. 1942;99:13–6.
11. Lessick M, Faux S. Implications of genetic testing of children and adolescents. Holistic Nursing Practice. 1998;12:38–46.
12. Petersen C, Francomano C, Kinzler K, et al. Presymptomatic direct detection of adenomatous polyposis coli (APC) gene mutation in familial adenomatous polyposis. Huts' Genet. 1993;91:307–11.
13. Puck J. Molecular and genetic basis of X-linked immunodeficiency. J Clin Immunol. 1994;14:81–8.
14. Raines D. Ethical implications of genetic testing. Nurs Clin North Am. 1998;33:275–86.
15. Singer P. Sanctity of life or quality of life? Pediatrics. 1983;72(1):128–9.
16. Strong L, Marteau T. Evaluating children and adolescents for heritable cancer risk. J Natl Cancer Inst Monogr. 1995;17:111–3.
17. Wertz D, Fanos JH, Reilly PR. Genetic testing for children and adolescents: Who decides? JAMA. 1994;272:875–81.
18. Williams J, Lessick M. Genome research: Implications for children. Pediatr Nurs. 1996;22:40–6.

CHAPTER 19

Genetic Conditions of Adolescents and Adults

Suresh Sharma, Kumar Satish Ravi

GENETIC STATISTICS

Some statistical terms are commonly used that describing genetic conditions and other disorders. These terms include the following:

- **Incidence:** The incidence of a gene mutation or a genetic disorder is the number of people, who are born with the mutation or disorder in a specified group per year. Incidence is often written in the form '1 in (a number)' or as a total number of live births. About 1 in 200,000 people in India are born with syndrome A each year. An estimated 15,000 infants with syndrome B were born last year worldwide.
- **Prevalence:** The prevalence of a gene mutation or a genetic disorder is the total number of people in a specified group at a given time, who have the mutation or disorder. This term includes both newly diagnosed and pre-existing cases in people of any age. Prevalence is often written in the form '1 in (a number)' or as a total number of people, who have a condition. Approximately 1 in 100,000 people in India have syndrome A at the present time. About 100,000 children worldwide currently have syndrome B.
- **Mortality:** Mortality is the number of deaths from a particular disorder occurring in a specified group per year. Mortality is usually expressed as a total number of deaths. An estimated 12,000 people worldwide died from syndrome C in 2002.
- **Lifetime risk:** Lifetime risk is the average risk of developing a particular disorder at some point during a lifetime. Lifetime risk is often written as a percentage or as '1 in (a number).' It is important to remember that the risk per year or per decade is much lower than the lifetime risk. In addition, other factors may increase or decrease a person's risk as compared with the average. Approximately 1% of people in India develop disorder D during their lifetimes. The lifetime risk of developing disorder D is 1 in 100.

NAMING GENETIC CONDITIONS

Genetic conditions are not named in one standard way (unlike genes, which are given an official name and symbol by a formal committee). Doctors who treat families with a particular disorder are often the first to propose a name for the condition. Expert working groups may later revise the name to improve its usefulness. Naming is important because it allows accurate and effective communication about particular conditions, which will ultimately help researchers to find new approaches for treatment.

Disorder's names are often derived from one or a combination of sources: The basic genetic or biochemical defect that causes the condition (e.g., α1-antitrypsin deficiency).
- One or more major signs or symptoms of the disorder (e.g., sickle cell anemia)
- The parts of the body affected by the condition (e.g., retinoblastoma)

- The name of a physician or researcher, often the first person to describe the disorder (e.g., Marfan syndrome, which was named after Antoine Bernard-Jean Marfan)
- A geographic area (e.g., familial Mediterranean fever, which occurs mainly in populations bordering the Mediterranean Sea)
- The name of a patient or family with the condition (e.g., amyotrophic lateral sclerosis, which is also called Lou Gehrig's disease after a famous baseball player, who had the condition).

Disorders named after a specific person or place are called eponyms. There is debate as to whether the possessive form (e.g., Alzheimer's disease) or the non-possessive form (Alzheimer disease) of eponyms is preferred. As a rule, medical geneticists use the non-possessive form, and this form may become the standard for doctors in all fields of medicine. Genetics Home Reference uses the non-possessive form of eponyms.

Genetics home reference consults with experts in the field of medical genetics to provide the current, most accurate name for each disorder. Alternate names are included as synonyms.

COMMON GENETIC CONDITIONS

Cancer Genetics: Familial Cancer

Cancer is a class of diseases or disorders characterized by uncontrolled division of cells and the ability of these to spread, either by direct growth into adjacent tissue through *invasion*, or by implantation into distant sites by *metastasis* (where cancer cells are transported through the bloodstream or lymphatic system). Cancer may affect people at all ages, but risk tends to increase with age.

Based on causative foundation (carcinogenesis); cancer is broadly classified in two major categories:

1. **Sporadic cancer:** Most of the cancers are caused by series of mutations that develop during a person's lifetime called acquired mutations. Acquired mutations are caused by tobacco, overexposure to ultraviolet (UV) radiation and other toxins, and chemicals. These mutations are not in every cell of the body and are not passed from parents to child. Cancer caused by this type of mutation is called sporadic cancer.
2. **Familial cancer:** For various reasons genes often undergo mutations. Some mutations have no effect on a cell, while other mutation is harmful or helpful to the cell. These are two basic kinds of genetic mutations. If mutation passes from one of the parents to the child; it is called germline mutation. When a germline mutation is passed on from a parent to the child, it is present in every cell of the child's body, including the reproductive cells; it is passed from generation to generation. Germline mutations are responsible for 5%–10% of cancer cases. This is also called familial cancer.

Familial Cancer

Most forms of cancer are 'sporadic' and have no basis in heredity. There are, however, a number of recognized syndromes of cancer with a hereditary component, often a defective tumor suppressor allele. For example, in medicine, the term syndrome is the association of several clinically recognizable features, signs, symptoms, phenomena or characteristics, which often occur together, so that the presence of one feature alerts the physician about the presence of the others.

It is believed that about 5% of the colorectal and breast cancer arise as a result of an inherited cancer susceptibility gene. There are a number of other features, which suggest an inherited cancer susceptibility syndrome in a particular family. Features include:
- Several first- or second-degree relatives show a common cancer
- Several close relatives have related cancer, e.g., breast and ovary or bowel and endometrial cancer
- An early age of onset
- Tumors in two different organs systems in one person
- Bilateral tumors in paired organs
- Two family members may have the same rare cancer.

Familial Cancer Predisposing Syndrome

Most cancer occurs at a specific site. There are some families in which the cancer occurs at different sites in various members of the family or at more than one site in an individual. The incidence is more common than would be expected. Such families are referred to have familial cancer predisposing syndrome. Most of them are with dominant inheritance. Some of them are (also summarized in **Table 19.1**):
- **Breast and ovarian cancer syndrome:** Certain inherited mutations in the genes *BRCA1* and *BRCA2* are associated with an elevated risk of breast cancer and ovarian cancer. *BRCA1* (named for breast cancer 1) is a human gene located on the long arm of the 17th chromosome (17q21). The *BRCA2* refers to either a gene (breast cancer susceptibility gene 2), located on human chromosome 13 (13q12–13) or the protein coded for by that gene. Breast cancer is cancer of breast tissue. Ovarian cancer is a malignant ovarian neoplasm (an abnormal growth located on the ovaries).
- **Multiple endocrine neoplasia (MEN types 1, 2A, 2B):** It refers to tumors of various endocrine organs. Multiple endocrine neoplasia (MEN) or multiple endocrine adenomas,

Table 19.1: Inheritance familial cancer predisposing syndromes.

Syndrome	Mutation in gene	Chromosomal location	Cancer	Inheritance
Breast and ovarian cancer	BRCA1 and BRCA2	BRCA1-17q21 BRCA2-13q12–13	Breast, ovary	Autosomal dominant (AD)
Multiple endocrine neoplasia (MEN types 1, 2A, 2B)	MEN2A and 2B	10q	Thyroid, pheochromocytoma	AD
Li-Fraumeni syndrome	p53	17q	Sarcoma of breast, brain, leukemia, adrenal cortex	AD
Turcot syndrome	—	—	Brain tumors, colonic polyposis	AD
Familial adenomatous polyposis	APC gene	5q	Colorectal, duodenal, thyroid	AD
Familial Retinoblastoma	Rb1	13q	Retinoblastoma	AD

or multiple endocrine adenomatosis (MEA) consists of three syndromes featuring tumors of endocrine glands, each with its own characteristic pattern.
- **Li-Fraumeni syndrome:** It is a rare autosomal dominant hereditary disorder, which occurs due to mutations of *p53*. Various tumors seen in this disorder are osteosarcoma, breast cancer, soft tissue sarcoma and brain tumors. Osteosarcoma is a common primary bone cancer. A brain tumor is any intracranial tumor created by abnormal and uncontrolled cell division, normally either found in the brain itself [neurons, glial cells (astrocytes, oligodendrocytes, ependymal cells), lymphatic tissue, blood vessels], in the cranial nerves (myelin producing Schwann cells), in the brain envelopes (meninges), skull, pituitary and pineal gland.
- **Turcot syndrome (brain tumors and colonic polyposis):** It is the association between familial adenomatous polyposis and brain tumors. A brain tumor is any intracranial tumor created by abnormal and uncontrolled cell division, normally either found in the brain itself [neurons, glial cells (astrocytes, oligodendrocytes, ependymal cells), lymphatic tissue, blood vessels], in the cranial nerves (myelin producing Schwann cells), in the brain envelopes (meninges), skull, pituitary and pineal gland.
- **Familial adenomatous polyposis:** It is an inherited mutation of the *APC* gene that leads to early onset of colon carcinoma in which numerous polyps form mainly in the epithelium of the large intestine. Colorectal cancer includes cancerous growths in the colon, rectum and appendix.
- **Familial retinoblastoma:** In young children, it is an inherited cancer. Retinoblastoma is a cancer of the retina.

Genetic Testing

Genetic testing for high-risk individuals is already available for certain cancer-related genetic mutations. Carriers of genetic mutations that increase risk for cancer incidence can undergo enhanced surveillance, chemoprevention or risk-reducing surgery. Genetic testing allows the genetic diagnosis of vulnerabilities to inherited diseases and can also be used to determine a person's ancestry. The **Table 19.2** presents the involved gens among different types of familial cancer.

Management of Familial Cancer

- **Cancer gene therapy:** It is one of the experimental area in field of cancer treatment. Some of the current areas of research in cancer gene therapy include RNAi approaches, drug resistance, hematopoietic gene transfer, homologous recombination, ribozyme technology, antisense technology, tumor immunotherapy and tumor suppressors, translational research, gene delivery systems (viral and nonviral), antigene therapy (antisense, siRNA and ribozymes), apoptosis; mechanisms and therapies, vaccine development, immunology and immunotherapy, DNA synthesis and repair. Some of the successful cancer therapy are as follows:

Table 19.2: Gene involved in familial cancers.

Cancer types	Gene
Breast, ovarian, pancreatic	BRCA1, BRCA2
Colon, uterine, small bowel, stomach, urinary tract	MLH1, MsH2, MsH6, PMs, PMs2

- Nanoparticle delivery of antimetastatic *NM23-H1* gene improves chemotherapy in a mouse tumor model.
- Expression of HBx, an oncoprotein of hepatitis B virus, blocks reoviral oncolysis of hepatocellular carcinoma cells.
- Adoptive immunotherapy using human peripheral blood lymphocytes transferred with RNA encoding *HER2*/neu-specific chimeric immune receptor in ovarian cancer xenograft model.

- **Chemoprevention:** For example, drug Tamoxifen can be given to a lady, who is vulnerable to develop familial breast cancer.
- **Risk-reducing surgery:** For example, if someone is susceptible for breast cancer and person finds a small lump during a regular breast self-examination (BSE); early breast surgeries can be performed.

Inborn Errors of Metabolism

The term *inborn error of metabolism* was coined by a British physician, Archibald Garrod (1857–1936), in the early 20th century (1908). He is known for the 'one gene, one enzyme' hypothesis, which arose from his studies on the nature and inheritance of alkaptonuria.

Inborn errors of metabolism comprise a large class of genetic diseases involving disorders of metabolism. The majority are due to defects of single gene that code for enzyme that facilitate conversion of various substances (substrates) into others (products). In most of the disorders, problems arise due to accumulation of substances, which are toxic or interfere with normal function or due to the effects of reduced ability to synthesize essential compounds. Inborn errors of metabolism are now often referred to as *congenital metabolic diseases or inherited metabolic diseases,* and these terms are considered synonymous.

In other words, IEM are conditions due to genetic defects related to synthesis, metabolism, transportation or storage of biochemical compounds.

Worldwide incidence of IEM has been estimated to be about 3–4/1,000 live births. More than 300 such defects are known. Most of the IEM are inherited in an autosomal recessive manner, some are through X-linked, though they can also arise out of spontaneous mutations.

Classification of Inborn Errors of Metabolism

Traditionally, the inherited metabolic diseases were categorized as disorders of *carbohydrate* metabolism, *amino acid* metabolism *organic acid* metabolism, or *lysosomal storage diseases*. In recent decades, hundreds of new inherited disorders of metabolism have been discovered and the categories have proliferated. Following are some of the major classes of congenital metabolic diseases, with prominent examples of each class. Many others do not fall into these categories:

- **Disorders of carbohydrate metabolism,** e.g., glycogen storage disease
- **Disorders of amino acid metabolism,** e.g., phenylketonuria, maple syrup urine disease, glutaric acidemia type 1
- **Disorders of organic acid metabolism (organic acidurias),** e.g., alkaptonuria
- **Disorders of fatty acid oxidation and mitochondrial metabolism,** e.g., medium chain acyl dehydrogenase deficiency (glutaric acidemia type 2)
- **Disorders of porphyrin metabolism,** e.g., acute intermittent porphyria
- **Disorders of purine or pyrimidine metabolism,** e.g., Lesch-Nyhan syndrome

- **Disorders of steroid metabolism,** e.g., congenital adrenal hyperplasia
- **Disorders of mitochondrial function,** e.g., Kearns-Sayre syndrome
- **Disorders of peroxisomal function,** e.g., Zellweger syndrome
- **Lysosomal storage disorders,** e.g., Gaucher's disease, Niemann-Pick disease.

Clinical Manifestations

Because of the enormous number of these diseases and wide range of systems affected, nearly every 'presenting complaint' to a doctor may have a congenital metabolic disease as a possible cause, especially in childhood. The following are examples of potential manifestations affecting each of the major organ systems **(Table 19.3)**.

Diagnosis

Because of the multiplicity of conditions, many different diagnostic tests are used for screening. An abnormal result is often followed by a subsequent "definitive test" to confirm the suspected diagnosis.

Common screening tests used:
- Ferric chloride test (turns colors in reaction to various abnormal metabolites in urine)
- Ninhydrin paper chromatography (detects abnormal amino acid patterns)

Table 19.3: System wise clinical manifestations in inborn errors of metabolism.

System involved	Clinical features
General	Growth failure, failure to thrive, weight loss, unusual facial features, congenital malformations
Genital	Ambiguous genitalia, delayed puberty, precocious puberty
Neurological	Developmental delay, seizures, dementia, encephalopathy, stroke
Sensory	Deafness, blindness, pain agnosia
Dermatology	Skin rash, abnormal pigmentation, lack of pigmentation, excessive hair growth, lumps and bumps
Hematological	Immunodeficiency, thrombocytopenia, anemia, enlarged spleen, enlarged lymph nodes
Gastrointestinal	Recurrent vomiting, diarrhea, abdominal pain
Hepatic	Hepatomegaly, jaundice, liver failure
Renal	Excessive urination, renal failure, dehydration, edema
Cardiovascular	Hypotension, heart failure, enlarged heart, hypertension, myocardial infarction
Respiratory	Excessive breathing (hyperventilation), respiratory failure
Musculoskeletal	Joint pain, muscle weakness, cramps
Endocrinal	Hypothyroidism, adrenal insufficiency, hypogonadism, diabetes mellitus
Behavioral	Abnormal behavior, depression, psychosis
Dental	Dental abnormalities
Others	Many forms of cancer

- Guthrie bacterial inhibition assay (detect a few amino acids in excessive amounts in blood) The dried blood spot can be used for multianalyte testing using tandem mass spectrometry (MS/MS)
- Quantitative plasma amino acids, quantitative urine amino acids
- Urine organic acids by mass spectrometry.

Specific diagnostic tests (or focused screening for a small set of disorders):
- Tissue biopsy or necropsy—liver, muscle, brain, bone marrow
- Skin biopsy and fibroblast cultivation for specific enzyme testing
- Specific DNA testing

Management

In the middle of the 20th century, the principal treatment for some of the amino acid disorders was restriction of dietary protein and all other care was simply management of complications.

In the last two decades, enzyme replacement, gene transfer and organ transplantation have become available and beneficial for many previously untreatable disorders. Some of the more common or promising methods are listed:
- Dietary restriction, e.g., reduction of dietary protein remains a mainstay of treatment for phenylketonuria and other amino acid disorders
- Dietary supplementation or replacement, e.g., cornstarch several times a day helps prevent people with glycogen storage disease from becoming hypoglycemic as quickly
- Vitamins, e.g., thiamine supplementation benefits several types of lactic acidosis
- Intermediary metabolites, compounds or drugs that facilitate or retard specific metabolic pathways
- Dialysis
- Enzyme replacement
- Gene therapy
- Bone marrow or organ transplantation
- Treatment of symptoms and complications
- Prenatal diagnosis and avoidance of pregnancy or abortion of an affected fetus.
Only commonly occurring inborn errors of metabolism are discussed in this chapter.

Phenylketonuria

Phenylketonuria (PKU) is an autosomal recessive genetic disorder characterized by a deficiency in the autosome phenylalanine hydroxylase (PAH). This enzyme is necessary to metabolize the amino acid phenylalanine to the amino acid tyrosine. When PAH is deficient, phenylalanine accumulates and is converted into phenylpyruvate (also known as phenyl ketone), which is detected in the urine.

Left untreated, this condition can cause problems with brain development, leading to progressive mental retardation and seizures. However, PKU is one of the few genetic diseases that can be controlled by diet. A diet low in phenylalanine and high in tyrosine can be a very effective treatment. There is no cure. Damage done is irreversible, so early detection is crucial.

Clinical Manifestations

- Early symptoms includes—seizures, albinism (excessively fair hair and skin), and a 'musty odor' to the baby's sweat and urine (due to phenylacetate, one of the ketones produced).

- Untreated children are normal at birth, but fail to attain early developmental milestones, develop microcephaly and demonstrate progressive impairment of cerebral function. Hyperactivity, electroencephalogram (EEG) abnormalities and seizures, and severe learning disabilities are major clinical problems later in life. A 'musty' odor of skin, hair, sweat and urine (due to phenylacetate accumulation); and a tendency to hypopigmentation and eczema are also observed.

Diagnosis (Screening)

Blood is taken from a 2-week-old infant to test for phenylketonuria. PKU is normally detected using the high performance liquid chromatography (HPLC) test, but some clinics still use the Guthrie test, part of national biochemical screening programs. Most babies in developed countries are screened for PKU soon after birth **(Fig. 19.1)**.

Treatment

- Diet low in phenylalanine for the rest of his/her life.
- Avoiding foods high in phenylalanine, such as meat, chicken, fish, nuts, cheese, legumes and other dairy products.
- Starchy foods, such as potatoes, bread, pasta and corn must be monitored.
- Infants may still be breastfed to provide all of the benefits of breast milk, though the quantity must be monitored and supplementation will be required.
- Many diet foods and diet soft drinks that contain the sweetener aspartame must also be avoided, as aspartame consists of two amino acids: Phenylalanine and aspartic acid.
- Supplementary infant formulas are used in these patients to provide the amino acids and other necessary nutrients that would otherwise be lacking in a protein-free diet. These can continue in other forms as the child grows up, such as pills, formulas and especially formulated foods (since phenylalanine is necessary for the synthesis of many proteins, it is required, but levels must be strictly controlled, usually being limited to 10 grams of protein. More severe forms of PKU, such as CPKU, require patients to be restricted to less than 5. In addition, tyrosine, which is normally derived from phenylalanine, must be supplemented).

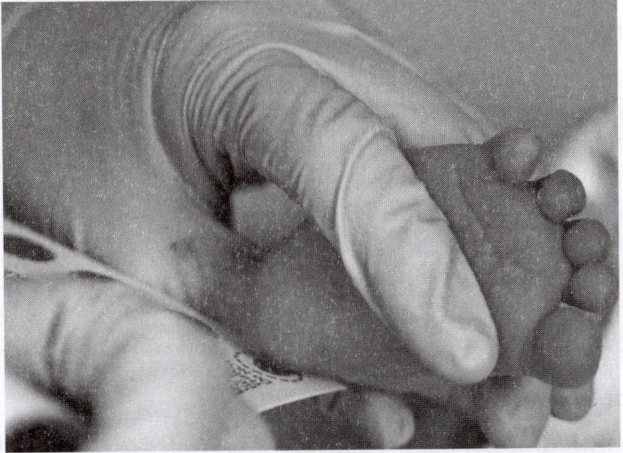

Fig. 19.1: High performance liquid chromatography (HPLC) test.

- The oral administration of tetrahydrobiopterin (a cofactor in the oxidation of phenylalanine) can reduce blood levels of the amino acid in certain patients.
- There are a number of other therapies currently under investigation, including gene therapy and an injectable form of PAH.
- Previously, PKU-affected people were allowed to go off diet after approximately 8, then 18 years of age. However, most physicians now agree that this special diet should be followed throughout life.

Maple Syrup Urine Disease (MSUD)

Maple syrup urine disease also called *branched-chain ketoaciduria*, is an autosomal recessive metabolic disorder affecting branched-chain amino acids. It is a type of organic acidemia. In this condition, the body is unable to process protein building blocks or amino acids properly. A rare genetic disorder that is characterized by deficiency of an enzyme complex, i.e., branched chain alpha keto acid dehydrogenase that is required to break down the three branched chain amino acids; leucine, isoleucine and valine. As a result of metabolic failure of these amino acids, they accumulate abnormally along many toxic by products.

Types

- **Classical or infantile MSUD:** It is the most common and severe type of MSUD. Symptoms usually appear within the first three days of birth. Babies born with this type either completely lack the necessary enzymes or produce very few of them.
- **Intermediate MSUD:** A type less severe than the classic one. Symptoms appear between 5 months and 7 years of age. In this type of MSUD, body makes more enzymes and can break the amino acids also.
- **Intermittent MSUD:** In this type, the symptoms appear only when any infection or stress occurs. People having this type of MSUD can tolerate the higher levels of amino acids in the urine and bloodstream.
- **Thiamine responsive MSUD:** Vitamin B1 boosts the enzyme activity so that the body can break the amino acids. People with this type responds to treatment with high doses of thiamine (vitamin B1) along with a restricted diet.

Clinical Manifestations

- From early infancy, symptoms of the condition include poor feeding, vomiting, dehydration, lethargy, hypotonia, seizures, ketoacidosis and neurological decline.
- The disease is characterized in an infant by the presence of sweet-smelling urine, sweat or ear wax, with an odor similar to that of maple syrup. Infants with this disease seem healthy at birth, but if left untreated suffer severe neurological damage, and eventually die.
- Developmental delay
- Sluggish, slow/tiredness and weakness
- Poor muscle tone, muscle tension
- Respiratory failure and coma

Diagnosis

Blood and urine biochemistry for presence of branched-chain amino acids (leucine, isoleucine and valine) and their toxic by products.

Management
- A diet with minimal levels of the amino acids leucine, isoleucine and valine must be maintained in order to prevent neurological damage.
- Monitoring of the patients for the level of amino acids. If it exceeds a person's tolerance level and begin to cause harm, IV glucose and insulin given to adjust the level of amino acids in the body.
- As these three amino acids are required for proper metabolic function in all people, specialized protein preparations containing substitutes and adjusted levels of the amino acids have been synthesized and tested, allowing MSUD patients to meet normal nutritional requirements without causing harm.

Gaucher Disease
Gaucher disease is a lipid storage disease, characterized by the deposition of glucocerebroside in cells of the macrophage-monocyte system. Deficiency of a specific lysosomal hydrolase, acid β-glucocerebrosidase, causes widespread accumulation of glucosylceramide-laden macrophages. Glucosylceramide accumulation is widespread and extends to the bone marrow, liver, spleen and lungs. Central nervous system involvement only occurs in patients with disease type 2 (acute neuronopathic) and type 3 (chronic neuronopathic) Gaucher's disease.

There are three clinical subtypes:
1. **Type 1**: Non-neuronopathic form. Often presents in childhood with hepatosplenomegaly, pancytopenia and skeletal disease. The severity of type 1 Gaucher disease is extremely variable, such that some patients present in childhood with virtually all the complications of Gaucher disease, while others are asymptomatic into the eighth decade. Patients diagnosed in the first 5 years of life are frequently non-Jewish and typically have a more malignant disease course.
2. **Type 2 (rare)**: Infantile form (acute neuronopathic). Causes rapidly progressive neurovisceral storage disease and death during infancy.
3. **Type 3**: Juvenile or Norrbottnian form (chronic or subacute neuronopathic). Less rapidly progressive neurovisceral storage disease, causing death in childhood or early adulthood.

Clinical Manifestations
Type 1: Gaucher Disease
- May present with chronic fatigue, hepatomegaly, splenomegaly (may become massive), bone involvement (bone pain due to bone infarcts or pathological fractures due to osteopenia) and may bruise easily or present with nosebleeds, bruising and petechiae (because of thrombocytopenia).
- Short stature and wasting occasionally are found in patients with massive organomegaly.
- Occasionally present with pulmonary infiltration or portal hypertension.

Type 2: Gaucher Disease
- Presents in infancy, with increased tone, strabismus, and organomegaly. Failure to thrive and stridor (due to laryngospasm) are also common.
- Rapid neurodegenerative course with extensive visceral involvement and death (usually caused by respiratory problems) within the first 2 years of life.

Type 3: Gaucher Disease

- Presents in infancy or childhood. In addition to organomegaly and bony involvement, neurological involvement is present, including developmental delay and abnormal neurological findings, e.g., increased tendon reflexes.
- Has been further classified as type 3a (with progressive myotonia and dementia) and 3b (with isolated supranuclear gaze palsy) based on the extent of neurological involvement.

Diagnosis

- **Acid β-glucosidase activity**: Diagnosis can be confirmed by measurement of acid. β-glucosidase activity in peripheral blood leukocytes. Heterozygotes have half-normal enzyme activity, but there is an overlap with non-affected controls.
- **Acid β-glucosidase genotyping**: Molecular diagnosis can be helpful, especially in Ashkenazi patients, in whom four mutations (N370 S, 84GG, L444P, IVS2 + 1) in the acid β-glucosidase gene account for nearly 97% of disease alleles.
- **Bone marrow aspiration**: Diagnosis may be suggested by the presence of classic glycolipid-laden macrophages (Gaucher cells). Not now the initial diagnostic test as the blood enzyme test is sensitive, specific and much less invasive.

General Assessment

- Full blood count and differential (assess the degree of pancytopenia), liver function tests (minor elevations of liver enzymes are common, but jaundice is a poor prognostic indicator).
- Skeletal radiography can detect and evaluate skeletal manifestations of Gaucher disease. Chest X-ray to evaluate pulmonary manifestations.
- Ultrasonography of the abdomen—determine extent of organomegaly.
- Magnetic resonance imaging (MRI) is more accurate in determining organ size and involvement.
- Patients with neuronopathic forms also need MRI scan of the brain, EEG and diagnostic brainstem evoked responses.
- Dual-energy X-ray absorptiometry (DEXA) scanning—evaluation of osteopenia.

Complications

- Bone—avascular necrosis of the hip, bone crises (secondary to infarcts)
- Splenic rupture (from trauma)
- Cirrhosis is rare
- Rarely, pulmonary infiltration by Gaucher cells may lead to overt lung disease
- Hematologic abnormalities (e.g., anemia, thrombocytopenia and leukopenia) are common
- Immunological abnormalities (e.g., hypergammaglobulinemia, T-lymphocyte deficiency in the spleen and impaired neutrophil chemotaxis) are also common.

Management

- Enzyme replacement therapy (ERT) with macrophage-targeted recombinant human glucocerebrosidase (imiglucerase) is administered as enzyme replacement therapy for non-neurological manifestations of type I or type III Gaucher disease. It is very effective in reversing the visceral and hematologic manifestations of Gaucher disease, but skeletal

disease is slow to respond. In patients with established acute neuronopathic disease, enzyme replacement therapy has had little effect on the progressively downhill course.
- Miglustat, an inhibitor of glucosylceramide synthase, is licensed for the treatment of mild to moderate type I Gaucher disease in patients for whom imiglucerase is unsuitable. It has been shown to help with the symptoms of mild to moderate type 1 Gaucher disease. Responses to miglustat are slower and less robust than those observed with ERT, and miglustat may produce significant side effects. Miglustat is currently in trials in combination with ERT to assess whether it will help to reduce some of the neurological deterioration in type 3 Gaucher disease.
- Bone marrow transplantation may be an effective treatment for neurological involvement in this disorder. However, there is significant morbidity and mortality, and therefore not currently recommended in the current management of neuronopathic Gaucher disease.
- Gene therapy may offer the possibility of definitive therapy in the future.
- Supportive treatment for specific organ involvement.
- There is evidence that, in neuronopathic Gaucher disease, complete or partial splenectomy is associated with increased severity and rate of progression of neurological and bone involvement and increased risk of infection.

Blood Group Alleles and Hematological Disorders

Blood Group Alleles

Blood group alleles came in existence through the discovery by Landsteiner in Vienna. According to this, there are two antigens on the red blood cells. They are antigen A and antigen B. Their presence or absence give rise to four phenotypes. They are A, B, AB and O. With the presence of an antigen, one can expect antibodies in the sera of these individuals. A person with blood group 'A' has an antigen A on his/her red cells and antibody anti-B in his/her serum. An individual with 'O' blood group has neither A nor B antigen on his/her red cells. So he/she possesses antibodies, anti-A and anti-B in his/her serum.

The ABO system forms an example of multiple allelism. The alleles are A, B, and O genes located at ABO locus on long arm of chromosome 9. Please note that gene O is recessive to genes A and B, while A and B are dominant. If both A and B genes are present, then both antigens (A and B) will be formed. The O gene is an amorph, i.e., it has no effect, thus leaving H-substance unaltered. So far, numerous subtypes of A and B have been detected. Significant among them are A_1 and A_2. As a result of this the AB group as also subdivided into A_1B and A_2B. Almost 85% of blood group A consists of A_1. Other variations of A and B although known and are rare **(Table 19.4)**.

Landsteiner and Wiener discovered Rh blood group system in 1940. The Rh system claims its place because of its role in hemolytic diseases of new born. There are both Rh-positive and Rh-negative individuals. Rh-positive persons are homozygous or heterozygous for gene specifying an antigen D, while Rh-negative persons do not have antigen D. The Rh locus is on chromosome 1. Fisher and Race suggested that there are five

Table 19.4: Alleles of the ABO blood group system.

Alleles	Protein
A1	A1 transferase
A2	A2 transferase
B	B transferase
O	Non-functional

Rh antigens designated as D, C, E, c and e. There are eight alleles. Their antigenic determinants are shown in **Table 19.5**.

Table 19.5: Alleles of the Rh blood group system.

Alleles	Antigen
R^0	D, c, e
R^1	D, C, e
R^2	D, c, E
R^z	D, C, E
r	c, e
r'	C, e
r''	c, E
r^v	C, E

Hematological Disorders

The common hematological disorders, which have genetic or hereditary associations are as follows:

Hemolytic Anemia

- Immune hemolytic anemia, e.g., hemolytic disease of newborn (Rh or ABO hemolytic disease)
- Hereditary red cell enzyme deficiency, e.g., glucose-6-phosphate dehydrogenase (G6PD) deficiency
- Hereditary defects of red cell membrane, e.g., hereditary spherocytosis, hereditary elliptocytosis
- Ineffective erythropoiesis, e.g., thalassemia (β or α)
- Hemoglobinopathies, e.g., sickle cell anemia, hemoglobin C, D or E disease
- Paroxysmal nocturnal hemoglobinuria
- Infantile pyknocytosis
- Diamond-Blackfan anemia

Hereditary Coagulopathies

- Hemophilia
- Von Willebrand disease
- Congenital amegakaryocytic thrombocytopenia (CAMT)

Hemolytic Disease of Newborn

In this disease, fetal red cells die earlier due to the action of antibodies formed by the mother against fetal Rh antigen. It begins in utero, but continue after birth for about 3 months, the time taken by maternal antibodies to get cleared from newborn's circulation. Although it is based on genetically determined antigenic disparity between mother and the fetus, it is an acquired hemolytic anemia, different from hereditary ones like hereditary spherocytosis.

Pathogenesis

In the natural course, there are no antibodies against Rh antigen in serum. During pregnancy, fetal and maternal blood pools are isolated by placental barrier. Toward the term, however, there are break occurring along this barrier. This permits transfer of fetal red cells to the mother's blood. When the mother is Rh negative and fetus is Rh positive, this transfer of Rh-positive red cells of fetus shall evoke an antibody response in the mother. These antibodies may get transferred across placenta to fetus circulation. They get attached to fetal red cells. Such anti-Rh coated cells are withdrawn from fetal circulation rendering it anemic. To compensate this, a large number of immature red cells called 'erythroblasts' are poured into fetal circulation. This offers it the name erythroblastosis fetalis.

Clinical Manifestation

Hyperbilirubinemia may follow after birth because of the rapid destruction of red cells of newborn. This leads to deposition of bilirubin in the brain and if not prevented by replacement transfusion, may cause cerebral damage. This may lead to mental retardation.

Management
- Usually Rh sensitization occurs at the time of delivery within 72 hours of delivery with Rh-immunoglobulin
- Replacement transfusion to newborn and phototherapy for management of increased bilirubin
- Regular monitoring of serum bilirubin
- Adequate hydration and infection prevention

Glucose-6-phosphate Dehydrogenase Deficiency

The G6PD deficiency is most common human enzyme defect. *Glucose-6-phosphate dehydrogenase deficiency* is an X-linked recessive hereditary disease characterized by abnormally low levels of glucose-6-phosphate dehydrogenase *(G6PD)*, a metabolic enzyme involved in the pentose phosphate pathway, especially important in red blood cell metabolism. Individuals with the disease may exhibit nonimmune hemolytic anemia in response to a number of causes, most commonly infection or exposure to certain medications or chemicals. The most common problem associated with G6PD deficiency is hemolytic anemia because the red blood cells are destroyed faster than the body can replace them.

The G6PD is the most common human enzyme defect, being present in more than 400 million people worldwide. African, Middle Eastern and South Asian people are affected the most.

Signs and Symptoms

Symptomatic patients are almost exclusively male, due to the X-linked pattern of inheritance, but female carriers can be clinically affected due to lyonization, where random inactivation of an X-chromosome in certain cells creates a population of G6PD deficient red blood cells coexisting with normal red cells. Abnormal red blood cell breakdown (hemolysis) in G6PD deficiency can manifest in a number of ways:
- Prolonged neonatal jaundice, possibly leading to kernicterus (arguably the most serious complication of G6PD deficiency)
- Paleness, dark urine, fatigue, shortness of breath and tachycardia.
- **Hemolytic crises in response to:**
    - Illness (especially severe infections)
    - Certain drugs (antimalarial, sulfonamides, aspirin, non-sulfa antibiotics)
    - Certain foods, most notably broad beans
    - Certain chemicals
    - Diabetic ketoacidosis
- Very severe crisis can cause acute renal failure.

Diagnosis

Generally, tests will include:
- Complete blood count and reticulocyte count; in active G6PD, Heinz bodies can be seen in red blood cells on a blood film
- Liver enzymes (to exclude other causes of jaundice)
- Lactate dehydrogenase (elevated in hemolysis and a marker of hemolytic severity)
- Haptoglobin (decreased in hemolysis)
- A "direct antiglobulin test" (Coombs' test)—this should be negative, as hemolysis in G6PD is not immune-mediated

- Beutler fluorescent spot test (identity NADPH produced by G6PD under ultraviolet light)
- Direct DNA testing and/or sequencing of the G6PD gene

Treatment

- Avoidance of the drugs, oxidative stressors and protein foods that cause hemolysis
- Vaccination against some common pathogens (e.g., hepatitis A and hepatitis B) may prevent infection-induced attacks
- In the acute phase of hemolysis, blood transfusions might be necessary
- Dialysis in acute renal failure
- Splenectomy, as this is an important site of red cell destruction
- Folic acid should be used in any disorder featuring a high red cell turnover. Although vitamin E and selenium have antioxidant properties, their use does not decrease the severity of G6PD.

Hereditary Spherocytosis

Hereditary spherocytosis is common cause of inherited disorder of red cell with varied clinical features that may present starting from the neonatal period to second decade of life. It is inherited as autosomal dominant with gene linked to short arm of chromosome 8 or 12.

Pathogenesis

Red cells' stromal protein spectrin and ankyrin are deficient because of reduced synthesis. Spectrin is also unstable and its binding to the red cell membrane is impaired. Due to this, red cells are sequestrated within the spleen. The stasis, hypoxia and metabolic acidosis decrease glycolysis of the red cells. As a result, less ATP is available. Phospholipids, cholesterol and protein are also lost. These metabolic changes cause loss of the red cell membrane, which reduces the surface area. As the cell volume does not concurrently decrease, the cells become more spheroidal or biconvex. Spheroidal cells are retained in the spleen and lysed.

Clinical Manifestations

- Anemia
- Hyperbilirubinemia
- Pale and mild jaundice
- Spleen enlargement
- Hepatomegaly
- Mild growth and developmental retardation

Diagnosis

- Peripheral blood smear show microspherocytosis
- High reticulocyte count and indirect bilirubin level
- Excessive fragile red cells

Management

- Phototherapy and exchange transfusion for newborns
- Blood transfusion to treat anemia in later childhood
- Folic acid to prevent megaloblastosis
- Splenectomy; preferable after 6 years of age to prevent risk of fulminating infection

Thalassemia

Thalassemia is an inherited abnormality of hemoglobin production. It is also known as Mediterranean anemia and Cooley's anemia. There are many forms and clinical severity varies enormously. The normal hemoglobin molecule has a heme base surrounded by 2 pairs of globin chains. The types of globin are called alpha (α), beta (β), gamma (γ) and delta (δ). Most types of hemoglobin have two α chains and two other identical types:
- The commonest form of adult hemoglobin is HbA, has two α and two β chains
- Fetal hemoglobin has two α and two γ components and is called HbF. This is the predominant type before birth
- The HbA2 is present in smaller amounts, with two α and two δ chains.

A decreased rate of production of any of these chains will lead to an imbalance between the amounts of the various forms of Hb in the erythrocytes leading to instability and hemolysis. The thalassemias are classified according to which chain of the globin molecule is affected. In α thalassemia, the production of α globin is deficient and in β thalassemia the production of β globin is defective. The classification of thalassemia major, thalassemia minor and sometimes thalassemia intermedia is based on clinical severity.

It is carried by 150 million or 3% of the world population. It is clinically apparent in 15 million people. The predominant type of thalassemia varies with geography. The β–thalassemia is the most common form around the Mediterranean, North Africa, Middle East, India and Eastern Europe. The α thalassemia is more common in Southeast Asia, India, Middle East and Africa.

Alpha Thalassemia

- Severe homozygous α thalassemia is usually lethal in utero. It should be considered when hydrops fetalis is diagnosed as rhesus incompatibility is a rare cause nowadays.
- Silent carrier α thalassemia is a fairly common type of subclinical thalassemia, usually found by chance among various ethnic African children being investigated for some other condition. There are two α genes on each chromosome 16, giving α thalassemia the unique feature of gene duplication. There is only one β-globin gene on chromosome 11. In the silent carrier state, one of the α genes is usually absent, leaving only three of four genes (aa/ao). Patients are hematologically normal, except for occasional low RBC indices. This diagnosis cannot be made on Hb electrophoresis, as results are usually normal in all α thalassemia traits. More sophisticated tests are necessary to confirm the diagnosis.
- The α thalassemia trait is characterized by mild anemia and low RBC indices. This condition is typically caused by the deletion of two α (a) genes on one chromosome 16 (aa/oo) or one from each chromosome (ao/ao). It is found mainly in Southeast Asia, the Indian subcontinent and some parts of the Middle East.
- Hemoglobin H (Hb H) disease results from the deletion or inactivation of three α globin genes (oo/ao). It represents a thalassemia intermedia, with mildly to moderately severe anemia, splenomegaly, jaundice and abnormal RBC indices. When peripheral blood films stained with supravital stain or reticulocyte preparations are examined, unique inclusions in the RBCs are usually observed. These inclusions represent β chain tetramers (Hb H), which are unstable and precipitate in the erythrocyte, giving it the appearance of a golf ball. These inclusions are called Heinz bodies.

Beta Thalassemia

- In β thalassemia, symptoms of anemia start when the γ chain production ceases and the β chains fail to form in adequate numbers. This is usually in the latter part of the 1st year of life, but sometimes they are 3–5 years old because of delay in stopping HbF production.
- In most patients with either α or β thalassemia traits, there are no signs or symptoms.

Clinical Manifestations

- In more severe forms, such as β thalassemia major, the symptoms vary from extremely debilitating in non-transfused patients to mild or absent in those on regular transfusion regimes and closely monitored chelation therapy.
- Ineffective erythropoiesis creates a hypermetabolic state with fever and failure to thrive.
- Overall manifestations varies with severity. Thalassemia minor rarely has any physical abnormalities with Hb over 9 g/dL. In patients with the severe forms, the findings on physical examination vary widely depending on how well the disease is controlled.
- Growth retardation is common even with well-controlled chelation therapy.
- Iron overload can cause endocrinopathy with diabetes, thyroid and adrenal disorders.
- **In severe, untreated cases there may be:**
  - Hepatosplenomegaly
  - Bony deformities including frontal bossing, prominent facial bones, and dental malocclusion are striking
  - Marked pallor and slight to moderate jaundice
  - Severe anemia causes exercise intolerance, cardiac murmur or even heart failure.

Diagnosis

Blood

- The FBC shows a microcytic, hypochromic anemia
- In the severe forms of thalassemia, the Hb level ranges from 2 to 8 g/dL
- The WBC count is usually elevated from the hemolytic process
- Platelet count may be depressed in splenomegaly
- Hemoglobin electrophoresis usually gives the diagnosis
- Serum iron level is elevated, with saturation as high as 80%
- Ferritin is also raised.

Imaging

- Skeletal surveys show classical changes in the bones, but only in patients, who are not regularly transfused. They result from expansion of marrow spaces and usually disappear when marrow activity is reduced by regular transfusions.
- Plain skull X-ray shows the classical 'hair on end' appearance. The maxilla may overgrow, with overbite, prominence of the upper incisors and separation of the orbit. These produce the characteristic facies of thalassemia major.
- Ribs, long bones and flat bones may be deformed.
- Chest X-ray to see cardiac size and shape.
- The CT or MRI scan can be used to evaluate the amount of iron in the liver in patients on chelation therapy.

Other tests
- The ECG and echocardiogram are used to monitor cardiac function.
- Human leukocyte antigen (HLA) typing is required where bone marrow transplantation is considered.
- Eye examinations, hearing tests and renal function tests are needed to monitor deferoxamine therapy.
- Bone marrow aspiration is sometimes needed at the time of diagnosis to exclude other conditions that may present as thalassemia major.
- Liver biopsy is used to assess iron deposition and the degree of hemochromatosis.
- Measurement of excretion of iron in the urine after a challenge test of desferrioxamine evaluates the need for chelation therapy.

Staging
A staging system has been developed, based on history of blood transfusions and cardiac symptoms, to decide when to initiate chelation therapy.
- **Stage I**—is patients who have received fewer than 100 units of packed RBCs. They are usually asymptomatic. The echocardiogram shows only slight left ventricular wall thickening, and both the radionuclide cineangiogram and the 24-hour ECG are normal.
- **Stage II**—patients have received between 100 and 400 units of blood and may have some fatigue. Echocardiograms may show some left ventricular wall thickening and dilatation but the ejection fraction is normal. The radionuclide cineangiogram findings are normal at rest but show no increase or fall in ejection fraction during exercise. Atrial and ventricular ectopic beats are usually found on the 24-hour ECG.
- **Stage III**—patients have symptoms ranging from palpitations to congestive heart failure. The ejection fraction on echocardiography is decreased. There is normal or decreased ejection fraction on cineangiogram at rest, and it falls on exercise. The 24-hour ECG reveals atrial and ventricular premature beats, often in pairs or in runs.

Complications
- Iron overload is one of the major causes of morbidity in severe forms of thalassemia even if they are not transfused.
- Bleeding tendency, susceptibility to infection and organ dysfunction are related to iron overload.
- Repeated transfusions increase the risk of blood-borne diseases including hepatitis B and hepatitis C although nowadays all blood is screened for these diseases.
- Infection with rare opportunistic organisms may cause pyrexia and enteritis in patients with iron overload. *Yersinia enterocolitica* thrives with the abundant iron. Unexplained fever, especially with diarrhea, should be treated with gentamicin and cotrimoxazole, even when cultures are negative.
- Osteoporosis is common and apparently multifactorial in etiology, but pamidronate is an effective treatment.
- Hyperuricemia sometimes produces gout.
- With increasing length of survival, hepatocellular carcinoma is becoming an increasing problem.
- Desferrioxamine can cause toxicity.

Management

- **Blood transfusion:** Transfusion improves both quality and quantity of life in severe cases. The target is not to let Hb fall below 9–9.5 g/dL. Transfused blood should be leucocyte poor. This is especially important if a bone marrow transplant is considered at some stage.
- **Neocyte transfusion:** Selecting and transfusion of younger red cells (neocytes), which will increase the interval between two transfusions and decrease the transfusion requirement.
- **Chelation therapy:** Desferrioxamine is given parenterally to aid iron excretion. The dose and means of delivery varies according to the needs of the patient. Oral chelating agents are being developed. Oral deferiprone used in combination with desferrioxamine produces a greater effect than either alone. Together they increase iron excretion, decrease ferritin levels and improve glucose tolerance in borderline cases, suggesting some reversal of damage to the pancreas by iron. Folic acid and vitamin E deficiency may both need treating.
- **Splenectomy:** When hypersplenism occurs splenectomy is often undertaken
- Cure can be achieved with a bone marrow transplant from a compatible, usually related donor.
- Recently embryo selection has been used to produce an immunologically compatible sib. While this induces horror in the expected quarters, the child is not simply a tissue culture, but will be a loved and wanted member of the family. The ethical and legal issues have been discussed.
- All families should be offered genetic counseling. In mild cases, no treatment is required, but anemia should not be treated with iron unless iron deficiency had been substantiated.
- Avoid food rich in iron. Extra vitamin E, folic acid and some vitamin C may be beneficial. Tea and coffee can reduce the absorption of iron.
- Gene manipulation and Gene therapy are under research.

Sickle Cell Anemia

Sickle cell disease or sickle cell anemia is a blood disorder characterized by red blood cells that assume an abnormal, rigid, sickle shape **(Figs. 19.2A and B)**. Sickling decreases the red cells' flexibility and results in a risk of various other complications. Life expectancy is shortened, with studies reporting an average life expectancy of 42 and 48 years for males and females, respectively.

Sickle cell anemia affects millions of people worldwide. Sickle cell disease occurs more commonly in people from parts of tropical and subtropical regions where malaria is or was common. It is particularly common among people whose ancestors come from Africa, Mediterranean countries (such as Greece, Turkey and Italy), the Arabian Peninsula, India and Spanish-speaking regions (South America, Central America and parts of the Caribbean).

Sickle cell anemia is the most common inherited blood disorder in the United States, affecting 70,000–80,000 Americans. The disease occurs in approximately 1 in 500 African-American newborns and 1 in 1,000 to 1,400 Hispanic-American births.

Causes and Pathology

- Sickle cell anemia is caused by a point mutation in the β-globin chain of hemoglobin, causing the amino acid glutamic acid to be replaced with the hydrophobic amino acid valine at the sixth position. The β-globin gene is found on the short arm of chromosome 11. The association of two wild type α-globin subunits with two mutant β-globin subunits

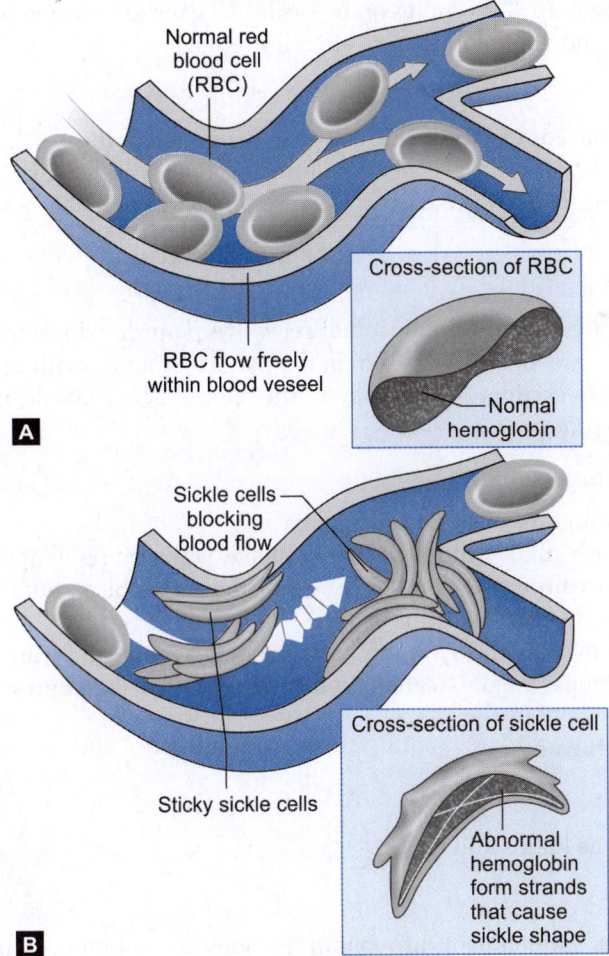

Figs. 19.2A and B: Sickle cell anemia: (A) Normal blood cells; (B) Abnormal, sickled, red blood cells (sick cells).

forms hemoglobin S (HbS). Under low-oxygen conditions, the absence of a polar amino acid at position six of the β-globin chain promotes the non-covalent polymerization (aggregation) of hemoglobin, which distorts red blood cells into a sickle shape and decreases their elasticity.
- The loss of red blood cell elasticity is central to the pathophysiology of sickle cell disease. Normal red blood cells are quite elastic, which allows the cells to deform to pass through capillaries. In sickle cell disease, low-oxygen tension promotes red blood cell sickling and repeated episodes of sickling damage the cell membrane and decrease the cell's elasticity. These cells fail to return to normal shape when normal oxygen tension is restored. As a consequence, these rigid blood cells are unable to deform as they pass through narrow capillaries, leading to vessel occlusion and ischemia.
- Sickle cell anemia is an inherited disease. People who have the disease inherit two copies of the sickle cell gene one from each parent. The sickle cell gene causes the body to make

abnormal hemoglobin. Two copies of the sickle cell gene are needed for the body to make the abnormal hemoglobin found in sickle cell anemia.

Sickle Cell Trait

If you inherit only one copy of the sickle cell gene (from one parent), you will not have sickle cell anemia. Instead, you will have sickle cell trait. People who have sickle cell trait usually have no symptoms and lead normal lives. However, they can pass the sickle cell gene to their children.

Inheritance Pattern

This condition is inherited in an autosomal recessive pattern, which means two copies of the gene in each cell are altered. Most often, the parents of an individual with an autosomal recessive disorder are carriers of one copy of the altered gene, but do not show signs and symptoms of the disorder.

Clinical Manifestations

- The signs and symptoms of sickle cell anemia vary.
- Some people have mild symptoms. Others have very severe symptoms and often are hospitalized for treatment. Sickle cell anemia is present at birth, but many infants do not show any signs until after 4 months of age.
- The most common signs and symptoms are linked to anemia and pain. The most common symptom of anemia is fatigue (feeling tired or weak). Other signs and symptoms of anemia include:
  - Shortness of breath
  - Dizziness
  - Headache
  - Coldness in the hands and feet
  - Pale skin
  - Chest pain
- **Sickle cell crisis:** Sudden pain throughout the body is a common symptom of sickle cell anemia. Sickle cell crises often affect the bones, lungs, abdomen and joints. A sickle cell crisis occurs when sickled red blood cells form clumps in the bloodstream. These clumps of cells block blood flow through the small blood vessels in the limbs and organs. This can cause pain and organ damage.
- Other signs and symptoms are linked to the disease's complications.

Diagnosis

- Prenatal screening through amniocentesis.
- Newborn screening/testing for sickle cell anemia as part of routine screening. If the test shows some sickle hemoglobin. Then a second blood test is done to confirm the diagnosis. The second test should be done as soon as possible and within the 1st month of life.
- Later diagnosis is usually based on clinical history and sickling in peripheral blood sample. Hemoglobin S is identified by electrophoresis and solubility studies. The HbS move slower than HbA on electrophoresis.
- DNA sequences can be amplified using polymerase chain reaction (PCR) technique.

Complications
- Hand-foot syndrome
- Acute chest syndrome
- Pulmonary arterial hypertension
- Delayed growth and puberty in children
- Ulcers on the legs
- Multiple organ failure
- Splenic crisis
- Infections
- Stroke
- Eye problems
- Priapism
- Gallstones

Management
Sickle cell anemia has no widely available cure. However, treatments can help relieve symptoms and treat complications. The goals of treating sickle cell anemia are to relieve pain; prevent infections, eye damage and strokes, and control complications (if they occur):
- Bone marrow transplants may offer a cure in a small number of sickle cell anemia cases.
- Researchers continue to look for new treatments for the disease. These include gene therapy and improved bone marrow transplants.
- Pain management through analgesics [non-steroidal anti-inflammatory drug (NSAIDs), and narcotics] and fluid administration to prevent sickling of red cells. Hydroxyurea is used to prevent painful crises, not to treat them when they occur.
- Blood transfusions are commonly used to treat worsening anemia and sickle cell complications. A sudden worsening of anemia due to an infection or enlargement of the spleen is a common reason for a blood transfusion.
- Routine vaccination and prophylactic antibiotic administration for prevention of infection.
- New drugs under research are—butyric acid, nitric oxide and decitadine. Butyric acid is a food additive that may increase normal hemoglobin in the blood, nitric oxide may make sickle cells less sticky and keep blood vessels open. People who have sickle cell anemia have low levels of nitric oxide in their blood. Decitabine increases hemoglobin F levels (this type of hemoglobin carries more oxygen). It may be a good choice instead of hydroxyurea.
- **Treating other complications:**
  - Acute chest syndrome is a severe and life-threatening complication of sickle cell anemia. Treatment usually requires hospitalization and may include oxygen, blood transfusions, antibiotics, pain medicine, and checking the body's fluids.
  - If you have leg ulcers due to sickle cell anemia, you may be given strong pain medicines. Ulcers can be treated with cleansing solutions and medicated creams or ointments. Skin grafts may be needed if the condition continues. Bed rest and keeping the legs raised to reduce swelling are helpful, although not always possible.
  - Gallbladder surgery may be needed if the presence of gallstones leads to gallbladder disease.
  - Priapism (a painful erection of penis in males) can be treated with fluids or surgery.

Diamond-Blackfan Anemia

Diamond-Blackfan Anemia (DBA) is a rare blood disorder that is caused by a failure of the bone marrow to generate enough red blood cells. It is characterized by deficiency of red blood cells at birth (congenital hypoplastic anemia) as well as slow growth.

Clinical Manifestations

Abnormal weakness and fatigue, paleness of the skin, heart murmur, low birth weight, irritability characteristic facial abnormalities, protruding shoulder blades (scapulae), webbing or abnormal shortening of the neck due to fusion of certain bones in the spine (cervical vertebrae), hand deformities, congenital heart defects, and/or other abnormalities. The symptoms and physical findings associated with Blackfan-Diamond anemia vary greatly from case to case.

Diagnostic Findings

- Hemoglobin and hematocrit levels
- Complete blood count
- Peripheral smear
- Bone marrow analysis

Treatment

Treatment includes medications, blood transfusions and bone marrow transplant. Corticosteroids improves red blood cell counts in about 80% patients. Stem cell transplant may cure DBA, but rejection and infection may also occur post-transplant. This is preferred only if the patient does not respond to steroids or blood transfusions.

Hemophilia

Hemophilia is a hereditary genetic disorders, where there is congenital deficiency of plasma coagulation factor that impair the body's ability to control blood clotting or coagulation. it is inherited in X-linked recessive pattern. Hemophilia is quite rare, with only about 1 instance in every 10,000 births (or 1 in 5,001 male births) for hemophilia A and 1 in 50,000 births for hemophilia B.

Types and Causes

- **Hemophilia A (classic hemophilia)** is an X-linked genetic disorder involving a lack of functional clotting factor VIII and represents 90% of hemophilia cases.
- **Hemophilia B (Christmas disease)** is an X-linked genetic disorder involving a lack of functional clotting factor IX. It is less severe, but more uncommon than hemophilia A.
- **Hemophilia C** is an autosomal recessive genetic disorder involving a lack of functional clotting factor XI.

Inheritance Pattern and Genetic Pathology

Females possess two X-chromosomes, whereas males have one X and one Y chromosome. Since the mutations causing the disease are recessive, a woman carrying the defect on one of her X-chromosomes may not be affected by it, as the equivalent allele on her other chromosome should express itself to produce the necessary clotting factors. However, the Y-chromosome in men has no gene for factors VIII or IX. If the genes responsible for production of factor VIII or factor IX present on a male's X-chromosome are deficient there is no equivalent on the Y-chromosome, so the deficient gene is not masked by the dominant allele and he will develop the illness.

Since a male receives his single X-chromosome from his mother, the son of a healthy female silently carrying the deficient gene will have a 50% chance of inheriting that gene from her and with it the disease; and if his mother is affected with hemophilia, he will have a 100% chance of being a hemophiliac. In contrast, for a female to inherit the disease, she must receive two deficient X-chromosomes, one from her mother and the other from her father (who must therefore be a hemophiliac himself). Hence, hemophilia is far more common among males than females. However, it is possible for female carriers to become mild hemophiliacs due to lyonization (inactivation) of the X chromosomes. Hemophiliac daughters are more common than they once were, as improved treatments for the disease have allowed more hemophiliac males to survive to adulthood and become parents. Adult females may experience menorrhagia (heavy periods) due to the bleeding tendency. The pattern of inheritance is criss-cross type.

A mother who is a carrier has a 50% chance of passing the faulty X chromosome to her daughter, while an affected father will always pass on the affected gene to his daughters. A son cannot inherit the defective gene from his father.

As with all genetic disorders, it is of course also possible for a human to acquire it spontaneously through mutation, rather than inheriting it, because of a new mutation in one of their parents' gametes. Spontaneous mutations account for about 33% of all cases of hemophilia A. About 30% of cases of hemophilia B are the result of a spontaneous gene mutation.

Classification of Hemophilia

See **Table 19.6**.

Clinical Manifestations

The major signs and symptoms of hemophilia are excessive bleeding and easy bruising.
- The extent of bleeding depends on the type and severity of the hemophilia. Children with mild hemophilia may not have symptoms until they have excessive bleeding from a dental procedure, an accident or surgery. Males with severe hemophilia may bleed heavily after circumcision. Bleeding can be obvious (external bleeding) or hidden within the body (internal bleeding). Signs of excessive external bleeding include:
  - Bleeding in the mouth from a cut or bite or from cutting or losing a tooth
  - Nose bleeds for no obvious reason
  - Heavy bleeding from a minor cut
  - Bleeding from a cut that resumes after stopping for a short time.
- Signs of internal bleeding include blood in the urine (from bleeding in the kidneys or bladder) and blood in the stool (from bleeding in the intestines or stomach).
- **Bleeding in the brain:** Internal bleeding in the brain is a very serious complication of hemophilia that can happen after a simple bump on the head or a more serious injury. The signs and symptoms of bleeding in the brain include:
  - Long-lasting painful headaches or neck pain or stiffness
  - Repeated vomiting

Table 19.6: Classification of hemophilia.

Hemophilia type	Percentage of normal factors present
Mild hemophilia	5–30% of normal factor
Moderate hemophilia	1–5% of normal factor
Severe hemophilia	<1% of normal factor

- Changes in behavior or being very sleepy
- Sudden weakness or clumsiness of the arms or legs or difficulty walking
- Double vision
- Convulsions or seizures

Diagnosis
- Blood tests for bleeding time, clotting time.
- Blood level of clotting factors. Hemophilia A and B are classified as mild, moderate or severe, depending on the amount of clotting factor VIII or IX in the blood.

Management
- **Replacement therapy:** Giving or replacing the clotting factor that is too low or missing. Concentrates of clotting factor VIII (for hemophilia A) or clotting factor IX (for hemophilia B) are given slowly by intravenous drip or injection.
- **Desmopressin:** Desmopressin (DDAVP) is a synthetic hormone used to treat people with mild-to-moderate hemophilia A. DDAVP cannot be used to treat hemophilia B or severe hemophilia A. It is administered intravenous or nasal spray, which stimulates the release of stored factor VIII.
- **Antifibrinolytic medicines:** Tablet tranexamic acid and aminocaproic acid may be used with replacement therapy. Usually given before dental work, for treatment of nasal or oral bleeding or mild intestinal bleeding.
- **Gene therapy:** Researchers are trying to develop ways to correct the defective genes that cause hemophilia to cure the disorder. But it is still under trial.
- Specific exercises to strengthen the joints, particularly the elbows, knees, and ankles, after an internal bleed occurs and on a daily basis to strengthen the muscles and joints to prevent new bleeding problems. Many recommended exercises include standard sports warm-up and training exercises, such as stretching of the calves, ankle circles, elbow flexions, and Quadriceps sets.
- Selected alternative therapies, such as self-hypnosis and certain herbs.

von Willebrand Disease

von Willebrand disease (vWD) is an inherited bleeding disorder that occurs due to qualitative or quantitative deficiency of von Willebrand factor (vWF), a multimeric protein that is required for platelet adhesion. In humans, the incidence of vWD is roughly about 1 in 100 individuals. Because most forms are rather mild, they are detected more often in women, whose bleeding tendency shows during menstruation. The actual abnormality (which does not necessarily lead to disease) occurs in 0.9–3% of the population. It may be more severe or apparent in people with blood type O.

Types
- **Type 1 vWD:** In this, person has a low level of the von Willebrand factor and may have lower levels of factor VIII than normal. This is the mildest and most common form of the disease. About 3 out of 4 people who vWD have type 1.
- **Type 2 vWD:** In this, the von Willebrand factor does not work the way it is supposed to work. Type 2 is divided into subtypes: 2A, 2B, 2M and 2N. Different gene mutations cause each type, and each is treated differently. This makes knowing the exact type of vWD that one have very important.

- **Type 3 vWD:** In this, usually person has no von Willebrand factor and low levels of factor VIII. Type 3 is the most serious form of vWD, but it is very rare.

Inheritance Pattern and Genetic Pathology

von Willebrand disease types I and II are inherited in an autosomal dominant pattern. von Willebrand disease type III (and sometimes II) is inherited in an autosomal recessive pattern. The vWF gene is located on chromosome twelve (12p13.2). It has 52 exons spanning 178kbp. Types 1 and 2 are inherited as autosomal dominant traits and type 3 is inherited as autosomal recessive. Occasionally type 2 also inherits recessively.

Clinical Manifestations

The signs and symptoms of von Willebrand disease depend on the type and severity of the disease. Many people have following mild-to-moderate bleeding symptoms in type 1 or type 2 vWD:
- Frequent large bruises from minor bumps or injuries
- Frequent or hard to stop nose bleeds
- Extended bleeding from the gums after a dental procedure
- Menorrhagia (heavy or extended menstrual bleeding in women)
- Blood in your stools from bleeding in your intestines or stomach
- Blood in your urine from bleeding in your kidneys or bladder
- Heavy bleeding after a cut or other accident
- Heavy bleeding after surgery

People with type 3 vWD may have all of the symptoms listed above, as well as severe bleeding episodes for no reason. These bleeding episodes can be life-threatening if not treated right away. They also may have bleeding into soft tissues or joints, causing severe pain and swelling.

Diagnosis

- Complete blood count (especially platelet counts)
- Activated partial thromboplastin time (APTT), prothrombin time, thrombin time and fibrinogen level. Testing for factor IX may also be performed if hemophilia B is suspected.
- A platelet function assay
- Blood plasma for quantitative and qualitative deficiencies of vWF
- Clotting factor VIII levels estimation
- Testing for factor IX may also be performed if hemophilia B is suspected
- Other coagulation factor assays may be performed depending on the results of a coagulation screen.

Management

Treatment is based on the type and severity of von Willebrand disease. Most cases of vWD are mild, and may need treatment only if have surgery, tooth extraction or an accident.

Specific treatments
- Desmopressin (DDAVP) is a synthetic hormone that is usually given by injection or nasal spray. It makes the body to release more von Willebrand factor and factor VIII into your bloodstream. The DDAVP works for most patients who have type 1 vWD and for some who have type 2 vWD.

- von Willebrand factor replacement therapy is an infusion of a concentrate of von Willebrand factor and factor VIII. This treatment can be used if:
  - The DDAVP is contraindicated or need extended treatment
  - Type 1 vWD that does not respond to DDAVP
  - In type 2 or type 3 vWD
- Antifibrinolytic drugs help prevent the breakdown of blood clots. They are mostly used to stop bleeding after minor surgery, tooth extraction, or an injury. They may be used alone or together with DDAVP and replacement therapy.
- Fibrin glue is medicine that is placed directly on a wound to stop the bleeding.

Treatments for women: Treatments for women who have vWD with heavy menstrual bleeding include:

- Combined oral contraceptives. The contraceptives can increase the amount of von Willebrand factor and factor VIII in bloodstream and reduce menstrual blood loss.
- A levonorgestrel intrauterine device. This is a contraceptive device that contains progestin. It is placed in the uterus.
- Aminocaproic acid or tranexamic acid. These antifibrinolytic drugs can reduce bleeding by slowing the breakdown of blood clots.
- DDAVP
- Endometrial ablation, who has completed the family.

Congenital Amegakaryocytic Thrombocytopenia

Congenital amegakaryocytic thrombocytopenia (CAMT) is a rare inherited disorder. The primary manifestations are thrombocytopenia and or low numbers of platelets and megakaryocytes, which may make a person potential for bleeding. There is an absence of megakaryocytes in the bone marrow with no associated physical abnormalities. The cause for this disorder appears to be a mutation in the gene for the TPO receptor, *c-mpl,* despite high levels of serum TPO. In addition, there may be abnormalities with the central nervous system including the cerebrum and cerebellum, which could cause symptoms. The primary treatment for CAMT is bone marrow transplantation. Bone marrow/stem cell transplant is the only thing that ultimately cures this genetic disease. Frequent platelet transfusions are required to protect the patient from bleeding to death until transplant is done, although this is not always the case.

Genetic Hemochromatosis

"Hemochromatosis is a disorder that causes the body to absorb too much iron from the diet. The excess iron is stored in the body's tissues and organs, particularly the heart, liver, pancreas and joints. Because humans cannot increase excretion of iron, the extra iron accumulates over time and eventually can damage the tissue or organ."

Normally an individual get 10–20 milligrams of iron a day in diet. However, of that amount the body typically only absorbs 1–2 milligrams. The rest of the iron is not absorbed and some is lost in any skin cells that are shed. Individuals with hereditary hemochromatosis absorb 3–4 milligrams of iron through the intestine and the body does not have any way to get rid of it. Over decades, this iron accumulates in organs including the heart, liver and pancreas. Iron accumulation results in organ damage and other conditions, such as diabetes and abnormal heart rhythms that signs that the organs are sick.

It takes a long time for organs to sustain enough damage due to excess iron before they begin to malfunction. Excess iron accumulation in the organs begins in childhood, but the symptoms of this disorder do not usually appear until adulthood. Symptoms of hemochromatosis begin to occur when the body has stored 20 grams or more of iron, which can take four to six decades.

Etiology and Genetic Basis

The most common cause of hemochromatosis is *genetics*; known as hereditary hemochromatosis, by definition, hereditary hemochromatosis is an iron overload disorder that runs in families: An individual develops the condition by inheriting altered or mutated, copies of the *HFE gene* (which regulates iron absorption in our bodies) from his/her parents. However, even though the disorder is clearly inherited, it is not always easy to spot a pattern of disease within families who have the mutation. This is because people can be carriers of a hemochromatosis mutation without having any symptoms or complications. Thus, the fact that no one in one's immediate or extended family has symptoms of hereditary hemochromatos does not mean he/she cannot develop this disorder.

In fact, everyone who carries mutated, copies of the *HFE gene* does not develop disorder, but a far smaller number of people develop fully symptomatic hemochromatosis. Others who carry a mutation, but do not have symptoms of hemochromatosis, may be at increased risk for other disorders, such as cardiovascular problems.

Inheritance Pattern

Although approximately 1 out of every 200 people is a carrier of one of the genetic mutations that cause hereditary hemochromatosis, not nearly that many people actually develop symptoms or complications from the disorder. This is because hereditary hemochromatosis is passed through families in what is known as autosomal recessive fashion, which means that an individual must inherit a mutated copy of the *HFE* gene from both parents to develop the disorder. A person who has inherited only one defective gene will most likely be a carrier of hemochromatosis and will not have the disease. A carrier can pass the defective gene on to his/her children:
- If only one parent is a carrier of a defective gene, the child will not have hemochromatosis; however, there is a 50% chance that the child will be a carrier
- If both parents are carriers, there is only a 25% chance that the child will have hemochromatosis, but a 50% chance that the child will be a carrier.

Clinical Manifestations

With over 30 different symptoms associated with hemochromatosis. Symptoms may begin anywhere from age 30 to age 60, although in some rare cases they occur as early as 20. Many of the early symptoms of hemochromatosis are nonspecific, including:
- Weakness
- Fatigue
- Abdominal pain
- General muscle aches
- Loss of sex drive
- Impotence
- Cessation of monthly menstrual cycles

- Joint pain in the fingers
- Shortness of breath on exertion
- Increased skin pigmentation (a bronze color)
- Loss of body hair
- Hepatomegaly

If untreated or not diagnosed early enough, hemochromatosis can lead to; diabetes, joint pain, dysrhythmias, heart failure, cirrhosis of the liver, liver failure, or (rarely) liver cancer, impotence or decreased sex drive in men and early menopause in women.

Factors Affecting clinical Presentation

Many factors affect clinical presentation of hemochromatosis:
- **Alcohol:** Because alcohol is an independent toxin to the liver, liver disease may be present earlier due to the combined effects of alcohol and iron.
- **Diet:** People who take vitamin supplements that contain iron or take vitamin C, which increases the body's effectiveness at absorbing iron, may have symptoms at a younger than average age.
- **Gender:** Men are twice as likely to go to their doctor with symptoms of hereditary hemochromatosis than women. In untreated men, symptoms usually begin between age 40 and 60. For women, the symptoms usually start later, between age 50 and 65. One reason is that women have regular episodes of blood loss through menstruation or childbirth.
- **Blood loss:** Individuals who lose iron through blood donation may also delay the onset of symptoms.
- **Mutation type:** There are two common mutations in a gene called *HFE*, which is known to cause hereditary hemochromatosis. One of these two mutations, H63D, is associated with a less severe and later onset form of hemochromatosis. People who have one or two copies of this mutation have a milder form of the disease compared to people who have two copies of the other common mutation (called C282Y).

Diagnosis

Screening diagnosis of hemochromatosis is done through the following:

Transferrin Saturation Test

The transferrin saturation test determines how much iron is held by the protein that carries iron in the blood. A fasting transferrin saturation of 60% or higher in men, or 50% or higher in women, on at least two occasions, is considered a sign of iron overload. However, factors in addition to hemochromatosis can cause iron overload. Values of greater than 45% are considered suggestive of hemochromatosis and deserve further evaluation.

Serum Ferritin Level Test

The serum ferritin test acts as an indirect measure of iron storage in the liver. Serum ferritin levels are considered in the normal range for males and postmenopausal females if they are between 20 and 300 mg/L, or between 20 and 200 mg/L for premenopausal females. People with advanced hemochromatosis may have serum ferritin levels as high as 15,000 mg/L. However, other factors besides hemochromatosis can cause high serum ferritin levels, including liver disease, infection, cancer, heart disease, AIDS, metabolic disorders and inflammatory conditions, such as arthritis.

If individuals have elevated serum ferritin levels, or fasting transferrin saturation levels, genetic testing for hemochromatosis may help to identify the reason for the increase in iron storage.

Liver Biopsy

Before the availability of genetic testing for hemochromatosis, a liver biopsy with measurements of hepatic iron was considered the 'gold standard' for diagnosing hemochromatosis. A liver biopsy is now rarely needed to make the diagnosis, and is usually only used in cases of apparent iron overload with a negative genetic test result and no other family history of hemochromatosis. However, a liver biopsy is the only test that can tell whether cirrhosis is present, which is the only complication that affects the lifespan of someone with hemochromatosis, since it increases the risk for liver cancer. A liver biopsy should be recommended for anyone with hemochromatosis who is also:
- Over 40 years old
- Has a ferritin level over 1000 mg/L
- Has abnormal liver function test results

Human Leukocyte Antigen Testing

Testing of HLA antigens was also once used to help make the diagnosis. This was because the gene for hemochromatosis was very close to the highly polymorphic HLA genes on chromosome six, and certain HLA gene alleles were often found in patients with hemochromatosis. This test had many false positive and false negative results, and is now obsolete (although still offered by some laboratories).

Genetic Testing

To identify affected gene.

Management

Management includes:
- Weekly phlebotomy until iron levels reach normal.
- **Chelation therapy:** The chelating agents deferoxamine and deferasirox bind to iron in blood and helps to remove excess iron present in body.
- Preventing further accumulation of iron through blood removal three to four times a year, and avoiding supplemental iron and high doses of vitamin C.
- Regular monitoring of the serum ferritin levels. For effective treatment serum ferritin iron levels are less than 50 nanograms (ng) per milliliter and transferrin saturation levels are less than 50% should be maintained.

Huntington's Disease

Huntington's disease (HD), also called Huntington's chorea, chorea major or HD, is a genetic neurological disorder characterized after onset by uncoordinated, jerky body movements and a decline in some mental abilities. These characteristics vary per individual, physical ones less so, but the differing decline in mental abilities can lead to a number of potential behavioral problems.

The disorder itself is not fatal, but as symptoms progress, complications reducing life expectancy increase. Research of HD has increased greatly in the last few decades, but its exact mechanism is unknown, so symptoms are managed individually. Globally, up to 7 people in 100,000 have the disorder, although there are localized regions with a higher incidence. Onset of physical symptoms occurs gradually and can begin at any age, although it is statistically most common in a person's mid-40s (with a 30 year spread). If onset is before age 20, the condition is classified as juvenile HD.

The disorder is named after George Huntington, an American physician who published a remarkably accurate description in 1872. In 1983 a marker for the altered DNA causing the disease was found, followed a decade later by discovery of a single, causal, gene. As it was caused by a single gene, an accurate genetic test for HD was developed; this was one of the first inherited genetic disorders for which such a test was possible. Due to the availability of this test, and similar characteristics with other neurological disorders, the amount of HD research has increased greatly in recent years.

Genetic Basis

Huntington's disease is one of several trinucleotide repeat disorders, caused by the length of a repeated section of a gene exceeding the normal range. The *huntingtin* gene (HTT) normally provides the information to produce huntingtin protein, but when affected, produces mutant huntingtin (mHTT) instead.

The *huntingtin* gene (HTT) is located on the short arm of chromosome 4 (4p16.3). The HTT contains a sequence of three DNA bases—cytosine-adenine-guanine (CAG)—repeated multiple times (i.e., …CAGCAGCAG…) on its 5′ end, known as a trinucleotide repeat. The CAG is the genetic code for the amino acid glutamine, so a series of them results in the production of a chain of glutamine known as polyglutamine or polyQ tract, and the repeated part of the gene, the *PolyQ region*.

A polyQ region containing fewer than 36 glutamines results in production of the cytoplasmic protein called huntingtin (HTT) **(Table 19.7)**. Generally, people have less than 27 repeated glutamines, however, a sequence of 36 or more glutamines, results in the production of form of Htt, which has different characteristics. This altered form, called mutant Htt or more commonly *mHtt*, increases the rate of neuronal decay in certain types of neurons, affecting regions of the brain with a higher proportion or dependency on them. Generally, the number of CAG repeats is related to how much this process is affected, and correlates with age at onset and the rate of progression of symptoms. For example, 36–39 repeats result in much later onset and slower progression of symptoms than the mean, such that some individuals may die of other causes before they even manifest symptoms of Huntington disease, this is termed 'reduced penetrance'. With very large repeat counts, HD can occur under the age of 20 years, when it is then referred to as juvenile HD, akinetic-rigid, or Westphal variant HD and accounts for about 7% of HD carriers.

Table 19.7: Huntingtin gene repeat count and severity of disease.

Repeat count	Classification	Disease status
<27	Normal	Unaffected
27–35	Intermediate	Unaffected
36–39	Reduced penetrance	± Affected
>39	Full penetrance	Affected

Inheritance Pattern

Huntington's disease is inherited autosomal dominantly, meaning that an affected individual typically inherits a copy of the gene with an expanded trinucleotide repeat (the mutant allele) from an affected parent. In this type of inheritance pattern, each offspring of an affected individual has a 50% chance of inheriting the mutant allele and therefore being affected with the disorder. **Figure 19.3** shows that if a father is a sufferer, there is 1 in 2 chances of the child having this disease.

Homozygous individuals, who have two affected genes, are very rare except in large consanguineous families. While HD seemed to be the first disease for which homozygotes did not differ in clinical expression or course from typical heterozygotes, more recent analysis suggests that homozygosity affects the phenotype and the rate of disease progression, but does not alter the age of onset, suggesting that the mechanisms for these factors differ.

Clinical Manifestations

- The most characteristic physical symptoms are jerky, random and uncontrollable movements called chorea. In a few cases, very slow movement and stiffness (called bradykinesia and dystonia) occur instead, and often become more prominent than the chorea as the disorder progresses. Abnormal movements are initially exhibited as general lack of coordination, an unsteady gait and slurring of speech, but as the disease progresses, any function that requires muscle control is affected, causing physical instability, abnormal facial expression, and difficulties chewing and swallowing. Eating difficulties commonly cause weight loss and may lead to malnutrition. Associated symptoms involve sleep cycle disturbances, including insomnia and rapid eye movement sleep alterations. Juvenile HD generally progresses faster, is more likely to exhibit rigidity and bradykinesia, instead of chorea commonly includes seizures.
- Selected cognitive abilities are impaired progressively. Especially affected are executive functions, which include planning, cognitive flexibility, abstract thinking, rule acquisition, initiating appropriate actions and inhibiting inappropriate actions. Psychomotor function, controlling muscles, perception and spatial skills, is also affected. As the disease progresses, memory deficits tend to appear. Memory impairments reported range from short-term memory deficits to long-term memory difficulties, including deficits in episodic (memory of one's life), procedural (memory of the body of how to perform an activity) and working memory.

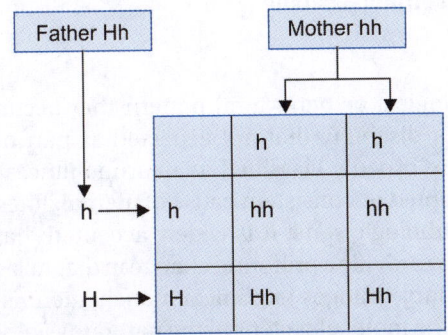

Fig. 19.3: Inheritance pattern in Huntington's disease.

- Psychiatric symptoms vary far more than cognitive and physical ones, and may include anxiety, depression, a reduced display of emotions (blunted affect), egocentrism, aggression and impulsive behavior, which can cause, or worsen addictions, including alcoholism and gambling, or hypersexuality. Difficulties in recognizing other people's negative expressions has also been observed.

Diagnosis
- **Prenatal screening through:**
  - Preimplantation genetic diagnosis in the setting of in vitro fertilization
  - Prenatal diagnosis in case of family history to decide about continuation of pregnancy.
- **Postnatal disease diagnosis through:**
  - A physical and/or psychological examination
  - Presymptomatic testing is possible using a blood test, which counts the numbers of CAG repeats in each of the HTT alleles, although a positive result is not considered a diagnosis, since it may be obtained decades before onset of symptoms. A negative blood test means that the individual does not carry the expanded copy of the gene.
  - A full pathological diagnosis can only be established by a neurological examination's findings and/or demonstration of cell loss in the areas affected by HD, supported by a cranial computed tomography (CT) or MRI scan findings.

Management
- Antidepressants, sedatives, and low doses of antipsychotics for cognitive and psychological symptoms.
- There is limited evidence for specific treatments aimed at controlling the chorea and other movement abnormalities, although tetrabenazine has been shown to reduce the severity of the chorea.
- High-caloric diet to maintain body weight.
- Thickening agent can be added to drinks as swallowing becomes more difficult, as thicker fluids are easier and safer to swallow.
- Percutaneous endoscopic gastrostomy, when eating becomes too hazardous or uncomfortable. A 'stomach PEG' greatly reduces the chances of aspiration of food, which can lead to aspiration pneumonia, and also increases the amount of nutrients and calories that can be ingested, aiding the body's natural defenses.
- As for any patient with neurologic deficits, a multidisciplinary rehabilitation approach is key to limiting and overcoming disability.

Mental Illness

Mental illness is a psychological or behavioral pattern that occurs in an individual and is thought to cause distress or disability that not expected as part of normal development or culture. Mental illnesses are broadly classified as neurotic illness and psychotic illness. As such there is not single accepted or consistent cause of mental illnesses.

Almost regardless of pathologic state, it is widely accepted that genetic information has started to provide or will soon provide a profound change in diagnosis and therapy in medicine. The potential for revolutionary changes in clinical management is based on the detail with which genetics is revealing the molecular steps of the pathophysiologic process. In psychiatric illness, this is also true, but there is a strong argument for predicting an effect that is even more fundamental than it is in other disease states. It is long been known that certain diseases tend to run in families. In fact, most of our understanding of mental illness comes from family, adoption and twin studies. Now, researchers have discovered a gene that can double the risk of depression, another that can increase the risk of schizophrenia, and others that may play a role in the risk of bipolar disorder.

Causes

There are several factor associated with causation of mental illness. However, there is no single accepted or consistent cause currently established. Some of the hypothesized theories are:

- **Genetic causes:** A most common opinion about the causes of mental illnesses is genetic vulnerabilities precipitated by environmental stressors. Genetic studies have indicated that genes often play an important role in the development of mental illness, via developmental pathways interacting with environmental factors. The reliable identification of connections between specific genes and specific categories of disorders has proven more difficult. However, researchers have uncovered more information about how genetics can determine the risk of schizophrenia and manic depression. Genes 'DISC1', and phosphodiesterase 4B (PDE4B) are found to be associated increased risk of mental illness.
- **Environmental causes:** Prenatal environment as well as postnatal environment found to be associated with increased risk of mental illness.
- **Biopsychosocial causes:** A number of biological, psychological and social factors are found behind the development of several mental illnesses. As biological factors; malfunctioning of selected neurotransmitters, such as serotonin, norepinephrine, dopamine and glutamate may cause mental illness.

Genetics of Depression

Each year an estimated 9.5% of American adults suffer from mood disorders. People suffering from depression experience symptoms of sadness, emptiness, or hopelessness that interfere with their lives. One of the questions scientists have been trying to answer is why some people become depressed in reaction to life stresses, while others do not.

One study sheds some light on this question. Researchers followed 847 New Zealanders over 5 years and charted their reaction to different life stressors. Stressors included things, such as loss of job, death of a loved one, broken relationships, or prolonged illness. What they found was that participants with a short version of a particular gene were more likely to become depressed than those who had the long version of the same gene. Specifically, 43% of people with the short form of the gene developed depression, in contrast to 17% of those with the long form. The findings suggest that some people, because of their genes are more vulnerable to depression when certain stressors activate the gene. Other researchers have found similar findings.

Genetics of Schizophrenia

The family link to schizophrenia is well established, but paring down the risk to one specific gene has proven difficult. For example, we each inherit two copies of the *COMT (catecho-O-methyltransferase)* gene, one from each parent. There are two *COMT* types possible: The *val* type (short for the amino acid valine) and the *met* type (short for the amino acid methionine). Research suggests that the *val* type may increase the susceptibility to schizophrenia by reducing dopamine activity.

One study tested the working memory of 181 schizophrenic patients, 219 of their well siblings and 75 controls. The researchers found that individuals who had two copies of the *val* type gene performed worse than those with only one copy, and those with the *met* type gene performed best of all. What this suggests is that the *val* type gene may increase an individual's susceptibility to schizophrenia.

Genetics of Bipolar Disorder

Bipolar disorder is a disease that causes extreme shifts of mood from depression to mania to a mixed state. While family and twin studies have shown that bipolar disease can be inherited, they have not yet pinpointed a particular gene. In fact, evidence suggests that bipolar disorder is affected by the presence and interaction of many genes.

In another study, researchers found that patients with bipolar disorder had a significantly higher frequency of the *COMT* and short *5-HTT* genes. Again, these findings suggest that genes may affect people's susceptibility to this condition.

Genetic Testing in Mental Illnesses

Despite the growing number of genetic tests available, there are no genetic tests for depression, schizophrenia or bipolar disorder. Genetic testing also causes concerns among many people, particularly in regards to privacy. Therefore, as new tests are developed, people who choose to be tested must weigh the benefits against the risks of finding out what their genes contain.

As exciting as these discoveries may be, researchers are quick to note that mental illness, such as other diseases, is an equation of sorts, with genetics being only one of the variables. For example, while genes may increase risk for a disease, other factors also play a role. These factors can be exposures to toxins, bacteria, and viruses during fetal development, as well as nutritional status, stress, emotional trauma, childhood development, environment and a history of other medical conditions.

Management

There is no gene therapy used to treat mental illness. Some of the traditional treatment modalities include:
- Cognitive behavioral therapy
- Psychoanalysis
- Systemic or family therapy
- Milieu therapy
- Psychoeducation
- Creative therapies
- Music therapy
- Art or drama therapy
- Psychiatric medications (antidepressants, anxiolytics, mood stabilizers, antipsychotics)
- Electroconvulsive therapy (ECT)
- Lifestyle adjustment and supportive therapy
- Dietary supplementations

THERAPEUTIC APPROACHES FOR GENETIC DISORDERS

Although prevention is the ideal goal for genetic disorders; genetic disorders can be detected early or prevented through preimplantation genetic testing, prenatal testing, newborn screening, effective required antenatal micronutrient supplementation, etc.

However, various types of therapeutic management approaches are available, such management approaches depends on the nature of defect, and how well it is understood or graded at the genetic and biochemical levels and the practical feasibility of correction. In some conditions, certain management approaches are now tailored to the specific genotype. The client being treated may be the fetus, the infant, the child or the adult. Treatment methods used in genetic disorders may involve surgical, cognitive/behavioral, pharmacological, dietary, environmental, avoidance, transfusion, plasma exchange, enzyme and cell or gene therapy. They are basically aimed at:
- Limiting the intake of a substrate or its precursor
- Depleting the accumulation or promoting the excretion of a substrate, precursor or product
- Directly or indirectly replacing or stimulating production of the enzyme, gene product
- Replacing, repairing or reprogramming the gene itself

For example, diet therapy may be based on the principle of limiting the amount of a specific substrate, which cannot be adequately metabolized by the appropriate enzyme, as in phenylketonuria, or it might be aimed at providing a product needed in order to circumvent a metabolic pathway, as in the provision of uridine in orotic aciduria. Gene product replacement might involve the administration of the product directly (e.g., insulin in type I diabetes mellitus) or indirectly by means of bone marrow transplantation (e.g., in severe combined immunodeficiency caused by adenosine deaminase deficiency). Toxic substances can be removed by chelation with drugs, plasmapheresis or surgical bypass procedures. The administration of pharmacological doses of vitamins, supplies the needed cofactor for holoenzyme function in certain vitamin responsive disorders.

Pharmacological approaches have taken advantages of underlying genetic mechanism in certain disorders; most notably in treating certain cardiac conditions and cancer. For example, it is known that for some disorders, multiple combinations of therapies are necessary. In Refsum disease (an autosomal recessive disorder with retinitis, pigmentation, ataxia, peripheral neuropathy and accumulation of phytonic acid), for example, both dietary restrictions of phytanic acid and plasmapheresis at weekly intervals are usual. Correction of birth defects, such as craniofacial anomalies or limb anomalies usually involve multiple phases of surgical treatment at various stages of the development of the individual, along with the use of prosthetic devices and long rehabilitation, such interventions require a skilled treatment group, that is prepared to deal not only with the physical correction by surgery, but with the nursing, psychological, speech, hearing and rehabilitative measures needed to achieve optimum results. Therapeutic approaches may range from a one time surgical correction of a birth defect to a long-term special diet, to an infant stimulation program to improve maximum potential, to experimental gene replacement. Some of the common therapeutic approaches for genetic disorders are as follows:
- **Promoting excretion of toxins:** The excretion of certain toxin metabolites can be promoted by chelating agents. For example, penicillamine promotes excretion of copper in patients with Wilson disease or desferrioxamine can be used to chelate iron in cases of thalassemia and hemochromatosis.
- **Reducing accumulation of toxins:** The intake of substance, which cannot be metabolized by the body, should be reduced, especially if their accumulation is potentially toxic. For example, in galactosemia, galactose cannot be metabolized adequately. As lactose in the milk is hydrolyzed in the body to glucose and galactose, milk in the diet of the affected infant is substituted by non-lactose-containing dietary formula to obviate damage due to

excess of galactose in tissue. The phenylketonuric infant is placed on the low protein diet to prevent irreversible neurological damage. Certain drugs, e.g., allopurinol inhibits xanthine oxidase and thus reduces the synthesis of uric acid and hence is useful in cases of gout.

- **Induction or stabilization of enzymes:** Certain enzyme systems, which may be immature or reduced at certain phases of life, may be induced or stabilized by the use of chemical agents, e.g., phenobarbitone is used for inducing the hepatic microsomal enzyme glucuronyl transferase, in cases of neonatal hyperbilirubinemia or Crigler-Najjar syndrome.
- **Administration of enzymes:** In a number of metabolic disorders, enzymatic block can be bypassed by administration of large quantities of the coenzyme. For example, pyridoxine in homocystinuria.
- **Avoiding drugs:** Certain drugs, which precipitate adverse symptoms in metabolic disorders, such as barbiturates in porphyria hepatica and oxidative agents in glucose-6 phosphate dehydrogenase deficiency, should never be administered in these patients.
- **Environmental protection:** Patients with hemophilia and osteogenesis imperfecta should be protected from trauma and other environmental hazards to prevent excessive bleeding and fractures respectively.
- **Surgery:** Surgery helps to reduce the structural, functional and cosmetic deformity in many of the congenital defects. For example, surgery is required for cleft lip and cleft palate or congenital heart defects.
- **Replacement therapy:** The deficiency of the metabolic end product may be made up by replacement or administration of the product. Thus, thyroxine restores the thyroid function in familial goiter erogenous cretinism, cortisone suppresses the adrenogenital syndrome and administration of factor VIII/IX prevents bleeding in cases of hemophilia. Enzyme replacement has been used in Gaucher's disease.
- **Gene therapy:** Gene therapy is the ultimate goal for genetic disorders. Though significant research has been done in this field, gene therapy has been effectively tried only for adenosine deaminase deficiency, familial hypercholesterolemia and some cancers. The aim is to introduce the normal gene in the affected individual. This is done by using viral or non-viral vectors for introducing normal functioning genes. The therapy can be in vivo (i.e., directly introduction in the body/tissue) or ex vivo (when cells with the normal functioning gene are grown outside and then introduced), which is the preferred mode. As the exact regulation of gene function of single gene disorder is very complex, so implementation of gene therapy is complicated.

NURSING MANAGEMENT IN GENETIC DISORDERS

Assessment

Family History

Blood relatives share the most similar genetic information and are thus at risk for acquiring characteristics or disease present in family members. Therefore, while dealing with a genetic case, the first step is recording the family history of the index case/proband. Proband is an affected person who has brought the family to the attention of a clinician. Proband is also called propositus, if male or proposita if female. The procedure starts with gathering information of the person's sociodemographic profile, information about disorder, age of onset, duration of complaints and any other major illness. The next step is to collect information regarding the

first-degree relatives, i.e., parents, siblings and offsprings of the proband. Following need to be collected in family history:
- Does any relative suffer from similar trait? This will help in deciding the pattern of inheritance and subsequently working out the recurrence risk of the disorder.
- Does any relative show any other disease, which is not present in, proband? For example, in case of dissecting aneurysm caused by Marfan's syndrome, ask about cardiac anomalies, ocular malformations or skeletal abnormalities in relatives.
- Ask for any condition with which any of the relatives suffered or is suffering. Or a condition that might have been unnoticed. For example, a propositus of pheochromocytoma can be suspected of having von Recklinghausen's disease, if patient's brother has scoliosis and mental retardation since both are manifestations of this disease.
- Is the proband an outcome of consanguineous marriage? Special attention should be given to this because consanguinity may lead to an autosomal recessive trait.
- What is the ethnic group of the family? This is important because certain traits are common in some ethnic groups. African blacks show hematological disorders, such as sickle cell anemia, β–thalassemia and conditions, such as glucose-6-phosphate dehydrogenase deficiency (G6PD) deficiency with much greater frequency.
- Some specific points need to be emphasized during family history, such as infant deaths, stillbirths and abortions to be noted with time of abortion, any obvious deformity in fetus or stillborn baby or in deceased infant, etc. This may significantly alter the risk to subsequent pregnancy.

Preparing and Analysis of Family Pedigree

Preparing and analysis of family pedigree depicts the family data. It is shortest method of providing relevant information and also the mode of transmission of the disorders in the family. Furthermore, preparing a family pedigree is useful in identifying classic inheritance patterns and potential conditions for referral. A family pedigree using standardized documentation symbols indicating familial relationships, gender, and living or dead status should be part of the patient's medical record. Notes from the interview relevant to particular family members can be added to the pedigree. A three generation display including the patient, parents, and grandparents is most useful in identifying patterns of inheritance. Pedigree symbols indicate whether the members are male or female, affected or unaffected by the disease of concern and living or dead; lines denote relationship to the patient. A pedigree should also include marginal notes regarding current health status or diseases, age of onset for serious conditions, age of death, cause of death, consanguinity, reproductive history, age of pregnant women and ethnicity. There are standardized symbols used in drawing up a pedigree. **Figure 19.4** shows symbols used in pedigree charting and **Table 19.8** presents aspects details about what should be included in pedigree.

Additional Areas of Assessment

Additional areas of assessment include:
- Environmental factors (exposure to teratogens, triggers, radiation and toxic substances)
- Lifestyle factors (substances use and abuse, prescription drug use and complementary therapies)
- Nutrition
- Psychosocial factors (emotional state, coping mechanisms, social support)
- Family system (cohesion, communication styles, resources) and family support system

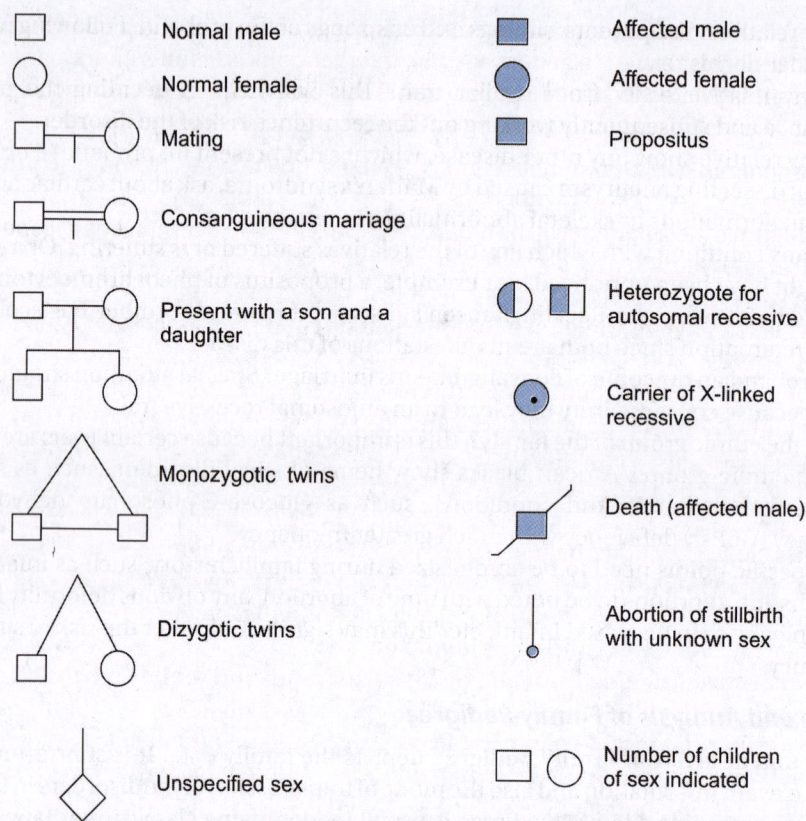

Fig. 19.4: Selected standardized symbols for use in drawing a pedigree.

Table 19.8: Specific facts and health information to be included in a pedigree.

• Age/birth date or years of birth	• Estimated date of delivery	• Relevant health information
• Age of death (year, if known)	• Infertility versus no children by choice	• Affected/unaffected status
• Cause of death	• Pregnancy complications with gestational age	• Ethical background
• Age at diagnosis	• Miscarriage	• Date pedigree taken or updated
• Full sibling versus half or stepsiblings	• Stillbirth	• Name of person who took pedigree
• Pregnancy with gestational age (LMP)	• Pregnancy termination (TOP)	• Key or legend

Nursing Diagnosis, Outcomes and Interventions

- Decisional conflict related to genetic testing or therapeutic interventions
- Anticipatory grieving related to genetic disorder diagnosis
- Anxiety related to genetic testing or therapeutic interventions
- Disturbed body image related to genetic defects
- Ineffective coping related to newly diagnosed genetic disorder
- Interrupted family process related to genetic disorder to family member(s)

CHAPTER 19: Genetic Conditions of Adolescents and Adults

- Ineffective health maintenance related to poor social support and genetic disorder
- Knowledge deficit related to genetic testing, interventions and inheritance pattern
- Powerlessness related to structural, functional and behavioral genetic defects
- Spiritual distress related to uncertainty of life secondary to genetic disorder.

1. **Nursing diagnosis:** Decisional conflict related to genetic testing or therapeutic interventions.
   Expected outcomes: Patient will be able to make an effective decision about genetic testing or medical interventions.
   Nursing interventions: As follows—
   - Provide relevant information about the genetic condition, associated genetic tests and interventions
   - Provide information about the alternatives of testing and not testing as a choice
   - Provide the information about consequences of having the genetic test and interventions or not having it
   - Provide specialized support
   - Recognize potential family resistance to pursuing genetic testing and interventions
   - Acknowledge the potential impact of information gathered from genetic tests on other family members
   - Acknowledge the risks of having genetic information after genetic tests as social, employment and insurance discrimination
   - Ensure active listening through paying a close attention to the verbal and nonverbal messages conveyed by the patient; clarify messages with follow-up questions
   - Provide for privacy and confidentiality during assessments and discussion
   - Provide information about alternatives and assist patient in identifying advantages and disadvantages of options
   - Facilitate discussions with other family members
   - Provide reassurance, acceptance and encouragement during the decision-making process; be nonjudgmental and convey empathy
   - Arrange for services of a genetic counselor if desired; contact provider

2. **Nursing diagnosis:** Anxiety related to genetic testing or therapeutic interventions.
   Expected outcomes: Patient will be able to have reduced anxiety state.
   Nursing interventions: As follows—
   - Assess for the level of anxiety and factors responsible for precipitating and reducing the anxiety
   - Encourage the patient to verbalize the feelings
   - Clarify patients' doubts in simple language carefully
   - Provide diversional therapy through family discussion, music, reading tools, etc.

3. **Nursing diagnosis:** Anticipatory grieving related to genetic disorder diagnosis.
   Expected outcomes: Patient will be able to pass through normal grieving process.
   Nursing interventions: As follows—
   - Assess the stage of grieving through which client is passing
   - Identify client's use of positive and negative defense mechanisms, boost positive defense mechanisms and discourage for negative mechanisms
   - Assess for support system available in family and community
   - Encourage the patient for ventilating the feeling loudly

- Listen the patient and family carefully and provide support as per need
- Provide crisis interventions as therapeutic tolls to manage crisis situation.

4. **Nursing diagnosis:** Disturbed body image related to genetic defects.
   Expected outcomes: Patient will come to terms with altered body image as evidenced by ability to verbalize feelings, participating in self care and reintegrate into activities of daily living as capable.
   Nursing interventions: As follows—
   - Note patient's ability to look at defect and reaction regarding same
   - Note frequency and tone of critical remarks directed toward self, regarding appearance and/or functions
   - Assess perceived impact of actual change on activities of daily living (ADL), social behavior, personal relationship and/or occupational activities
   - Listen and share presence
   - Acknowledge normalcy of emotional response to actual or perceived change in body structure or function
   - Assist the patient in identifying frightening or worrisome potential situations; role-play responses
   - Encourage attendance at support group.

5. **Nursing diagnosis:** Ineffective coping related to personal vulnerability, secondary to genetic disorders.
   Expected outcomes: Patient will be able to identify own maladaptive coping behavior, available resources/support system and alternative coping strategies.
   Nursing interventions: As follows—
   - Assess patient's ability to openly express feelings about disorder
   - Assess family and significant other's support system during disorder management
   - Set aside time to talk to patients when patient is comfortable to do so
   - Assist patient in understanding the chronicity of disorder(s) and the need to follow suggested testing and management instructions
   - Provide information on coping strategies
   - Establish a working relationship with patient through continuity of care
   - Involve social services, psychiatric liaison, and or pastoral care for additional and ongoing support resources
   - Inform patient and/or family about existing community resources.

6. **Nursing diagnosis:** Interrupted family process related to genetic disorder to family member.
   Expected outcomes: Family will identify resources available for problem solving.
   Nursing interventions: As follows—
   - Assess for precipitating events and family members perception about problem
   - Evaluate strengths, coping skills and current support system in their community
   - Provide opportunity to express concerns, fears, expectations and questions
   - Explore feelings, identify loneliness, anger, worry and fear
   - Encourage the family members to empathize with other family members
   - Assist family in setting realistic goals
   - Assist family in breaking down problems into manageable parts. Assist with problem-solving process, with delineated responsibilities and follow through

CHAPTER 19: Genetic Conditions of Adolescents and Adults

- Encourage family members to seek information and resources that increase coping skills
- Refer family to social services or counseling.

7. **Nursing diagnosis:** Ineffective health maintenance related to presence of physical disabilities and mental retardation secondary to genetic disorder.
   Expected outcomes: Patient/family will describe positive health maintenance behavior, such as keeping scheduled appointments, making diet and exercise changes, improve home environment and use available resources effectively.
   Nursing interventions: As follows—
   - Assess the patient's knowledge about health maintenance behavior
   - Determine patient's specific questions related to health maintenance
   - Assess for patient's economic, cultural and resources related barriers for positive health maintenance
   - Compliment patient on positive accomplishments
   - Ensure regular follow-up programs
   - Involve family and friends in health planning discussion, so that later they can ensure adherence with advices.

8. **Nursing diagnosis:** Knowledge deficit related to genetic testing, interventions and inheritance pattern.
   Expected outcomes: Patient/family will verbalize understanding of condition, testing procedure, treatment and inheritance pattern.
   Nursing interventions: As follows—
   - Assess understanding of genetic disorder(s) and usual expected genetic testing, management and their inheritance pattern
   - Teach about etiology, inheritance pattern, signs and symptoms, and also discuss about medical and nursing management
   - Teach importance of genetic testing, continuous medical care and follow-ups
   - Instruct about dietary modifications and things to be avoided.

9. **Nursing diagnosis:** Powerlessness related to structural, functional and behavioral genetic defects.
   Expected outcomes: Patient will have improved power as evidenced by patients accomplishment of self-care activities.
   Nursing interventions: As follows—
   - Promote self-care and self-awareness
   - Advise the client to avoid coffee, tobacco and alcohol any of which increase fatigue further
   - Promote adequate sleep each day; reduce amount of sleep cycle interruptions by preparing for sleep and keeping needed items at the bedside
   - Promote rest and activity by developing a written 24 hours schedule of daily activities that alternates short activities with rest periods
   - Identify activity priorities, such as eating breakfast and then resting before bathing in the morning, as opposed to the reverse
   - Evaluate the client needs and point out ways to conserve energy, such as sitting down, while dressing, shaving or preparing food, sitting on shower chair, while bathing

- Prepare an exercise schedule (immobilization may decrease endurance and increase fatigue) and plan exercise at peak of energy times (after a rest period). Follow exercise with rest.

10. **Nursing diagnosis:** Spiritual distress related to uncertainty of life secondary to genetic disorder.
    Expected outcomes: Patient/family will express hope in and value of his/her own belief system and inner resources.
    Nursing interventions: As follows—
    - Assess history of religious affiliation and desire for religious contact. Also assess cultural beliefs
    - Assess for hope and spiritual meaning of illness and treatment
    - Display an understanding and accepting attitude, encourage verbalization of feelings of anger or loneliness
    - Structure nursing interventions in terms of patient's belief system
    - Develop an ongoing relationship with patient and family
    - When requested by patient or family arrange for clergy, religious ritual or display of religious objects, especially when the patent is hospitalized
    - Acknowledge and support patient's hope
    - Do not provide logical solutions for spiritual dilemmas
    - Facilitate communication between patient and family, clergy and other caregivers.

MULTIPLE CHOICE QUESTIONS

1. **Acquired mutations are caused by:**
   a. Tobacco
   b. Overexposure to UV radiation
   c. Exposure to toxin and chemicals
   d. All of the above
2. **When the mutation passes from one of the parents to the child is termed as:**
   a. Chromosomal mutation
   b. Point mutation
   c. Germline mutation
   d. Frameshift mutation
3. **Name an autosomal dominant hereditary disorder, which occurs due to mutations of p53.**
   a. Turcot syndrome
   b. Li-Fraumeni syndrome
   c. Edward syndrome
   d. Patau syndrome
4. **Which of the following is an organic acid metabolism disorder?**
   a. Phenylketonuria
   b. Alkaptonuria
   c. Maple syrup urine disease
   d. Glycogen storage disease

Answer Key

1. d   2. c   3. b   4. b

FURTHER READING

1. Beauchamp TL, Childress JF. Principles of Biomedical Ethics. New York: Oxford University Press; 1994.
2. Billings PR, Kohn MA, de Cuevas M, et al. Discrimination as a consequence of genetic testing. Am J Hum Genet. 1992;50(3):476–82.
3. Borgna-Pignatti C, Vergine G, Lombardo T, et al. Hepatocellular carcinoma in the thalassemia syndromes. Br J Haematol. 2004;124(1):114–7.
4. Bove CM, Fry ST, MacDonald DJ. Presymptomatic and predisposition genetic testing: ethical and social considerations. Semin Oncol Nurs. 1997;13(2):135–40.

5. Burke W, Press N. McDonnel SM, et al. Hemochromatosis: Genetics helps to define a multifactorial disease. Clin Genet. 1998;54(1):1–9.
6. Cao A, Rosatelli C, Galanello R, et al. The prevention of thalassemia in Sardinia. Clin Genet. 1989;36(5):277–85.
7. Caspi A, Sugden K, Moffitt T, et al. Influence of life stress on depression: Moderation by a polymorphism in the 5-HTT gene. Science. 2003;301(5631):386–9.
8. Clarke GM, Higgins TN. Laboratory investigation of hemoglobinopathies and thalassemias: Review and update". Clin Chem. 46 (8 Pt 2):1284–90.
9. De Virgiliis S, Cossu P, Toccafondi C, et al. Effect of subcutaneous desferrioxamine on iron balance in young thalassemia major patients. Am J Pediatr Hematol Oncol. 1983;5(1):73–7.
10. Edwards CQ, Griffen LM, Goldgar D, et al. Prevalence of hemochromatosis among 11,065 presumably healthy blood donors. New Engl J Med. 1988;318(21):1355–62.
11. Egan MF, Goldberg TE, Kolachana BS, et al. Effect of COMT Val108/158 Met genotype on frontal lobe function and risk for schizophrenia. Pro Natl Acad Sci USA. 2001;98(12):6917–22.
12. Egan MF, Kojima M, Callicott JH, et al. The BDNF val66met polymorphism affects activity-dependent secretion of BDNF and human memory and hippocampal function. Cell. 2003;112(2):257–69.
13. Farmaki K, Angelopoulos N, Anagnostopoulos G, et al. Effect of enhanced iron chelation therapy on glucose metabolism in patients with beta-thalassaemia major. Br J Haematol. 2006;134(4):438–44.
14. Fucharoen S, Ketvichit P, Pootrakul P, et al. Clinical manifestation of beta-thalassemia/hemoglobin E disease. J Pediatr Hematol Oncol. 2000;22(6):552–7.
15. Gaba AM, Zhang K, Marder K, et al. Energy balance in early-stage Huntington disease. Am J Clin Nutr. 2005;81(6):1335–41.
16. Gill JC, Endres-Brooks J, Bauer PJ, et al. The effect of ABO blood group on the diagnosis of von Willebrand disease. Blood. 1987;69(6):1691–5.
17. Gladwin MT, Sachdev V, Jison ML, et al. Pulmonary hypertension as a risk factor for death in patients with sickle cell disease. N Engl J Med. 350(9):886–95.
18. Haldane JBS. The rate of mutation of human genes. In: Proceedings of the VIII International Congress on Genetics and Heredity. 1949; p. 267.
19. Hariri AR, Drabant EM, Munoz KE, et al. A susceptibility gene for affective disorders and the response of the human amygdala. Arch Gen Psychiatry. 2005;62(2):146–52.
20. Havens DM, Kovner R. Genetic testing: How it is transforming the role of health professionals and the implications for pediatric nurse practitioners? J of Pediatr Health Care. 1997;11(4):193–7.
21. Holtzman NA, Watson MS. Promoting safe and effective genetic testing in the United States: Final report of the task Force on genetic testing. [online]. Available http://www.nhgri.nih.gov/ELSI/TFGT_final. [Accessed September, 1997].
22. Imarisio S, Carmichael J, Korolchuk V, et al. Huntington's disease: From pathology and genetics to potential therapies. Biochem J. 2008;412(2):191–209.
23. James P, Notley C, Hegadorn C, et al. The mutational spectrum of type 1 von Willebrand disease: Results from a Canadian cohort study. Blood. 2007;109(1):145–54.
24. Jenkins J. Educational issues related to cancer genetics. Semin Oncol Nurs. 1997;13(2):141–4.
25. Johnson SA, Stout JC, Solomon AC, et al. Beyond disgust: Impaired recognition of negative emotions prior to diagnosis in Huntington's disease. Brain. 2007;130(Pt 7):1732–44.
26. Kieburtz K, MacDonald M, Shih C, et al. Trinucleotide repeat length and the progression of illness in Huntington's disease. J Med Genet. 1994;31(11):872–4.
27. Lippman-Hand A, Fraser FC. Genetic counseling: provision and reception of information. Am J Hum Genet. 1979;3(2):113–127.
28. Love RR, Evans AM, Josten DM. The accuracy of patient reports of a family history of cancer. J of Chronic Dis. 1985;38(4):289–93.
29. Lucarelli G, Galimberti M, Polchi P, et al. Marrow transplantation in patients with thalassemia responsive to iron chelation therapy. N Engl J Med. 1993;329(12):840–4.

30. MacDonald DJ. The oncology nurse's role in cancer risk assessment and counseling. Semin Oncol Nurs. 1997;13(2):123–8.
31. Matloff ET, Peshkin BN. Complexities in cancer genetic counseling: Breast and ovarian cancer. Principles and Practice of Oncology Updates. 1998;12:1–11.
32. McDonnell S, Preston BL, Jewell SA, et al. A survey of 2,851 patients with hemochromatosis: Symptoms and response to treatment. Am J Med. 1999;106(6):619–24.
33. Merikangas KR, Risch N. Will the genomics revolution revolutionize psychiatry? Am J Psychiatry. 2003;160(4):625–35.
34. Michie S, Bron F, Bobrow M, et al. Nondirectiveness in genetic counseling: An empirical study. Am J Hum Genet. 1997;60(1):40–7.
35. National Society of Genetic Counselors: Code of Ethics. 1992.
36. National Society of Genetic Counselors: Position Statements. 1991.
37. Offit K: Clinical Cancer Genetics: Risk Counseling and Management. New York: Wiley-Liss; 1998. p. 249.
38. Olivieri NF, Brittenham GM, Matsui D, et al. Iron-chelation therapy with oral deferipronein patients with thalassemia major. N Engl J Med. 1995;332(14):918–22.
39. Pearson H. 'Sickle cell anemia and severe infections due to encapsulated bacteria'. J Infect Dis. 136: S25–30.
40. Peters JA, Stopfer JE. Role of the genetic counselor in familial cancer. Oncology. 1996;10(2):159–75.
41. Platt OS, Brambilla DJ, Rosse WF, et al. Mortality in sickle cell disease. Life expectancy and risk factors for early death. N Engl J Med. 330(23):1639–44.
42. Points to consider: Ethical, legal, and psychosocial implications of genetic testing in children and adolescents. American Society of Human Genetics/American College of Medical Genetics. Am J Hum Genet. 1995;57(5):1223–41.
43. Powars DR, Elliott-Mills DD, Chan L, et al. Chronic renal failure in sickle cell disease: Risk factors, clinical course, and mortality. Ann Intern Med. 115(8):614–20.
44. Powell LW, George DK, McDonnell SM, et al. Diagnosis of hemochromatosis Ann Int Med. 1998;129(11):925–31.
45. Reilly PR, Boshar MF, Holzman SH. Ethical issues in genetic research: disclosure and informed consent. Nat Genet. 1997;15(1):16–20.
46. Rieger PT. Overview of cancer and genetics: Implications for nurse practitioners. Nurse Practit Forum. 1998;9(3):122–33.
47. Rothenberg K, Fuller B, Rothstein M, et al. Genetic information and the workplace: Legislative approaches and policy changes. Science. 1997;275(5307):1755–7.
48. Rothenberg KH. Genetic discrimination and health insurance: A call for legislative action. J Am Med Womens Assoc. 1997;52(1):43–4.
49. Rowland LP. Molecular basis of genetic heterogeneity: Role of the clinical neurologist. J Child Neurol. 1998;13(3):122–32.
50. Sadler JE. A revised classification of von Willebrand disease. For the Subcommittee on von Willebrand Factor of the Scientific and Standardization Committee of the International Society on Thrombosis and Haemostasis. Thromb Haemost. 1994;71(4):520–5.
51. Salonen JT, Tuomainen TP, Kontula K. Role of C282Y mutation in haemochromatosis gene in development of type 2 diabetes in healthy men: prospective cohort study. BMJ. 2000;320(7251):1706–7.
52. Sandyk R. L-tryptophan in neuropsychiatric disorders: A review. Int J Neurosci. 1992;67(1–4):127–44.
53. Savage R, Armstrong D. Effect of a general practitioner's consulting style on patients' satisfaction: A controlled study. BMJ. 1990;301(6758):968–70.
54. Scanlon C, Fibison W. Managing genetic information: Implications for nursing practice. Washington, DC, American Nurses Association; 1995.
55. Schneider KA. Counseling About Cancer: Strategies for Genetic Counselors. Dennisport, MA: Graphic Illusions; 1994.
56. Shiloh S, Saxe L. Perception of risk in genetic counseling. Psychological Health. 1989;3:45–61.
57. Thomas C. Preimplantation genetic diagnosis: Development and regulation. Med Law. 2006;25(2):365–78.

58. Van Duijn E, Kingma EM, van der Mast RC. 'Psychopathology in verified Huntington's disease gene carriers. J Neuropsychiatry Clin Neurosci. 2007;19(4):441–8.
59. Voskaridou E, Terpos E, Spina G, et al. Pamidronate is an effective treatment for osteoporosis in patients with beta-thalassaemia. Br J Haematol. 2003;123(4):730–7.
60. Walker AP. Historical perspective and philosophical perspective of genetic counseling. In: Emery AEH, Rimoin DL, Connor JM, et al (Eds): Principles and Practice of Medical Genetics, 3rd edition. New York: Churchill; Livingstone; 1996.
61. Walker FO. Huntington's disease. Lancet. 2007;369(9557):218–28.
62. Wertz DC, Fanos JH, Reilly PR. Genetic testing for children and adolescents. Who decides? JAMA. 1994;272(11):875–81.
63. Wong W, Powars D, Chan L, Hiti A, et al. Daily assessment of pain in adults with sickle cell disease. Ann Intern Med. 1992;148(2):94–101.

CHAPTER 20

Services Related to Genetics

Suresh Sharma, Mohd Salahuddin Ansari

INTRODUCTION

Genetic services provide genetic information, education and support to patient and families with genetic-related health concerns. Genetic professionals, including medical geneticists, genetic counselors, and advanced practice nurses in genetics provide specific genetic services to patient and families who are referred by their primary healthcare providers. A team approach is often used by genetic specialists to obtain and interpret complex family history information, evaluate and diagnose genetic conditions, interpret and discuss complicated genetic test results, support patients throughout the evaluation process and offer resources for additional professional and family support. Patient participates as team member and decision-maker throughout the process. Genetic services encompass an evaluation and communication process by which individuals and their families come to learn and understand relevant aspects of genetics, to make informed health decisions and to receive support, as they integrate personnel and family genetic information into daily living.

GENETIC TESTING

The task force on genetic testing defines a genetic test as *"the analysis of human DNA, RNA, chromosomes, protein and certain metabolites in order to detect heritable disease-related genotypes, mutations, phenotypes or karyotypes for clinical purpose"*. **Such purposes include predicting risk of disease, identifying carriers, establishing prenatal and clinical diagnosis or prognosis.**

Genetic testing identifies changes in chromosomes, genes or proteins. Most of the time, testing is used to find changes that are associated with inherited disorders. The results of a genetic test can confirm or rule out a suspected genetic condition or help determine a person's chance of developing or passing on a genetic disorder. Several hundred genetic tests are currently in use and more are being developed.

Genetic tests are performed on a sample of blood, hair, skin, amniotic fluid or other tissue. The sample is sent to a laboratory where technicians look for specific changes in chromosomes, DNA or proteins depending on the suspected disorder.

Some genetic tests are diagnostic, while others are predictive or inform individual of an increased risk of acquiring a disease or condition. A 'positive' genetic test may indicate that the asymptomatic individual will develop a genetic condition, but a prediction of the onset or severity of the condition cannot be made. A negative test result cannot guarantee the disease or its development in the future, often because environmental influence cannot be measured or controlled. Also, the genetic test may have only been able to detect the most common gene mutations and not all of the disease-producing gene alterations are available for inclusion in clinical testing. Clients may learn they will develop a genetic condition such as Huntington's disease for which there is no treatment. Client may find out through testing that they are a carrier and they have unknowingly passed the altered disease-producing gene on to their children.

Purposes of Genetic Testing

Genetic tests can provide information about a person's genes and chromosomes from conception throughout the life. Basically genetic testing may be used for clinical management, making personal decision or for assisting in reproductive choice. Some of the basic purposes of genetic testing is as following:
- Finding possible genetic diseases in unborn babies
- Finding out if people carry a gene for a disease and might pass it on to their children
- Screening embryos for disease
- Testing for genetic diseases in adults before they cause symptoms
- Confirming a diagnosis in a person who has disease symptoms.

Types of Genetic Testing

The nurses should understand that genetic testing can be classified into two categories, i.e., screening and diagnostic. A positive screening genetic test result notifies the client of an increased risk or probability, but must always be confirmed by diagnostic testing. Screening genetic tests are most commonly completed in prenatal, newborn and carrier circumstances. In contrast, a diagnostic test can definitively validate a genetic disorder in a symptomatic client and then direct clinical management.

Several categories of genetic tests included as subcategories of screening and diagnostic genetic tests are as follows (techniques used in these tests may be seen in **Table 20.1**):

Preimplantation Genetic Diagnosis
- The diagnosis involves the detection of disease-causing gene alteration in human embryo just after in vitro fertilization and before implantation in the uterus, thus providing an opportunity for preselection of unaffected embryo for implantation.
- This type of genetic testing is most often used by parents who are both carriers of a single gene recessive disorder and who wish to implant into the uterus only the embryo(s) without the disease causing alteration.
- PGD is usually very costly and is available at only a small number of centers and for only a small number of disorders.
- More recently, it has also been used to determine tissue type for donation of tissue such as bone marrow to a sibling or parent.

Prenatal Testing
- Prenatal testing is used to detect changes in a fetus's genes or chromosomes before birth.
- This type of testing is offered to couples with an increased risk of having a baby with a genetic or chromosomal disorder.
- In some cases, prenatal testing can lessen a couple's uncertainty or help them decide whether to abort the pregnancy. It cannot identify all possible inherited disorders and birth defects.

Table 20.1: Genetic test techniques.

Type of genetic tests	Description	Examples of genetic conditions
Molecular genetic tests		
Direct deoxyribonucleic acid (DNA) testing	Tests for presence of genes known to cause disease	Hemophilia Huntington's disease Polycystic kidney disease Familial adenomatous polyposis
Linkage testing	Tests for genetic material from several family members for presence of genetic markers believed to be located near affected gene	Huntington's disease Malignant hyperthermia susceptibility Neurofibromatosis Polycystic kidney disease
Methylation studies	Examine attachment of methyl groups to DNA molecule	Angelman syndrome Beckwith-Wiedemann syndrome Prader-Willi syndrome
Protein truncation test (PTT)	Tests for proteins that have been shortened and whose function has been altered	Rett syndrome Breast cancer Familial adenomatous polyposis
Uniparental disomy (UPD)	Tests for two chromosomes from same parent rather than one from each	Angelman syndrome Prader-Willi syndrome
X-linked inactivation studies	Tests for carrier status in women with some X-linked disorders	Fragile X syndrome Rett syndrome X-linked severe combined immunodeficiency
Cytogenetic test		
Fluorescence in situ hybridization (FISH)	Identifies presence or absence of chromosome segments using fluorescein-tagged DNA probes	Angelman syndrome Aniridia Williams syndrome
Chemical genetic tests		
Analyte testing	Assesses presence of substance in body indicative of genetic disorder	Homocystinuria
Enzyme assay	Measures the rate of chemical reaction of an enzyme in presence of a particular protein associated with genetic disorder; can identify affected individual or carrier	Gaucher's disease Lowe syndrome Galactosemia
Protein analysis	Tests for structure of proteins known to be associated with genetic disorders	Marfan's syndrome Spinocerebellar ataxia

Newborn Screening
- Newborn screening is carried out on large section of the newborn population and provides a means to identify infants who have an increased risk for developing a genetic disorder such as phenylketonuria, congenital hypothyroidism and sickle cell disease or maple syrup urine disease.

- It is used just after birth to identify genetic disorders that can be treated early in life to prevent disorders. For example, phenylketonuria with protein-free diet.

Predictive Genetic Testing

- Predictive types of testing are used to detect gene mutations associated with disorders that appear after birth, often later in life.
- This is usually made available to the asymptomatic individual and includes both predispositional and presymptomatic testing.
- A positive predispositional testing results will indicate there is an increased risk that the individual might eventually develop the disease. For example, an individual with a mutation in *BRCA1* has a 65% cumulative risk of breast cancer, similarly hereditary nonpolyposis colorectal cancer.
- Presymptomatic testing can determine whether a person will develop a genetic disorder, such as hemochromatosis and hypercholesterolemia, before any signs or symptoms appear.
- The results of predispositional and presymptomatic testing can provide information about a person's risk of developing a specific disorder and help when making decisions about medical care. In addition, life planning and lifestyle choice can be influenced by predictive testing.

Carrier Testing

- This test is completed on asymptomatic individuals who may be carrier of one copy of a gene alteration that can be transmitted to future children in an autosomal recessive or X-linked pattern of inheritance.
- This may be part of couple's premarriage or preconception planning, if they belong to a particular ethnic group with known incidence to genetic disorders such as sickle cell anemia and Tay-Sachs disease.
- It may be necessary to determine the exact gene mutation from affected family member prior to carrier testing.
- This is often completed through lineage analysis.

Diagnostic Testing

- Diagnostic testing is used to diagnose or rule out a specific genetic or chromosomal condition.
- In many cases, genetic testing is used to confirm a diagnosis when a particular condition is suspected based on physical mutations and symptoms.
- Diagnostic testing can be performed at any time during a person's life, but is not available for all genes or all genetic conditions.
- The results of a diagnostic test can influence a person's choices about health care and the management of the disease.

Forensic Testing

- Forensic testing uses DNA sequences to identify an individual for legal purposes.
- Unlike the tests described above, forensic testing is not used to detect gene mutations associated with disease. This type of testing can identify crime or catastrophe victims, rule out or implicate a crime suspect, or establish biological relationships between people, e.g., paternity.

Research Testing
- Research testing includes finding unknown genes, learning how genes work and advancing our understanding of genetic conditions.
- The results of testing done as part of a research study are usually not available to patients or their healthcare providers.

Other Genetic Testing

Other uses of genetic testing include organ transplantation tissue typing and pharmacogenetic testing, which involve predicting or studying the client's response to particular medication. For example, pharmacogenetic testing has shown that individuals who have Alzheimer's disease and carry two copies of a particular altered gene do not respond well to a drug frequently used in the treatment of Alzheimer's disease. However, if the individual only has one copy of the altered gene, the drug is effective in showing the progression of the disease.

Benefits of Genetic Testing

Provide for
- Early screening and preventive measures
- Future planning and life preparation
- Lifestyle adaptations
- Decreased confusion, uncertainty and anxiety
- Psychological stress relief
- Reproductive choice
- Informed extended family members
- Cost medical follow-up reduced (if negative result).

Negative Outcomes of Genetic Testing
- Emotional, social or financial consequences of the test results
- Angry, depressed, anxious or guilty about their results
- Tension within a family because the results can reveal information about other family members in addition to the person who is tested
- Genetic discrimination in employment or insurance
- Survivor guilt
- Loss of identity
- No treatment may exist
- Confusion about accessing health care and resources
- Risk for invasion of confidentiality and privacy
- Social stigmatization.

Interpreting Genetic Test Results

- The results of genetic tests are not always straightforward, which often makes them challenging to interpret and explain. When interpreting test results, healthcare professionals consider a person's medical history, family history and the type of genetic test that was done.

- A *positive test result* means that the laboratory found a change in a particular gene, chromosome or protein of interest. Depending on the purpose of the test, this result may confirm a diagnosis, indicate that a person is a carrier of a particular genetic mutation, identify an increased risk of developing a disease (such as cancer) in the future or suggest a need for further testing. Because family members have some genetic material in common, a positive test result may also have implications for certain blood relatives of the person undergoing testing. It is important to note that a positive result of a predictive or presymptomatic genetic test usually cannot establish the exact risk of developing a disorder. Also, health professionals typically cannot use a positive test result to predict the course or severity of a condition.
- A *negative test result* means that the laboratory did not find a dangerous copy of the gene, chromosome or protein under consideration. This result can indicate that a person is not affected by a particular disorder neither a carrier of a specific genetic mutation; nor have an increased risk of developing a certain disease. It is possible that the test missed a disease-causing genetic alteration because many tests cannot detect all genetic changes that can cause a particular disorder. Further testing may be required to confirm a negative result.
- In some cases, a negative result might not give any useful information. This type of result is called uninformative, indeterminate, inconclusive or ambiguous. Uninformative test results sometimes occur because everyone has common, natural variations in their DNA, called polymorphisms that do not affect health. If a genetic test finds a change in DNA that has not been associated with a disorder in other people, it can be difficult to tell whether it is a natural polymorphism or a disease-causing mutation. An uninformative result cannot confirm or rule out a specific diagnosis and it cannot indicate whether a person has an increased risk of developing a disorder. In some cases, testing other affected and unaffected family members can help clarify this type of result.

Ethical, Legal and Social Issues in Genetic Testing

Advances in technology have presented numerous ethical challenges and concerns. Humans exist within the same society; however, subcultures with their own values, beliefs and moral perspectives influence the individual's decision. Ethical questions raised by genetic testing, screening and analysis vary considerably depending on the specific condition identified. Numerous issues exist in the obstetric and neonatal areas. Confidentiality in screening and counseling has become a major concern with regard to potential employer and insurance discrimination. Informed decision-making is another issue that arises frequently. At what point is an individual truly informed? When does the family understand the risk/benefit considerations? How is autonomy in decision-making most enabled? Some people ask why test if there is no intent to abort, whereas other people contend that genetic information facilitates adequate preparation or that knowing is better than not knowing. There is also concern about efficient resource allocation, potential for suffering, arid the cost of maintaining life. Issues such as pro-choice and pro-life are raised frequently along with issues of quality of life versus sanctity of life.

Currently, genetic screening before implantation is possible with in vitro fertilization techniques using blastomere analysis. Such testing provides a couple with genetic information before transfer of the blastomere to the womb. The couple can make an informed decision whether to attempt pregnancy or stop at this point. Numerous legal and ethical issues have been raised regarding this practice. Who should pay for this service? Is this a form of legitimate diagnosis, prevention and possible treatment of disease? Is this a vehicle for phenotype selection? If the pregnancy is continued, are there grounds for a 'wrongful life' suit later if a genetic problem that should have been identified was not? Recently, the concept of 'meaningful life,' meaning dependent on individual perception and cultural beliefs, also has been introduced. Also raised are issues concerning who has rights, the mother, father, fetus, extended family or society?

Information from genetic testing can affect the lives of individuals and their families. In addition to personal and family issues, genetic disease or susceptibility may have implications for *employment* and **insurance**. Therefore, careful consideration in the *handling* of this information is very important. Critical issues include:

- **Privacy:** The rights of individuals to maintain privacy. Some genetic tests are required or strongly encouraged for developing fetuses and newborn babies. If an infant is found to be a carrier or likely to develop or be affected by an inherited disease, these findings may affect the future employability or insurability of the individual.
- **Informed consent:** Obtaining permission to do genetic testing. One must have knowledge of the risks, benefits, effectiveness and alternatives to testing in order to understand the implications of genetic testing.
- **Confidentiality:** Acknowledgment that genetic information is sensitive and access should to limited to those authorized to receive it. Future access to a person's genetic information also should be limited.

Role of Nurses in Genetic Testing

- With knowledge, available genetic tests and the many implications related to genetic testing, the nurses can assist client, as they weigh choice regarding genetic testing.
- Nurses should inform about following aspects when considering a client for genetic testing:
    - The reason that testing is appropriate for this person.
    - What is being tested for?
    - How much can be predicted about disorder without genetic testing.
    - What the procedure being considered entails, including description, cost, length of time, where it is to be done.
    - What can and cannot be tested, if relevant, this should include the information that while some mutations will be looked for and detected, other rare ones might not be and that negative results refer only to whatever was being tested or screened for and to every genetic disorder, for example, if one is testing for cystic fibrosis (CF), the most common mutations in that will be tested, but not every rare mutation will be tested for.
    - What would both positive and negative results mean, including that negative results do not necessarily translate to a zero risk that a positive tested may result in fear and anxiety, whereas negative results can also have emotional and relationship impact.
    - The accuracy, validity and relationship of the test, including the likelihood of false-negative or false-positive results and the suitability of this test for the information the client is seeking.
    - The possibility that testing will not yield additional risk information.
    - The length of time between the procedure and when results will be obtained.
    - How the result will be communicated to the client.
    - What will be analyzed?
    - What happens to the sample used for testing who owns it, what uses are possible?

- A discussion of the possible risk of life and health insurance coverage and/or employment discrimination after testing results are positive, although there may be benefit, such as if a person is free of a certain mutation, better insurance rates or coverage might result.
- The level of confidentiality of results and what this means (who can know or find out the results).
- Risk of psychological distress and negative impact not only on the individual but also on the family including stigmatization and altered self-image.
- Risk of passing on the mutation in the disorder being tested to children and the meaning of the risk.
- What discloser might the client consider for other family members.
- Provision for referral for periodic surveillance, further testing, lifestyle changes and/or treatment after testing, if needed.
- What these mean in the context of both positive and negative test results?
- The nurses are responsible for alerting clients of their rights to make an informed decision prior to any genetic testing with considering of the special circumstances arising from the family, culture and community life.
- All genetic testing should be voluntary and it is the nurse's responsibility to ensure that the consent process include discussion of the risk and benefit of the test, including any physical harm as well as potential psychological discrimination and emotional stress.
- Nurses need to ensure client's confidentiality and privacy of genetic testing.
- Nurses should address psychological, social and economic issues of person and family undergoing for genetic testing.

GENE THERAPY

In gene therapy, a 'correct copy' or 'wild type' gene is provided or inserted into the genome. Generally, it is not an exact replacement of the 'abnormal,' disease-causing gene, but rather extra, correct copies of genes are provided to complement the loss of function. A carrier called a 'vector' must be used to deliver the therapeutic gene to the patient's target cells. Currently, the most common type of vectors are viruses that have been genetically altered to carry normal human DNA. Viruses have evolved a way of encapsulating and delivering their genes to human cells in a pathogenic manner. Scientists have tried to harness this ability by manipulating the viral genome to remove disease-causing genes and insert therapeutic ones. Target cells such as the patient's liver or lung cells are infected with the vector. The vector then unloads its genetic material containing the therapeutic human gene into the target cell. The generation of a functional protein product from the therapeutic gene restores the target cell to a normal cell.

Gene therapy is the insertion of genes into an individual's cells and tissues to treat a disease, and hereditary diseases in which a defective mutant allele is replaced with a functional one. Although the technology is still in its infancy, it has been used with some success.

In other words gene therapy is the process of inserting genes into cells to treat disease. The newly introduced gene will encode proteins and correct the deficiency that occur in genetic diseases. Thus, gene therapy primarily involves genetic manipulation in animal or humans to correct a disease and keep the organism in good health.

Gene therapy is a technique for correcting defective genes responsible for disease development.

Researchers may use one of several approaches for correcting faulty genes:
- A normal gene may be inserted into a nonspecific location within the genome to replace a nonfunctional gene. This approach is most common.
- An abnormal gene could be swapped for a normal gene through homologous recombination.
- The abnormal gene could be repaired through selective reverse mutation, which returns the gene to its normal function.
- The regulation (the degree to which a gene is turned on or off) of a particular gene could be altered.

Although gene therapy is a promising treatment option for a number of diseases (including inherited disorders, some types of cancer and certain viral infections), the technique remains risky and is still under study to make sure that it will be safe and effective. Gene therapy is currently only being tested for the treatment of diseases that have no other cures.

Types of Gene Therapy

Basically gene therapy may be classified into the two types. **Figure 20.1** shows the steps of germline gene therapy and somatic gene therapy.
1. **Somatic gene therapy:** In the case of somatic gene therapy, therapeutic genes are transferred into the somatic cells of a patient. Any modifications and effects will be restricted to the individual patient only, and will not be inherited by the patient's offspring.
2. **Germline gene therapy:** In the case of germline gene therapy, germ cells, i.e., sperm or eggs, are modified by the introduction of functional genes, which are ordinarily integrated into their genomes. Therefore, the change due to therapy would be heritable and would be passed on to later generations. This new approach, theoretically, should be highly effective in counteracting genetic disorders. However, this option is prohibited for application in human beings, at least for the present, for a variety of technical and ethical reasons.

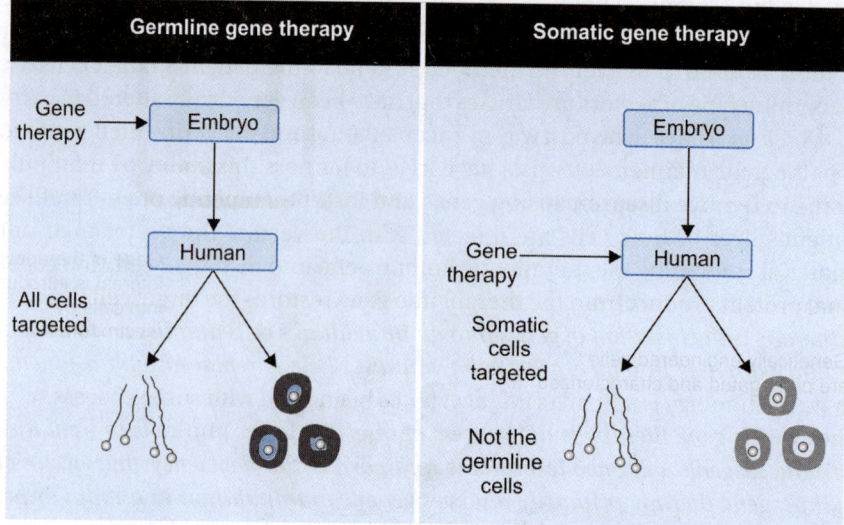

Fig. 20.1: Germline gene therapy versus somatic gene therapy.

Approaches of Gene Therapy

- **Ex vivo gene therapy:** This is accomplished by transfer of genes in cultured cells (e.g., bone marrow cells), which is then reintroduced into human body **(Fig. 20.2)**. In this approach, following steps are followed:
    - Cells with genetic defect are isolated from patients
    - These cells are cultured to grow in laboratory
    - Introduction of therapeutic gene to correct gene defect
    - Select the genetically corrected cells and grow them fully
    - Ultimately transplant the modified cells into the patients.
- **In vivo gene therapy:** In this approach of gene therapy, therapeutic gene is directly delivered into target cell of particular tissue of a patient. Generally, targeted tissues include liver, muscles, skin, spleen, lungs, brain and blood cells. Gene delivery can be carried out by viruses or non-viral vector system **(Fig. 20.3)**. The success of in vivo therapy depends on:
    - The efficiency of the uptake of the therapeutic gene by the target cells
    - Intracellular degradation of the gene and its uptake by nucleus
    - The expression capability of the gene.

A new gene is injected into an adenovirus vector, which is used to introduce the modified DNA into a human cell. If the treatment is successful, the new gene will make a functional protein.

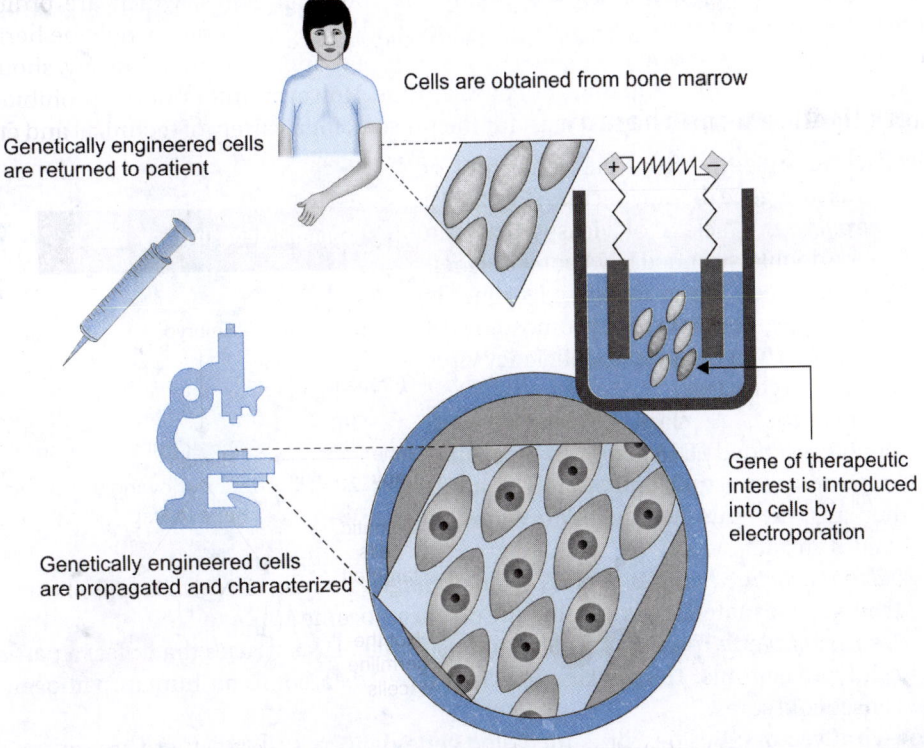

Fig. 20.2: Ex vivo gene therapy.

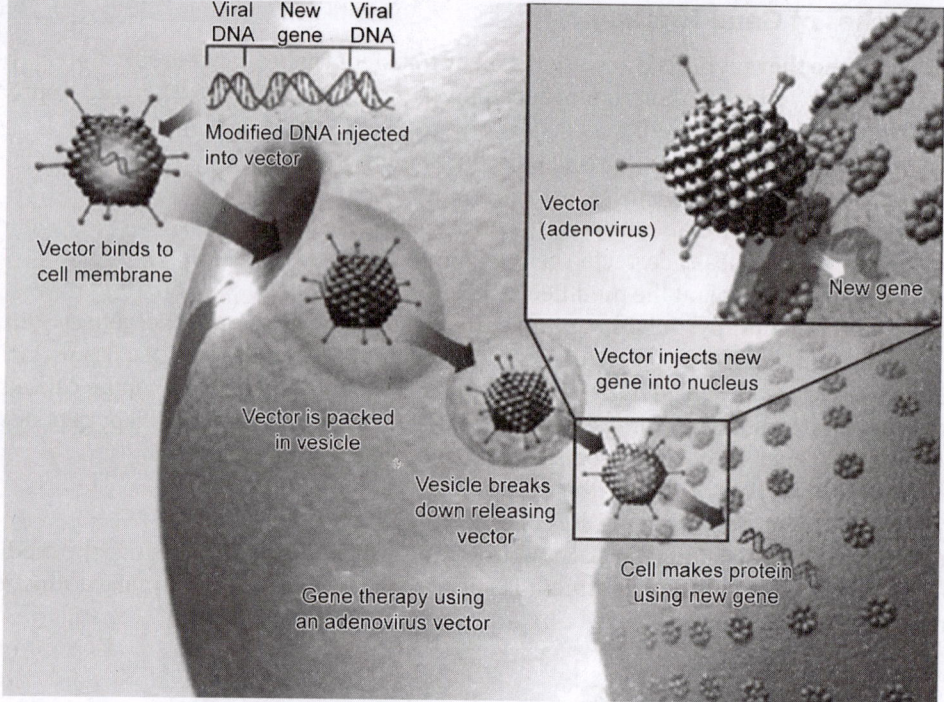

Fig. 20.3: In vivo gene therapy approach.

Vectors Used in Gene Therapy

- **Viral vectors**: Some of the different types of viruses used as gene therapy vectors (**Fig. 20.4**):
    - *Retroviruses*: A class of viruses that can create double-stranded DNA copies of their RNA genomes. These copies of its genome can be integrated into the chromosomes of host cells. Human immunodeficiency virus (HIV) is a retrovirus.
    - *Adenoviruses*: A class of viruses with double-stranded DNA genomes that cause respiratory, intestinal and eye infections in humans. The virus that causes the common cold is an adenovirus.
    - *Adeno-associated viruses*: A class of small, single-stranded DNA viruses that can insert their genetic material at a specific site on chromosome 19.
    - *Herpes simplex viruses*: A class of double-stranded DNA viruses that infect a particular cell type, neurons. Herpes simplex virus type 1 is a common human pathogen that causes cold sores.
- **Non-viral vectors**: Besides virus-mediated gene-delivery systems, there are several non-viral options for gene delivery:

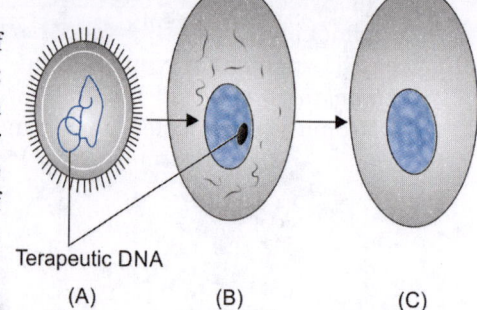

Fig. 20.4: Illustration showing use of vector in gene therapy.

- *Naked DNA:* The simplest method is the direct introduction of therapeutic DNA into target cells. This approach is limited in its application because it can be used only with certain tissues and requires large amounts of DNA. This success, however, does not compare to that of the other methods, leading to research into more efficient methods for delivery of the naked DNA such as electroporation, sonoporation and the use of a 'gene gun', which shoots DNA-coated gold particles into the cell using high pressure gas.
- *Human artificial chromosome:* It is synthetic chromosome (an artificial lipid sphere with an aqueous core) that can replicate with other chromosome besides encoding a human protein. This liposome, which carries the therapeutic DNA, can pass the DNA through the target cell's membrane. Since retroviruses as a vector in gene therapy are associated with enormous risks, these risks can be prevented with the use of human artificial chromosomes. However, this is still under research.
- *Bone marrow cells:* Bone marrow contains totipotent embryonic stem cells. These cells are capable of dividing and differentiating into various cell type (e.g., red blood cells, platelets, macrophages, osteoclasts, B- and T-lymphocytes). For this reason, bone marrow stem cells are used a vector in ex vivo gene therapy **(Fig. 20.5)**.
- *Oligonucleotides:* The use of synthetic oligonucleotides in gene therapy is to inactivate the genes involved in the disease process. There are several methods by which this is achieved. One strategy uses antisense specific to the target gene to disrupt the transcription of the faulty gene. Another uses small molecules of RNA called siRNA to signal the cell to cleave specific unique sequences in the mRNA transcript of the faulty gene, disrupting translation of the faulty mRNA, and therefore expression of the gene. A further strategy uses double-stranded oligodeoxynucleotides as a decoy for the transcription factors that are required to activate the transcription of the target gene. The transcription factors bind to the decoys instead of the promoter of the faulty gene, which reduces the transcription of the target gene, lowering the expression. Additionally, single-stranded DNA oligonucleotides have been used to direct a single base change within a mutant gene.
- *Lipoplexes and polyplexes:* To improve the delivery of the new DNA into the cell, the DNA must be protected from damage and its entry into the cell must be facilitated.

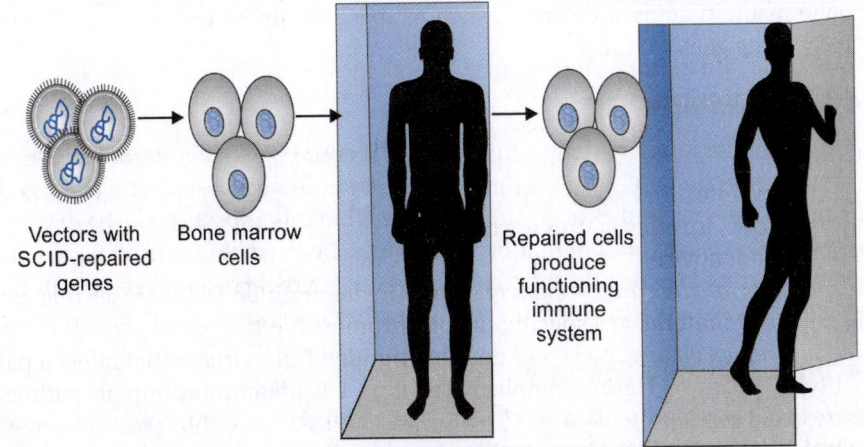

Fig. 20.5: Use of bone marrow cells as vector in gene therapy.

To this end, new molecules of lipoplexes and polyplexes have been created that have the ability to protect the DNA from undesirable degradation during the transfection process.

- **Hybrid methods**: Due to every method of gene transfer having shortcomings, there have been some hybrid methods developed that combine two or more techniques. Virosomes are one example; they combine liposomes with an inactivated HIV or influenza virus. This has been shown to have more efficient gene transfer in respiratory epithelial cells than either viral or liposomal methods alone. Other methods involve mixing other viral vectors with cationic lipids or hybridizing viruses.

Shortcomings of Gene Therapy

- **Short-lived nature of gene therapy:** Before gene therapy can become a permanent cure for any condition, the therapeutic DNA introduced into target cells must remain functional and the cells containing the therapeutic DNA must be long-lived and stable. Problems with integrating therapeutic DNA into the genome and the rapidly dividing nature of many cells prevent gene therapy from achieving any long-term benefits. Patients will have to undergo multiple rounds of gene therapy.
- **Immune response:** Anytime, if a foreign object is introduced into human tissues, the immune system is designed to attack the invader. The risk of stimulating the immune system in a way reduces gene therapy effectiveness, which is always a potential risk. Furthermore, the immune system's enhanced response to invaders, it has seen before makes it difficult for gene therapy to be repeated in patients.
- **Problems with viral vectors:** Viruses, while the carrier of choice in most gene therapy studies, present a variety of potential problems to the patient like toxicity, immune and inflammatory responses, and gene control and targeting issues. In addition, there is always the fear that the viral vector, once inside the patient, may recover its ability to cause disease.
- **Multigene disorders:** Conditions or disorders that arise from mutations in a single gene are the best candidates for gene therapy. Unfortunately, some of the most commonly occurring disorders, such as heart disease, high blood pressure, Alzheimer's disease, arthritis and diabetes, are caused by the combined effects of variations in many genes. Multigene or multifactorial disorders such as these would be especially difficult to treat effectively using gene therapy.

Facts of Gene Therapy

Gene therapy is under study to determine whether it could be used to treat disease. Current research is evaluating the safety of gene therapy; future studies will test whether it is an effective treatment option. Several studies have already shown that this approach can have very serious health risks such as toxicity, inflammation and cancer. Because the techniques are relatively new, some of the risks may be unpredictable; however, medical researchers, institutions and regulatory agencies are working to ensure that gene therapy research is as safe as possible.

Pharmacological Gene Therapy

Pharmacological gene therapy is a new field that combines pharmacological therapy and gene therapy. It is used either to prevent a defective gene from producing its protein or to increase the concentration of normal protein produced in the body by insertion of DNA or

RNA fragments. It can also be to generate immunity from contagious disease such as TB, via the process of DNA vaccination.

Gene therapeutics can be used to treat such conditions as cystic fibrosis (via the addition of a normal *CFTR* gene), hemophilia A or even some of the complications of AIDS. It uses a number of methods including *gene augmentation, targeted inhibition* (using antisense or antigen technology), *cell killing* (either direct or assisted) and *DNA vaccination*.

Ethical Issues Regarding Gene Therapy

Because gene therapy involves making changes to the body's set of basic instructions, it raises many unique ethical concerns. The ethical questions surrounding gene therapy include:
- How can 'good' and 'bad' uses of gene therapy be distinguished?
- Who decides which traits are normal and which constitute a disability or disorder?
- Will the high costs of gene therapy make it available only to the wealthy?
- Could the widespread use of gene therapy make society less accepting of people who are different?
- Should people be allowed to use gene therapy to enhance basic human traits such as height, intelligence or athletic ability?

Current gene therapy research has focused on treating individuals by targeting the therapy to body cells such as bone marrow or blood cells. This type of gene therapy cannot be passed on to a person's children. Gene therapy could be targeted to egg and sperm cells (germ cells), however, which would allow the inserted gene to be passed on to future generations. This approach is known as germline gene therapy. The idea of *germline gene therapy* is controversial. While it could spare future generations in a family from having a particular genetic disorder, it might affect the development of a fetus in unexpected ways or have long-term side effects that are not yet known. Because people who would be affected by germline gene therapy are not yet born, they cannot choose whether to have the treatment. Because of these ethical concerns, the governments of different countries does not allow research units to be used for research on germline gene therapy in people.

Role of Nurses in Gene Therapy

Gene therapy is one of the complex medical procedures in which the nurses have following responsibilities represented in **Figure 20.6**:
- Assess the patient's family, health and other related history
- Collect all the relevant genetic testing records

History/data collection	Support	Regular monitoring/ and follow-up	Coordination/record keeping
• Family history, relevant genetic testing records • Collect other related health history	• Psychological support, clarification of information, provide relevant information regarding gene therapy • Provide supportive services	• Monitor for any adverse effects of therapy • Regular evaluation and follow up	• Coordinate between individual and genetic specialist, assist in implementation of gene therapy • Maintain patients records related to therapy

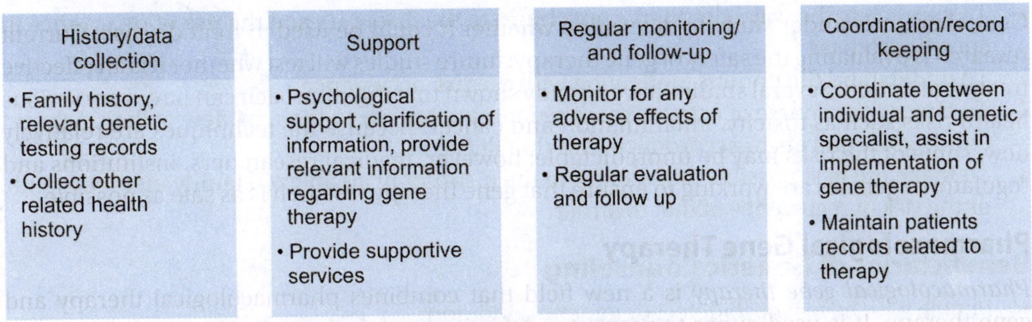

Fig. 20.6: Role of nurses in gene therapy.

- Provide psychological support during gene therapy procedure
- Ensure that all the physical needs of individual are fulfilled
- Provide relevant information regarding gene therapy to individual and family
- Coordinate between the individual and genetic specialist
- Assist the genetic specialist in implementation of gene therapy procedure
- Regularly monitor individual for any adverse effect of the gene therapy
- Provide information and supportive services for individual and family
- Maintain all the records of patient related to gene therapy
- Provide regular evaluation and follow-up care.

GENETIC COUNSELING

In response to increasing knowledge of the role of genetics in health and disease, Reed proposed the term 'genetic counseling' in 1947, although giving of genetic advice and the transmission of certain traits were not new ideas.

"*Genetic counseling is a communication process, which deals with the human problems associated with the occurrence or the risk of occurrence of a genetic disorders in a family.*"

In other words, "*genetic counseling is the process by which patients or relatives, at risk of an inherited disorder, are advised of the consequences and nature of the disorder, the probability of developing or transmitting it, and the options open to them in management and family planning in order to prevent, avoid or ameliorate it. This complex process can be seen from diagnostic (the actual estimation of risk) and supportive aspects*".

Genetic counseling is offered to people with genetic or inherited diseases and their families and to individuals (often children with birth defects or developmental delays) who are suspected of having a genetic condition. These services help families and their healthcare providers make informed decisions about their health care. In some cases, families use the information they get in a genetic evaluation to help them make reproductive decisions.

Purpose of Genetic Counseling

Genetic counselors provide supportive counseling to families, serve as patient advocates and refer individuals and families to community or state support services. Counseling process involves an attempt by one or more appropriately trained person to help the individual or family:

- To comprehend the medical facts, including diagnosis, the probable course of the disorder and the available management
- To appreciate the way hereditary contributes to the disorders and the risk of recurrence in specific relatives
- To understand the options for dealing with the risk occurrence
- To choose the course of action, which seems appropriate to them in view of their risk and family goals and act in accordance with that decision
- To make the best possible adjustment to the disorder in an affected family members and/or the risk of recurrence of that disorder.

Beneficiaries of Genetic Counseling

- People who have a birth defect or genetic condition
- Parents who have had a child with a birth defect or genetic condition

- Parents who have a child with developmental delay, mental retardation or other problems with growth and development
- Women who have had three or more miscarriages or infertility from an unknown cause
- Pregnant women or couples considering having children in which:
  - The mother will be 35 years or older at the time of delivery
  - The couple are blood relatives (second cousins or closer)
  - Testing during the pregnancy indicated that the baby may have a birth defect or genetic condition
  - There is a family history of birth defects, mental retardation or genetic disease.
- People concerned may have inherited a tendency to develop cancer
- People concerned may have inherited a tendency to develop a neurologic condition such as Huntington disease (Huntington's chorea)
- A person whose doctor or healthcare provider has recommended a genetic evaluation or genetic testing.

Phases of Genetic Counseling

Genetic counseling generally involves five phases **(Fig. 20.7)**.

1. **Assessment phase:** This is primary beginning phase of counseling in which following tasks are accomplished:
   - Initial interview with counselee and family for preparation of counselee for genetic counseling
   - Collect family history, and other relevant histories; prepare and analyze pedigree
   - Carry out primary assessment of counselee, i.e., physical examination, etc.
   - Considering potential diagnosis based on collected information.
2. **Diagnostic phase:** In some cases, the goal of a genetic evaluation is to make a diagnosis of a particular genetic condition or syndrome. This is commonly the case when a child is born with multiple birth defects or problems with growth and development. In other cases, the diagnosis already is known, and the genetic counselor or geneticist probably will confirm the established diagnosis to proceed for next phases of the counseling. Therefore, this phase include following steps:
   - Confirmatory or supplementing tests or procedure such as:
     - Chromosomal analysis
     - Biochemical tests
     - Molecular DNA testing
     - X-rays, biopsy
     - Linkage analysis
     - Developing testing

Assessment phase

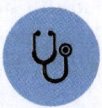
Diagnostic phase

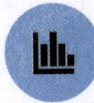
Analysis phase

Communication phase

Referral and support phase

Fig. 20.7: Phases of genetic counseling.

- Dermatography
- Prenatal diagnosis
- Immunological tests, etc.
- Establishment of an accurate diagnosis.
3. **Analysis phase:** This phase includes following tasks:
   - Literature search and review of information
   - Consultation with other experts.
   - Compiling of information and determination of recurrence risk.
4. **Communication phase:** This phase includes:
   - Communication of the results and risk to the counselee and to the family, if appropriate
   - Discussion of natural history of disorder, current treatment options and anticipatory guidance, if relevant
   - Discussion of options and review of questions
   - Assess the counselee's understanding about facts and relevant hereditary pattern, diagnostic and management options for disorder
   - All explanation should be culturally appropriate for counselee and appropriate for their education.
5. **Referral and support phase:** In this phase, counselor offers following services:
   - Refer the individual to genetic specialist for further interventions, for example, referral for prenatal diagnosis or treatment modalities for different disorders
   - Support of decision made by counselee
   - Psychological support should be provided throughout the process
   - Follow-up and evaluation.

Role of Nurses in Genetic Counseling

Nurses work as members of a healthcare team and act as a patient advocate as well as a genetic resource to physicians. Genetic nurses are present at high risk or specialty prenatal clinics that offer prenatal diagnosis, pediatric care centers and adult genetic centers. Genetic counseling can occur before conception (i.e., when one or two of the parents are carriers of a certain trait) to adulthood (for adult onset genetic conditions such as Huntington's disease or hereditary cancer syndromes). Following are the main roles that a general genetic nurse have to accomplish during genetic counseling:

- Receive the client and family, and make them comfortable in assessment room for genetic counseling
- Obtain prenatal, family and other health histories from individual and family
- Conduct a primary physical examination and collect other relevant information
- Identify families at risk, investigate the problems present in the family, interpret information about the disorder, analyze inheritance patterns and risks of recurrence and review available testing options with the family
- Prepare and analyze a pedigree, to establish information about hereditary pattern
- Provide psychological support to individual and family throughout the counseling
- Collect other related information from individual and family, for example, any prior test report or documents
- Obtain an informed written consent for any planned genetic test or intervention
- Encourage the individual and family to ask question as much as they can understand about all aspects of disorder, about genetic testing, management, inheritance pattern and natural course of disorder

- Provide all explanation about all the questions related to genetic testing, treatment modalities and inheritance pattern of disorder, which should be culturally appropriate for counselee and appropriate for their educational level
- Genetic nurses provide information and support to families who have members with birth defects or genetic disorders, and to families who may be at risk for a variety of inherited conditions
- Establish a plan of care with the family and coordinate care with other healthcare professionals
- Maintain privacy and confidentiality of all the information related to individual and family only disclose the information as per individual's wish and permission
- Provide the referral guidance to individual for genetic specialist for further interventions
- Coordinate for available community resources to help individual and family to provide available help
- Be available for the individual and family for any genetic services through the course of disorder
- Ensure follow-up and supportive services to individual and family during entire course of need.

MULTIPLE CHOICE QUESTIONS

1. Which of the following is the benefit for gene testing?
    a. Early screening
    b. Future planning
    c. Lifestyle adaptation
    d. All of the above
2. Name the test for presence of genes known to cause disease.
    a. Linkage testing
    b. Direct DNA testing
    c. Methylation studies
    d. PTT
3. Which is NOT a negative outcome of genetic testing?
    a. Loss of identity
    b. Genetic discrimination
    c. Early screening
    d. Social stigmatization

Answer Key

1. d
2. b
3. c

FURTHER READING

1. Allingham-Hawkins D. Successful genetic tests are predicated on clinical utility. Genetic Engineering and Biotechnology News. 2008;28(14):6.
2. Harmon A. Insurance Fears Lead Many to Shun DNA Tests. The New York Times; 2008.
3. ANA. Comments on the HIPAA Regulations Submitted to the Department of Health and Human Services (February 17, 2000). http://www.nursingworld.org/gova/federal/agencie/dhhs/dhanacmt.htm
4. ANA. State Legislative Tracking of Telehealth Legislation. Washington DC, ANA; 1998, 1999, 2000.
5. Andrews LB, Fullarton JE, Holtzman NA, et al. Assessing Genetic Risks: Implications for Health and Society (TOM Report). Washington DC: National Academy Press; 1994.
6. Begley S. Decoding the Human Body. Newsweek; 2000.
7. Bowles BB, Marteau TM. The future of genetic counseling: An international perspective. Nat Genetics. 1999;22(2):133-7.
8. Colby JA. An analysis of genetic discrimination legislation proposed by the 105th congress. American Journal of Law and Medicine. 1998;24(4):443-80.

9. Cooper RA, Henderson T, Dietrich CL. Roles of nonphysician providers as autonomous providers of patient care. JAMA. 1998;280(9):795-802.
10. Cooper RA, Laud P, Dietrich CL. Current and projected workforce of nonphysician clinicians. JAMA. 1998;280(9): 788-94.
11. Fuetz-Harter SA. Nursing and the Law. Eau Claire, Wisconsin, Professional Education Systems, MC; 1993.
12. Hallowell C. Playing the odds: health insurers want to know what's in your DNA. Time. 1999;153(1):60.
13. Holtzman NA, Murphy PD, Watson MS, Barr PA. Predictive genetic testing: from basic research to clinical practice. Science. 1997;278(5338):602–5.
14. https://web.ornl.gov/sci/techresources/Human_Genome/project/5yrplan/5yrplanrev.shtml
15. https://web.ornl.gov/sci/techresources/Human_Genome/research/elsi.shtml
16. Brandon K. Genetic Discrimination by Insurers, Employers Becomes a Crime, Wired.com. Retrieved on 28 May 2008.
17. Kotval JS. Market-driven managed care and the confidentiality of genetic tests: The institution as double agent. Albany Law Journal of Science and Technology;1998.
18. Mehlman MJ. How will we regulate genetic enhancement? Wake Forest Law Review. 1999;34(3):671-714.
19. Roth RL, Jarquin JB, Palmer AJ. Confidentiality issues affecting practitioners in telemedicine: what someone else does not know could hurt you. In: Gosfield AG (Ed): Health Law Handbook. Saint. Paul MN, West Group; 1999.
20. Scanlon C. The legal implications of genetic testing. RN. 1998;61(3):61-5.
21. Schneider KA. Counseling about cancer: Strategies for Genetic Counselors. Massachusetts: Graphic Illusions; 1994.
22. Serbaroli FJ. Telemedicine and the internet. New York Law Journal: 1999.
23. Swindler RN, Rothstein MA. Discrimination based on genetic information. Jurimetrics. 1992;33(1):13-8.
24. Wakitsch DJ. New York's legal restrictions on the employer's collection and use of an employee's genetic information. Albany Law Journal of Science and Technology. 1998;39:102.
25. Waller AA. Computers and Health Care Integration: Mapping the New Legal. Landscape. In Gosfield AG (Ed). Health Law Handbook. Deerfield, Illinois, Clark Boardman Callaghan; 1996.
26. Waller AA. Preparing for the complexities of administrative simplification under HIPAA. In: Gosfield AG (Ed). Health Law Handbook. Saint Paul: MN West Group; 1999.

Index

Page numbers followed by *b* refer to box, *f* refer to figure, and *t* refer to table

A

ABO blood group system 349, 349*t*
  alleles of 461*t*
Abortion 417
  clinical spontaneous 418
  complete 418
  early pregnancy 138
  incomplete 418
  inevitable 418
  missed 418
  septic 418
  spontaneous 241, 375, 394, 417
Abscess, perinephric 217
Acetazolamide 18, 29, 30, 107
Acetic acid derivatives 37
Acetyl salicylic acid 33
Achondroplasia 337, 383
Acid 164
  phosphatase test 281
Acidifiers 26
Acidosis 31
  metabolic 27, 28, 152
Acid-Schiff stain 213
Acne 124, 245
Acquired immunodeficiency syndrome infection 373
Acrivastine 4
Acrodysostosis 383
Actinomycin D 175
Acupuncture 417
Acute pyelonephritis 216, 218*f*
  etiopathogenesis of 217*f*
Acyclovir 24
Addison's disease 46
Adenine 355*f*, 356*f*, 358*f*, 359, 359*f*
Adenocarcinoma 223, 235, 238, 239
Adenoid cystic carcinoma 254
Adenoma
  cortical 223
  oncocytoma 223
Adenosine 153
Adenoviruses 506
Adrenal cortex 452
Adrenal disease 411
Adrenal gland hyperactivity 27
Adrenaline 95, 153
Adrenergic antagonist 131

Adult polycystic kidney disease 337, 414
Adverse drug reaction 83, 85, 201*t*
Agoraphobia 80
Agranulocytosis 66, 67, 77
  leukopenia 66
Akathisia 67, 77
Albright osteodystrophy 342
Albumin 155
Albuminuria 73
Alcohol 391, 392, 478
  consumption 252
  intoxication, acute 158
  withdrawal symptoms 82, 89
Aldostrone antagonist 16
Aliphatic carboxylic acid 87
Alkalinize urine 152
Alkalosis
  metabolic 26, 27
  systemic 29
Alkaptonuria 454
Alleles 461
  homozygous 295
Allergenic foods 379
Allergic effects 77
Allergy 17
Allylestrenol 118
Alpha-fetoprotein 401, 424
Alpha-thalassemia 465
Alport's syndrome 216
Alprazolam 54, 84
Alter taste 9
Alzheimer's disease 124
Amantadine 94
Ambisome 24
Amenorrhea 66, 227, 245
American Academy of Pediatrics 378, 379
American College of Medical Genetics 437
Amikacin 24
Amiloride 16, 17
Amino acid 328*f*
  metabolism, disorders of 454
  synthesis 325
Aminoglycosides 387
Aminopeptidase 276
Aminopterin 387

Amitriptyline 75
Ammonium chloride 26, 27
Amnesia 262
Amniocentesis 400, 400*f*, 425
  analysis of 401
  complications of 402
  early 402
  indications for 401
  mid trimester 402
  procedure of 401
  risks of 402
Amnionitis 402
Amniotic fluid
  diagnostic testing of 402
  leakage 402
Amoxapine 80
Amphetamine 103
  mechanism of action of 103*f*
Amphotericin B 24
Amyloid angiopathy 261
Amylolytic amylase 276
Analgesia
  obstetrical 44
  stage of 43
Analgesic 33, 38
Anaphylactic shock 96, 152
  treatment of 96
Anaphylaxis 150, 152
Androgens 386
Anemia 66, 105, 136, 225, 241, 373, 455, 460, 464
  hemolytic 462
  megaloblastic 88
Anencephaly 421, 422, 422*f*
Anesthesia 42, 44, 98
  classification of 42, 42*f*
  epidural 49
  induction 44
  infiltration 48
  intravenous regional 49
  local 47*f*
  spinal 48
  surface 48
  surgical 43
Aneuploidy 333*t*
Angelman syndrome 498
Angina 150, 152
  acute episodes of 151
  pectoris 151

Anginal attacks 105
Angiokeratoma, diffuse 345
Angiomyolipoma 224
    medullary interstitial tumor 223
Angiotensin-converting enzyme
    inhibitors 12, 73, 386, 387
Anion gap 28
Aniridia 337, 498
Annulus, calcification of 259
Anorexia 25, 104, 226
Anorexiant 103, 103f, 104
Antacid 152
Antiandrogens 231
Antianxiety drugs 81, 81t
Antibiotics 175
Antibody reagents 180
Anticancer drugs 171, 387
    classification of 171
Anticholinergic
    central 94
    effects 77
Anticoagulants 387
Anticonvulsants 71, 74, 86, 387, 392
    drugs, classification of 86t
Antidepressants 387, 484
    atypical 76, 80
    classification of 75, 75t
    mechanism of action of 75f
Antidiuretic hormone 12, 20
    doses of 20t
Antidote 39, 40
Antiepileptics 52
Antiestrogens 116
Antihistamines 3, 82
Anti-hypertensive 151, 387
Antimetabolites 173, 387
Antineoplastics 386
Antiparkinsonian drugs 92
    classification of 92f
Antiprogestins 119
Antiproliferative drugs 179
Antipsychotics 63, 71, 484
    atypical 65
    drugs
        classification of 64f
        doses of 66t
        side effects of 67t
Antipyretics 38
Antirabies serum 170
Antiseptic 108
    urinary 24
Antisnake venom polyvalent 170
Anti-tetanus serum 170
Antithyroid 387
Anuria 14, 17
Anxiety 79, 81, 83, 105, 151, 261
    endogenous 81
    exogenous 81
    generalized 77, 78, 80, 82

moderate 83
preoperative 82
severe 83
Aortic aneurysm rupture 277
Aortic valve disease 259
Apert syndrome 383
Aphasia 261, 262
Apnea 59
Apoptosis 315f
Appendicitis 277
Appetite 66
    loss of 77
Armanni-Ebstein lesions 216
Arrhythmias 59, 77, 98, 100, 104, 105, 108, 259
    cardiac 89, 167, 278
    ventricular 96, 99, 100
Arteriosclerosis 104, 231
    cerebral 68
Artery, splenic 277
Artificial insemination 127, 415
Artificial reproductive technique 417
Ascaris lumbricoides 274
Ascorbic acid 26, 27
    dose of 28, 28t
Aspergillus flavus 161
Aspiration 50
Aspirin 33, 152
Assisted reproductive technique management 415
Asthenospermia 281
Asthma 40, 150, 152
    acute bronchial 107
Astrocytoma 265
Asystole 150
Ataxia 22, 77, 258, 262, 267
    cerebellar 412
Atherosclerosis 231, 260
    risk of 21
Atosiban 131
Atracurium 56
Atrial fibrillation 259
Atrial septal
    aneurysm 259
    defects 428
Atrioventricular canal defects 428
Atrophic vaginitis 123
Atrophy
    testicular 231, 231f
    urogenital 123
Atropine 150, 153
    poisoning 157
Atypical antidepressants 76, 80
    mechanism of action of 80f
Autosomal dominant 336
    inheritance 337t, 351
Autosomal recessive 336, 338
    inheritance 340t, 351

Ayurveda 183
    drugs for 185
Azapirones 82
Azathioprine 179
Azoospermia 281
    factor 411
    gene 413
Azosemide 12

B

Bacille Calmette-Guerin 168
Backache 124
Baclofen 56, 62
Bacteria 285
Bacteriuria 25, 217
Bamford classification 261
Barbiturates 52, 86, 157
    mechanism of action of 52, 53f
Bardet-Biedl syndrome 412
Barium enema 249
Basal cell nevus syndrome 383
Battelle developmental inventory screening test 444
Bayley infant neurodevelopmental screener 444
Beckwith-Wiedemann syndrome 498
Behavior
    abnormal 455
    problems 428
    therapy, cognitive 484
    warning signs 443
Bendroflumethiazide 15
Benzodiazepines 15, 45, 53, 54, 81, 82, 151
    antagonist 54
    mechanism of action of 83f
Beta-thalassemia 412, 466
Bevacizumab 176
Bile salts 276
Biliary colic 40
Bilirubin 284
Biopsy
    endometrial 242
    testicular 415
Biotin 165
Biotinidase deficiency 436
Bipolar disorder 71
    genetics of 484
Bladder
    compression 241
    irritation 25
Blastocyte transfer 416
Bleeding
    disorders 261
    intracranial 51
    menstrual 128
    per vaginal 420
    vaginal 242, 243, 419

Index

Blepharitis 7
Blindness 373, 455
    cortical 262
Blood 113, 153, 276, 466
    agar 287
    analysis 210
    biochemistry 442, 447
    brain barrier 92
    cells, normal 469f
    count, complete 472
    dyscrasias 66
    group 348, 349, 350t
        alleles 461
        genes 351t
        system 349
    loss 478
    pressure 38, 85, 105
    products 153
    sampling, procedure of 405
    tests 406, 407b, 415
    transfusion 468
    urea 46
    vessels 219, 231
    volume 40
Bloodstream infection 109
Blue sclera 381
Blurred vision 6, 67, 73, 78, 84, 85
Body hair, loss of 478
Bone
    marrow
        analysis 472
        aspiration 460, 467
        cells 507
        depression 68, 90
        mass 113
        resorption 113, 227
Boric spirit drop 8
Botulinum antitoxin 170
Bowel obstruction 241
Bradycardia 146, 150
Brain 452
    abscess 256, 272
    cyst 372
    infarct 272
    trauma 72
    tumors 452, 453
Breast 251, 266, 452
    cancer 124, 252, 498
        syndrome 452
    carcinoma of 123, 249
    disease of 251, 252
    engorgement 66, 138
    malignancy 128
    sarcoma of 452
    tenderness 124
Breastfeeding 109
Breathing
    excessive 455
    shortness of 470, 478

Brenner tumor 247
Bromocriptine 93, 127, 140
Bronchial casts 274
Bronchial smooth muscle 40
Bronchodilators 152
Broncholiths 274
Bronchospasm 59, 108, 150, 152
    management of 96
Bronchus 266
Brudzinski's and Kernig's signs 256, 257
Bruits 262
Bulimia nervosa 78, 79
Bumetanide 12-14
Bupivacaine 48
Buprenorphine 149
Burning sensation 6, 7
Buspirone
    hydrochloride 85
    ispapirone 82
Busulfan 172
Butyrophenone 66

C

Cabergoline 127
Caenorhabditis elegans 322
Caffeine 19, 102
    mechanism of action of 102f
Calcineurin inhibitor 179
Calcium 162
    channel blocker 131, 151
    chloride 27
    gluconate 145
    stones 219
Cancer 452
    cervical 237
    endometrial 124
    forms of 455
    gene therapy 453
    genetics 451
    induction 394
    ovarian 245, 246
    types 453
Candida albicans 221
Cap contraceptive 125f
Captopril 24
Carbamazepine 22, 86, 90, 386
Carbidopa 93
Carbimazole 386, 387
Carbohydrate metabolism, disorders of 454
Carbon
    dioxide 49, 51
    monoxide poisoning 50
Carbonic anhydrase inhibitors 18
    dose of 18t
Carboplatin 24, 173
Carboxypeptidases 276

Carcinoma 115, 174, 233, 234, 237, 238, 249, 255, 278
    endometrial 115, 123, 240f
    epidermoid 238
    inflammatory 255
    intraductal 253
    latent 234
    lobular 252, 254
    medullary 254
    metastatic 267, 279
    papillary 254
    prostatic 235
    secretory 255
    tubular 254
Cardiac arrest 96, 99, 100
Cardiac disease 11, 30, 51, 128, 130, 259
Cardiomyopathy 151, 259
    hypertrophic 151
Cardiovascular disease 46, 72, 104
Cardiovascular system 39
Carisoprodol 56, 62
Carotid sinus 100
Carpenter syndrome 447
Cataracts 428
Catechol-O-methyltransferase 483
    inhibitors 93
Caudal agenesis 421
Cavity, buccal 5
Cefotaxime 24
Ceftazidime 24
Cefuroxime 24
Celecoxib 38
Celiac disease 428
Cell
    cycle 303
    killing 509
Cellular division 302
Centchroman 120, 121
Central nervous system 33, 39, 87, 256, 374
    classification of 102f
    disorders 372
    effects 67
    problems 392
    stimulants 102
Cephaloceles 423
Cerebral palsy 381
Cerebrospinal fluid
    analysis 271
Cervical
    cap 125
    penetration test 415
Cervix 113
    carcinoma of 237, 238f
Cetirizine 5
Cheesy masses 274
Chelation therapy 468, 479
Chemical genetic tests 498

Chemotherapy, failure of 177
Chest syndrome, acute 471
Chhaya 121
Chiari malformation 424, 425
Chickenpox 372
Chills 104, 217, 221
Chlorambucil 171
Chloramphenicol 5, 387
Chlordiazepoxide 54
Chlorhexidine mouthwash 9
Chloride-sweat test, abnormal 414
Chlorine 276
Chloroquine 387
Chlorothiazide 15
Chlorpromazine 64-66
Chlorpropamide 21
Chlorthalidone 15
Cholecystitis 277
Cholera 168
Cholesterol 124, 276
Choriocarcinoma 243, 244f, 248
Chorionic villus sampling 402, 403f, 419, 429
    contraindications of 403
    indications of 403
Christmas disease 345, 472
Chromosome 329, 330, 330f, 381
    abnormalities 382t
    functions of 330
    homologous 294
    structure of 329f, 333t
Chymotrypsin 276
Cidofovir 24
Circulatory system 191
Cirrhosis 277
    hepatic 278
Cisplatin 24, 173
Citalopram 76
Clavulanic acid 24
Clear cell tumor 247
Cleft
    lip 347
    palate 347, 381
Clobazam 81
Clofibrate 23
Clomiphene citrate 127
Clonazepam 81
Clonidine 149
Clopamide 15
Clostridium
    difficile 288
    tetani 135
Clozapine 65, 66
Clozaril 66
Cocaine 47, 391, 392
Codeine 40, 41
Colistimethate 24
Colloid 153
    carcinoma 254
    types of 155, 155t

Colon 266
Color blindness 343, 345
Coma 22, 51, 78, 104, 258, 262
    hepatic 14
Combined pills 120
Complex genetic syndromes 246
Condom, female 125, 125f
Confusion 84, 85, 104, 109, 226, 262
Conjunctivitis
    allergic 3
    bacterial 6, 7
    perennial 3
Consanguinity
    atopy 375
    genetic aspect of 376
    negative effects of 377
Constipation 22, 67, 76-78, 80, 84, 191, 226
Contraceptive
    emergency 120
    hormonal 119
    postcoital 120
    vaginal 125
Contraction stress test 138
Convulsions 104
    cerebral 98
Cooley's anemia 465
Cornea, pigmentation of 97
Coronary artery 278
    bypass graft surgery 259
    disease 100, 150, 152, 259
    spasm 151
Coronary syndrome, acute 150, 152
Corpus luteum 112, 181
Corticosteroids 152, 387
Cough 108, 191
    suppression 40
Coxsackie 371
Cramps 104, 455
Cranial dysraphism 422
Cranial nerve dysfunction 267
Craniofacial dysmorphism 447
Craniosynostoses syndrome 447
Crouzon craniofacial dysostosis 383
Cryotherapy 51
Cryptorchidism 229, 231
    etiopathogenesis of 230f
Crystalloid 153
    types of 154, 154t
Crystals 285
Cyanide 159
Cyanocobalamin 162
Cyclic gaba analogues 87
Cyclopenthiazide 15
Cyclophosphamide 171
Cyclosporine 24, 179
Cypionate 114
Cyproheptadine 5

Cystadenocarcinoma
    mucinous 247
    serous 247
Cystadenoma, serous 247
Cystathionine-B-synthase 436
Cystic fibrosis 339, 414, 437
Cystine stones 220
Cystitis 25, 104, 221
    acute 222
    chronic 222
    cystica 222
    etiopathogenesis of 221, 221f
    follicularis 222
    interstitial 222
    types of 221
Cystoscopy 225
Cysts 244, 415
    ovarian 244
Cytarabine 174
Cytogenetic test 498
Cytokinesis 307, 308f
Cytomegalovirus 371, 372, 374
    infection 258
Cytosine 355f, 356f, 358f, 359, 359f
    adenine-guanine 337, 480
Cytotoxic drugs 175, 179

D

Dacarbazine 173
Danazol 386
Dantrolene sodium 56, 61
Dapsone 24
Deafness 373, 455
Death
    neonatal 393
    prenatal 393
Decamethonium 59
Deep vein thrombosis 120
Dehydration 72, 455
Deletion mutation 358f
Delirium 43, 77, 257
    stage of 43
Dementia 124, 267, 455
Dental
    abnormalities 455
    analgesia 44
    problems 428
Denver developmental screening test 445
Deoxybarbiturate 86
Deoxyribonuclease 276
Deoxyribonucleic acid 304, 305, 320, 328f, 329, 507
    replication 324f
    structure of 323f
Depression 84, 85, 105, 124, 455
    bipolar 77
    circulatory 58
    cyclic 72

genetics of 483
major 77, 82
respiratory 58, 88, 91
secondary 77
severe respiratory 59
Dermal hypoplasia, focal 342
Dermal sinus, congenital 421
Dermatitis 66, 105
contact 66
Desamino-oxytocin 137
Desipramine 75
Desmopressin 20, 474
Desogestrel 116, 118, 122
Dextran 155
Dextromethorphan 40
Dextrose 152
Dhaka method 144
Diabetes 72, 115, 238, 259
insipidus 15, 19, 21
mellitus 128, 215, 411, 455
Diabetic nephropathy 209, 215, 215f
Diakinesis 312
Dialysis 456
Diamond-Blackfan anemia 462, 472
Diaphragm 125, 125f
Diarrhea 22, 23, 25, 40, 73, 88, 104, 108, 128, 143, 191, 226, 455
Diastematomyelia 424
Diazepam 54, 56, 62, 81, 83, 87, 91, 149, 151
Dibenzoxazepine 66
Diclofenac sodium 37
Dienestrol 114
Diet, high-fat 252
Diethylstilbestrol 386
Digestive system 191
Digitalis 157
intoxication 96
toxicity 100
Dihydroergotamine 140
Dihydrogesterone 118
Diphenhydramine 5
Diphtheria 168
antitoxin 170
Diplopia 22, 84, 261, 262
Diplotene 312
Direct deoxyribonucleic acid testing 447, 498
Distress, respiratory 98
Disulfiram 148, 149
aversion therapy 148
Dittrich's plug 274
Diuresis 104
Diuretics 12
classification of 13f
site of action of 12f
Dizziness 22, 84, 85, 96, 104, 105, 108, 109, 261, 262, 470

Dobutamine 100, 153
mechanism of action of 100f
Dopamine 64, 98, 150, 153
mechanism of action of 98f
precursor 92
Dopaminergic agonists 93
Dorsal dermal sinuses 424
Dorzolamide 18
Down syndrome 335, 336, 380, 381, 382, 398, 426, 426f, 428t, 434
neonatal features of 427b
Doxapram, mechanism of action of 106f
Doxepin 75
Doxorubicin 175
Drama therapy 484
Drosophila melanogaster 348
Drowsiness 3, 5, 9, 77, 79, 84, 105, 145, 258
Dry mouth 5, 67, 73, 76-78, 80, 100
Dual-energy X-ray absorptiometry scanning 460
Duchenne muscular dystrophy 343, 345, 383, 437
Duct carcinoma 253
Duodenal atresia 407, 428
Duodenal ulcer, perforated 277
Dydrogesterone 116
Dysentery 40, 191
Dysgerminomas 248
Dyslexia 262
Dysmenorrhea 115
Dysmorphism, types of 446
Dyspareunia 221, 245
Dysphagia 262
Dysphasia 261
Dyspnea 40, 96, 104, 108, 209
Dysrhythmia 138
cardiac 23, 143
Dystonias 68
Dysuria 25, 104, 191, 217, 221

E

Ear
disorders of 3
drop 6f
dryness in 8
surgery 8
topical application for 5, 7
Eating disorder 77
Ecchymosis 227
Echinococcus granulosus 274
Echocardiography 442, 447
Eclampsia 141
management of 144, 151
Eczema photosensitivity 66
Edema 3, 15, 73, 76, 78, 100, 191, 455
acute pulmonary 14, 150, 152
angioneurotic 66

cerebral 14
fluid, mobilization of 21
pulmonary 96, 151, 226
Edwards syndrome 335, 336, 447
Eiperazines 66
Elapid bite 155
Electrocardiogram 442, 447
Electroconvulsive therapy 484
Electroencephalogram 457
Electron microscopy 216
Embolism, pulmonary 108, 225
Emphysema 40
Empty sac 418
Empyema 256
Enalapril 24
Enalaprilat 24
Enanthate 114
Encephalitis 256, 257
bacterial 258
types of 258
viral 258
Encephalocele 421
Encephalopathy 455
Endocarditis 256
Endocrine 66, 92
disorders 428
Endometriosis 115, 127
Endometrium 112
carcinoma of 238
Enolic acid derivative 36
ENT disorders 5t, 428
Entamoeba histolytica 161
Enuresis, childhood 77
Envenomation, level of 160t
Enzyme
administration of 486
assay 498
digestive 276
proteolytic 276
replacement therapy 456, 460
stabilization of 486
Eosinophilia 77
Ependymomas 265
Epididymis 415
Epilepsy 18, 107, 128, 191
risk of 372
Epinephrine 95, 150
mechanism of action of 96f
Epirubicin 175
Epithelium, vaginal 113
Erectile dysfunction 227
Ergometrine 140
Ergot alkaloids 130
mechanism of action of 130f
Ergotamine 140
Ergotoxine 140
Erlotinib 176
Erythema 58, 105
infectiosum 374

Escherichia coli 221, 256, 284, 286
Esophageal atresia 407, 428
Estradiol benzoate 114
Estramustine 174
Estriol succinate 114
Estrogen 112, 123, 176
    conjugated 114
    effects of 113
    exogenous 252
    natural 112
    synthesis of 112, 113*f*
Ethacrynic acid 12, 15
Ethamivan 107
    mechanism of action of 107, 107*f*
Ethanol 386
Ether 43
Ethinylestradiol 114, 122
Ethosuximide 86
Ethyl alcohol 131
Etoposide 174
Etoricoxib 38
Euphoria 104
Ewing's sarcoma 174
Ex vivo gene therapy 505, 505*f*
Excretion 114
Expectorants 27
Extracellular fluid 19, 162
Eye 187
    defects 372
    disorders of 3
    injury, penetrating 59
    problems 471
    topical application for 5
Eyelashes, shedding of 97
Eyelids, pigmentation of 97
Ezy pill 120

F

Fabry's disease 216, 343, 345
Face, arm speech test (FAST) 264
Failure to thrive 455
Fallopian tubes 113
Fallot tetralogy 407, 428
Familial cancer 451
    management of 453
    predisposing syndrome 452
Family pedigree
    analysis of 487
    preparing of 487
Family therapy 484
Fatigue 5, 76, 78, 84, 477
Fatty acid 276
    oxidation, disorders of 454
Febrile convulsions 151
Fecal occult blood 287
Fenamate 36
Fentanyl 41
Fentanyl derivatives 40
Fertility 416*f*

Fertilization
    abnormal 242
    tests 415
Fetal
    abdominal wall problems 407
    abnormalities 385
    alcohol effects 392
    anomaly screening 398
    blood sampling 405, 406
        indications of 405
        risks of 406*t*
    chromosomal abnormalities 418
    death 130, 373
    development 394*f*
        stage of 386*b*, 394
    distress 130, 138
    echocardiography 399, 399*f*
    growth, period of 390*f*
    kidney disease 407
    radiology 400
    tissue sampling 406, 407, 408*b*
Fetoscopy 407
Fetus, malposition of 241
Fever 22, 105, 143, 217, 221, 225, 257
    acute rheumatic 34
Fexofenadine 4
Fibrillation 151
Fibroadenoma 251
Fibroids 240
Fibroma 249
Fibromyomas 240
Fibrosis
    interstitial 231
    peritubular 231
Fistula, tracheoesophageal 428
Fits 191
Flatulence 8
Flubiprofen 35
Fluid retention 124
Flumazenil 54
Fluorescence in situ hybridization 409, 442, 447, 498
Fluorouracil 174
Fluoxetine 76
Fluphenazine 64
Fluvoxamine 76
Folic acid 136, 136*t*, 162, 165, 380
Follicle-stimulating hormone 412
Food allergy, prevention of 379
Food poisoning, causes of 160
Foot deformities 428
Foscarnet 24
Fosphenytoin 86
Fragile X syndrome 447, 498
Frame-shift mutation 357
Frontonasal dysplasia sequence 447
Fructose test 281
Frusemide 13, 152

Fungal
    infection 8
    meningitis 272
Fungi 161
Furosemide 12, 13

G

Gabapentin 87
Gadopentetate dimeglumine 24
Gadoxetate disodium 24
Gait disturbances 267
Galactorrhea 77
Galactosemia 436, 498
Gallbladder, perforated 277
Gallstones 471
Gamete in vitro fertilization technique 127
Gamete intrafallopian transfer 416
Gamma
    aminobutyric acid 54, 87
    globulin 170
Ganciclovir 24
Ganglia 108
Gas gangrene antitoxin 170
Gastric constituents
    abnormal 275
    analysis of 275
Gastric juice examination 275
Gastroesophageal reflux disease 59, 428
Gastrointestinal
    bleeding 226
    disorders 428
    disturbances 14, 35
    system 226
    tract 39, 249, 438
Gastroschisis 407
Gaucher's disease 455, 459-461, 498
Gene 294, 316
    augmentation 509
    functions of 318
    locus 294
    mutation 353, 354, 419, 452
        causes of 354
        effects of 358
        types of 355
    proportion of 376*t*
    structure of 316, 317*f*
    therapy 456, 474, 486, 503, 506, 506*f*, 507*f*, 509, 509*f*
        approaches of 505
        facts of 508
        pharmacological 508
        shortcomings of 508
        short-lived nature of 508
    types of 318, 318*t*
General anesthesia 42, 98
    stage of 43

Genetic 371
  code 327, 327f
  concept of 293
  conditions 298, 411-413, 450
  counseling 510
    beneficiaries of 510
    phases of 511, 511f
    purpose of 510
  diseases 411
  disorders 297, 337t, 340t, 342t, 345t, 351, 383t
    categorization of 438f
    diagnosis of 296
    hereditary 472
    nursing management in 486
    prevention of 380
    therapeutic approaches for 484
  emerging paradigm of 362
  factor 443
  hemochromatosis 476
  nursing practice milestones 363
  services 496
  statistics 450
  testing 415, 420, 437, 442, 447, 453, 479, 484, 496, 500, 502
    benefits of 500
    negative outcomes of 500
    purposes of 497
    types of 497, 498
Genital bleeding 115
Genital system
  female 237
  male 229
Genital tract 249
Genitalia, ambiguous 455
Genitourinary tract 104
Genome 295
Gentamicin 7, 24
Germ cell
  elements 231
  tumors 247, 248
German measles 372
Germline 354
  gene therapy 504, 504f
Gestation, multiple 407
Giardia lamblia 161
Gingivitis 9
Glaucoma 18, 104, 105
  congenital 428
Gliomas 265
Glomerular disease
  secondary 214
  types of 211
Glomerular filtration rate 19, 209, 210
Glomerulonephritis 209, 212f
  acute 211, 211f
  chronic 128, 214, 215f

etiopathogenesis of 209, 210f
focal 213
membranoproliferative 213
membranous 212
primary 209t
rapidly progressive 211
secondary 209t
Glomerulosclerosis, focal segmental 209, 213, 214f
Glossitis 104
Glucocorticoids 176, 180
Glucose
  6-phosphate dehydrogenase deficiency 345, 462, 463
  agar 287
  estimation of 273
  intolerance 113
Glutamate antagonist 94
Glutamine 359f
Glutaric acidemia 454
Glycerol 19
Glyceryl trinitrate spray 152
Glycogen storage disease 454
Glycosuria 66, 217
Goiter 73
Goldenhar syndrome 447
Gonadal dysgenesis 246
Gonadoblastoma 249
Gonadotropin 127
  releasing hormone 127, 181, 411
  agonists 176
Grand mal seizures 89
Grand multipara 130
Gray baby syndrome 6
Gross motor warning signs 443
Growth
  delayed 471
  failure 455
  retardation 392
Guanine 359, 359f
Guillain-Barre syndrome 273
Gynandroblastoma 249
Gynecomastia 66, 77

H

Haemophilus influenzae 168, 256
Hair loss 245
Hallucinations 104
Haloperidol 64
Halothane 44, 131
Hand-foot syndrome 471
Head injury 40, 51
Headache 3, 5, 9, 22, 27, 79, 84, 85, 99, 104, 105, 108, 124, 257, 261, 262, 470
Healthcare systems 193
Hearing
  loss
    congenital 437
    mixed 428

services 446
warning signs 444
Heart
  anomalies, congenital 373
  block 99
    complete 89
  disease 141
    congenital 347
    coronary 124
    pulmonary 50
  enlarged 455
  failure 77, 455
    chronic 175
    congestive 259, 277
    uncompensated 108
  surgery 99
  valves, artificial 259
Hematogenous infection 216, 217
Hematological disorders 89, 428, 461, 462
Hematopoietic malignancies 249
Hematuria 25, 225
Hemianopia 261, 267
Hemiparesis 262, 267
Hemochromatosis 437
Hemodynamic insufficiency 50
Hemoglobin 472
  C disease 462
  D disease 462
  E disease 462
  H 465
Hemoglobinopathies 462
Hemoglobinuria, paroxysmal nocturnal 462
Hemolytic crises 463
Hemolytic disease 462
  screening for 398
Hemophilia 343, 345, 462, 472, 498
  A 383, 472
  B 472
  C 472
  classification of 473, 473t
  mild 473
  moderate 473
  severe 473
  type 473
Hemorrhage
  cerebral 96l, 98
  intracerebral 261
  intracranial 78
  postpartum 138
Hemorrhoids 191
Henoch-Schonlein purpura 213
Heparin 158
Hepatic
  disease 27
  disorders 72
  dysfunction 31, 89
  failure 115

insufficiency 40
    vein obstruction 277
Hepatitis 22
    A 169
    B 169, 172
        immunoglobulin 170
        virus 372
Hepatosplenomegaly, congenital 372
Hereditary breast and ovarian cancer syndrome 362
Herpes simplex virus 374, 506
Heterozygous alleles 294
Hiccup 108
High performance liquid chromatography test 457f
High-potency antipsychotic drugs 64
Hip dislocation 347, 428
    congenital 347
Hirschsprung's disease 428
Hirsutism 245
Histidine 358f, 359
Hodgkin's disease 174
Homeopathy 183
    fundamental principles of 187
Homocystinuria 436, 498
Hormonal drugs 176
Hormonal replacement therapy 114, 119, 122, 124t
Hormone, antidiuretic 12, 20
Human chorionic gonadotropin 427
    testing 420
Human genome project 293, 437
Human immunodeficiency virus 371-373, 506
    encephalitis 258
Human leukocyte antigen 467, 479
Human parvovirus B19 372
Hunter syndrome 343, 345
Huntingtin's gene 480, 480t
Huntington's disease 337, 437, 479, 481f, 498
Hybrid methods 508
Hydantoin 86
Hydatidiform mole 242, 243f
Hydrocephalus 425
Hydrochloric acid 275
Hydrochlorothiazide 15, 21
Hydrocortisone 152
Hydrophids 155
Hydroxyprogesterone 118
Hydroxyurea 175
Hydroxyzine 82
Hyperbilirubinemia 462, 464
Hypercalcemia 146
    acute 14
    chronic 167
Hypercalciuria 15
Hypercarotenemia 271

Hypercholesterolemia, familial 337
Hyperflexibility 428
Hypergammaglobulinemia 460
Hyperglycemia 21, 27, 66, 73, 77, 98
Hyperkalemia 14, 17, 145
Hyperlipidemia, familial 259
Hypermagnesemia 145
Hyperphenylalaninemia 436
Hyperphosphatemia 18, 167
Hyperplasia
    benign prostatic 77
    congenital adrenal 436, 455
    endometrial 123
    prostatic 231, 232f, 233f
Hyperprolactinemia 127, 411
Hyperpyrexia 78
Hypersensitivity 5-9, 21, 38, 51, 66, 91, 100, 138, 141, 146
    reactions 22, 25
Hypersomnia 78
Hypertension 14, 15, 30, 78, 96, 99, 100, 104, 109, 130, 225, 238, 259, 261, 455
    intraoperative 151
    malignant 128
    mild-to-severe 210
    persistent pulmonary 50
    pulmonary arterial 471
    severe 96, 107
    systemic 151
Hyperthermia, malignant 44, 59, 498
Hyperthyroidism 77, 99, 104
Hyperventilation 455
Hypervolemia 209
Hypnotics 52, 54t
    classification of 52f
    effect 82
Hypocalcemia 27, 145
Hypochloremia 27
Hypochondriasis 79
Hypoglycemia 22, 77, 152
Hypogonadism 455
Hypokalemia 21, 27
Hypomania 72
Hyponatremia 22, 73, 138, 145, 166
    dilutional 22
Hypoperfusion, systemic 259
Hypophosphatemia 146
Hypopituitarism 411
Hypoplastic nose 373
Hypotension 46, 58, 59, 84, 103, 130, 138, 455
    orthostatic 67, 75, 78
    postural 77
    severe 69
Hypothalamic-pituitary factors 411
Hypothermia 109
Hypothyroidism 73, 428, 455
    congenital 436

Hypovolemia 99, 152
Hypoxanthine-guanine phosphoribo-syltransferase 345
Hypoxemia 50, 259
Hypoxia 98
Hypoxic respiratory failure 50
Hysterectomy 123
Hysterosalpingography 242
Hysteroscopy 242

I

Ibuprofen 24, 35
Ichthyosis, X-linked 345
Ifosfamide 24, 171
Imatinib 175
Iminostilbene 86
Imipramine 75
Immature teratomas 248
Immotile cilia syndrome 413
Immune hemolytic anemia 462
Immunity
    active 167
    impaired cellular 428
Immunization 171
Immunoglobulins 170t, 171
Immunostimulants 94, 178
Immunosuppressants 178
Imperforate anus 428
Impotence 104, 477
In utero strokes 392
In vitro
    fertilization 408, 415, 416f
    maturation 416
In vivo gene therapy 505, 506f
Indapamide 15
Indigestion 79, 124
Indomethacin 37, 131
Infarction, acute myocardial 151, 259
Infection 22, 241, 371, 471
    ascending 216
    bacterial 8, 375
    maternal 371, 372t
    neonatal 373, 398
Infertility 126, 227, 245, 280, 410
    causes of 127t, 410
    diagnosis of 415
    drugs for 126
    female 127
    genetic basis of 411
    male 231, 410
    medical
        management of 415
        treatment for 127t
    primary 126, 410
    secondary 126, 241, 410
    treatment of 126, 127, 127t, 128
    types of 126f
    unexplained 410

Infestations, parasitic 278
Inflammation, corneal 3
Influenza 169
Injury, pulmonary 50
Insomnia 79, 82, 84, 85, 151
Insulin 158
    secretion, inhibition of 21
Integumentary system 191
Interferons 178
International Society of Nurses in Genetics 363
Interstitium 219
Intestine, perforated 277
Intoxication, acute 22
Intracranial pressure 46
Intractable hyperemesis gravidarum 128
Intracytoplasmic sperm injection 127, 416
Intraocular pressure 59
Intrauterine
    fetal death 375
    growth retardation 393
Intubation procedures 59
Invasive tests 400
Iodides 387
Iodine overdosage 159
Iohexol 24
Iopamidol 24
Ioversol 24
Ipratropium 152
Irinotecan 175
Iron 136, 159
    deficiency disorder 191
    supplementation 381
Irritation
    bronchial 100
    conjunctival 97
Ischemic asthmaticus 107
Isocarboxazid 76
Isoimmunization 407
Isoleucine 358f, 359
Isoproterenol 99
    mechanism of action of 99f
Isosorbide 19
Isotretinoin 386
Itching 58, 66

J

Jacobsen syndrome 335
Japanese encephalitis 169, 172
Jaundice 68, 77, 455
    cholestatic 22, 66
    mild 464
    neonatal 130
    pale 464
Joint pain 88, 455, 478
Juxtaglomerular cell 11
    tumor 223

K

Kallman's syndrome 411, 412
Kartagener's syndrome 413
Kearns-Sayre syndrome 455
Keratitis 3
Keratoconus 428
Ketamine 45
Ketone 209, 285
    bodies 284
Ketonuria 217
Ketoprofen 35
Kidney 11, 266
    disease 7, 11
    disorders 72
Killed vaccine 167
Kimmelstiel-Wilson lesion 216
Klinefelter's syndrome 335, 336, 412
Klonopin 81
Krukenberg's tumor 249
Kussmaul's breathing 226

L

Labor
    augmentation of 137
    preterm 241
Lactation 8
    abnormal 66
Lactic acidosis 96
Lacunar infarct 261
Lamotrigine 87
Language 446
    disorders 267
Laser vaporization 127
Lavertiracetam 87
Leber's hereditary optic neuropathy 346
Leiomyoma
    signs of 240
    symptoms of 240
Leptotene 311
Lesch-Nyhan syndrome 345, 454
Lethargy 226
Leucine 359
Leukemia 272, 452
    acute 428
    chronic myeloid 175
Leukocyte esterase 285
Leukocytosis 66, 73, 77
Leukopenia 460
Leukorrhea 191
Levocetirizine 4, 5
Levodopa 92
Levonorgestrel 116, 118, 121, 122
Leydig cell 231, 413
Lidocaine 48
Li-Fraumeni syndrome 452, 453
Light headedness 80, 84, 85
Lignocaine 150

Limb
    deformities 373
    hypoplasia 372
    reduction 392
Lipid
    cell tumors 249
    metabolism 124
Lipolytic lipase 276
Lipomyelomeningocele 424
Lipoplexes 507
Lisinopril 24
Lithium 24, 71, 386, 392
    carbonate 72
    chloride 72
    mechanism of action of 72f
Live attenuated vaccine 167
Liver 277
    biopsy 479
    cirrhosis 15
    damage 68
    diseases, alcoholic 109
    dysfunction 22
    failure 455
    function 22
        tests 225
Local anesthesia
    mechanism of action of 47f
    use of 48
Locasamide 87
Lodixanol 24
Loop diuretics 13
Lorazepam 54, 81, 85, 87, 149, 151
Lowe syndrome 498
Lower back pain 245
Low-potency antipsychotic drugs 64
Loxapine 64
Lucontincotia pigmenti 342
Lumbar
    puncture 256, 257, 272
    tenderness 217
Lung, carcinoma of 174
Lupus nephritis 209, 214
Luteinizing hormone 412
Lymph nodes, enlarged 455
Lymphoma 272, 278
Lynestrenol 118
Lypressin 20
Lysosomal storage diseases 454, 455

M

MacConkey agar 287
Magnesium 166, 381
    deficiency 166
    sulfate 131, 144, 144t
    toxicity of 145
Major depressive disorder 80
Malaise 143, 221
Malakoplakia 222
Malaria 178

Malformations, congenital 455
Mammary glands 113
Mandibulofacial dysostosis 383
Mania, recurrent 72
Manic depressive psychosis 71
Manual physical therapy 417
Maple syrup urine disease 436, 454, 458
Maprotiline 76
Marfan syndrome 381, 383, 498
Marijuana 391
Marshall-Smith syndrome 447
Maternal drug therapy 384
Mature teratoma 248
Measles 169
Mechlorethamine 171
Meckel's diverticulum 428
Medical radiation procedures 394
    minimizing risk of 395
Medicine
    alternative systems of 183
    antifibrinolytic 474
Medroxyprogesterone 116
    acetate 118
Medullary interstitial cell tumor 224
Meiosis 308, 309f, 310, 314, 316, 316t
Melancholia 77
Melanoma
    malignant 266
    meningeal metastatic 271
Melphalan 172
Meningeal irritation 256, 258
    signs of 256
Meningiomas, characteristics of 264
Meningitis 256, 273
    aseptic 256
    bacterial 272
    parasitic 272
    signs of 256
    tuberculous 272
    viral 272
Meningocele 421, 423
Meningococcal vaccine 168
Meningoencephalitis 272
Meningomyelocele 421
Menkes disease 345
Menstrual disorders 191
Mental
    illness 482, 484
    retardation 372, 373, 428
    status, altered 50
Meperidine 41
Mephenamic acid 36
Meprobamate 82
Mercaptopurine 174
Mesalamine 24
Mesoblastic nephroma 223, 224
Mesoridazine 64
Messenger ribonucleic acid 321

Mestranol 114
Metabolism 114, 117, 385
    inborn errors of 454, 455t
Metallic taste 73
Metaplasia 255
Methadone 149
Methamphetamine 391
Methanol 157
Methazolamide 18
Methenamine 24, 25
    doses of 25t
    hippurate 25
    mandelate 25
    mechanism of action of 24, 24f
Methergin 140
Metherone 140
Methionine synthetase 436
Methohexitone sodium 45
Methotrexate 24, 173, 179, 387
Methyl alcohol poisoning 94, 108, 109
    treatment of 109
Methylation studies 498
Methylergometrine 140
Methylphenidate 103, 103f, 105
Methylxanthines 19
Methysergide 140
Metolazone 15
Metronidazole 161
Mianseril 76
Microcephaly 372
Micturition, frequency of 217
Midazolam 54, 151
Middle ear surgery 51
Mifepristone 121, 128
Milieu therapy 484
Milk-alkalosis syndrome 29
Milky pericardial fluid 279
Minerals 161, 162
    supplementation 161
Mini pill 120
Mirtazapine 76
Miscarriage 392, 417
    delayed 418
    recurrent 418
Misoprostol 136, 139, 139t, 386
Missense mutation 357, 358f
Mitochondrial function, disorders of 455
Mitomycin C 175
Mitosis 304, 305f, 316, 316t
    phases of 305
Mitral valve
    disease 259
    prolapse 381
Moebius sequence 447
Molecular genetic tests 401, 442, 447, 498
Molindone 64

Monoamine oxidase inhibitor 74, 77, 90
Monodermal teratoma 248
Mood
    elevators 74
    stabilizers 70, 484
Morning after pill 120
Morphine 39, 152, 153, 156
    poisoning, acute 40
Mountain sickness, acute 18
Mouth wash 9
Multicystic nephroma 223, 224
Multigene disorders 508
Multiple endocrine
    adenomatosis 453
    neoplasia 452
Mumps 169, 371, 373
Muscle
    aches, general 477
    pain 88
    relaxant
        classification of 55f
        mechanism of action of 57, 57f
    weakness 59, 455
Musculoskeletal system 191
Music therapy 484
Myasthenia gravis 46, 145
Mycophenolate mofetil 179
Mydriasis 67, 108
Myelitis 256
Myeloma, multiple 272
Myelomeningocele 421, 423, 423f
Myeloproliferative disorder 428
Myocardial infarction 34, 40, 77, 150, 152, 259, 455
Myocardial infection 99
Myoclonic jerks, generalized 88
Myomas 240
Myotonic dystrophy syndrome 414, 447
Myxedema 46, 278

N

N-acetylcysteine 39
Nafcillin 24
Nail-patella syndrome 216, 337
Naloxone 40, 41
Naltrexone 42
Naproxen 35
Narrow angle glaucoma 31, 59
Nasal congestion 67
Nausea 9, 22, 73, 77, 84, 88, 99, 104, 108, 128, 138, 143, 145, 226
Necrospermia 413
Negri bodies 258
Neisseria meningitis 256
Nephritic syndrome 213
Nephritis, hereditary 216

Nephrosis 407
Nephrotic syndrome 277, 278
Nephrotoxic drugs 24, 24t
    effects of 24f
Nephrotoxins 221
Nerve
    block 48
    neurolysis of 108
Nervous system 33
    classification of 33f
Neural tube defect 347, 401, 407, 420, 421, 422f
    etiology of 422f
    types of 421t
Neuralgia 23
    trigeminal 90, 108
Neuroblastoma 174
Neurodegenerative disorders, drugs for 92
Neurofibromatosis 498
Neurological deficit, focal 258
Neurological disorders 428
Neuromuscular disorder 108
Neuron 75
Neurosyphilis 273
Niacin 161, 164
Nicotinic acid 161
Niemann-Pick disease 455
Nifedipine 131-133, 151
Nikethamide, mechanism of action of 107, 107f
Nimesulide 37
Niotin 162
Nitrates 131
Nitrazepam 54
Nitrites 285
Nitrofurantoin 25
Nitroglycerin 151
Nitrous oxide 43, 49, 50
Nocturia 221
Non-depolarizing blocker muscle relaxants, side effects of 56t
Nonsense mutation 357, 359f
Non-steroidal anti-inflammatory drug 33, 34, 131, 387, 471
    classification of 33, 34f
Noonan's syndrome 413
Norepinephrine 75, 97
    mechanism of action of 97f
Norethindrone 122
Norethisterone 116, 118
Norgestrel 122
Norpramin 75
Nortestosterone derivatives 116
Nortriptyline 75
Nose
    disorders of 3
    topical application for 5

Nucleic acid 320
Nucleus 276
Nystagmus 262, 267, 428

O

Obesity 40, 72, 238, 240, 252, 259
Obsessive compulsive disorder 78, 80
Obstruction
    idiopathic epididymal 414
    respiratory 88
    severe pulmonary 31
Obstructive sleep apnea 428
Occupational therapy 446
Odor 284
Oestrogel 114
Olanzapine 66
Oligodendrogliomas 265
Oligomenorrhea 245
Oligonucleotides 507
Oligospermia 191, 281
Olopatadine 4
Omphalocele 407
Oncocytoma 223
Ophthalmic eye drops 4f
Ophthalmological disorders 428
Opioid 39, 41, 152, 387
    analgesics 39
    antagonist 41, 150
    classification of 39f
Oral contraceptive 119, 120, 122t, 252
    types of 120
    use of 259
Organ failure, multiple 471
Organic
    acid metabolism 454
        disorders of 454
    acidurias 454
    brain damage 96
    psychoses 258
    solvent chemicals inhalants 391
Ormeloxifene 121
Ornithine transcarbamylase deficiency 342
Orofaciodigital syndrome 342
Orthopedic disorders 428
Orthopnea 209
Osmotic diuretics 19
Osteogenesis imperfecta 337
Osteomyelitis 256
Osteo-onychodysplasia 216
Osteopenia, evaluation of 460
Osteoporosis 227
Otitis media 4, 8, 256
Ovarian cancer 245, 246
    syndrome 452

Ovulation
    disorders 127
    induction 127
    problems 410
Oxaliplatin 173
Oxcarbamazepine 86
Oxygen 49, 150
Oxytocic drugs 98
Oxytocin 129, 136, 137, 137t
    antagonist 131
    challenge test 130
    mechanism of action of 129f
    sensitivity test 138
    types of 137f

P

Pachytene 311
Pain 34, 77
    abdominal 25, 105, 109, 191, 455, 477
    agnosia 455
    anginal 104
    chest 98, 100, 108, 143, 470
    chronic 150
    postoperative 40
    precordial 104
    relief of 90
Pale skin 470
Palpation, abdominal 398
Palpitation 75, 85, 191
Pancreatic juice, composition of 276
Pancreatitis, hemorrhagic 277
Pancytopenia 66
Panencephalitis, subacute sclerosing 273
Panic
    attack 77, 82
    disorder 77, 78, 80
Pantothenic acid 161, 164
Pap test 249
Para-aminophenol derivatives 38
Paracentesis, abdominal 277
Paracetamol 38
    poison 39, 156
Paradoxical excitation 88
Paragonimus westermani 274
Paralysis 258, 262
    absence of 262
    medullary 43
    periodic 18
Parasites 274, 285
Paratyphoid 168
Paresthesias 77, 108, 146
Parkinson disease 78
Paroxetine 76
Paroxysmal atrial fibrillation 259
Parvovirus 371
Patau syndrome 335, 336, 447
Patellar subluxation 428

Patent foramen ovale 259
Pelvic
    discomfort, mild 245
    hematoma 138
    pain 221
Pelvicalyceal system 219
Pelvis, contracted 130, 138
Penfluridol 65
Penicillamine 386
Penicillium islandicum 161
Penis, carcinoma of 233, 234f
Pentazocine 41, 150
Peptic ulcer 77, 191
Peptidases 276
Percutaneous umbilical blood sampling 405
Pericardial fluid, analysis of 278
    aspiration
        complications of 278
        indications for 278
Pericarditis
    bacterial 279
    idiopathic hemorrhagic 279
Periodic acid-Schiff 255
Periodontitis 9
Peripheral decarboxylase inhibitors 93
Peripheral nervous system effects 67
Peritoneal fluid, analysis of 277
    color of 277
Peritonitis, biliary 277
Peroxisomal function, disorders of 455
Perphenazine 64
Pertussis 168
Pethidine 41, 153
Peucine 358f
Peutz-Jeghers syndrome 246
Pharmacokinetics 384
Pharmacopoeia commission 190
Phenazopyridine 27
Phencyclidine 391
Phenelzine sulfate 76
Phenobarbitone 52, 86, 88
Phenothiazines 66
Phenotype 295, 349
Phenylalanine 435
    hydroxylase 456
Phenylketonuria 435, 436, 454, 456
Phenyltriazine 87
Phenytoin 86, 88, 386, 387
Pheochromocytoma 99
Phlebitis 108
Phospholipase 276
Phosphorus
    deficiency 167
    use of 167
Photophobia 3, 67, 98
Phyenylketonuria 341

Physical therapy 446
Phytonadione 136
Pipecuronium 56, 57
Piperacillin 24
Piretanide 12
Piroxicam 36
Placenta previa 138
Plague 168
Plasma
    protein-A, pregnancy associated 427
    pseudocholinesterase, deficiency of 59
Pneumococcal vaccine 168
Pneumonia 256, 428
Pneumothorax 51, 107, 278
Poisoning
    management of 153
    organophosphorus 156
    treatment of 153
    type of 156
Poliomyelitis 169
Polycystic kidney disease 498
Polycystic ovarian
    disease 246f
    syndrome 244
Polycythemia 225, 428
Polydactyly 337
Polymerase chain reaction 409
    technique 470
Polyplexes 507
Polypoid cystitis 222
Polyposis
    colonic 452, 453
    familial adenomatous 452, 453, 498
Polythiazide 15
Polyuria 6, 104
Porphyria 6
Porphyrin metabolism, disorders of 454
Postcoital pill 120
Postcoital tests 415
Postejaculatory urine sample 415
Post-myocardial infarction syndrome 278, 279
Post-pericardiotomy syndrome 279
Potassium 166, 276
    citrate 29, 30
    sparing diuretics 16, 17t
Potency antipsychotic drugs, moderate 64
Prader-Willi syndrome 412, 447, 498
Pre-eclampsia, severe 141, 144
Pregabalin 87
Pregnancy 8, 51, 72, 77, 104, 115, 129, 191
    early 31
    first trimester 51

loss
    early 418
    recurrent 418
    medical termination of 112, 126, 128
Preimplantation genetic
    diagnosis 408, 415, 497
        indications of 408
    screening 408
Premenstrual dysphoric disorder 79
Prenatal diagnosis 396
    purposes of 397
Prenatal nutrition 378, 378f, 380
    facts of 378
Prenatal screening 398, 424
Prenatal testing 377, 396, 497
Prethcamide 106
    mechanism of action of 106f
Priapism 471
Primidone 86, 89
Pritchard method 144
Progeris progeria 383
Progesterone 112, 116, 118, 131
    doses of 118t
    effects of 117
    only pill 120
    synthesis of 113f, 116
Progestin 123, 176
    cyclic 123
    therapy 123
Prolactin suppressing agents 127
Prolixin 64
Propanediols 82
Prophylaxis 26
Propionic acid derivatives 35t
Propofol 45
Prostaglandins 141
    classification of 142, 142t
    types of 142t
Prostate
    carcinoma of 115, 234, 235, 235f
    hypertrophy, benign 231
Protein 284, 461
    analysis 498
    biosynthesis 325
    estimation of 272
    synthesis 325, 327
        steps of 325
    truncation test 498
Proteinuria 25, 210, 217, 227
Proteus vulgaris 286
Protriptyline 75
Pruritus 3, 108
Pseudomonas aeruginosa 286
Psoriasis 72
Psychiatric disorders 51
Psychoanalysis 484
Psychoeducation 484
Psychosis 455

Index

Psychotic disorders, childhood 373
Ptosis 261, 262
Puberty
    delayed 455, 471
    precocious 455
Pulmonary disease, severe 27
Pulseless ventricular tachycardia 150
Purine, disorders of 454
Pyelonephritis 25, 216
    acute 216, 218f
    chronic 218
Pyknocytosis, infantile 462
Pyloric stenosis 428
Pyonephrosis 217
Pyridoxine 162, 164
Pyrimidine metabolism 454
Pyuria 217

Q

Quinine 56, 61, 387

R

Rabies 169
    immunoglobulin 170
Radiation
    effects of 389, 393
    exposure 396
    genetic aspect of 393
    high-energy 354
    quality of 394
Rasagiline 93
Rasayana therapy 185
Raynaud's phenomenon 151
Rebound hypersecretion 29
Red blood cell 49, 210, 272, 285, 288
Red cell
    antigen 349
    enzyme deficiency, hereditary 462
    membrane, hereditary defects of 462
Refractive errors 428
Refractory angina 151
Rehydration therapy 152
Renal angiography 225
Renal artery 225
Renal calculi 219
Renal cell carcinoma 223, 224, 224f
Renal disease 17
    end-stage 5
    severe 27
Renal dysfunction 31
Renal failure 99, 225, 455
    acute 14, 226
    chronic 226
    etiopathogenesis of 226, 226f
    severe 14

Renal impairment 22, 72
Renal insufficiency 68
Renal parenchyma, epithelial tumors of 223
Renal pelvis, epithelial tumors of 223
Renal toxicity 73
Renal tumor
    etiopathogenesis of 223, 223f
    types of 223t
Renin-angiotensin aldosterone
    system 11, 11f
    physiology of 11
Reninoma 224
Replacement therapy 474, 486
Reproductive system 113, 117, 130, 191, 227
Respiratory failure 50, 108, 109, 455
Respiratory stimulant 51, 94, 106
    classification of 106f
Respiratory system 191, 226
Restless sleep 41
Retardation, severe 428
Retinitis 372
Retinoblastoma 452
    familial 452, 453
Retinopathy 128
Retroviruses 506
Rett syndrome 498
Rhesus system 351
Rheumatic disease 259
Rheumatoid arthritis 34, 191
Rhinitis, allergic 4, 191
Rhinorrhea 41
Rhythm, cardiac 96
Riboflavin 161, 164
Ribonuclease 276
Ribonucleic acid 317, 320, 328f
    ribosomal 322
    structure of 323f
    synthesis of 323
Rifampicin therapy 271
Risperidone 65
Ritodrine 131
Robertsonian translocation 410
Rocuronium 56, 57
Rotavirus 172
Rubella 169, 371, 372, 373
    infection 374

S

Salbutamol nebulization 152
Salicylate 33, 152
    overdose 35
    poisoning 156
Sarcoidosis 146
Sarcomas 223
Schizophrenia
    genetics of 483
    high risk of 372

Sclerosis
    multiple 273
    tuberculous 337, 437
Scoliosis 428
Sedation 22, 67, 77, 80, 84, 85
Sedative 52
    classification of 52f
    effect 82
Seizures 68, 258, 267, 428, 455
    disorder 82, 105
    maternal 138
    mixed 90
    neuroleptic malignant 68
    prevention of 151
    psychomotor 89, 90
Selective estrogen receptor
    modulators 116
Selective serotonin reuptake
    inhibitor 76, 79
    mechanism of action of 79f
Selegiline 93
Semen
    analysis 279, 281, 413, 415
    purposes of 280
    sample, collection of 280
Seminal vesicles 415
Senile vaginitis 115
Sensory loss 267
Septicemia 99
Serine 359
Serotonin 75
Sertoli-Leydig cell tumors 249
Sertraline 76
Serum ferritin level test 478
Sex
    chromosome
        abnormalities 336
        disorders 336
    cord-stromal tumors 248
    determination 330
    drive, loss of 477
    linked inheritance 336, 341
Sexual dysfunction 76, 78
Sexually transmitted infections 121
Shamana therapy 185
Shock 99, 150
    anaphylactic 152
    cardiogenic 150
    hypovolemic 98, 150
    septic 150
Shodhana therapy 185
Sibai method 144
Sick sinus syndrome 259
Sickle cell
    anemia 341, 412, 462, 468, 469f, 471
    crisis 470
    disease 468
    trait 470

Siddha
  drugs for 187
  system 186
Single gene disorders 347f
Sinus arrhythmias 257
Sinusitis 256
Sirolimus 24
Skeletal muscle 65
  relaxants 55, 59
  spasm 82
Skin
  disorders 191
  rash 23, 77, 88, 105, 373, 455
  reactions 3
Skull fracture 256
Sleeplessness 79
Snake bite, treatment of 154
Social phobia 78
Soda glycerine 7
Sodium 113, 162, 276
  acetate 29
  bicarbonate 29, 152
    mechanism of 29f
  chloride 166
  citrate 29, 30
  overload 29
  valporoate 87
Softened ear wax 8
Somatic cell 304f
Somatic gene therapy 504, 504f
Sorbitrate 151
Sore throat 4, 9
Speech 264, 446
  blockage 77
  difficulties 261
  slurred 84, 262
Sperm
  antibody test 415
  count 281
  infantile 88
  morphology 281
  penetration 113
Spermatogenesis 412
Spherocytosis, hereditary 464
Spina bifida 381, 421
  occulta 421, 424
Spinal cord tumors 273
Spinocerebellar ataxia 498
Spironolactone 16, 17
Spleen 277
  enlargement 455, 464
Splenectomy 468
Splenic crisis 471
Spontaneous abortion 241, 375, 394, 417
  diagnosis of 420
  management of 420
  types of 418

Sporadic cancer 451
Sputum
  examination of 273
  normal 274
Squamous cell 285
  carcinoma 223
Staphylococcus saprophyticus 286
Status asthmaticus 46
Status epilepticus 88, 150, 151
  seizures 89
Steroid metabolism, disorders of 455
Stimulants 94
Stomach cramps 8
Stomatitis 25
Stool 187
  culture 288
  specimen, collection of 287
Strabismus 428
Streptococcus pneumoniae 256
Streptomycin 387
Stress disorder, post-traumatic 78, 80
Stroke 258, 259, 455, 471
  embolic 260
  hemorrhagic 261
  ischemic 260
  symptoms of 261
  thrombotic 260
Struma ovary 248
Subcortical brain damage 69
Subfertility 410
Succinimide 86
Succinylcholine 56, 59
Sudden infant death syndrome 392
Sulfa allergy 31
Sulfasalazine 24
Sunitinib 176
Supportive therapy 160
Suprapubic aspiration 282, 283
Suxamethonium 59
Sweating 41, 75
Swelling 124
Sympathomimetic drugs, classification of 95, 95f
Symphysis-fundal distance, measurement of 398
Syncope 104, 146
Synthesis 117
Systemic infectious diseases 209
Systemic lupus erythematosus 210, 279

T

Tachycardia 5, 58, 67, 77, 84, 85, 96, 99, 100, 104, 105, 138, 191
  supraventricular 151
Tachypnea 226
Tacrolimus 24, 179

Tandem mass spectrometry 435
Tardive dyskinesia 68, 77
Tartar, formation of 9
Taste perversion 5
Tay-Sachs disease 339, 437
Tazobactam 24
Telophase 307, 313
Temazepam 54
Tenacious sputum 226
Tension 105
  headache 143
Teratogenic drugs 386
Teratomas 248
Terbutaline 131
Terlipressin 20
Testis
  blood vessels of 231
  prevent overheating of 415
  undescended 229, 229f, 230f
Tetanic uterine contractions 138
Tetanus 168
  antitoxin 170
  immunoglobulin 170
  prophylaxis 135
  toxoid 135, 135t
  vaccine 135, 135f
Tetracycline 386, 387
Thalassemia 339, 465
Thalidomide 178, 386, 392
Thecoma 249
Theophylline 19
Thiamine 149, 161, 164, 458
Thiazide 15
  diuretics 21
Thin gauge embryo fetoscopic technique 407
Thiopentone sodium 45
Thioridazine 64-66
Thiouracils 387
Thioxanthenes 66
Thorazine 64, 66
Throat
  disorders of 3
  irritation 9
Thrombocytopenia 66, 455, 460
  congenital amegakaryocytic 462, 476
Thromboembolic disorders 115
Thymine 355f, 356f, 358f, 359, 359f
  replaces adenine 356f
Thyroid
  disorders 411
  pheochromocytoma 452
  stimulating hormone 436
Thyrotoxicosis 107
Ticarcillin 24
Tinnitus 73
Tizanidine 56, 62
T-lymphocyte deficiency 460

Tobramycin 24
Tocolytics 131
Tonic-clonic seizures, generalized 88
Topfer's test 276
Topiramate 24, 87
Topoisomerase inhibitors 174
Topotecan 174
Torn mesenteric vessels 277
Torsemide 12, 13, 15
Total radiation dose 394
Toxemia, symptoms of 242
Toxicity 6, 50
Toxins 160
    promoting excretion of 485
    reducing accumulation of 485
Toxocara canis 274
Toxoids 167
Toxoplasmosis 371, 372
Trabecular bone density 213
Transabdominal fetal ultrasound 399*f*
Transcervical cannula 403*f*
Transdermal estradiol 114
Transfer ribonucleic acid 321, 328*f*
Transferrin saturation test 478
Transient ischemic attacks 34, 259
Transversion mutation 356, 356*f*
Tranylcypromine sulfate 76
Trauma 261
Treacher Collins syndrome 383
Tremors 77, 78, 104
Tretinoin 175
Triamterene 16, 17
    amiloride 17
Triazolam 54
Tricyclic antidepressants 75, 76
    mechanism of action of 76*f*
Trifluoperazine 64
Triflupromazine 65, 66
Trimethadione 387
Triple-X syndrome 335
Trisomy 382, 447
Trypsin 276
Tubal
    abnormality 127
    blockage 410
    ligation 410
Tuberculosis 178, 278, 279
Tubo-tubal anastomosis 127
Tumors
    benign 223
    borderline
        mucinous 247
        serous 247
    carcinoid 248
    embryonal 223
    endometrioid 247
    invasion 266
    malignant 224

    metastatic 223, 247, 249, 272
    mucinous 247
    non-epithelial 223
    ovarian 245
    primary 264
    secondary 265
    serous 247
Turcot syndrome 452, 453
Turner's syndrome 335, 336, 413, 447
Typhoid 168
Tyrosinemia 436

U

Ulcers 471
Ultrasonography 442, 447
Unani system 189
Unipolar depression 77
Unstable angina 151
Uric acid stone 220
Urinary bladder 11, 39, 277
Urinary calculi 191
    etiopathogenesis of 219*f*
    types of 219, 220*f*
Urinary flow, obstruction of 225
Urinary retention 5, 67, 77, 96, 108, 225
Urinary system 11, 191, 209
Urinary tract infection 24, 285
Urine 187, 283*t*, 284*t*
    analysis 210
    culture 286
    dipstick test 286, 286*f*
    examination 282
    sample collection of 282
Urobilinogen 284
Urticaria 66, 104
Usher's syndrome 413
Uterine
    abnormality 127
    bleeding 402
        abnormal 245
    contraction 128
    cramping 143, 402
    endometrium 113
    fibroids 240
    inertia 138
    leiomyomas 241*f*
        causes of 240
    problems 410
    relaxants 129, 131, 131*t*
    rupture 130, 138, 143
    scar 138
    stimulants 94, 129
        classification of 129*f*
    tetany 143
Uterus 113
    hyperactive 138
    hypertonic 138
    intact 123

V

Vagina 113
Vaginal contraceptives 125
    types of 125*f*
Vaginal disorder 191
Vaginal ring 125, 125*f*
Valacyclovir 24
Valganciclovir 24
Valine 359
Valporic acid 87, 90, 387, 386
Valvular disease 259
Van der Woude syndrome 337
Vancomycin 24
Varicella 169, 371, 372
    infection 372
    zoster virus 372
Vas deferens, congenital absence of 414
Vasectomy, previous 410
Vecuronium 56, 57
Venezuelan equine encephalitis 371
Venous thromboembolic disease 124
Ventilatory support 50
Ventricular septal defects 428
Verapamil 151
Vertigo 22, 76, 78
Vesicular mole 242
Vestibulary dysfunction 7
Vigabatrin tiagabine 87
Villi, absence of 244
Vinblastine 174
Viper bite 155
Viral vectors 506, 508
Viscosity 280
Vision
    disturbances 3, 261
    warning signs 443
Visual field deficit 262
Vital force, theory of 188
Vitamin 161, 163
    A 163, 386, 392
    B1 161, 164
    B12 162, 165
    B2 161, 164
    B3 161
    B5 161
    B6 162
    B7 162
    B9 162
    B-complex, types of 161
    C 165
    D 163
    E 163
    fat-soluble 163*t*
    K 163
    K1 supplement 136, 136*t*
    supplementation 161
    types of 161*f*
    water-soluble 163*t*

Index

Voice 186
Vomiting 9, 22, 25, 77, 88, 98, 99, 103, 104, 108, 128, 138, 143, 145, 191, 226, 258
  recurrent 455
von Willebrand disease 337, 462, 474

W

Waardenburg syndrome 383
Warfarin 158, 386, 387
Water retention 22, 113
Weakness 78, 85, 96, 191, 262, 477
Weaver-Smith syndrome 447
Wegner's granulomatosis 213
Weight
  gain 22, 23, 67, 73, 76-78
  loss 104, 455
Wheezing 58
White blood cell 272, 285, 288

Williams syndrome 498
Wilms' tumor 174, 223, 225, 225f
Wilson's disease 381
Wolf-Hirschhorn syndrome 332
Worm infestation 191
Wurn technique 417

X

Xanthine 220
Xanthochromia 271
Xipamide 15
XX male syndrome 413
XYY syndrome 335, 413

Y

Yawning 41
Yeast cells 285
Yellow fever 169
Yersinia enterocolitica 288, 467

Yolk sac tumor 248
Young's syndrome 414

Z

Zaleplon 54
Zellweger syndrome 455
Zepines 87
Zidovudine 373
Zinc supplementation, therapy 381
Zolpidem 54, 55
Zonisamide 24, 87
Zopiclone 54, 55
Zuspan method 144
Zygote
  in vitro fertilization technique 127
  intrafallopian transfer 416
Zygotene 311